Creative Tools and Techniques of Multidimensional Educational Methods in Nursing

Creative Tools and Techniques of Multidimensional Educational Methods in Nursing

Cecy Correia
Nursing Tutor
Uday General School of Nursing
Cardinal Gracias Memorial Hospital
Sandor, Bangli, Vasai (W)
Thane, Maharashtra, India

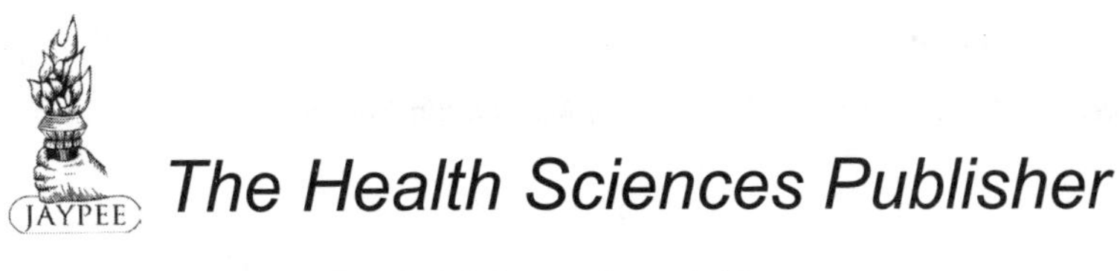

New Delhi | London | Panama

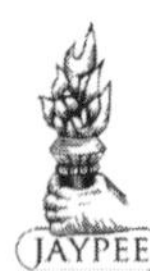

Jaypee Brothers Medical Publishers (P) Ltd

Headquarters

Jaypee Brothers Medical Publishers (P) Ltd
4838/24, Ansari Road, Daryaganj
New Delhi 110 002, India
Phone: +91-11-43574357
Fax: +91-11-43574314
Email: jaypee@jaypeebrothers.com

Overseas Offices

J.P. Medical Ltd
83 Victoria Street, London
SW1H 0HW (UK)
Phone: +44 20 3170 8910
Fax: +44 (0)20 3008 6180
Email: info@jpmedpub.com

Jaypee-Highlights Medical Publishers Inc
City of Knowledge, Bld. 235, 2nd Floor, Clayton
Panama City, Panama
Phone: +1 507-301-0496
Fax: +1 507-301-0499
Email: cservice@jphmedical.com

Jaypee Brothers Medical Publishers (P) Ltd
17/1-B Babar Road, Block-B, Shaymali
Mohammadpur, Dhaka-1207
Bangladesh
Mobile: +08801912003485
Email: jaypeedhaka@gmail.com

Jaypee Brothers Medical Publishers (P) Ltd
Bhotahity, Kathmandu, Nepal
Phone +977-9741283608
Email: kathmandu@jaypeebrothers.com

Website: www.jaypeebrothers.com
Website: www.jaypeedigital.com

Inquiries for bulk sales may be solicited at: jaypee@jaypeebrothers.com

Creative Tools and Techniques of Multidimensional Educational Methods in Nursing

First Edition: 2017

ISBN: 978-93-86150-73-8

Printed at Sanat Printers

Dedication

I humbly dedicate this book to my Father Thomas Correia and Mother Santan Correia. May they continue to live through this book. May God bless them.

Our Body, no matter how much time and effort we lavish in making it look good, it will leave us when we die.

Our possession, status and wealth, when we die, will go to others.

Our family and friends, no matter how close they had been there for us, when we are alive, and the furthest they can stay by us is up to the grave.

And our Soul, neglected in our pursuit of our material wealth and pleasure. It is actually the only thing that follows us wherever we go.

Preface

The textbook *Creative Tools and Techniques of Multidimensional Educational Methods in Nursing* has 62 chapters in total. It is based on 'Community Health Nursing' syllabus. This book is helpful for students and teachers to prepare health educational topics for rural and urban areas and to carry out procedures in the field area as a guide.

The layout is unique and simple. It is useful for the students to learn theory and practice at the same time. The book has many figures explaining the work carried out in the field. The students will find it helpful to see the pictures and it will remain in their memory. The contents of the chapters will give the students the idea of the book.

Cecy Correia

Acknowledgments

With gratitude in my heart, I convey my sincere thanks to Jaypee Brothers Medical Publishers (P) Ltd, New Delhi, India for their efforts and suggestions, especially Shri Jitendar P Vij (Group Chairman), Mr Ankit Vij (Group President), Ms Chetna Malhotra Vohra (Associate Director–Content Strategy), and Ms Ruby Sharma (Project Manager) for helping me through my idea. They have worked tirelessly in completing this title. I want to acknowledge the entire team which has done wonderful layouting and designing of the book. May God bless all their efforts, time, energy, and commitment towards this task.

Contents

CHAPTER 1

Change with Changing Times

PURPOSE

To walk towards the 21st century, where today there are new and diverse approaches to nursing profession. Today with high-tech and scientific revolution world has developed with latest technologies, one can ever imagine few years ago. With internet, satellite, websites, email, and computers, which in olden times people could never think of, is taking over human mind.

ADVANCED EQUIPMENT

Digital monitors and microscopes help to grasp nursing concept better than before—computer presentation, advanced technological aids, facilities like laser projector, laptops, on line education courses and knowledge-orientated technology.

Now We Faced the Following Questions

Where are we?
Where is nursing profession reached today?
Do we feel outdated/or lost?
Do we feel confident enough to practice our skill and knowledge at home and abroad?

Challenges that Nurse Has to Face Today

- Human needs are varied that creates stressful situation.
- Nurses who have to be with the patients round the clock.
- She has to play a vital role in safeguarding the health of the people.
- Nursing needs to develop in its potentialities as millions are in need of expert nursing care.
- There is always a shortage of nurses for high quality care.
- Her ability, intelligence, aptitude, initiative, particular knowledge is considered in favors in promotion.

Value of Trained Nurse

A technical knowledge in her field enables her task to become dynamic, creative and innovative.

- More assisting with highly technologic medical care.
- They work in number of specialty and super-specialized departments.
- Her practice requires her to fulfill professional responsibilities.
- With the use of computer clinical investigations, advanced in scientific knowledge the role and function of a nurse has been extended.
- Techniques which were formally regarded as the doctors' province may be carried out by her.
- She has collective responsibilities, which include all dimensions of holistic health.
- A nurse provides multipurpose nursing care to families and individuals at their homes, work place, schools and in the community.

SELF-FORMATION

- To be responsible for updating one's knowledge and skills,
- To be an efficient team leader.
- To be a manager, a coordinator, a trainer an advocator a key person.
- A communicator, a change agent, a teacher, a decision maker, a care giver, a researcher, an administrator, an advisor and a counselor.
- This can only be successfully achieved if she can communicate and put her message across.
- She should be able to interact with her team members.
- She needs to be a link between the patient, the family and the doctor.

Nurse in the Community

How

She is an important pillar providing health education to the individual, groups and community.

- To mobilize community involvement, to provide integrated health care including the treatment of emergencies and making referrals.
- Maintaining epidemiological surveillance.
- Training and supervising health workers.
- Collaborating with other developmental sectors, monitoring progress.
- She has to provide health care in scientific and relevant manner.
- She has significant role in carrying out preventive, promotive, curative, and rehabilitative services.

Nurse in the Hospital

- Is to provide nursing care to the client, to administer medications and treatment.
- To observe clients' illness, to prevent any complications.
- To teach the client and his family regarding prevention of diseases and promotion of health.
- To participate in research works related to health.
- She should be quick in making decisions and should be knowledgeable—because delay may cause the life of the client.
- To keep proper recording of every details of the patient.

Marching Ahead

- The nurse of today will be the citizen of the 21st century.
- The change is associated with tremendous speed.
- If we have to survive, we have to keep the pace with it.
- We have to bring competitive change in our thinking, feelings, behavior and system of functioning.
- We have to adopt new technologies, new knowledge and skills.

To be Creative

- Creative people show their creativity in everything and do not wait for a particular cause of action or event.
- The best way to start is to start working in the area that we are so passionate about and to stop evaluating others' work.
- However, the success or failure of an individual largely depends on our performance.
- Conviction will inspire confidence in our abilities;
- Let our creative personality surface.
- We do not know how much power we have deep within us until we try to discover it.

Factors Affecting Nursing

- Aging nurse workforce
- Aging population
- Increased demand for nurses
- Work place issues
- Inadequate staffing
- Heavy workloads
- Increased use of overtime
- Lack of sufficient support staffs
- Inadequate wages
- Difficulty recruiting and retaining nurse's.

Standards of Professional Performance

- Systematically enhances the quality and effectiveness of nursing practice.
- Evaluates ones own practice in relation to professional guidelines.
- Attain knowledge and competency that reflects current nursing practice
- Interactions, contributes collaborate in nursing practice
- Integrates research findings into practice
- Provides leadership in professional practice setting.

6 Cs of Caring in Nursing

1. Compassion—sharing joys, sorrows, pain and particularly in the experience of another.
2. Competence—having the knowledge, judgment, skills, energy, experience and motivation to respond adequately to others within the demand of professional responsibilities.
3. Confidence—the quality that fosters relationships, comfort with self, patient and family.
4. Conscience—morals, ethics and informed sense of right and wrong awareness of personal responsibility.
5. Commitment—convergence between ones desire and obligations and the deliberate choice to act in accordance with them.
6. Comportment (attitude)—appropriate bearing demeanor (manner or character), dress and language that are in harmony with a caring presence. Presenting oneself as someone who respects others and demands respect.

I-value

- Helping others
- Work ethics
- Honesty
- Creativity
- Good character
- Stability
- Safety
- Inner harmony
- Trustworthiness
- Challenge
- Caring
- Spirituality

To Believe in Self

- Believing in the power we have within us.
- Believing in the strength that we have deep inside,
- Believing in tomorrow and what it will bring—if we trust and believe, there is no limit to what we can do.
- Overcoming setbacks in life is an art in itself. Determination and perseverance make it possible. When we look to future with hope, the horizons becomes larger and brighter.
- Nursing field is dynamic and challenging.
- To match the pace, we need to invest our time in improving knowledge.

- We need to clear many misconceptions before arriving at any decision for our profession.
- Napoleon Hill, the well known motivator-educator said,

'Whatever mind can conceive and believe, it can be achieved'.

Therefore, we need to believe in ourselves.

Our profession is in no way less than any other profession, it also has wide variety of openings to go ahead.

'Go Set Go': The world of tomorrow belongs to the nurse who has vision today. Get the edge.

Keywords

Purpose, advanced equipment, challenges that nurse has to face today, value of trained nurse, self-formation, nurse in the community, nurse in the hospital, marching ahead, to be creative, factors affecting nursing, standards of professional performance, to believe in self.

CHAPTER

2

Educational Aids and Principles in Nursing

Abstract

Ones entire life is continuous process of learning. However, today; technologies are rapidly transforming—the way we live, work and spend our leisure time. Change taking place rapidly and on such a vast scale that globalization is becoming reality. The greatest need of today is to educate our generation to the highest standard possible. For this, self-training is must. We are on threshold of having a high-resolution to video and personal computers tied to networks. While globalization has brought with it technological advances and newer tools of communication, it has also opened up a number of avenues in the field of nursing education. To equip people with skills, knowledge and attitudes to enable them solve their health problems by their own action and efforts. Today you have many opportunities to get trained in different skills and be creative and innovative to become a future orientated and to be excellence.

INTRODUCTION

Let us look into ourselves and try to see where we are today in advanced education? What are the challenges we will have to face if we do not walk with the sings of the time?

Education is an essential part of the development, then that may be information technology or medical advances. New ideas need to be designed constantly and creatively through good education into the birding generation, who are architect of society and worthy citizens of tomorrow.

Real knowledge, as everything else is of the highest value, which cannot be obtained easily. It must be worked for, studied for, and thought for. Familiarity with books is not knowledge. Ones entire life is continuous process of learning. As the heat of the fire reduces wood into ashes, the fire of knowledge burns ignorance and gives wisdom. Therefore, strive towards to get best of knowledge in the world.

The greatest need of today is to educate our generation to the highest standard possible. For this, self-training is must and it needs to face harsh realities of life, which will meet the challenges of the external world.

Learning is as if rowing upstream, not to advance is going backward. A man learns in two ways: by reading, practicing and by association with smarter people. So to get such education one has to look backward with gratitude, upward with confidence and forward with hope.

Today's age is known as an information age. Today technologies rapidly transforming the way we live, work and spend our leisure time. It has extended to spread knowledge immensely and made its sharing easy, promising almost near universal empowerment of the people, provided we make innovative uses of these new technologies. As a result, a wind of change now sweeping across and much of the world is paving way for an open world. Today's advances made by man are fundamentally transforming the organized human life to see the dawn of a new era. Today any events that are taking place in any corner of the planet become known to the world over almost in no time. Change taking place rapidly and on such a vast scale that globalization is becoming reality.

Other features of the present day situation which is microprocessors and the "chips" have not only made possible in physical terms, but economic terms, its technologies and computer is transforming business operations, broadcasting, telephone system and human interaction. We are on threshold of having a high resolution two way video and personal computers tied to net works, so that sitting at home or office, one can receive information from anywhere in the world and engage in a two way video conversation across the world.

Today information technology media has assumed significance, which we never had before; media has become a mechanism to govern our lives. It has become a way of life itself. Many of the societies are already changing from being advanced industrial societies to "information societies" their network and other enhanced forms are major force. Companies are in process of building a vast web of electronic network, information super highways of fiber optics and computers. This network will deliver an abundance of goods and services at your offices and homes. A user or customer requires video images, phone calls, enormous amount of data on various fields. They promise to change the way people think, work, live and use their leisure time.

In the last few years break through in satellite and high speed computing have given leading users an overwhelming economic advantages over those who have not kept pace.

The "pull" for the "lasts" and the "best", there have been revolutionary changes in IT, which both provides challenges and opportunities. Amazing times acquired new meanings. What used to be distant is no more that far away, what used to be local has become global.

While globalization has brought with it technological advances and newer tools of communication, it has also opened up a number of avenues in the field of nursing education. Once confined to the four walls of a classroom, learning has now moved beyond the traditions format on to the virtual medium.

In the seamless world of tomorrow mind would matter. The wireless web further facilitates connectivity. The quality of images and the speed of downloads will improve significantly multimedia; mobile message will be the next rival of e-mail.

E-learning or online learning is fast emerging as a popular mode in various fields such as computer, science, biotechnology, commerce, arts, psychology, etc. Online learning is also a viable mode to pursue further education without disrupting your regular professional life, e.g. MBA. In India e-learning not yet popular but will hopefully take centre stage in the next 10 years. The internet is like just a world passing around notes in a classroom.

The uses of Audio Visual aids are related to learning. Their direct experiences consist in getting immediate sensory contact with actual object. It is rich and tested, touched and felt and smelled through the careful selections of the pictures. We can bring them all to the classes.

Today, information is being transmitted across organizations in seconds. The gap between theory and practice can be made easy by these methods. Rapid changes in health care technology diversity in the workforce, organizational restructuring and changing work system can place stress on nurses.

What are the advantages of audio-visual (AV) aids?

1. AV aids give reality to learning situation.
2. AV aids gives vividness to learning situations.
3. AV aids give clarity to learning.
4. AV aids motivates learning.
5. AV aids concreteness to abstract ideas.
6. AV aids help various sense organs to work jointly.
7. AV aids help to reduce verbalization.
8. AV aids provides variety.
9. AV aids promote human values.
10. AV aids promotes national integration and understanding.

What are the general principles of AV aids?

1. They are used for learning task or reinforcing the values during learning process.
2. It must be suitable to age and intellectual capacity of the people.
3. They should not be confused with entertainment.

What are the principles of education?

Principles of health education is like interest, participation, comprehension, motivation, reinforcement, learning, human relationships, etc.

1. **Forward looking**—should have an insight into the future life and enable students to prepare for a worthy life, equip them with the caliber to meet the challenges of life.
2. **Motivation**—should be tailored to suit the needs of interest of the students, it must be goal directed.
3. **Creative**—enable students to exercise her creative power.
4. **Flexible**
5. **Cultivate critical sense**—problem solving and decision making
6. **Prepare a student** for all round development, to develop wholesome personality, to develop intellect, the physique and the mind
7. **Should not be bookish** and theoretical
8. **Should not be examination oriented** only but character building, a nation building, a person building, a life support building.

How is the format on which health educational lesson plan prepared?

Health education format points are as follows—

1. Select appropriate topic
2. Subject
3. Date
4. Place
5. Time
6. Aim
7. Specific objectives
8. Self-introduction

Topic Objectives	Subject Matter	Method of Teaching	AV Aids	Evaluation

What are the important points to be kept in mind by the person who gives health education?

The points are as follows—

1. The student has to plan and submit it in time
2. She has to take initiative and interest
3. She has to select apt topic
4. Have to have a relevant group in mind for the topic selected to be delivered
4. Up to date knowledge
5. Reliable matter
6. Interesting presentation that is appropriate

7. Communicate her ideas correctly
8. Use the language appropriately
9. Effective and satisfactory
10. Get positive response from the participant
11. Control the group
12. Correct visual aids at right time used.

What are the areas and the examples of topics on which health education is focused?

There are number of topics according to the different situations and group of people. **Some of the examples are as follows—**

1. Human biology
2. Nutrition/balanced diet
3. Hygiene
4. MCH/family planning
5. Prevention of communicable diseases
6. Prevention of accidents
7. Mental health
8. Immunization
9. Skin problems like scabies
10. Cancer
11. Diabetes
12. Hepatitis
13. HIV/AIDS
14. Malnutrition
15. Breastfeeding.

What is the objective of health education?

1. It gives public information to create awareness and dispel misconceptions, doubts and ignorance.
2. Help people achieve health by their own actions and efforts; people are motivated to face the problem intelligently and take rational decisions concerning health. It needs sincere desire and active efforts in the part of the individual to change his habits and behavior.
3. To induce people to make use of the health services available.

What are the aims of health education?

It aims to ensure health as a value and asset. To equip people with skills, knowledge and attitudes to enable them solve their health problems by their own action and efforts.

What are its stages?

1. Create awareness.
2. Motivate people.
3. Create an interest—The individual begins to take interest in subject.
4. Evaluation—He then evaluates the information received, decides whether wants to adopt or not.
5. Action—Conviction leads to action, adoption or acceptance of the idea.

What are the different levels of health education?

1. Individual health education.
2. Group health education.
3. General public.

How do you classify AV aids?

No health education can be effective without audio-visual aids. **Audio-visual aids can be classified into 3 groups—**

1. Auditory aids
2. Visual aids
3. Combined audio-visual aids.

Auditory aids

1. Tape recorders
2. Microphones
3. Amplifiers
4. Ear phones.

Visual aids

1. Blackboard
2. Flannel graph
3. Models
4. Specimens
5. Posters
6. Slides
7. Film strips
8. Epidiascope
9. Overhead projector.

Combined audio-visual aids

1. Sound films
2. Slide tape combination
3. Television
4. Computer and internet

Methods of group teaching

1. One way-lecture
2. Films
3. Charts
4. Flannel graph
5. Exhibits
6. Flash cards.

Two ways

1. Group discussion
2. Panel discussion
3. Symposium
4. Workshop

5. Role play
6. Demonstration.

There are other ways like—Individual counseling, group instructions, use of mass media communications, community action programed, informal health education, posters, leaflets, booklets, charts, puppets, and cinemas.

As today nurses walk towards 21st century, where today there are new and divers approaches has been developed in nursing profession' and if one has to do well in the career, one has to update. Where we have to change with changing times and keep abreast with things that are evolving, How to be a new way of becoming a nurse? Or How to improve our profession? Today you have many opportunities to get trained in different skills and be creative and innovative to become a future orientated and to be excellence.

Keywords

Architect of society, highest value, self-training, learning, information age, innovative, information technology media, satellite and high speed computing, e-learning or online learning, audio-visual aids, principles of education, aims and objective of health education, stages and different levels of health education, classify and methods of health education.

CHAPTER

3

What is Education in Nursing?

Abstract

Emphasizing the worth and dignity of the individual as human bring. Education helps, realization of the highest values of life. The education today revolves around ideas and innovations. Knowledge is learning something every day. The aim of education is to produce good efficient nurses to serve humankind. Education leads a person from darkness to light, he grows from within, and builds innate power, and capacities that leads forth or to unfold the hidden talents of man. Education draws out and stimulates the spiritual and intellectual faculties. Philosophy has influence on education. Learning is like rowing upstream. Teachers are the storehouse of knowledge and wisdom, and they contribute with their dedicated work beyond the blackboard.

INTRODUCTION

In Latin—the meaning of education is to bring up, to lead, to lead out of or to all knowledge inherent in students. So that the student can be helped to develop habits, interest, attitudes and skills to lead a full life. It is all round drawing out of the best, training of the human soul, givers inner light, development of all the capacities, to have a complete living.

The aim of education is knowledge, vocational development and completes living.

How the education enables?

It helps one to lift the mind from blind alleys. It teaches to dispel error and discovers truth and positive changes in life, giving power to the people. Emphasizing the worth and dignity of the individual as human being.

Today science and technology have caused radical changes on the lives of the people. With help of radio, TV, computer, internet, FB, mobile teachers have eliminated all physical barriers of communication.

There is formal and informal education system. In formal education, it is well-planned system of education, which envisaged bringing about specific behavioral changes in education. It has fixed curriculum. Formal education is based on certain rules, customs and procedures.

Informal education—it is not systematically planned and not well-defined curriculum, non-formal education adopts a midway. Non-formal education is life long. Exhibiting open system, it has self teaching pattern. It helps in eradication of illiteracy, enables pupils to learn and earn simultaneously, enables drop out to continue studies and enables them to refresh knowledge and provides the educational facilities to neglected sectors. This includes correspondence courses, open schools, satellite instructional TV programers, etc.

Primary education should aim at preparing children for higher education. Public education among masses has practical application in day today life. Education in vernaculars or Indian languages or indigenous education, also be promoted and those who have exceptional aptitude for higher education can go ahead for higher level.

Educational planning in India is an attempt to shape the future by deliberate action. Its objective is to get the most and best educational results for the effort expended and to maximize the contribution policy and education adapted by the Parliament in 1968.

It stressed

1. Free compulsory education
2. Improve status, emoluments and education of teachers
3. Investment of 6% of national income in education
4. Equalization of education especially in science and research, etc.

The new education policy of 1986 a total of 205 schools have been opened up in 1987–1988.

National Council of Educational Research and Training (NCERT) has established in 1961. It has taken up Central Board of Secondary Education (CBSE).

Modernization is the process by which fundamental social and cultural changes take place as a result of the adoption of science based technology. It implies a wide explosion of knowledge, rapid social change and a re-orientation of moral and spiritual values.

Main tasks are to enable children to keep pace with rapidly growing knowledge. Children should have progressive and harmonious development of all the faculties of the individual—head, heart and hand. This goal and task can be fulfilled by Education that finds out the means to achieve the goal.

Teachers have to be acquainting themselves with a new concept of education technology for the challenges that the children will have to face in rapidly changing society. Develop critical thinking and balanced moral spiritual values. All round drawing out best educational philosophies, Plato said, "one who has a taste for every sort of knowledge, who is curious to learn, is never satisfied". A teacher must possess a sound philosophy. He must be a lover of wisdom, a seeker of knowledge and a man of values.

Education helps, realization of the highest values of life. The divine in man is to be un-folded and brought to his consciousness by education. In methods of teaching, he gives them an insight into deeper experience, infuses confidence in them and brings out their talents and potentials through stimulating experience. Education for life and through life the psychological principles or known to unknown, simple to complex, concrete to abstract.

Knowledge is learning something every day, wisdom is letting go off something every day. An investment in knowledge always pays the best interest.

Education is only after having finished a course of study that the real learning begin as we start to unravel some of the new ideas and transfers new knowledge in to the realities of our practice. Nursing education has become increasingly complex. The increasing diversity of students, the restructuring of institution of higher education, the redesigning of health care delivery system and the continuing explosion of the use of information technology in education practice.

The education today revolves around ideas and innovations. We are moving in an era of accelerating change in all walks of life. We are moving towards newer educational activities based on technology so that we are ready to face the challenges of tomorrow. Today competencies have become essential to the implementation of the educator's role hence it is important to learn to develop a way of thinking, to seek information, and to learn to convert whatever you grasp into practice.

The principle and habit of thinking are universal. A scientific approach is necessary and essential for public safety. The giving of care and the overcoming of obstacle to care needs imagination, creativity, vertical thinking and innovations. The aim of education is to produce good efficient nurses to serve humankind.

Education leads a person from darkness to light, he grows from within, and builds innate power, and capacities that leads forth or to unfold the hidden talents of man. Education is something which makes a man self-reliant and selfless, through education one enjoys life. Education is that which makes a man of good character and useful to the society.

Education draws out and stimulates the spiritual and intellectual faculties of the children. Knowledge is considered as the accumulated experience of the human race. We receive education many a times even when we are not conscious of the fact, as all experience is said to be educative in the formation of new ideas. It is a process of development from infancy to maturity. It begins at birth, continuous through life and ends with death—from womb to the tomb as a life long journey. It teaches to live life to all its manifestation. It helps to mould and modify child's behavior and character. Intelligent and bright students can learn things in better way, as motivated pupil learns more readily.

It is ongoing, goes on forever, without any break or barrier. However, knowledge should not end in itself and should always be related to life experience. Scope of education is wide, and it is limitless and fathomless ocean, which knows no end.

What are the fundamental principles of idealism?

1. Spirit and mind constitute reality
2. Man being spiritual, is supreme
3. God is the source of all knowledge
4. Values are absolute and unchanging
5. What is ultimately real is not the object itself but the idea behind it
6. Man is not the creator of values.

Philosophy is search for wisdom and truth, so it is a philosophy of life, which embraces the body, mind, and carrier. Philosophy has influence on education. There is a relationship between both. All great philosophers of the world have also been great educators. There is a philosophy of nurse. The education is like a sailor who does not know his destination and the pupil is like a rudderless vessel which may be drifted alone somewhere a shore.

Education helps to develop social, moral and spiritual values, democratic citizenship, democratic personality, democratic leadership, vocational efficiency, initiating person to the art of living, increases productivity, social and national integration, and modernization.

What education is, what education does; and what education should do. Train people for integrated growth. Life is not static; it is continuously growing and changing. Education should conserve and preserve all the old traditions, values ideas worthwhile customs and way of living. It will have to transmit the cultural heritage to the younger generation and reconstructuring new experiences unfolding new dimensions of knowledge developing new capacities in the individual and furthering civilization and cultures.

Nurses should be technically trained in hospital and associated with a medical school. The nursing school should be affiliated with a teaching hospital but independent of it. The curriculum should include both theory and practical experience.

Intellectual development is concerned as mastery of subject matter achieved primarily through teacher expositions, drills tests, etc. the primary purpose is to build a storehouse of information, skills, values which may be useful to the individual in his future life. Intellectual development is important, but development for effective functioning in all areas of living is important in itself.

Knowledge is the quickest and safest path of success in any area of life. Lack of knowledge in nursing profession may give rise to unforgiving mistakes. So nurse has to acquire knowledge and transfer it to future generations. Nurses working in clinical area are cream of profession in healthcare system.

By virtue of birth itself, man is endowed with hidden potentials and education will develop all those capacities and enables him to fulfill his possibilities. Drawing out the vitality education is a purposeful activity is a deliberate process, planned activity based on objective. Education provides knowledge and skills, and helps it earn livelihood.

The goal of learning and living is to transform the natural man into an ideal man by attaining all round perfection. School as a garden, the teacher as a gardener and students as tender plants intended to grow to beauty and perfection. Education should give importance to scientific methods of observation and verification. Nursing is a healing science.

Higher education today is undergoing a radical change posing new age challenges to universities. The role of teachers and educators has gone through a metamorphosis as technology and globalization redefine the contours of the world; with access to information-anywhere anytime-knowledge today is no longer restricted to physical classroom. Re-investing higher education, most of the learning now takes place outside the classroom, through the internet and social medical sites.

Considering the way technology has changed the education landscape, the traditional mindset, has to change. That can help the academic community to perceive the future needs of a student going through this transition. In digital age most of the learning takes place through video games, we need to see things differently. The future roadmap of higher education, the academic world agree, need's to include blended methodology, lifelong learning, collaborative efforts in research and curriculum development, introduction to transnational accreditation agencies and increased student mobility.

While students today are well versed in new technologies, thus are acquiring new skills and attitudes towards learning. Technology and globalization are reshaping the way in which knowledge has traditionally been generated and disseminated teaching student to work in multiple geographies, among others. In this new landscape, is there a need to re-invent higher education.

The dynamics of a traditional class-room has under gone a major change. With the online space coming in students have a broader knowledge source today.

Focus on Child's Aptitude and Interest

As city's school education system churns the class room too is changing. Where it was once a functional space hemmed in by four walls, today it is a concept. Schools frequently hold lectures in gardens, museums or on beaches. The blackboard has been replaced by a projector screen, notepads swapped for iPads.

We want that education by which character is formed, strength of mind is increased, the intellect is expanded and by which one can stand on ones own feet.

How did this transformation take place? And how is it benefiting our kinds?

Many schools in the city have introduced innovations in their methods of teaching—

1. Classes are held in parks, libraries to help the children multisensory development.
2. Computers and overhead projectors are used as supplementary teaching tools in classroom to enhance the understanding of subjects.
3. Separate rooms have been created for music, dram, recreation among other things, students can walk into these rooms as any time to destress.
4. Children are made to sit at round tables instead of in the more typical rows to initiate discussions and spur interaction.
5. Several subjects are taught through iPads to teach languages. Every classroom is equipped with smart class accessories such as TV sets, projectors and the like.
6. The library is being digitized to present easier search and cataloguing.

A new dawn—shift in perspective—100% education means 100% progress, education is more, much more, than for economic benefit of an individual. It is a universal human right for education. Empower a person by helping him achieve other basic human rights building a spiral of power in his life. The right to education at the right time education that has to be met if future opportunities are to be seized, not just for better livelihoods, but for better civic and social consciousness.

We spend a lot of time acquiring intelligence at the expense of developing intellect. Intelligence is built by gaining information, knowledge from external agencies, from schools and universities, teachers and test books. The intellect is developed thorough your individual effort by exercising the faculty of questioning, thinking and reasoning. Not accepting anything that does not admit logic or reasons, know the difference between the two.

The intelligence acquired from external is as if data fed into a computer. All the knowledge stored in its memory cannot help the computer action its own. If the room catches fire, it will go up in flames.

The knowledge you acquire is of no use to you without intellect. This knowledge gained has to be practical use in life. That explains why among millions of doctors graduating only a few have discovered life saving procedures, cures and remedies.

Some with engineer only few design something unusual. It is there intellect that renders their predominance outstanding. People sometimes make no attempt to develop this thus education lost the meaning and purpose, without awareness human being becomes robots. That explains why highly educated business persons, professionals and scholars become alcoholics and short tempered when intellect is underdeveloped and weak unable to control mind.

Strike balance between acquired intelligence and developing intellect will lead mind under perfect control and people live in peace and prosperity.

Real knowledge, like everything else of the highest values, is not to be obtained easily. It must be worked for, studied for, thought for. Familiarity with books is not knowledge; the entire life is continuous process of learning. As the heat of the fire reduces wood to ashes the fire of knowledge burns ignorance and gives wisdom.

The greatest need of our generation was to be educated to the highest standard possible self-training, face harsh realities of life, meet the challenges of the external world.

Learning is like rowing upstream, not to advance is to drop back. A man only learns in two ways by reading and by associating with smarter people. Your expression is the most important thing you wear. Do things that the others say you cannot do.

Today, people are living in an "audio-visual culture", as information catering to their five senses which rule the minds of the people, media that is people friendly, people based, goal oriented yet powerful in communicating the intended messages to the propel.

Street theatre is one media to educate masses with health and social messages. It is powerful highly economic, effective and easy to use. What we require is a good blend of imagination and creativity and physical body to perform the same. A combination of interest, motivation, enthusiasm and commitment, imagination, creativity, will make you effective street theater artist and effective communicator. Street theater also known as earth theater since plays are performed on the ground also called body theater as body used maximum due to overwhelming presence of electronic media, the traditional art forms are pushed to the back seat. To perform a proscenium theater, we need an auditorium with stage, sound system, costumes, properties, make up light, publicity, etc. which means a large sum of money for a single performance.

How do we do it?

Live-communication—face-to-face communication can never replace any kind of communication for meaningful transaction.

Earth is our stage—has advantage both sender and the receiver are on the same platform creating a sense of equality between both. We go close to the people, play are performed during daylight, where actors and the audience are in lighted area. Good use of voice the last person in audience. Voice adds more power to the action and the character, e.g. when a person is cutting a wood with axe, he produces the sound of a woodcutter, he has no axe, no wood to cut, imagination, hand position, creative sound. Imagination is the key and simple costume, e.g. Towel on the shoulder, one becomes property owner, when held under arm he becomes a servant. Songs always help to reach hearts of the people as they have emotional appeal.

It means transmitting and sharing of ideas, opinions, facts and information and have common understanding is important. If helps to improve relationships, doubts and misunderstanding; it clarify gossip rumors and one gets objective feedback. In addition, an act is a great force to control life. Get influenced, inspired, etc.

Teachers open the door, but you must enter by yourself. Education is the transmission of civilization. The mind is not a vessel to be filled but a fire to be kindled. Learning is a treasure that will follow its owner everywhere. I am learning all the time; the tombstone will be my diploma. Education is a progressive discovery of our own ignorance. Teaching is the profession that teaches all other profession. The highest result of education is tolerance. Only the educated are free.

Creativity in education leads to evolution of self-reliant youth with knowledge and action. It is more about motivation, than money, its not only about 100% education; it is about the right kind of education. If we release the locked potential in every child, there is nothing that India cannot achieve. Creativity leads to thinking, thinking provides knowledge, and knowledge makes you great. India is heralded as the land of opportunity and considered among the emergent economies of the 21st century. The right kind of education alone can empower our young in the toughest battle—a ballet they must never stop fighting until they arrive at the destined place that is discovers their own unique identity. What will be the weapons to fight this battle? have a great aim in life, continuously acquire the knowledge needed to achieve it, work hard and persevere to realize your goals. Therefore, it is important to create confidence that 'I can do it'.

Influence of life time—Henry brooks Adams once said "a teacher affects eternity; he can never tell where his influence stops".

Teachers can bring about a sea change in the life of their students. It's very important to have good teachers in ones education time. So that students will have life changing influence on them. A teacher helps develop student's personality. Teachers inspires love for the subject, they change our outlook towards life. Her confidence and the view she shares makes lot of difference into ones life. She influence you a lot, and inspires them with their behavior teachers instill confidence in students. Quenching thirst for knowledge, focus on better future. Youth has immense potentials; they have to be influenced in making world a better place. Teachers are the storehouse of knowledge and wisdom, and they contribute with their dedicated work beyond the blackboard. What is taught in class helps students think best of their abilities, trains future leaders.

Technology and its impact on teaching—today's generation is known as technology natives and it has become the integral part of their lives. Children are exposed to technology from mobiles to computers and all sorts of devices on one hand accelerated growth in global economy has been challenging the aspirations of young students. Students are advanced in gathering information and knowledge due to the availability of various technology tools, and that is imperative for educators to realize the change that is talking place in the role of students and teachers. When technology is used as a tool with appropriate guidance students are in a position of defining their goals and also evaluating their progress. There is a feeling of self worth as they are given freedom to explore and they gain a sense of empowerment to real world and handle more complex assignments of higher skills. Today educators have to take an approach that transforms educations system in order to reasons to the diversity of learners and their varied expectations. The call for a change is the role of teachers, teachers need to realize their new role and accordingly equip themselves to positively work towards the change. 21st century educators need to have a global mindset, understanding the power of technology and its impact on teaching and learning, transformative learning process where students to make good decisions will use technology tools, expand their worldview, acquire employability skills and leads a successful life based on values and ethics. While introducing technology we must remember if there is no proper ecosystem to support it, it can be disruptive in nature. Therefore developing of digital pedagogies and professional development of teachers is vital to leverage the use of technology in classroom.

Aristotle said: 'Those who educate children well are more to be honored than they who produce them; for these only gave them life, the art of living well'. Unfortunately most of the teachers are forgotten after learning is acquired.

Nurse have to practice a good human relationship; which adds value to her profession. They have to respect everyone who are exposed to them. We cannot run down anyone, but we have to respect social sentiments, and develop skills in our profession.

Conclusion—Education implies act of drawing out, act of extracting out, act of learning forth, act of leading out, act of teaching and act of training. Education should be a student centered process, life long process, it is more than instruction and teaching, it is more tan giving information's it is developing knowledge, skills and attitudes. Their philosophy is to develop body and soul, creation of sound mind in sound body. It prepares you for complete living, controlling the mind and making life harmonious and whole. It gives knowledge, transforms character, enriches spiritual and moral values, develops individual, and develops your personality to live in fullness. It stimulates teacher and makes the individual to act with meaning and intelligence.

Self-reflections

What responsibility does the nurse have towards society?

What are our beliefs with regard to education?

What are the factors that will make a nurse and nursing noble?

What are the factors that will attract the youth to choose this noble profession?

What is our individual role—to safeguard the nobility of nursing and the image of our profession?

Keywords

The aim of education—education enables science and technology, formal and informal education system, primary education, educational planning, modernization, and education helps. Nurses should be intellectually developed, hidden potentials, nursing profession. Higher education today, focus on child's aptitude and interest. A new dawn-shift in perspective, intellect and intelligence, creativity in education, influence of a life time, technology and its impact on teaching.

CHAPTER

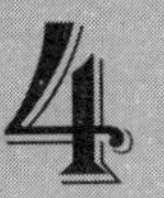

Importance of Education in Nursing

Abstract

Knowledge is power. It motivates force, unites, and binds people and nations. It makes people think for themselves. It is the greatest wealth today. Action is an ongoing journey, education is a life-long process, you can never say enough I have learnt and I know all that I wanted and now I stop. Education is life and life is education because education brings modification of behavior, makes person responsible for life, makes life dynamic and gives direction, helps to improve the quality and personality, provides opportunity for improving, healthy attitudes and values are formed.

What is education?

- Education is to acquire knowledge and learning
- Education is to understand this environment; and search for security and safety
- Education is to develop ones mental faculties
- Education is to acquire knowledge and experience
- Education is to learn from the past history, tradition, customs, rich heritages
- Education helps in the development of the personality of the individual
- Education foresees and prepares individual for a future life
- Education creates a desire to strive hard to cope with changing phase and ultramodern life that is jet age that is every changing
- Education helps in expand learning as the demands increase
- Education creates awareness in various multiple aspects that touch life complexities
- Education is essential to improve ones quality of life
- Education brings about a transformation of behavior. It provides training to take up responsibilities
- Education involves thinking, reasoning, and judgment to face the problems and challenges of life
- Education moulds our character and morals
- Thus making life dynamic and progressive
- Education leads to integrated growth, new power, and functions
- Education directs the attitude to desirable channel
- Education liberates, free people from ignorance, superstitious beliefs, prejudices
- Lads to the light of knowledge and self-realization
- Develops personality and modifies behavior
- Education enables to make correct choices in life
- Education develops nation
- Education is a life long process
- From the womb to the tomb
- Education is from Cradle to grave life long onward journey.

What is health education?

It is a process, which effects changes in the health practices of people and in the knowledge and attitudes related to such changes.

What education does?

It is an essential tool which effects changes in the attitude. It helps people to solve their problems by their own way. It promotes good health and discards certain habits that are harmful to self and others. It modifies existing practices. It motivates force and unites and binds people and nations. It makes people think for themselves. It tells them how to keep fit and adopt and maintain healthy practices and lifestyles.

What is the changing concept?

Historically health education has been committed to disseminating information and changing human behavior. After Alma Ata declaration in 1978, the emphasis has been shifted from prevention of disease to promotion of healthy lifestyle. It is from the modification of individual behavior to modification of 'social environment' in which the individual lives. Community participation to community involvement and promotion of individual and community self-reliance.

What are the points on which health education is given?

Health education can be given on number of topics relevant to the group in front of you. There are different topics to the different groups. Like industrial workers take a topic on accidental injured, safety and working conditions, first aid, etc. School children personal hygiene, skin problem, dental caries, etc. as the set up like rural or urban, educated or not educated. And choose the method that you know and is effective. Nurse can take the education to the houses, schools, health centers, industries and variety of public places.

What are the points to be kept in mind while giving health education?

- Prepare your topic carefully.
- Create friendly atmosphere by greeting the target group.
- A talk should include introduction, teaching points, summary.
- Never teach too many ideas at a time, it is difficult to retain.
- Look at the audience and do not look at the point all the time.
- Do not talk too fast.
- Include local stories, songs to catch interest of the audience.
- Have time for discussion and answer the quarries.
- Do not make the talk too long, out of focus and boring.
- Stand in place where you have eye contact on the audience and they are able to see you.
- Make them comfortable.
- Use simple language and not technical words they do not understand.
- Make frequent pauses.
- Facial expression communication skill be developed.
- Use audio visual aids that are attention capturing.

What is goal of education?

The goal of education is to encourage people to adopt and sustain health promoting lifestyle and practices. To promote the proper use of health services available to them. To arose interest, provide new knowledge, improve skills and change attitude in making national decisions to solve their own problems and to stimulate individual and community self-reliance and participation to achieve health development through individual and community involvement at every step from identifying problems to solving them.

What is the importance of education in today's scenario?

Today education is a treasure. If you are well educated you can reach to any corner of the globe. You will develop confidence and you will enjoy high positions and security of life. You will learn the art of living. You will always have constructive things to do in life. You will feel the intellectual hunger as you feel for the food. You want to grasp all that is new and interesting. One life is not enough for the things to learn that are so interesting. It is the greatest wealth today. You will be respected and people will flock to get substantial knowledge and wisdom from you. You will feel worth living and you will make the difference in your life and the life of the people in the society. Today sky is not the limit, there is always scope for those who have desire to learn and can climb the ladder of success and fulfillment. To get quality education you have to work hard honestly, lot of time and energy will be consumed, good education is very expensive but worth. The more you know the more you feel you do not know that vast is the knowledge. You are like a drop in the ocean trying to dive deep in to it and never gets quenched. It will build your character and will make you a better human being.

What are the characteristics of education?

Education is an ongoing journey what you learn from your birth by the family, society, and people around you that is just the formal education.

Education is a life-long-process, you can never say enough "I have learnt and I know all that I wanted and now I stop". No, you need to keep abreast to the latest discoveries, researches, updated renovate ideas, every day something new is discovered so you have to acquaint to all fields and all round knowledge.

To have integral development person needs a training to develop his mental faculties along with other faculties to bring about the balance, harmony in development. Otherwise, he will be bookworm and dull person.

Education is tri-polar process: meaning teacher gives—individual receives and he imparts all he has received in environment and society in which he lives.

Education is not only changing your present but helps in future change and will help the future generation to adapt to the changing situation.

Education transmits values, creativity and makes you practical person not just theoretic but all round development which is based on skill and makes you self-reliant and self-sufficient.

Education unlocks the door of modernization, opens the new avenues, new horizons, in creating better world to live.

What are the important factors in education?

1. Education gives you direction, education keeps you on right track.
2. You develop your philosophy of life that is sound.
3. You are highly educated but rooted and ground on the reality of human element of nature.
4. You understand better religion, politics, problems of nation.
5. Culture in which you are born, heritage you belong to, tradition that our forefather hold, and continue to explore

the knowledge at the same time know the meaning and purpose of education, these are the factors once you get good education.

How education helps a person in his life?

- Education prepares the person to earn his livelihood and economic security.
- You have healthy adjustment in life, modification in behavior and awareness of society in which you live and have your being.
- Makes you capable for complete living.
- Your powers are developed in harmonious manner.
- It helps to realize who you are—self-realization.
- Civilized, mannered, courtesy you live with others.
- You become good citizen.
- Your individuality blooms by realizing physical, moral, intellectual, emotional, spiritual capacities and abilities.

What is the importance of nursing education?

- Nurse becomes capable and confident to give care to the patient in all phases.
- She becomes expert bed side care giver in all settings in all situations.
- She integrates theory and practice.
- Every care she gives has a scientific principle that she keeps in mind and understands the functioning of the body and mind in health and disease.
- Human body is a complex, so nurse has to be observant and vigilant, as what agrees one patient may not agree with another, because body chemistries differ.
- Works in team spirit in cooperation.
- Takes initiative, responsibilities.
- Purpose of good nurses is to get qualified professionally, becomes a role modem.
- Imparting up to date scientific principle based knowledge where she gets theory and practical knowledge.
- Has a leadership quality in decision making.
- Keeps professional ethics and code of conduct.
- Develops her personality, self-motivated, holding herself in public with respect and dignity of her profession.
- Does nursing research.
- Has democratic citizenship.

Education is life and life is education because education brings—

- **Modification of behavior**—giving a new shape to man
- **Makes person responsible for life**—involves thinking, reasoning and judgment to face the problems and challenges of life. It models character and morals
- **Makes life dynamic** and progressive
- **New powers** and functions are developed
- **Gives direction** to life
- **It liberates** one within
- **Helps to improve the quality and personality**—self-expression, creative thinking and critical awareness and improves quality of life
- **Creates awareness,** awareness leads to awareness-to-awareness
- **Provides opportunity for improving** vocational efficiency
- **Healthy attitudes and values** are formed, way at looking at things change, all is well in my world feeling
- Creates conscious of ones duties and responsibilities
- Develops leadership qualities
- Contributes in progress and prosperity of the nation building
- Develops discipline.

What is the nurse's role as health educator?

She has multiple roles to play such as she is a key person and a team leader; she is a trainer and teacher; she is change agent; rehabilitator; researcher; sheet anchor; decision maker and care provider- she is an important pillar providing health education to the community, individual, school, factory.

1. Provide opportunities for people to learn how to identify and analyze health and health related problems and how to set their own target and priorities.
2. Make health and health related information easily accessible to the community.
3. Indicate to the people alternative solutions for solving the health and health related problems they have identified.
4. People must have access to proven preventive measures.
5. The health problem must be identified in terms of its public importance.
6. The objectives should be clear stated before under talking health education.
7. All possible information regarding the problem should be collected. This includes vital statistics of the diseases or condition age groups involved geographically and climatic factors, health facilities.
8. Collect information about the community this includes knowledge and understanding of people about the problem misconception and tradition, communication barriers, other social programed, operation in the area and attitude of people towards the program and availability of personnel.
9. Plan is made about the knowledge and the be imparted, facts that need emphasis.
10. AV aids are prepared.
11. Local leaders and local voluntary agencies are approached and good rapport must be maintained.

12. The nurse has to coordinate the various sectors of the community.
13. She has to impart health education to the people.
14. Evaluation of the health education to be done.
15. She has top clarify the doubts and misconception of the people.
16. She has to maintain good communication skill with community.
17. All the all she is a counselor, advocate, promote, guide.

What are the functions of a nurse?

1. Identify health problem
2. Survey and collect vital statistics
3. Knowledge and understanding of the people
4. Planning and organization
5. Preparation of AV aids
6. Maintain good communication skills
7. Use peoples language
8. Place peoples health in peoples hand by awakening, motivating
9. Mobilize, train and monitor, supervise other health workers.

How is your health teaching evaluation done?

- On basis of planning
- Submission of plan in time
- Showed initiative and interest
- Selection of proper topic
- Relevant matter to the relevant group
- Up to date knowledge
- Reliable subject matter
- Method used appropriately
- Ideas communicated correctly
- Language used appropriately
- Was it effective
- Group participation and response of the people
- Got involved
- Control of the group
- Use of appropriate AV aids
- Handling and placement of education material.

Life is always knocking on your door every day, every minute, it is telling to change, get courage to change, if you want peace, joy, harmony work towards it. You get thorough working knowledge. Have a burning desire. It is not desire that makes one a successful, it is wide field and it takes time to learn its aspects.

You are wet mud in the hands of a teacher

One fish said to the other; do you believe in this ocean that they talk about. How narrow our vision of the world and the universe can be. We see the world from our limited perceptual framework and our sight is limited.

With scientific knowledge we know that many things are not what they appear to be, e.g. the sky is not blue, only the scattering of the blue light absorbed by the atmosphere makes it appear so. The moon does not rise in the night, and the house we live is not stationary but orates along with the earth. Essentially, we see, hear and we process what we can not what reality is; our perceptions are clouded by our personal thoughts.

Life is a combination of ignorance and knowledge. It needs fine training. You have knowledge but it is not polished with humility and understanding, then such knowledge will not bless you. Look at life with awareness. Courage is the power to let go of the familiar.

What is memory is a re-creating of things already perceived by the mind. Daily we are constantly re-collecting things perceived in the past. How does one activate memory? Brain is noting more than a worldly machine for mental recollection. Its various parts assist the mind in various ways. Even though an impression has faded from the nerve cells the mind can recreate the impression by its own power. 'Cerebral memory' the memory of its past life remains awake for approximately first 5 years of its new life. To re-experience past events one does not need the cooperation of the old brain 'Extra-cerebral memory'.

God has given an intelligent but we have to log on to it. It is hidden in us. Wake up, a problem is an alarm system act on it and be creative to solve it. Every problem is an invitation for us to be creative. It is not the load that breaks you, it is the way you carry it.

Knowledge is flooding day by day and we live in era of knowledge of explosion.

The proverb 'to teach is to learn twice' Teacher's unique style of teaching will make her efficient positive feed back, re-enforcement. The human mind is like a parachute and it works only when it opens, knowledge does not simply flow, receptive elicit interest in student, pay attention to individual student using creativity to motivate them.

What are the components of teaching skills?

1. Selecting the content
2. Selecting AV aids materials
3. Introducing the lesson
4. Questioning skills
5. Fluency in questioning
6. Probing questions
7. Response management
8. Pacing explanation
9. Discussions, demonstration
10. Illustration, teaching aids
11. Reinforcement and management of the class planned recitation, giving assignments, evaluation progress

12. Skill of promoting students participation, skill of using examples
13. Purpose to arose interest and curiosity focus, attention, stimulate pupil provide opportunities to assimilate and reflect
14. Maintain intellectual climate and establishing appropriate level of motivation help to revise earlier learning
15. A good teacher demands constant and conscious effort
16. Education stands between poverty and prosperity, education opens the door of opportunities
17. Use encouraging words and avoid criticism, be around but not over involved. Give it your best shot. Take charge now for a better tomorrow. It is time for a new wave of young leadership. With power comes responsibilities, limitation are challenges.

Lack of education leads to lack of wisdom, which leads to lack of morals, which leads to lack of progress, which leads to lack of money, which leads to oppression of vulnerable classes, see what havoc lack of education can cause.

Nothing great can be achieved without enthusiasm. The basic principles of education is to empower self and discover infinite potential through self-realization.

Education is the most powerful weapon, which you can use to change the world. Today education has become very expensive, and with the increasing competition, high fees and inadequate attention of the government towards education, the future is quiet uncertain. Education should be freely and easily available to everyone.

You can create your own success story—success is not the same as hard work. Traditionally a good academic qualification along with hard work was seem as pre-requisites for success. Things have changed in the new age competitive world. It is sum total of many things which prepare you. And when the preparation meets the opportunities one becomes successful, to get competitive age despite their background and high academic profiles. It is the fight for growth or survival to stay in the job. While millions of young graduates passing out of universities do not get appropriate jobs while the industry is craving for talents, what most need I the ability to deal with people, building high self-image, attitudes, skill of effective working in teams, managing difficult situations, managing change, resolving conflicts.

Catch them young—empowering the students with the relevant life skills thus youth who have got trained and mastered the life skills shall experience success as a by-product. Going beyond personality development, total human transformation, everything is possible if you think.

Curriculum for professional nursing—as defined "all the planned opportunities subject matter (body of knowledge, skills, values and attitudes) and learning activities that the faculty plans and implements in all settings (classrooms, laboratories, hospitals) for a particular group of students for specified time period" the curriculum in nursing also reflects the changes nature of society and its emerging themes. Curriculum should not be rigid and static, not neglecting mother tongue, not only book centered, narrow, limited and single track but progressive. Presence of technical and vocational studies and centered in learners to build a socially creative individuality and giving continuous intelligent growth process based on principle of child centered, activity centered, elasticity an variety, integration and based on principle of organization, willingness to receive and response.

Reflection and personal learning by asking the following:

1. How do you think you would respond in a similar situation? Why? What does it tell you about your skills and practice? How will you respond? Explain why? Why not? (skills technical, ethical legal, interpersonal) meet the criteria for successful outcome.
2. Bridging the gap to evidence based practice incorporate knowledge of the health related effects of the practice.
3. Researching in nursing—disclosing genetic test results to family members, all are composed of genes, how genes affect both growth and development—nurses can integrate this knowledge into care and counseling of patients in a variety of diverse settings.

The one trend to look forward to that will change education in India is to make the education system more practical oriented rather than theoretical. Right from kindergarten child should be instilled with practical knowledge and skill to apply the theory. In the present age of technology with everything only a click away use of good technology can bring in a big leap in the education system. Education needs to be upgraded at every level. Technology has taken an important place as far as teaching is concerned and future for learning. Education should inculcate value which will produce complete human being and not mere professions. Education is responsible for creating entrepreneurs who can generate job, at the same time, creative abilities should find their way in academics. Academics should produce individuals who are crisis managers, problem solvers and wealth creators.

Health education is an powerful tool in helping to solve India's multifarious health problem. Health education is an vaccine. It is as effective as an immunization if it is carried out with purpose and meaning.

Important role of a nurse in educational programme where she is an educator as well as a learner a liaison between community, home, hospital, doctors and other members of the team. The nurse should use her voice, ears, eyes and enhance knowledge to carry out the program. It requires skill and ability. At every opportunity, she should feel responsible to talk to patients and family. It you an educator are well prepared on the contents, you will be respected. Explain with definite reasoning why you are teaching a particular topic. For example, when you are advising a mother to eat green leaf vegetables, fruits, why she has to include this in her diet explain convincingly. She should remember that all these should be a continuous process involving the participation of community. Several obstacles like ignorance, poverty, beliefs, customs and habits are present before the result seen.

What are the different techniques of modern interviews?

With growing technology, the interview techniques have also attained a new modus operation. The olden techniques are now replaced by more modern technique like audio video online interviews, telephonic interview, intervention of new gadgets of Sci-Fi technology for too busy and speedy world of employers. AV interviews seems bit easier as compared to other modus. In such interviews, the panel of experts is seating at far and district places across the country or many times overseas as the candidates has to connect with the panel through AV peripheral and software. This mode of interview more suitable

Tips interviews—check out the internet and telephone access along with AV compatibility soft ware as well as hard ware configured to your computer system. A trial of all is highly expected prior to the actual commencement of interviews. Power back up sources like ups to ensure they re working. The back of seating pleasant background to produce better video profile the webcam with better resolution and focus point properly adjusted to get clear and visible picture. You should sit bit inclined in front of the webcam. With the light source illuminating your entire face. You should have pen, pencil and plain paper to jot down some calculations, keep calculator at your disposal. Sit with all your credentials and gist of your achievements on a single paper in chronological order. Keep cell phone away on salient mode, feel motivated, you should be positive and confident, get relaxed and wait for your call. Start with. Zeal and zest to convince the interviewer, and start with manner with wishing interviewer, while speaking at the microphone, the distance should not be far less or far more. it should be adjusted so that the interviewer at other end listens to each and every single word of your audio intonation. Ask, excuse me, am I audible to you or not? If not adjust your setting, avoid coughing or sneezing directly over the mouthpiece of microphone. If it happens, say sorry sir, keep physical and mental health support, which helps in many ways in interview.

Knowledge is power. One life is not enough for those who want to dive deep into it. The journey is long but your intellectual thirst will be satisfied. Then only you will experience the power and the confidant of having knowledge that is up to date and how far it will take you, it will make a world of difference in your life, it is worth.

Keywords

What is education—What education does, changing concept, goal of education, importance of education in today scenario, characteristic of education, nurse's role as health educator, functions of a nurse, components of teaching skills, curriculum for professional nursing different techniques of modern interviews.

CHAPTER

5

Value of Education in Nursing

Abstract

Value of education remains same to any profession you take. It helps to live our life harmoniously, builds our character, and makes us better human beings. It increases the strength of mind and trains, disciplines ones interior being which radiates, reflects exterior aspect of life.

A nation's strength lies in its intellectual property, which needs border vision and intellectual quality research in terms of our innovation.

The nurse plays a vital role in health education of the people who come daily in her contact. She can give good amount of reliable health information. She can be an instrument in implementing and interpreting various levels of education through teaching and learning process.

Nurse can create conducive atmosphere and environment to facilitate critical thinking and self-learning curiosity. She is a good mediator and a link that connects like an umbilical cord to the client and self, people and community.

What is education?

Education means to cause learning where knowledge and skills can be actively acquired. It makes people think for themselves. Health education is an essential tool of education which helps to influence people in order that they may attain best of health. It is a process which effects changes in the health practices of people and in the knowledge and attitudes related to such changes. Health education helps to bridge the gulf between the health knowledge and the health practice of the people. Health education is "cement" that binds together the "bricks" of the health programed.

Real education will not teach you to compete. It will teach you to cooperate. It will not teach you to fight and come first. It will teach you to be creative, to be loving, blissful, without any compares with the other. It will not teach you that you can be happy only when you are first, it will form your character and make you a fine human being. The highest education is that which does not merely give us information but makes our life in harmony with all existence.

Today education is must for first to the last, it is a fundamental duty of the state that its people get basic education. If the poor cannot come to education, education must reach them at the plough, in the factory, everywhere.

India is moving at a fast pace towards globalization and hence there will be an ever increasing demand of qualified professionals with an exclusive skill set and international exposure which will empower nurses to face the challenges to the future through your quality education. We have to improve higher education in terms of quality of our innovation and research.

Let us understand this meaningful and purposeful story to get the moral of wisdom how.

Wisdom, food and wealth set out on a journey. Soon, they met a man who asked, where are you going? They said, looking for a place to live. The man said, oh God, I want wealth to live with me. Wealth said, oh foolish man, you would not have me around for long.

Soon they met another who also asked where they all were going. They answered hunting for a place to live. The man said in that case, I invite food to live with me. Food said even if I come with you today, you could not keep me for long.

Further along them met a third man. He too asked where they are going, seeking a place to live, they said. The man said wisdom can live with me. Food and wealth said, you have chosen wisdom, so you will be able to take good care of us too. All three moved to his place.

Our experience tells us that too much human conflict, distress and suffering comes from lack of wisdom. Wisdom consists of making the best use of knowledge, and real knowledge comes from education.

While intelligence, cleverness or the ability to appear dynamic is something a man is born with, wisdom is not. One way to increase in wisdom is to move from raw to refined thinking, feeling, reflecting and acting.

Refined thinking involves becoming aware, informed, interested, discerning, from right to wrong. They learn what truly is important.

Communication skill is a core and essential of health education. Our ability to influence others depends on the skill of communication; therefore, it is very important. The health message how is it communicated, do the public understand, it is clear and accurate will depend on your communication skill, and the channels of communication that you are using. All efforts and attempt must be made through creativity of channels to reach to the targeted group. All the barriers overcome by good communication skill.

Throughout the world, people are seeking better health and better education. Never before have such high priorities been given to these two attributes. From the smallest village to the most complex urban center, new hopes exists for improving the health of individuals, families and communities. At the same time education, which is suitable to the locality and the times, has become a matter of major importance. Vast resources, both human and financial, are now directed towards bringing about better health and better education at local, state, regional, national and international levels. Education is increasingly recognized as an essential part of all health efforts-education which will evoke understanding, support and willing participation of the people themselves.

The term health education means many things to many people. Nurses exert their influence on patents or individuals in such a way as to affect their health behavior. It is an attempt to improve both personal and community health attitudes and habits by involving the individual or a group, so that they learn how to apply available knowledge to meet their needs. Thus, the health education makes the difference between what people know and what they do with what they know. Education must help the interest of the people in improving their conditions of living and health betterment as member of the families.

Education supplies a person with enough new and correct knowledge about a disease to make the preventive measures required by scientific medicine, makes person keen in importance of his own health and adopts these preventive measures.

Education is a delightful moment and is a part, i.e. integral part of ones life, which enhances to make right choice and gives clarity of perception, makes life worth to live and develops mental and innate powers. Education is a complete development of a child into full human life with its potentials, talents and God given capacities and strengths. Education therefore known as a manifestation of divine into the core of man that is hidden comes to enlightenment.

Due to the education strength of mind increased and sharpened where one can stand on his own feet rooted and grounded happen what may, in all seasons and in all climates and all the ups and downs of life it gives forbearance, endurance and firmness as strong rock unmoved untouched by any eventuality. Making within and outside environment harmonious with contentment and self satisfaction to the fullness. It trains and disciplines ones interior being; which radiates and reflects exterior aspects of life. From core to core relating, human to divine realization of atman, transformation of self.

Intellect and intelligence—we spend a lot of time acquiring intelligence at the expenses of developing intellect. Intelligence is built by gaining information, knowledge from external agencies, from schools and universities, teachers and textbooks. The intellect is developed through your individual effort by exercising the faculty of questioning, thinking and reasoning. Not accepting anything that does not admit logic or reason—know the difference between the two.

The intelligence acquired from external is like data fed in to a computer. Not all the knowledge stored in its memory can help the computer to act its own. If the room catches fire, it will go up in flames.

The knowledge you acquire is of no use to you without an intellect. This knowledge gained should have practical use in life. That explains why among millions of doctors graduating only a few have discovered life saving procedures, cures and remedies.

It is same with engineer they have only a few designs-something unusual. It is their intellect that makes their performance outstanding. People sometimes do not attempt to develop this, thus education lost the meaning and purpose, without this type of awareness human being becomes robots.

That explains why highly educated businesspersons, professionals and scholars become alcoholics, and short-tempered when intellect is under developed and weak. Unable to control mind, strike balance between acquired intelligence and developed intellect will lead mind under perfect control, and people live in peace and prosperity.

In education E-books have arrived with a big bang. Electronic form is easy and economical to fix a mistake. It is easy to read with appealing title, draws an audience to read the book. Lower the price of e-book the more the chance of it getting downloaded. It helps to reach out to larger audiences, it is technical in nature, and it has to be up to date in electronic form.

Life is never constant. It varies continuously, just as the flow of river. If it comes to a standstill, it starts to stagnate, no adventure and no activity. Find newfound sense of living with a purpose.

Value of Importance

Some of the most brilliant, most successful people are forgotten in their own lifetime. That is the problem with fame, power, success, and money. They do not stay in the hearts and minds of people.

1. Name a few teachers who helped you along during your growing up years in school and college.
2. Name some friends who saw you through your difficult days.
3. Name a few people you loved and who loved you.
4. Think of some people who made you feel appreciated and special.
5. Think of 5 people you enjoy spending time with.
6. Moral of the story is people who make a difference to your life are not the ones with the best credentials, the

most money or the most awards, you admire them, but they never impact your life in the way those closet to you. We tend to forget this. We believe the rich, the famous, and the successful inspire us, but we actually cherish those who touch our lives, even if they move on.

In education E-books—distance learning is gaining more popularity since it is cost effective as well as convenient education. Pursuing higher education in abroad is considered a big boost for career growth, it involves a lot of finance, and however, if one has to climb the corporate ladder, upgrading knowledge is important weapon in the armory. Distance learning requires you to read, think and express your thoughts on your own. Education provides the foundation for development of individuals and nation.

It is easier to blame the system than self-introspect, how does system change? There are 378 universities, 18,064 colleges us, 4.92 lakh teachers, 140 lakh students, one of the largest in the world, despite the country has maximum number of illiterate. Equitable access to education to remote corners, using education as a growth driver the education that developing nation desperately need and constantly seek, is one which equitable opportunities for the poor.

In youth the days are short and the years are long, in old age the years are short and the days are long.

Medical Quiz

1. When is national voluntary blood donation day observed in India–October 1st?
2. How many vertebrates are present in human neck–07?
3. Which is the main artery that carries oxygenated blood from the heart to the body–aorta?
4. Which is the gland in the human body that acts both as exocrine and endocrine gland–pancreas?
5. What does the term Brady-cardiac mean–slow heart rate?
6. What is the average life span of blood platelets–5 to 90 days?
7. Which endocrine gland takes an active part in body's immune system–thymus gland?
8. What is the chemical name for vitamin B_{12}–cyanocobalamin?
9. What is the cause of hypokalemia–potassium?
10. What is the common name for schizophrenia–spilt personality?

Gaining education is a slow process—Do not be in a hurry—e.g. A man who was very fond of trees wanted to see a green tree in the courtyard of his home. He thought that if he planted a sapling, it would take a long-time to grow into the tree. So he went to a garden and selected a fully grown tree. He then employed several laborers to dig it up and then transplant it to his courtyard where he had it planted.

The man was very happy. He thought to himself, I have traveled a long journey in a single day. Planting sapling or a seed would have been a lengthy business and how I have found quick way of having lush green tree. However, the next morning when he looked at the tree, he found that its leaves had begun to wither and after a few days, the whole tree dried up. He was disappointed. I am in hurry, but God is not.

The law of nature is based on gradual development and not sudden leaps. This law applied to every profession, every business and tree is no exception. Constructing a really solid foundation requires a long period of time; you cannot have foundation by just talking wild leaps, final results uprooted.

In today's world, is it possible for a teenager to follow Gandhian principles of ahimsa and truth.

1. Some values that Gandhi spoke about can be implemented today. Especially the value of personal hygiene and is perennially relevant across the length and breath of our country.
2. Ahimsa can be implemented today where there is a lot of violence across all segments of the society.
3. He was the chief architect of India's freedom movement. He was an inspiration for his principles and ideologies which he professed till his last breath.
4. He is very much lives among us, he is not just the person, but a way of life that brings perfect harmony in body, mind and soul.
5. His life of modesty and discipline and ability to plan with precision, he always practiced what he preached, he believed in simple living and high thinking. His wisdom became his weapon. The ideas of the Mahatma are timeless.
6. Rural development—if the village perishes, India will perish too. It will be no more India. In other words, if villagers are independent and strong both economically and politically, states will boom and so will the center.
7. Fearless or fight for truth—no one can defeat us, despite all the hardship. Fearless is the first requisite of spirituality.
8. There is a sufficiency in the world for mans need but not for mans greed.
9. You must be the change you wish to see in the world.
10. He had a habit of a silence on the issue which he did not want to talk.

Literature increases the perspective of students by exposing them to different cultures and lifestyles. They learn to be sensitive to the problems of others and also learn to appreciate other cultures and ideology.

Today nanotechnology is seen as the way of the future and many people feel that it will revolutionize the world. Its benefits are cheap and powerful energy generation, improved formulation of drugs, interactive smart appliances. Education will play key role in achieving high growth. Science and technology competitions are tough.

Leadership is largely a behavioral skill. It cannot be taught, only learnt. The key to leadership is to accept responsibilities. To be a leader you have to be at one with the people you lead. Leaders need a clear vision; they should know where they are going. Leaders set high standards and inspire people to achieve. Leaders should understand the needs of their followers.

Swami Vivekananda (1863–1902): It is time we reflect on the educational aspects with our life. We are what our thoughts have made us; so take care about what you think. Words are secondary. Thoughts live; they travel far. Have faith that you are all, my brave lads, born to do great things. Let not the barks of puppies frighten you-no, not even the thunderbolts of heaven. So long as millions live in hunger and ignorance. I hold every man a traitor who, having been educated at their expense, pays not the least heed to them. I want each one of my children to be a hundred times greater then I could ever be. Every one of you must be a giant, obedience, readiness, and love for the cause—if you have these three, nothing can hold you back. Take up one idea. Make that one idea your life—think of it, dream of it, live on that idea. Let the brain, muscles, nerves, every part of your body, be full of that idea, and just leave every other idea alone. This is the way to success. Always hold on to the highest. Be steady. Avoid jealousy and selfishness. Be obedient and eternally faithful to the cause to truth, humanity, and your country, and you will move the world.

Keywords

What is education—communication skill, education is a delightful moment, education supplies, the strength of mind, intellect and intelligence, the knowledge you acquire, an investment in knowledge pays the best interest. An investment in knowledge pays the best interest. E-books, life is never constant, distance learning, literature, today nanotechnology, leadership.

CHAPTER

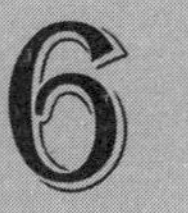

Education in Practice

Abstract

Education is the power to think clearly, the horizons of the students have to be widened which is relevant and life oriented with the revolution brought about by computers, connectivity through the internet focus on new value system which can enable to create a new world. Exposure to the latest technologies, gadgets, gimps, television, computer has developed keener learner then ever before, today parents wants their children excel in all kinds of activities so that they develop confidence. The aim of education must be to earn for his livelihood and become self-sufficient, stand on his own feet, do healthy adjustment in life, modify his attitudes, morals, behavior, and life in its fullness.

What you learn in theory the nurse has to practice it in the field correlating the theory and practice and closing the gap between the two. For example, a theory helps her to understand the procedure and procedure helps her to understand theory. They are two sides of the same coin.

Beyond classroom—Your expression is the most important things you wear. Do things that others say you cannot do. Sci-tech example—a student from national institute re-design the tanpura to make a modern day version of the ancient musical instrument. It is a digital tanpura with sensory pads as part of a classroom project. Although not a musician himself, he is inspired, and has observed the playing postures and finger movements of the musician use when they play the tanpura. The original posture itself had a lot of drawbacks.

He looked at the point which comes in contact with the human body while playing and tried to create a stable but similar posture. He added sensory pads for better sound output. He design, despite having a simplified form, does achieve its purpose of bridging the gap between the electronic and acoustic tanpura in terms of function, while maintaining the tactile and emotional relationship between the instrument and its player, it is light in weight. This is the important difference with people with wisdom and knowledge. Adding something new to existing things using unique capacity and talents with creativity.

Education is the process that enables you to have knowledge. Education allows us to access the collected wisdom, learning and conclusion of the human race since methods of knowledge transmission began.

A goal without plan is just a wish.

Education costs money, but then so does the ignorance.

'We want that education by which character is formed, strength of mind is increased, the intellect is expanded and by which one can stand on ones own feet.'

—Swami Vivekananda

The goal of mankind is knowledge. Now this knowledge is inherited in man. No knowledge comes from outside. It is all inside, he discovers, unveils. We are responsible for what we are, and whatever we wish ourselves to be. We have power to make ourselves.

New Trials in Mumbai Schools

Schools will now make teachers answer all the papers they set for their pupils to gauge how easy or difficult it would be for them. A unique move, in the new system the teacher will set the question paper which will be send for moderation to the examination committee consisting of subject and department heads after questions are finalized, the teachers will appear for the paper before the students do.

The idea is to make the teacher appreciate the paper critically. The teacher will know how much time it actually takes to answer the questions, of course, they will tackle faster than the pupil will cope with, the teachers answers will be reviewed by the committee and approved cope set as benchmark for the students. The new process is aimed at introducing complete transparency in the examination system and to improve the quality of education

A teacher will know the answer to the questions set by him. But it is different thing to sit and answer it like a student. This will give them an idea of how balanced is paper in terms of application and theory. It will also help them understand if it is good enough for both the bright and the weak students.

Focusing on academic and theory alone is not enough, schools today realize the importance of practice education and are laying more stress on the same.

A clear vision is developed in the minds of students after practical teaching. These are pursuits taken to meet the needs of the students, as they have to face stiff market competing when the time comes for them to exercise their career option. In today's competitive world, progress and advancement is going on at a fast pace and one, therefore, cannot afford to lag behind. Hence, the new technologies of practical teaching should be adopted regularly keeping in mind that a balance of modern technology.

Practical teaching helps even the dull students to come up to the level of bright students.

Exposure to the latest technologies, gadgets, gimps, television, computer has developed keener learner then ever before, today parents wants their children excel in all kinds of activities so that they develop confidence.

Innovating ways of teaching makes person all rounder when he comes out as product. It makes learning more fun, they are taken for education visits, different specialty departments, encouraged to participate competitions, quiz, debates leaves deeper impact and develops their analytical skills. Practical teaching is beneficial for both the teachers and the students it makes learning easier.

Knowledge is Supreme Strength

1. The very essence of education is concentration of mind, not the collecting of facts
   'Literary education is of no value if it is not able to build up a sound character. If we are to teach real peace in this world, and if we are to carry on a real war against war, we shall have to begin with the children'—Gandhi
2. 'The product of education should be free creative man, who can battle against historical circumstances and adversities of nature. The highest achievement of the human mind and spirit are not limited to the past. The gates of the future are wide open'—Dr Sarvepalli Radhakrishnan
3. 'The object of education is to give the man unity of truth'—Rabindranath Tagore
4. Physical education of the body to be effective must be rigorous and detailed, farsighted and methodological. This will be translated into habits. These habits should be controlled and disciplined while remaining flexible enough to adapt themselves to circumstances and to the needs of growth and development of the being.

The future of education in India is intrinsically linked to the improvement in quality of education encompassing its availability for all. It is also crucially dependent on its ability to equip our youth with the capacity to meet future challenges. Today countries across the world are mobilizing resources towards establishing knowledge based societies.

Education in India, therefore should be similarly geared to achieve these objectives by inculcating scientific temper, positive activities integrated development of individual personality, pursuit of knowledge and excellence synthesizing Indians cultural ethos and cherished human values, which will strengthen and reinvigorate future of education in India.

Students never regard your study as a duty, but as the envisaged opportunity to experience freedom of your capabilities. Education enables you to experience the spirit of your personal joy and also enables you to work toward the profit of the country, to which your later work belongs.

The dream of India be accomplished by giving a strong foundation to our youth. What should remain constant is our value, our culture and our philosophy. Education in India will have to provide a dynamic, broad based curriculum in an intellectually stimulating environment aimed at meeting the challenging needs of tomorrow's world.

The younger generation who will step into a school today will face the real world in future. Education should be combination of four core factors which are—

1. Academics
2. Sports
3. Extra-curricular activities
4. Values.

Thus leading to an over all development of a child which in turn will lead to the over all; development of our nation in the future.

India is a land of diverse social and economic statues. **Education begins from** the school and we have various systems of education to offer to the schoolchildren. However, the basic aim of all systems of education should be create strong foundation of education to make children of rich human resource for the country. For third, analytical attitude must be developed in children from the very beginning, creativity has to be encouraged in children and they should not be given a chance to express their views. Education is not merely the memorization of facts but the learning of fundamental principles to guide us to face life.

Education is what remains after one has forgotten everything he leant in the school.

The education extends beyond classroom, books and structured learning, molding, mixing. Though the digital gap between haves and have not become less, because of rapidly advancing technology, the emphasis should be good educational facilities. The horizons of the students have to be widened which is relevant and life-oriented with the revolution brought about by computers, connectivity through the internet focus on new value system which can enable to create a new world. Class room teaching and learning is an enjoyable activity.

Education is the power to think clearly, the power to act well in the world of work and the power to appreciate life. It takes half of life before you, to discover life is to do it yourself project.

For effective and relevant education needs good infrastructure.

Quality Institutions

Working towards preserving and perpetuating the arts.

The whole purpose of education is to turn mirror into window.

Knowledge determines attitudes and an attitude determines behavior. It is the power that drives a person from within to act. Persuasion is an art, a conscious attempt which can change lifestyle and modify the risk factors of disease.

Health education can help to increase knowledge and to reinforce desired behavior patterns. The goal is to make realistic improvements in the basic quality of life. Effective health education has the potential for saving many more lives. For this people must be educated through planned learning experience what to do, informed, educated and encouraged to make their own choice for a healthy life. The results are slow but enduring.

We all have the extraordinary talents within us waiting to be released and education is the wise path to unleash the power within. Education and knowledge gives us wisdom. Wisdom knows what to do and virtue is doing it.

Where there is righteousness in the heart, there is beauty in the character, where there is beauty in character, there is harmony in the home, there's order in the nation. Where there is order in the nation, there is peace in the world. To provide righteousness in the heart of young minds, we should have environment of great education and spiritual way of life. The combination of creativity and courage is knowledge.

—Shri APJ Abdul Kalam

Continuous effort—not strength or intelligence is the key to unlocking our potential.

Learning is a treasure that will follow its owner everywhere. We are learning all the time. The tombstone will be our diploma. Education is a progressive discovery of our own ignorance. Teaching is a profession that teaches all the other professions. The highest results of education are tolerance. Only the educated are free.

Education is a social process by which the innate capacities of an individual are drawn out and he is adjusted to the society in which he lives. Thus, it is a two fold process of growth of personality and enhancement of the degree of adjustability to the surrounding. The basic aim of education is to modify behavior.

Intelligent is the ability to give response that are true, carry out abstract thinking is a goal directed behavior, it is a creativity, concrete. Learning takes place best when a person is ready to learn.

Education is the ability to listen to almost anything without loosing your temper or your self-confidence.

The ancient masters did not try to educate the people, but kindly taught them know-how.

Formal education will make your living; self-education will make your a fortune.

Education plays a vital role in developing country. Education is not just about text books, exams, assignments and projects. To be educated means to be enlightened, to be aware of your surrounding and to be conscious of your rights. Education is tool towards better future to make your presence felt in today's fast paced domain. Education is a turning point in people's life. It helps to march ahead with the changing times and proves worth against all odds. It is your attitude, not your aptitude, which determines your altitude.

Education is our passport to the future. For tomorrow belongs to the people who prepared for it today.

E-CLASS

A revolutionary teaching and learning methodology—chapter wise audio video content in a pen drive. E-class comprises of a pen drive that has the entire syllabus for standard 8, 9, 10th in English. It has innovative features like world class animations, demo of science lab experiments, learning techniques like mind maps and important questions after very chapter.

It helps students to understand what they learn and not just memorize them for the exams. Students are taught each subject, chapter by chapter, by a real teacher in virtual classroom, something their mind can relate to; the content is exactly as per test book.

It helps students to write their paper confidently, thus giving them more marks in their exams. It is a perfect educational solution for schools, coaching classes, teachers, parents and students.

Benefits

1. Increases success rate in board examination.
2. Stronger intuitional image in society.
3. Bridging the digital, divide among the students and building better bonds between teacher and students.
4. A generation teaching aid with a plethora of reference.
5. Comprehensive lesson plan.
6. An energy format for better student learning and hassle free teaching environment.
7. Exciting audio videos which help the students to remember chapter better as compared to just by hearing it from books.

Various Devices to Play E-class

1. **E-box**—portable pen drive player comes with a remote control can be used to play other versions and see photographs on your TV.
2. **E-screen**—digital screen comes with a remote control and ear phones; can be used to play other videos and see photographs too.

3. **E-projector**—high luminous projector with key good clarity and result on screen.
4. **Pullable screen**—best quality screen available I standard sizes and also can be made as per customized measurement.
5. **E-board**—interactive white board you can connect to internets and show web pages well as write on e-board. Use option one—attaché's pen drive on e-box and view content on your TV. Option two—you can also directly load the content on your laptop/computer.

We can use in nursing this above method, e.g. to show on line operation, procedures, lectures, video conferences with new methodology, new technique and new inventions, even sitting in India international level video conferences can be attended.

In today's fast forwards ultramodern life, nurses too have to progress in her day today knowledge and get access to the internet to make a world of difference to her skill and personality, which is the need of the hour. She cannot just be satisfy herself with whatever she knows but get in touch with the advances made in science. If she wants to be component with the world of medicine, she will have to plunge into the updated knowledge. That not only will make her self-confidant but much more efficient and capable in her field.

There are client-oriented sites as well as medico-specific ones. With increasing usage of the www by everyone all over the world, telemedicine, client support groups and health-focused information has become freely available to everyone. Clients more than ever before, are better informed and have access to various databases. It therefore becomes important to keep abreast of the various health-info sources available on the net. It offers tremendous opportunities for the medical profession to serve humankind. We get latest information.

The internet has already changed the way we live. It has changed the way every important activity, weather commercial or academic, is translated. For the health professionals, it represents a big opportunity, not only to stay updated on the latest in the world of medicine, but also to get connected to the medical fraternity across the world as never before. A person with wide experience in both the field of health care and computer is important. It is a powerful tool. In the earlier days when a doctor could do nothing more for a critically ill person, the family would start praying. Now they turn to the internet, which provides a wealth of information for clients that can be very useful for the care of a critically ill client. People with medical conditions use the internet to communicate with each other in support groups and to compare experiences. Therefore, Internet is a resource that should not be ignored today.

Medical education on the internet—medicine is the only discipline, which requires a formal continuing education process. With advance of the internet, the newest modality of learning is the information technology you can participate in continuing medical education at websites. There you find visuals on the human body; research reports and lets you explore the amazing world of senses, nervous system, brain imaging and scanning techniques.

Learn about your topic as you search. It gives you subject categorization or you may be able to find a database on your subject. Multiple database searching lets you search in all of info mines categories at once. It is very convenient, searchable database, very worthwhile for many topics and for references. To see alphabetical list on everything available through search com; which is comprehensive, informative and useful, easily found.

General sites of medical and pharma interest you have health and medical news, information on hypertension, dialysis and clinical nephrology, the alternative and complementary medicine center, hospital sites directory-international and national, anesthesiology, ayurveda, cardiology, clinical, dentistry, dermatology, emergency, to name them few health care professionals providing for the exchange of ideas and opinions with experienced professionals.

Today nurse is not merely attendant in the ill room but also a educator and researcher. It is applied science to establish certain laws and principles. It requires sound knowledge. The better the scientific background the safer and more intelligent care provider she becomes. Thus, she utilizes the skills and techniques to meet the whole person in its totality that is considering all the aspects of physical, psychological, spiritual, social, economical, and intellectual.

Her profession promotes human and social welfare. She has to be up-to-date with the knowledge of physical and biological sciences, social science, and medical science, etc. to become a good nurse.

Today's nurses do various functions in the hospital as well as in the community for this she needs to be adequately prepared and learn new ideas by lot of in-depth extensive reading, and attending latest conferences to fulfill her responsibility of the nurse who is responsible to conserve life and promote health, nature and nourishes her profession on continues research work. This will help her to maintain health, promote health and prevent diseases. That will help her to come up the level of accuracy and able to respond to the challenges. When she keeps her knowledge up-to-date, she can maintain a highest standard of care, current in the nursing practice. She will be able to plan her work in a purposeful way. Thus, she will do her work skillfully to provide relief and comfort to the client.

While caring the patient when she comes across a confusion terminology or a diagnosis or diseases she can turn to the net and get the information to have better understanding of the condition as well as she will be better equipped to respond to the client. Knowledge is a power and an asset. It is the greatest weapon of our times. Good sound knowledge of a subject one can deals with situation in apt manner and it will take the person to the high-test ladder of achievement.

Today we are served with so many good things only one has to have interest and access to right kind of information to know where and how to get it. Medical health is a vast giant subject and one can never dive into its depth, the more one knows the more thirst felt as there is so much to explore it is never enough . So together with your work and study go on and on getting in touch with the latest.

Keep informed yourself everyday, because, even after few years of study, one knows something yet you are just like a drop in the ocean. Due to vast subject, you specialize in particular subject you are more interested in and go on exploring into that line to develop your specialty and your identity. Internet provides students and there teachers to easy to implement educational materials to spark an interest an interest in all manner of subject. You are a new age nurse with challenges and opportunities to gain skills.

Nurses with today's rapid and unprecedented changes, new urgency has been added to the critical need for a body of knowledge specific to nursing. Knowledgeable nursing services are indispensable to public safety. Humanitarian values add a further imperative to the search for understanding man and his world. True focus of the profession is on patient health care needs. Applying and teaching all we know for patient's highest potential for healthful living.

Nurse is a person who has completed a program of nursing education, qualified, and authorized to provide responsible and competent professional service. Her responsibility is to promote health to prevent illness, to restore health and to alleviate suffering. Public health nurse most directly concerned with giving health education and care to individual and families in the community. To shoulder new tasks and responsibly and to much wider role she plays in society. She acts as a sheet anchor of total health care system. For the purpose of promoting, maintains, monitoring and restoring health. She is a key person and the back born of health care delivery system.

There is growing need for community-based health care. As more and more health care delivery shifts into the community, more nurses are working in a variety of community-based settings, such as public health department, ambulatory health clinics, long-term care facilities, prenatal and well baby clinics, hospice agencies, and industrial settings as occupational nurses, homeless shelters and clinics and clients homes.

Here they must be self-directed, flexible, adaptable and tolerant of various lifestyles and living conditions. Here often it is an independent decision-making, critical thinking, assessing, and health education. It focuses in maintaining the health of the population and of preventing and minimizing the progression of diseases. Here direct care is given to the entire community. So here she needs added knowledge to deal with multidimensional situations and problems that arise in health field.

In critical thinking—using ones own reasoning or though process while thinking refine-thinking skills, high level critical thinking within nursing process. Goal orientated activity, truth seeker with an open mindedness to the alternative solutions that might surface. Reflective, insightful, analyze information, questioning all findings, creative methods of proceeding. Knowing to interpret information and knowing what it tells her.

Today sophisticated technology can prolong life well beyond the time when death would have occurred in the past. Expensive experimental procedures and medication are available for use in attempting to preserve life, this has an influence on all stages of life, e.g. genetic screening in vitro fertilization, the harvesting and freezing of life, premature infants are given a chance for survival because of technical support. Children and adult who would have died a result of organ failure are living longer because organ transplantation. Technological advances have also contributed to increase life expectancy and better quality of life. The nurse as a teacher is challenged to focus on the educational needs of society. Nurses must seize opportunities both inside and outside of health care settings to facilitate wellness. Talking responsibilities for oneself is the key to successful health promotion. The possibilities are endless and the opportunities are countless. In addition, for people with drive and ambitions the world is truly is not enough.

Nursing is a profession is much wider and greater than the world ever knows. Today they are sheet anchor. It has transformed the narrow confines of traditional nurses to professional nurses with wider responsibility. We have to equip them with better skill and higher education. Today curriculum is reviewed, revised and restructured for improving the quality of human life. In this new dispensation they will become resource to people is the essence of community health. Nurses works like magic and give client considerable relief from mental anxiety. As hungry man needs food and water, so a sick client needs care and medicines. And the mediator and bridge, link, forming chain is this great nurse a key force in providing.

Folded computer and television screens come closer to reality. Computers that can be folded up to be in the pocket and televisions sets that can be ended to view may soon be a reality, thanks to the efforts of researchers from Sony, beginning of a technological revolution for screen display. Such technology can also lead to the mass production of moving image posters for display systems that let readers to upload daily news to an easy to carry display contraption, the researches say. For example, no mean feet—researchers helped create prosthesis for an athlete who competed at the paralympics; plans include similar devices for other disabled people. For example, follow the A, B, C, D, E—that is avoid alcohol, smoking, blood pressure control, cholesterol, diabetes, and exercise. Before they seek you, you seek them with early detection. Due to globalization, all advance technology of west available in India but cost factor is more.

Remote diagnosis—on a computer monitor with high tech hub radiologist examines a scan of the skull of a six-year of boy who fell off his bicycle. A few minutes later, thousands of miles away, doctors at a hospital in Philadelphia prepared the boy for surgery after receiving an urgent e-mail diagnosing a sub-dural hemorrhage in the child's brain. India faces an acute shortage of radiologists even as teleradiology clinics sprout up. We can act as extended arm, teleradiology is just the beginning, telecardiology, telepathology, teledermatology, and robotic telesurgery are possible in the very near future.

New artificial intelligence dupes people into thinking they are talking with fellow humans–bridging the divide between man and machine. All this only means computers are getting better in conversing with humans, reducing the gap between man and machine.

There was a time not so long ago when getting a second opinion almost always meant going to another qualified doctor that is spending more money, time and effort. Today internet is available at home to look for health information at home on line. Up to 75% of online patients with chronic problems have search and taken decision to treat illness or conditions. Recent surge in high speed, always on broadband connectivity has enabled much more frequent and in depth in formation searches which is particularly attractive if something important is at state. Patient go back to doctor with new questions regarding drug, diets or alternative procedures, they also post-technical advice on line about managing a certain diseases beside offering advice on how to communicate with health care providers.

Such expanded level mean patient empowerment and more democratization of health care with information no longer flowing only one way from an erudite doctor to an untaught sufferers. It is certainly better than being very dependent on a physician, surgeon or specialist praising clinician who. Largely because of time constrains makes patient full fledged and equal participation in the entire treatment procedure and the system as a whole? Causation, misinformation generated this way can harmful specially taking decisions without supervision or worse self-medication.

The mind is meant to absorb information, transform it into knowledge and lead it into action. Action and speech determine the quality of life. Wise men say that most peoples minds are as hard as rock. Just as rock is impervious to water, information that falls on a hard mind bounces off without trace. A hard mind offers immense resistance. It is full of previously absorbed information that prevents the flow of new knowledge and action. Our mind must be soft as sponge for maximum absorption; just as water, can easily absorb.

Moreover, computer improves efficiency, decrease expenditure; convey a modern image to patients.

Modern health care delivery system has become very complex and there is need to obtain continuously up dated information that is efficient information transmission. Used in right time for the purpose of solving patients care problems. The development of electronic devices has given added impetus in problems that are difficult to tackle earlier; now detect accurately and rapidly. Today's nurse needs to communicate with people as well as with machines.

Computer technology has undergone significant changes from its inception. Health care institutions must also keep pace with the changes constantly with the invasions of internet essential latest technology. Because it improves efficacy at work, improves the services to the patient, provides netter professional care to the patient, and improves profitability, efficient utilization of staff resources, time management.

In clinical too it helps in professional work, data handling, diagnosis and decision, prescriptions, statistics and reference and number of ways. It is useful in mental health and psychiatric nursing. Its technology is widely used. It has potential in continuous medical education and distance learning program. With the help of internet, worldwide latest information with regard to diagnosis, treatment modalities and other therapeutic measures can be made available. In addition, for clinical conference, storage of information for long and the gigantic database that it can hold and allow to access in variety of formats, helps to undertake any future activity. It is time saving and money saving by reducing stationary costs, better planning of resources information of new drugs, materials and therapies with advancement of science, with the help of internet and multimedia detailed information obtained. It helps to improve the skills or levels of knowledge so that each employee is better equipped. It helps in desired medications in the skills, attitudes to perform job efficiently and effectively.

Many of the places nurses are isolated and feeling all alone, aloof working in a place where she has no opportunity to update herself. In this case she can approach internet and she will be united to the rest of the world and she will come to know what is happening latest in nursing field and where she stands and she needs to pay attention and can improve. Rather than get stagnated and be satisfied with old ways of doing things and not open to see the world around wherein has reached. If she wants to widen her horizons she needs to make personal effort to inform herself with such knowledge.

So many machines and monitors are equipped in certain areas of her department but nurse who works knows only the routine function and if she does not explore the possibility that this same machine can be operated differently and has many more information to provide.

If she does, she will be enriched and will be assets to her working place. So nurses need to update and be in touch with internet and all that is happening in and around the medical field. Because it is everyday new challenges and new discoveries and researches are being done which are useful for her to know and save life entrusted to her. Because world is moving in fast space and there is so much to know that perhaps one life is not enough only for those who thirst for such knowledge. Knowledge is greatest weapon and the power in today's world and if nurses develop nursing profession will grow and will change radically. Nursing field is progressing yet it needs to progress still faster rate and that will happen if all the nurses develop in the areas of there work with skill and technology.

Self-knowledge is not a thing to be bought in books, nor is it the outcome of a long painful practice and discipline, but it is awareness from movement to movement.

Knowledge born of the finest discrimination takes us to live furthest shore. It is intuitive, omniscient and beyond the divisions of time and space.

Your mind is a tool for you to use in any way you wish. Train your mind and you will be deeply fulfilled by all that you do. You will get good position, it is stepping stone.

Purpose of the mind—our mind must be as soft as sponge for maximum absorption. Absorb the information and allow free flow of knowledge into action closed mind can be soft gather information in mind and transformation into knowledge. A pure soft mind is a gateway to divine living. Self review will free our mind.

Education consumption in India to grow more than 500 million of population is below 25 years. Education is the 3rd largest expenditure group of an average Indian household. With 55 of the 1:7 billion Indian population under the age of 25, the demand for education and related supply indicate the need for Hugh capacity supply creation. Fees, books, private coaching, has an attractive rates of return and the growth potential. Today Indians education sector is experiencing radical change due to the introduction of new technology ad the globalization of education. Think globally and act locally with spirit of innovation, get intellectual stimulation for higher rise of your true potential.

What is the status of teachers today? Indian society has always respected these called gurus, where traditionally hailed as guru transferred the knowledge they had. In modern times it is diluted. Intellect had developed but reverence is lacking. Ideals that inspired education in ancient India must be rediscovered and introduced in our educational institutions. we are to make our contributions to civilized and to the freshness of human life. Numbers of schools, colleges and universities are multiplying graduates and holders of doctorates are increasing. Knowledge has spread, but have we grown in freshness, vitality and strength? Have we become more appreciative of the deeper values which alone give meaning and significance to life?

A new type of education is needed—an education which will not merely develop brain power, but an education which will give a triple training of the head and heart. What is wanted is not mere intellectual improvement but education that helps us become whole. The final end of education is not the gain of scholarship or power or financial independence. For all these without self-discipline and self control could well transform to be closing anti social forces. The object of education would be to form character. The education is not dead knowledge. It is pulsating with life. Education is the search for the spiritual centre of life and is possible with mental and physical discipline. Teach head, hand and heart.

Teachers love your subject and keep your drive to learn intact. Knowledge is the only thing that doubles on sharing. To teach youngsters remember you need to stay young at heart. Keep reading about what is happening around the world. Keep yourself abreast of change. What drives and motives them as teachers is fulfillment, overcome self-prejudices and pre-occupation, and gives transformative and creative experience.

High quality education—high quality career—this is what education often does. The aim of education not merely the acquisition of information or technical skills through essential in modern society, but the development of that bent of mind, that attitude of reasons, that spirit of democracy which will make us responsible citizens. The goal is commitment of knowledge and the advancement of learning. The aim of education is to emphasize not really earning power but learning power.

Education that ignores moral and spiritual values cannot quality as a quality education. What inspires teachers today is tremendous sense of fulfillment in being able to touch so many innocent young, wonderful lives. Teaching in that sense is a mission, task that one carries on with full satisfaction. In innovative world of computer still can not replace a teacher, as computer does not have warmth of heart.

Education should be related to life, real life. It is not merely academic or abstract; it must not aim at stuffing the students with information acquired from dead books or a set of sterile moralities and superficial values. True education should equip the student to cope adequately with life, with what lies ahead of hum so that he may become a worthy participant in the adventure of life.

Thinking

1. Reasoning—the rearrangement of concept so as to derive a new truth from an old valid conclusion.
2. Critical thinking—the rearrangement of concepts to evaluate something.
3. Problem solving—the assessment of concept so as to overcome a difficulty.
4. Creative thinking—the rearrange of concept so as to reproduce something that has not previously existed.

Elements of Learning Process

Goal, stimulus, perception, response, consequence, integration.

Types of Learning

Learning the administration of medication by hypodermal injection as nursing activity requires through knowledge of drug; and their actions, patient's risks to drug and what to do in unexpected reaction; and giving safely and without unnecessary pain; and synthesis of all above and adaptive thinking; for each patient. For the skill to acquire the practice is necessary in development in skill. The complexity of the skill, the ability of the learner and the attention and the effort put forth by the learner.

Characteristics of Learning

1. Learning is unitary (whole person, total)
2. Learning is individual and social
3. Learning is self-active
4. Learning is purposive
5. Learning is creative
6. Learning is transferable.

Three Main Functions to Fulfill

1. **Instructional** or the teaching of knowledge
2. **Training and practice** or the teaching of skills
3. **Inspirational and creative** or the instillation and the inculcation of ideals.

Growth in knowledge cannot be separated from growth in being for both growth and the self that grows are basically a while. What one knows affects the quality of ones being and also what one is influence the nature and quality of ones knowing and knowledge.

Characteristics of the Creative Individual

1. Creative person is sensitive to her surroundings, she stretches her perceptual powers, has the ability to see things to which the average person is blind.
2. Creative person is able to adjust quickly to new and changed situations.
3. Possess independence of judgment, has courage to be herself, willingness to be different, to take chance and risk failure and fine worth.
4. Ability to tolerate uncertainty even in the face of pressure.
5. Be creative, do not be worried about what you are doing, one has to do many things, but do everything creatively with devotion. Then your work becomes worship. If the atom can have so much energy, what to say about man. Every moment of your life is infinitely creative and the universe is endless.
6. Knowledge cannot be handed over ready made to the learner, nor does it exist in the human mind ready made, therefore, the awakening of the intellect, the utilization of the individuals inner resources and creativity—waking in them new dreams, new visions.

Nature is the storehouse of all ideas—it is a and mother of all inspiration resources has inspired poets, painters, musician and they have created masterpieces. Each time a seed drives its way through the soil in order to survive. Each time a river overcomes a big rock on its path. Each time a wiggly caterpillar transforms itself into a beautiful butterfly. Nature is inspiring you to excel. Deep look into nature and hear the secret messages nature sends. The root and shoot of a germinating seed exert force to burst open the seed coat and break through the hard ground to begin its life.

Though education in nursing is entirely different from other general fields of education, it deals with care of humankind, in other fields we may deal with machinery but in this field we deals with human lives. Therefore, to give efficient nursing care with total ability of understanding nurses have to follow rules.

Education—an unstable global economy is soon creating a competitive space for specialization, qualification and special experience. The proverb—the early bird catches the worm with range of new opportunities. As youngsters yearn for global exposure.

An exceptionally knowledgably person with his deep knowledge and wide ranging subjects has the capability to provide solutions to almost every problem. He has the intelligence required to understand the basic nature of the problem and then towards finding its solution. He always gives right advice to the right people are right time.

You are what you want to become. Why search anymore? You are wonderful manifestation. The whole universe has come together to make your existence possible. Plato said "he who has a taste for every sort of knowledge and who is curious to learn and never satisfied" may be just termed as philosopher.

What is life? What is man? What is man's origin? What is man's destiny or goal? Philosophers try to answer these questions as per their reflection and thinking.

Philosophy sets the ideals, principles, goals, standards, values thus it is in reality and truth. Education works out those values, explains how to achieve the goals. Education is the best mean for the propagation of philosophy. As all great philosophers were great educators. It determines the broad aspects of education. It determines the nature and forms of discipline. Importance of educational philosophy to a teacher is to understand values, develop intellect, improve standards of life, and reform society. According to Christian philosophy, nursing is considered as "profession of charity" nurse has to apply right conduct, in various situations of her daily life based on a sound moral character and right conscious. Judge wisely, reason soundly and develop communication skills. Nurse should have knowledge of how to guide the others, who need assistance in learning, how to improve health. Nursing is a service to individual, families and the society. Body-mind and spirit unity. Nursing is a dynamic, therapeutic and educative process which brings behavioral changes in person. To provide quality care nurse as a educator has to develop skilled and efficiency. Nurse must have the up to date knowledge, based on sound principles in her practice.

The aim of education must be to earn for his livelihood and become self sufficient, stand on his own feet, do healthy adjustment in life, modify his attitudes, morals and behavior and life in its fullness, in totality for the purpose he was created. develop balanced personality that is harmonious, to become what he is meant to be, so that he can think and judge independently and effectively where he has all round development, that is he gives his 100% BEST. It can help his to bring out is individual uniqueness that is he alone has and no other human is able to do it as he does. It must help him to highlight his innate powers and possibilities that he is capable off; where he can have harmonious, mental, emotional, moral, and physical, character development, his complete self-realization. Nursing education should also focus to prepare good leaders, inculcate values to tolerance, forgiveness, endurance, patience, forbearance, cooperation etc. Education is man's third eye, it opens man's inner eye and protects person like a mother.

By Daniel Webster (Speech in Farewell Hall)

1. If we work upon marble it will perish
2. If we work upon brass time will effaced it
3. It we rear temples they will crumble to dust
4. But if we work upon men's immortal mind
5. If we imbue them with high principles
6. With just fear of god and love of the fellow men
7. We engrave on those tablets something which no time can efface and will brighten and brighten to all eternity.

Keywords

Beyond classroom, education is the process, new trials in Mumbai schools, practical approach is must: practical approach, a clear vision, innovating ways of teaching, knowledge is supreme strength, the product of education, the future of education in India, the dream of India.

CHAPTER

7

Mental Health

Abstract

Mental health helps determine how we handle stress, relate to others, and make choices. Mental health is important at every stage of life. Mental illnesses are serious disorders which can affect your thinking, mood, and behavior. There are many causers of mental illness. Your mental health is affected by numerous factors from your daily life.

A nurse during their training is trained to give education on many topics and it depends on her interest and areas of specialization. She can select any topic that is relevant to the situation and the area and the types of people and there background. She will have to give at least fifteen to twenty minuets on a selected topic and explain what the illness means, how it is caused, what are its signs and symptoms, how it is diagnosed and treated and last most important point is the prevention and control of it. Then only her topic is completed, with discussions and clearing people's doubts.

Nurse is a first teacher her role in health education is to have clear objectives, collect correct information on topic to eliminate misconception and to clarify doubts. Health education is a vaccine, which helps to improve quality of life, unlocks the door of modernization, satisfies intellectual hunger, one comes to know good and, right from wrong and helps in scientific reasoning. God is disguise as a sick, injured and hungry. Give your knowledge to motivate people into action. One situation occurred in Mumbai on busy skywalk, no one has time to pick up dead man. Body lay for 9 hours on Kalian foot overbridge while railway and city police fought over jurisdiction, thought for reflection and action in deeds.

Mind is at place of soul—look within, observe internal activities. (psychology is scientific study of behavior and mental process).

Health psychology explains the relationship between psychological stress and physical ailments. One has to promote healthy ways of behavior. Psychological sickness needs psychological remedies. The nurse has to deal with different people having different problems both physical and mental. With having scientific knowledge of human nature, she will understand them better and thus achieve greater success in interpersonal relationship. She will become sympathetic, alert, and hardworking and love humanity. And will become emotionally mature. It will help her to improve situation by helping others solve problems. She will recognize how her emotions affect her body and she will recognize the same in her patients.

Body–mind relationship is inborn and surrounding in which we live. Mind is regarded as a function of body. It does not exist apart from the body. Mind is subtotal of various mental processes such as observing, knowing, thinking, reasoning, feeling, wishing, imagining, remembering, and judging, etc. human behavior involves both body and mind. They interact on each other. Mental functions and physical states affect each others. Mind motivates all physical and mental activities. Our emotions and strong feelings affects the body inwardly and outwardly like fear, anger and worry causes headaches, insomnia, indigestion, etc. various neurotic illness are caused by emotional conflicts. Deep thinking and concentration can cause physical fatigue. Persons psychology should be considered, he is an individual and not a machine. Each personality is highly individualistic and complex.

Action of Body Upon Mind

1. Rise in blood pressure which leads to mental excitement
2. Fatigue retards intellectual activity
3. Sudden emotions causes mental imbalance
4. Constipation makes people irritable
5. Dyspepsia makes people gloomy
6. Headache reduces concentration
7. Exam fear gives loose motion
8. Changes in the rate of respiration when excited, breath comes short, quick gaps, when depressed, breathing is slow
9. Dilatation of pupil
10. Sweating, decreased secretion of saliva
11. Increased blood pressure, blood sugar
12. Erect hair on the skin, tremors, giddiness, shock, hysteria.

Positive Emotions and Its Effect

1. Love has remarkable healing potential in major illness like cancer, colitis. Babies who get lots of love grow up healthier than children deprived of it
2. Forgiveness brings good health
3. Laughter ha benefited physically
4. Hope, purpose, meaning in life makes a person happier and healthier

5. Optimism and self-confidence, strong determination, will power helps to face any difficult challenges in life with ease
6. Sense of humor
7. Balance in work-relaxation
8. Philosophy of life helps coping with frustration and conflict
9. Acceptance of situation that cannot be changed, compromise, seek help, delay lack of recourses, failure, guilt, hassles of life leads to stress.

Re-adjustment

1. Death of a spouse
2. Divorce
3. Marital separation
4. Personal injury, illness
5. Fired at work
6. Retirement
7. Pregnancy
8. Change in financial state
9. Change in living condition
10. Trouble with boss
11. Change in sleeping habits, eating habits.

Coping Balancing Your Life Activities Through

1. Exercise
2. Yoga
3. Meditation
4. Slow down your pace of life
5. Make your goals realistic
6. Organize your life with priorities
7. Wait for a movement
8. Time will heal.

Common Defiance Mechanisms that People Use

1. Suppression
2. Reaction
3. Denial
4. Isolation
5. Projection
6. Fantasy.

Promoting Mental Health

1. Accept your personal feeling of fear, anger and find way of release tension
2. Know your weakness, what upsets you, hurts you
3. Recognize unhealthy behavior in you
4. Recognize the problem
5. Do not jump to any possible solutions
6. Listen to all solutions suggested by others
7. Be aware of your own prejudices
8. Get along with people
9. Your reaction affects
10. Think and reason
11. Adjustment
12. Development of the wholesome personality
13. Religious ethic
14. Strong mind, strong body
15. Everyday, have some undisturbed time to calm the mind, when your mind is cluttered, there is a higher possibility of going wrong. Use this undisturbed time to sort out your thoughts, concerns or simply relax, consider your lifestyle priorities
16. An unrestrained mind alone is the cause of degeneration while a controlled mind causes progress. The mind is like an poisonous snake sitting with its hood raised in the forest of the heart
17. Every one wants to lead a happy, blissful and peaceful life forever, but unless we learn to control the mind, happiness and peace would be impossible to achieve. If you over come your mind, you over come the world.
18. Some times physical illness can be detected and treated but if mental illness not detected remain invisible hidden for long. Mind also can become sick
19. Breaking bad undesirable habits such as carelessness, negligence etc. to remove the bad habits a new good habit must be formed in place of old bad ones. These habits are an important part of our character. The good habit of hard working, speaking in friendly manner, being honest. Accurate thinking in logical way, reasoning, perception are intellectual good habits.

Each Individual is Different Because of

1. Heredity, genetic chromosomal abnormalities
2. Environment in which he is brought up
3. Race, culture
4. Sex
5. Age
6. Personality
7. Educational level
8. Abilities and disabilities
9. Disturbing neighbors, etc.
10. Levels of aspirations
11. Functioning of sex urge
12. Emotional conflicts
13. Attitude to work
14. Outlook towards life
15. Biological factors—thyroid gland, sex gland
16. Physiological changes internal and external.

Mental illness can occur at any time, to anyone. It occurs when a state of physical, mental, social and spiritual well being is disturbed.

According to WHO report 24 million people worldwide suffer mental illness like schizophrenia, depression, etc. Mental disorders are great source of distress, impaired productivity and diminished quality of life for several people and families.

Lack of awareness about the illness and related information may affect the coping process of patient and family with the illness.

Adequate knowledge and negative attitude towards mental illness among family members as well as mentally ill patient we have to assess the knowledge, mental illness has been always looked down as a separate entity associated with anger, resentment, and matter of shame by public as well as family. Lack of awareness about the illness leads to different adverse consequences related with treatment and acceptance of the illness as well as the patient.

By asserting knowledge of the family members, different intervention needs to be planed.

Alcoholism, drug dependence, juvenile delinquency, crime and violence are also special areas where health education is needed.

It is concerned not only with early diagnosis and treatment of mental disorders, but also with the preservation and promotion of good mental health and prevention of mental illness. Mental health and physical health are interrelated. Good physical health is the basis of mental health. Proper functioning of all the systems of the body is essential. Person who suffers from physical defects, deformities, disabilities and chronic incurable diseases, fall an easy victim of mental illness. Therefore, good physical health is vital for good mental health.

Persons basic needs for food, shelter, clothing, rest, sleep, etc. is important. Psychological needs for affection, recognition; social needs for security, status all promote towards mental health.

Check if the Person is Mentally Healthy by following Parameters

- A mentally healthy person feels satisfied with himself
- He does not condemn or pity himself
- He feels happy, calm and cheerful
- There are no conflicts within himself
- The person is not at war with himself
- He is well adjusted
- He is able to get along well with others
- He accepts criticism and is not easily upset
- He understands the emotional needs of others and tries to be considerate in his dealings
- Has good self-control
- He is not dominated by fear, anger, love, jealousy, guilt or worries
- Has integrated personality
- Well adjusted
- Not frustrated, feels secure, mental tension sap vitality and upset mental balance; broken homes, death of a partner, separation of parents, disturbed home, poverty, alcoholism, parental neglect, severe punishment, lack of discipline, lack of moral teaching are stress factors needs to be identified and promote positive adaptation.

How to Do Primary Prevention

- Genetic counseling
- Happy pregnancy, happy and wanted, accepted, awaited child
- Physical touch and contact
- Feeling of belongingness
- Loving relatives gain satisfaction
- Receive recognition
- Emotional needs, love, security.

Secondary prevention—early identification and prompt treatment.

- Early detection
- Counseling services to motivate them.

Tertiary Prevention

- Vocational training and rehabilitation
- Prevention of progression to the point of disabilities
- Brief hospitalization and long term follow-up.

Build good health habits like adequate diet, enough sleep, and exercise, maintain weight, avoid harmful lifestyle activities, and submit oneself to periodic medical examination and screening. Accepting immunization and carrying out other specific diseases prevention measures of cleanliness, recreation, reporting early sickness. Avoid use of tobacco, alcohol and drugs. Maintain in regular surveillance of blood pressure, glucose, cholesterol and some of the parameters of health status. Prevention of accidents is also important health promotional measurers.

Mental health in different stages of life—life begins with conception and continuous through birth, childhood, adolescent, adulthood and ends in death. So, human life is a cyclic one. Life has a series of cycles through which all living being evolve. Development is a set of process through which person interacts to produce consistency and change in the characteristic of the person over the life span. Development never ends; each stage of physiologic development is different from the one before it. Physiological development is the result of a combination of maturation and learning factors. The rate of development may vary considerably. It occurs in a predicable sequence. The genetic code serves as the physiologic blue print for future growth. This genetic code sets parameters for physical development. Environment can influence in physical skills and learning, e.g. a child is born with a genetic potential for high intelligence but if raised in an environment with improper nutrition and lack of stimulation of the IQ he may reach only to average range. In infancy developmental task child gains control over body movement, adjust to adult's schedule of feeding, elimination and sleep. Develops an ego, develops trust in the environment, learns to communicate needs, begin to develop self care skills such as toileting and dressing and explores his surroundings. In childhood he increases social skills, increase in co-ordination and physical strength. Develops self-control and initiative. Achieves autonomy of self care skills, communicates and express needs. Forms a healthy self-concept, increases knowledge, shows initiative, learns to read, write, calculate and uses effective coping strategies. Person does not develop in fragmented section but as a whole human being. Certain tasks are not accomplished according to guidelines mile stones exact time suggested. Human development is complex; consider variations to understand it better.

Crucial Points in the Life Cycle of Human Beings

1. **Prenatal period**—pregnancy is a stressful period of some women. They need help not only for their physical but also emotional needs. Happy pregnancy, child welcomed, wanted, accepted and awaited guess.
2. **First 5 years of life**—the roots of mental health are in early childhood. The infant and young child should experience a warm intimate and continuous relationship with his mother and father. Broken homes are likely to produce behavior disorders in children.
3. **School child** (school age 6 to 12 years)—everything that happens in the school affects the mental health of a child. The program and practices of the school may satisfy or frustrate the emotional needs of the child. Children who have emotional problems may need child guidance clinic or psychiatric services. Proper teacher-pupil relationship and climate of the class room are very important.
4. **Adolescence is transitional, often a stormy period**—They have basic needs to be needed by others, increasing independence, need to achieve adequate adjustment to the opposite sex, etc. failure to recognize and understand these basic needs may prevent sound mental development. Young age is 18 to 25 years, adulthood is 25 to 65 years, and later maturity is 65 to death. Adolescent is a stage of transition from childhood to adulthood that is end of childhood and beginning of adulthood. He is not free from secure environment of a childhood yet heading towards adulthood that is unknown. Therefore, it is a stage neither down the stairs nor up the stairs. It is in-between which needs proper handling of physiological changes of rapid body growth and hormonal changes. Psychological reactions, specific problems of family adjustment, separation from family, choice of vocation, academic discipline, sexual behavior, societal adjustment. Visible and invisible changes that happen within the body. They have nutritional problem, self-esteem related problem to establish meaningful values, goals, ideas, personal standards, satisfying relationship with parents, peer, teachers, special qualities approval by others. Depression due to loosening the ties to their parents become independent, difficulty in concentration, restless, gloominess, tendency towards violence and accidents. Body's are very energetic at this age and are prone road accidents because of fast and negligence driving. They are adventurous, drug, alcohol and tobacco abuse. Emotional turmoil, identity crisis, teen age pregnancy and sexual related problems. Accept them as a unique individual, respect their ideas, likes and dislikes, be open to their views, allow them to do and learn by doing, provide clear reasonable limits, respect their privacy, be available to answer their questions. Be willing to apologies when mistaken. Provide unconditional lore and understanding.
5. **Old age**—causes can be organic conditions of the brain, economic insecurity, lack of home, poor status. Adjust to slower physical and cognition response, living alone, adjusting too possibly of moving to nursing homes. Adjusting to ones own deaths, and view life as worthwhile.

There is need for affection, belonging, independence, achievement, recognition and approval, personal worth and self-actualization is common to all seven stages.

Factors Contributing to Self-esteem

1. Parents acceptance of their children
2. Clear limits regarding behavior
3. Respects his individuality
4. Helps him to recognize that he is unique and special gift
5. Avoid constant criticism
6. Tap their talents, creativity
7. Correction and counseling
8. Avoid parental disputes before him
9. Eater variety of foods, maintain healthy weight
10. Sense of importance to him, to be truthful in answering, provide space and opportunity to grow, not over-protective
11. Handles thump sucking, bed wetting, telling difference
12. Discipline, avoid comparison, accepts individual difference
13. Smart age, he feels he knows everything
14. Needs attention, recognition, security, to develop wholesome intergraded personality.

Contributing factors—endocrine dysfunction, neurological disease, chronic infection, genetic inheritance, physical handicap, worry, anxieties, emotional stress, tension, frustration, broken homes, unhappy marriage, poverty, cruelty, etc.

1. Physical traits of a person, e.g. height, weight, color, facial expression.
2. Emotional are the feelings we have, e.g. fear, anger, love, jealousy, guilt, etc.
3. Intelligence also affects once personality.
4. Behavior is reflection of ones personality. It is partly dependent upon our feelings and partly on the expectations of the society. Behavior is described in terms as gentle, kind balanced, submissive, aggressive, affectionate, etc.
5. Personality is extrovert and introvert.

Mental hygiene deals with human adjustment. It promotes wholesome and socially adequate personality. Personality is a growing thing each person is helped to develop his full potentialities, to attain emotional stability and effective coping behavior. Frustration and conflicts produce by daily life leads to varying degree of mental ill health. Often we meet people who are laboring under emotional stress deeply upset, emotionally imbalanced and if can't do positive adjustment, situation continuous needs in time advice. Mind is like physical body becomes sick and get polluted with pent up emotions, anger, depression, loneliness, feat, misunderstanding, etc. sometimes physical illness can be detected easily but mental one remains hidden invisible for long.

Community mental health is an integral component of health, which is different by as an positive state of well being and methods of adopting various levels of prevention in order to improve the mental health of the community. It is shift from hospital to community or from specialist to generalist, it aims to bridge the wide gap between need and available services in the field of mental health feasible alternative approaches to extend care had to be developed and evaluated. Community mental health is a process, aim is to reduce the number of these suffer from mental disorders by primary, secondary and tertiary level prevention. Early detection and treatment continuity of care, environmental and social support and intervention, community participation, support and control. Urban areas mental health tends to be complex and different types or intensity of services. Patient should not be hospitalized specially against there will in lack of facilities if their illness can be treated in a more open settings. Goals are promote and maintain mental health and family system and their members through prevention, counseling and use of intervention. Teach families to recognize tensions, coping and communication pattern that have an adverse impact that behavior has sociocultural influence, so self-care.

Role of a nurse in community psychiatry—all activities undertaken in the community in the name of mental health

1. Responsible to a population of mental health care delivery
2. Treatment close to the patient in community based center, applies her knowledge of the nursing process in assessment planning. Implementation and evaluation to provide comprehensive care to the patients
3. Providing continuity of care
4. Avoidance of unnecessarily hospitalization
5. Plays an important role in preventive psychiatry
6. Primary prevention—identification of high-risk groups
7. Reeducation of incidence of new cases
8. Antenatal care to the mother
9. Ensure timely efficient gynecological assistance
10. Correction of endocrinal disorders
11. Training program for mentally handicapped children
12. Extruding mental health education services in child guidance clinics
13. Secondary prevention—reeducation of the duration of mental illness
14. Early diagnosis and case finding
15. Early referral
16. Screening program, early effective treatment
17. Crisis intervention, consultation services
18. Tertiary prevention—rehabilitation and follow-up services
19. Social reintegration
20. Utilization resources of family and community
21. Administering medications at door step
22. Health education
23. Community awareness program
24. Re-equipping the mentally restored with daily living care abilities.

Keywords

Nurse is a first teacher, mind is at place of soul, health psychology, body mind relationship, Action of body upon mind-positive emotions and its effect-coping balance your life activities through-re-adjustment, common defiance mechanisms, each individual is different because of, parameters, primary, secondary, tertiary prevention-mental health in different stages of life-crucial points in the life cycle of human beings, factors contribute to self esteem: components of personality components of personality, mental hygiene, community mental health, role of a nurse in community psychiatry.

CHAPTER 8

Dental Health

Abstract

Disorders of the mouth are numerous; it may be of local origin or may be secondary to disease elsewhere in the digestive system. Disorders of the mouth include discomfort or toothache when talking food as a result people take inadequate nutrition. Care of the teeth, oral hygiene is important. Tell them the importance of having good set of healthy teeth which is also sign of beauty and health, once you have it take care or else you will face endless other health problems if you do not take care of it in time

Your dental health is an essential part of your general health. Neglect of your teeth is most likely to reflect on your general well beings. So take good care of your health and they will take good care of you.

Dentine is an ivory like substance; it forms the second layer of a tooth and is softer than enamel. Gum is coral pink fibrous tissue covers the teeth and roots and supports the bone below, it absorbs the pressure exerted while chewing. Nerve is a cord-like structure with fibers which carry messages such as pain, touch from the tooth to the brain. Enamel is the hardest tissue in our body and forms the outer layer of a tooth. Pulp is the most vital part of a tooth; it contains nerves and blood vessels. Root is hidden part of a tooth beneath the gums which contains root canals which contain the pulp.

TYPES OF TEETH

Incisors teeth that help to cut food into small particles; cannes pointed and sharp for tearing food; premolars for crushing food particles, molars to grind food for better digestion. There are two types of dentition in the early years a child has 20 milk teeth, 8 incisions, 4 canines and 8 molars. These are also called primary teeth. Children lose their milk teeth between the age of 6 and 11 and their permanent or secondary teeth appear as the primary teeth are shed. An adult has 32 permanent teeth, 8 incisions, 4 canines, 8 premolars and 12 molars. The last 4 molars are commonly known as wisdom teeth as they appear much later during the teens or even adult years.

Disorders of the mouth are numerous; it may be of local origin or may be secondary to disease elsewhere in the digestive system. Primary lesions may be due to bacterial, viral or fungal infection, chemical irritation, congenital malformation, poor dietary habits, poor oral and dental hygiene, dehydration, emotional stress and mouth breathing

Disorders of the mouth include discomfort or toothache when talking food as a result people take inadequate nutrition. There may be a palpable mass or a swollen area evident within the oral cavity. Bleeding of the gums may be present. An offensive breath may indicate sordes or infection. Excessive salivation or dryness may be present. The individual may experience difficulty with clear speech or with swallowing.

Care of the teeth—oral hygiene is important, healthy teeth, healthy gums helps in food mastication and prevents dental caries, bad breath, cavity and other dental problems. It can be prevented by tooth brushing regularly, regular dental check ups, proper diet, and good habits, and care of dentures.

Mastication disorders—food is taken into the mouth where it is broken up, mixed with saliva, lubricated and then swallowed the act of chewing is partly voluntary and partly reflex. The teeth serve to break up the food and jaw and tongue movements shift the bolus of food around in the mouth.

Plaque is a sticky, almost invisible film of bacteria or germs that is constantly forming on your teeth and gums. If it is not brushed off after you eat, it contains with sugars present in food particles to produce acids which attack and harm your teeth. Plaque is the real villain behind both tooth decay and gum diseases.

How teeth decay—plaque turns food particles stuck between the teeth into acid which attacks the tooth enamel with repeated acid attacks, the enamel wear away and a cavity is formed. Once a cavity forms the decay spreads to the next layer—the dentine, but if the cavity is filled the decay can be stooped. If the cavity is not treated at the dentine stage, the decay spreads deeper into the pulp an can be very painful. If the last stager it decays spreads to the root and causes an abscess, accompanied by severe pain. At this stage, only root canal treatment can save the tooth. In some cases, the tooth may have to be extracted.

Gum disease, technically known as periodontal disease, is the major cause of tooth loss in adults. Here is how the disease starts and progresses. Healthy gums closely grip the sides of the teeth anchoring them firmly in placer, with the help of bone. Unresolved plaque produces acids and bacterial irritants. It also hardens into calculus commonly called tartar which passes around the gum line. As the gum becomes inflamed, it may bleed, this condition is known as gingivitis. If untreated the infection spreads to the bone supporting the tooth. Pus is formed, the bone begins to erode, and eventually, the tooth may be lost. The condition is called periodicities or pyorrhea.

Tooth enamel cannot be replaced by your body, so you must protect it. Regular brushing after every meal will help keep your teeth free of plaque and prevent tartar formation.

Halitosis—bad breath is caused by improper oral hygiene, sometimes it is due to the hormonal changes. It is caused by abnormal chewing habits, vitamin deficiency, and dehydration, cancer and chemotherapy drugs, etc.

Dental caries—tooth decay is a major health problem caused by the action of organisms on ingested refined carbohydrates, acids are produced which eventually destroy the enamel surface of the teeth. Tooth decay, cavity formation, inflammation and eventual loss of teeth result if measures are not initiated to prevent progression of the process. Prevention during childhood is regularly brushing of the teeth following eating, restriction of refined carbohydrates foods and the use of fluoride in topical applications, toothpaste and drinking water and adjoining gum and the effects of build up of debris on the tooth and gums. Dental caries can be prevented by decreasing the amount of sugar in the diet. Treatment for dental caries includes filling, extraction, dental implants and dentures.

Periodontal disease affects the tissues that support the teeth. It is developed due to built up of plaque on the teeth, poor nutrition, poor oral hygiene, malocclusion of the teeth and by some metabolic disorders. Symptoms include inflammation, bleeding and tenderness of the gum and loosening of the teeth. Formation of the plaque is prevented by regular use of dental floss and regular examination and care by a dentist.

Acute tooth infection—of the pulp or development of an abscess at the root of a tooth is very painful and may cause an elevated temperature and general malaise. The person should be advised to seek prompt treatment by a dentist. An opening or canal is made to provide drainage and an antibiotic preparation may be prescribed or the tooth may be extracted. Frequent antiseptic mouth wash is recommended.

Dental decay begins with small hole a break in the tooth's enamel or the area that is hard to clean. Left unchecked, the affected area penetrates the enamel into the dentin. Decay progress rapidly and reached the pulp. When the blood, lymph vessels and nerves are exposed, they become infected and an abscess formed either within the tooth or at the tip of the root. Soreness and pain felt, it may get swollen, if not treated extraction is necessary.

Mouth care—healthy teeth must be effectively cleansed on a daily basis. Brushing helps breaking up the bacterial plaque that collects around teeth.

Abscessed tooth involves the collection of pus which produces a dull, gnawing, continuous pain, fever and malaise. In the early stage dental surgeon may drill an opening into the pulp chamber to relieve tension and provide drainage.

Tips

1. Drink adequate water that is 8–10 glasses/day
2. Every two hours eat low calorie, small quantity meals
3. Brush teeth twice
4. Use tongue cleaner
5. Get investigated for systemic condition like gastritis, hiatus hernia, diabetes, liver diseases. If the condition is not caused by bleeding gums and gum diseased needs to be looked into it
6. Replaced the toothbrush at first sings of wear
7. Maintain adequate nutrition and avoid sweets
8. Avoid alcohol and tobacco product, including smokeless tobacco
9. Floss at least once a day
10. Visit the dentist at least every 6 months.

What is the Sensitive Tooth?

If you feel a mild electric current in upper tooth when you bite into ice cream or sip hot tea that is teeth sensitivity condition? It is a common condition. Some have mild discomfort for a belief moment to few hours. Tooth sensitivity is tooth discomfort. It occurs when the dentin or the middle layer of the tooth is exposed, the dentin can get exposed due to a variety of reasons mostly build up of plague on the teeth, prolonged usage of mouth wash intake of acidic food and routine dental procedures, touching the teeth with other teeth or tongues, and eating sweets. Sometimes old filling with crack or leak can also cause teeth sensitivity.

Reason can be like untreated cavities, decay or infection in the teeth or poor oral hygiene, when the underlying layer of your teeth becomes exposed as a result of receding gum tissue. The roots that are not covered by hard enamel, contains thus and of tiny tubules leading to the toothed nerve center. These dentinal tubules allow the stimuli, for example, hot, cold or sweet food to react the nerve in your teeth which results in pain, other reason is like brushing too hard or using a hard bristled tooth brush over time, can wear down enamel and cause dentin to be exposed of the gums. Inflammation and sore gum tissue may curve sensitivity due to the loss of supporting ligaments which exposes the root surface that leads directly to the nerves of the tooth. Some times chipped or broken teeth may fill with bacteria from plague and enter the pulp causing inflammation long-term use of certain mouth wash which contains acids can worsen the sensitivity. If you have exposed dentin, then the acid further damages the dentin layer of the tooth.

Doctor can check the sensitivity that which can determine if not canal treatment is needed may prescribe fluoride gel or tooth past containing fluoride and either potassium nitrate or strontium chloride. The ingredients help block transmission to the nerve. It also might help to massage the special paste onto your gums with your finger after brushing. Follow oral hygiene instructions.

Tips

1. Use a soft bristled toothbrush as there is lesser amount of pressure on the teeth while brushing them
2. Use a desensitizing toothpaste
3. Refrain from using alcohol base mouthwash, they tend to damage the teeth
4. Avoid eating foods that are highly acidic in nature, e.g. spicy food, red meats
5. Use a fluoride-based toothpaste
6. Avoid ice cream, hot/chilled beverages
7. Visit your doctor regularly.

Ask the Questions and Prepare the Answers to the Questions

1. How often do you brush your teeth?
2. Do you floss? How often?
3. Do you use a mouth wash? When?
4. Do your gums ever bleeding?
5. Do you get sores in your mouth? When? Where?
6. How often do you go to the dentist?
7. How often do you have your teeth professionally cleaned?
8. Do you have any loose teeth?
9. Do you have false teeth, bridges, partial plates
10. Do you have any problem with mouth drying
11. What medication do you talk
12. Can you chew all kinds of foods
13. Have you notice any change in sense of test
14. Are you able to do your own mouth care
15. What type of tooth brush you use, soft, hard
16. Your brushing technique

The beauty of natural teeth is tremendous, treatment of teeth is expensive affair, daily message and gargle every meal. **Cosmetic dentistry** is gaining popularity waves advanced technology has radically altered the field of dentistry cosmetic/esthetic dentistry focus on reconstruction and other esthetic dental procedures it offers—

1. **Dental whitening**—making teeth 8 times whiter-procedure through laser or applying gel trays gives immediate results and is popular today.
2. **Dental reshaping and resizing**—meant for those who wish to have their teeth perfectly aligned. Everyone wants a million dollar smile.
3. **Dental veneering** to correct irregularity dentist makes crowns and porcelain veneers and places them over the irregular teeth brightening them in just a coupe of sittings.
4. **Root canals and dental bonding**—for restoration of a decayed tooth. The root of the tooth—cleaned and cut from its nerve which causes inflammation. The bounding process involves the application of enamel like dental composite material to the tooth's surface. This material is sculpted into a particular shape, hardened and then polished.
5. **Gum lift**—this involves raising and sculpting the gum line. The procedure involves reshaping the tissue and underlying bones to create the appearance of longer or more symmetrical teeth.

You can demonstrate and re-demonstrate the technique of brushing teeth, brush teeth using a soft toothbrush at least two times daily. Hold toothbrush at a 45 degree angle between brush the gum and teeth. Gums and tooth surface should be brushed.

You can teach the people home made practice of using Neem and other medical plants chewing and cleansing teeth which is healthy practice too.

Tell them the importance of having good set of healthy teeth which is also sign of beauty and health, once you have it take care or else you will face endless other health problems if you do not take care of it in time.

You can use different AV aids to show and demonstrate your topic in clear manner.

Five Golden Rules for Healthy Teeth

1. Eat foods that have vitamins and minerals, they are not always costly.
2. Don't eat sweets or sticky foods between meals.
3. Brush your teeth after every meal to remove plaque.
4. Visit your dentist regularly.
5. Use a good toothpaste and toothbrush.

Keywords

Dentine, gum, nerve, types of teeth: care of the teeth; mastication disorders; plaque, how teeth decay, gum disease, halitosis; dental caries, periodontal disease, acute tooth infection, dental decay, tips; sensitive tooth, cosmetic dentistry, dental whitening, dental reshaping and resizing, dental veneering, root canals and dental bonding; gum lift, five golden rules for healthy teeth.

CHAPTER 9

Eye Care

Abstract

Hygienic care of the eyes prevents infection and helps maintain the functions. to prevent infections like conductivities, injuries, errors of refraction, blindness. Good diet with vitamin A is necessary to prevent eye problems like night blindness. Proper hygiene of the eyes should be maintained by keeping skin around eye clean by washing. Like the mind and body; our eyes too require some workout, therefore it is a wise thing to exercise your eyes too.

Eyes are important organs which require care in daily life. Hygienic care of the eyes prevent infection and help maintain the functions. Common problems of the eyes are secretions that dry on the lashes as crusts. This may need to be softened and wiped away under sterile conditions. In newborns, the eyes are treated soon after the baby is born to prevent ophthalmic neonatorum.

Common normally care that each individual has to observe to keep the good healthy sight. So teach the people the dos and don'ts of the eye care.

Care of the eyes—to prevent infections like conductivities, injuries, errors of refraction, blindness. Good diet with vitamin A is necessary to prevent eye problems like night blindness. Proper hygiene of the eyes should be maintained by keeping skin around eye clean by washing with soap and water, regular habit of washing at bed time will remove the dirt collected during the day. Do not touch eyes with unclean fingers, should not exposed to dust, very bright light, and do not practice harmful things like applying kajal which will make eye irritant. The care of the eye is more than mere medical attention.

Find Out if You Have Any of the following Complaints

Do you have any difficulty in seeing?
Do you have any eye pain?
Do you have redness or swelling in the eye?
Do your eyes water excessively?
Do your eyes discharge?
When was your last vision checked?
Do you have trouble with night vision?
Do you find difficulty while driving, climbing stairway?
Do your eyes feel dry and burn?
Do you use any eye medications?
Do you wear eye glass, artificial eye, lenses?

What is Sleep Hypersomnia or Excessive Sleepiness?

It is a condition in which a person has trouble staying awake during the day. They can fall asleep at any time, e.g. at work, while they are driving, they may have lack of energy and trouble thinking clearly.

Causes—not getting enough sleep at night that is sleep deprived; drug or alcohol abuse; a head injury or neurological diseases such as multiple sclerosis, prescription drugs such as tranquillizers, genetic.

Diagnosis done by talking history, habits, any emotional problem, blood test, CT scan, sleep test called polysomnography, EEG.

Treatment

Doctor may prescribe various drugs to treat including stimulants, antidepressants. Apnea doctor may prescribe CPAP (continuous positive airway pressure); you wear a mask over your nose while you are sleeping. A machine that delivers a continuous flow of air into the nostrils is hooked up to the mask. The pressure from air flowing into the nostrils helps keep the airways open, eliminated alcohol and caffeine change the medicines that cause drowsiness.

Normal Sleep Requirement

1. Neonate 3 months to 16 hours/day.
2. Infant 10 hours/day.
3. Toddlers 2 years to 12 hour/day.
4. Preschool 12 hours/day.
5. School age 11–12 hours/day.
6. Adolescent 7½ hours/day.
7. Youth 6–8½ hours/day.

Exercise your vision—like the mind and body; our eyes too require some workout. Our eyes are one of the most sensitive parts of our bodies and just like we sweat it out the gum, play sports and follow a diet in order to keep ourselves fit and healthy, we need to pay special need to the well being of eyes too. Our eyes constantly perform visual imagery for us and they are subjected to strain due to long hours spent in front of the computer, TV, dust and pollution and they only get rest when we sleep. Some people suffer from frequent headaches, blurred vision due to strain on the eyes. More and more youngsters are having eye problems and need to wear glasses or contact lenses. Therefore, it is a wise thing to exercise your eyes too, and unlike a work out at a gym, it does not involve any sweating or doing weights and is relatively easy.

Here is How You Can Exercise Your Eyes

1. One of the best eye exercises is to rub your palms together till they get warm, now close your eyes and lightly cover them with your cupped palms, without putting pressure on your eyeballs. As you are doing this, think about your happiest moment in life and breathe slowly, talking deep breaths. Practice this for a minimum of 3 minutes and gradually increase the repetitions.
2. Just close your eyes tightly for about 5–10 seconds and open them. Repeat 5 times.
3. Massaging your eyelids will give eye your eyes a relaxing feel. Close your eyes and gently using your finger tips massage your eyelids in the circular motion. Alternatively you can soak and drench a soft cloth in hot and cold water alternately after applying it softly on your eyes.
4. Roll your eyes clockwise, blink and then anti-clock wise.
5. Focus your attention on a distant object for about 10–15 seconds and then slowly re-focus your attention on a near by object without moving your head or neck.
6. Move your pupils from left to right and up to down. Repeat at 5–10 times.

Sleepy at work?

How many times have you felt yourself yawning while working?

How many times have you reached out for the coffee machine to give kicks?

Sleepiness at work could be due to poor sleeping habits, do you spend at night long hours of working behind a desk, try to get up frequently for short walks. At lunch time, try to take a 10 minutes walk around your building. This will make you more alert as well as refreshed. Avoid looking at your computer screen for hours at a time without any break. It causes eye strain and worsens sleepiness. Look away from the screen for a few seconds regularly to relax your eyes.

Nature of sleep—sleep is a relaxed state that is necessary to all humans. It is universal and natural at process. It is a state of composure, which restores cerebral function. More than body parts the brain is affected by sleep. During wakeful hours, the brain is constantly active on alert awaiting instructions. Sleep is a sensory experience. Sleep is influenced by an individual biologic clock, cyclic.

Sleep disorders—sleeplessness is common for millions of individuals. Feeling drowsy, heavy after meals—why? 8–9 hours daily.

Insomnia—difficulty falling asleep—Sleep is important for recovery from critical illness, unpleasant noisy sound, light, visitor's disturbances, and dim light.

As body needs food and air to keep alive, eyes needs rest and sleep to maintain body functions. Time of bed, place, age, and all these factors are important—work, lifestyle, habits like alcohol, coffee at night—all affect body function. Illness, drugs talking like narcotic, opium, Climate too hot and too cold.

Sleep Questionnaire

- Difficulty with sleep at home hospital
- Sleep more at home than hospital
- When awaken feel fatigued and groggy
- Take longer tine to fall asleep
- Awake frequently at middle of the night
- Hospital staff awake me while I am asleep and awaken at night for treatment
- Hospital timing—change-pattern disturbs
- Awaken by noise, light, that bothers sleep
- Room mate in hospital disturbs
- I have pain at night
- The medicines keeps me awake
- Illness keeps me awake
- Drink tea, cola around sleep time
- I exercise during the day for sleepy time
- I smoke, I drink alcohol
- Unpleasant conversation before sleep
- Negative thoughts during the day
- Keep thinking what happiness during the day and what I will have to do tomorrow
- I read during sleeping time
- I eat during sleep time, watch TV.

What to do?

- Stick to a regular time to bed and to wake up in time. Make a positive transition to bedtime, read, listen to soothing music or take a warm bath.
- Avoid the intake of coffee, drugs, alcohol.
- Do not watch violent, tragic or horror movies at night before sleep. These can emotionally disturb the mind and in turn your sleep as well.
- Brief afternoon naps can relieve fatigue and stress in people who are overworked and stressed throughout day.
- Do yoga, meditation—it helps to relax.
- Avail of counseling to deal with anxieties and emotional; turmoil.
- Consult a sleep specialist.
- When you are constantly feeling sleepy during the day and are unable to concentrate on the task at hand, it could be a signal for bigger problem.

- Recurrent sleepiness makes people want to nap repeatedly, even when you are at work. Therefore, sleep in full 8 hours—getting adequate sleep is extremely important. Do not cut sleep and do something else. You can thus recover from whole day fatigue.
- Avoid destruction like watching TV, reading, playing, games, etc.
- Wake up on time—that is going to bed and getting up in time. This will program your body into knowing its time to be awake even off days.
- Eat on time maintaining your regular meals time, good breakfast to get body energetic to last fore the day, avoid skipping meals which can cause sleepiness. Dinner should finish 2–3 hours before bed time. Avoid sugar based food and snacking at mid night.
- Work out—go for a walk and exercise 20 to 30 minutes.
- Do not go to bed until you are ready—avoid lounging around your bed prior to feeling sleepy. Avoid napping during the day that can disturb night time sleep.
- Destress—do not do so much racing through your head that you can not sleep, get your mind unwind and relax. Bath, calming music helps.
- See a doctor—do not take it lightly, and get medicines.

Snore sleep apnea—untreated can be risk factor for high blood pressure and other cardiovascular diseases, watch out for—

- Do you snore at night?
- Do you get sound sleep at night?
- Do you feel sleepy and lethargic during the day?
- Avoid heavy calorie meal at night—body should be properly hydrated.

Now a laser surgery that improves vision—British surgeons claim that they can now give people who are shortsighted better vision than they wee born with, by using a pioneers laser technology. Experts estimate the human eye is potentially capable of 20–10 vision. But the new treatment can give people up to 20-16 vision, thus enabling them to read a ca number plate 80 yards away, almost four times better than the minimum standard required for diving the treatment is due to new cool laser that precisely cuts flap in the cornea at the start. And a second laser then reshape the cornea to correct short sight, the results being achieved with thee new machines are simply among.

Diseases of eye caused by bad food habits, excess acidic and alkalis juices in the system, drug abuses, unhealthy sleeping positions, cold baths while the bodies are still sweating shifting vision focus abruptly from far to near objects, exposure to dust, fumes, smoke and excessive laughter.

Move your eyes upward as far as you can and then downward as far as you can. Repeat 4 more times. Blink quickly a few times to relax the eye muscles. Close your eyes as tightly as possible, really squeeze the eyes, so the eye muscles contract. Hold for 3 seconds and then let go quickly. This exercise causes a deep relaxation of the eye muscles.

A diet rich in fruits and vegetables, herbs, spices and fish contributes directly by supplying certain vitamins, carotenes, minerals and essentially fatty acids to your eyes. Include green beans, broccoli, sprouts, tomatoes, turnip greens, dried apricots, blue berries, mango, salmon, mackerel, sardines, dairy produces, etc.

Conjunctivitis—a virus infection with sudden onset of pain or the sensation of a foreign body in the eye. The diseases rapidly progresses to the full clinical picture of swollen eyelids, common in tropics and warm climate. Health teaching is essential especially personal hygiene, environmental; hygiene, sterilization of clothes, utensils, fomites, and child kept away from school and playmates, disinfection of clothes.

Keywords

Care of the eyes, complains, excessive sleepiness, causes: diagnosis, treatment, normal sleep requirement, exercise your vision, nature of sleep, sleep disorders: sleep apnea, laser surgery that improves vision, a diet.

CHAPTER

10

Tobacco Smoking

Abstract

Tobacco smoking and tobacco chewing or snuffing of any form is injurious to ones health. Cancer of the oral cavity, which may occur in any part of the mouth or throat due to this bad habit of tobacco. This type of cancer is associated with the use of tobacco. Tobacco has carcinogenic effect. If one develops lesion or irritation in areas of the mouth, tongue or throat, bloody sputum, discomfort caused by certain foods, one needs to consult the doctor without delay.

May 31st is celebrated as 'No Tobacco Day'.

The scary picture:

1. **Oral health**—tobacco use greatly increased the risk of oral cancer, a disease that progresses rapidly and can be deadly if not diagnosed and treated early. Smoking stains the teeth and affects gum and born supporting the teeth. Products in cigarette smoke decreases the blood supply to the gum, accumulation of plaque on leading to teeth decay. The chemicals found in it like tar and nicotine also stick to teeth, gum and have bad breath. It also causes dry mouth, stopping the flow of saliva and allowing bacteria to flourish.
2. **Cardiovascular health**—smoking is the direct cause of 255% of heart attacks and directly linked 80% of all heart disease death in India each year. Smoking increases stiffness of the arteries, this is known as endothelium therapy, creating blockage in arteries. Also, it increases cholesterol level in blood and makes the blood thicker leading to clotting of blood. It also causes coronary spasms leading to chest pain, angina or even heart attack. It plays a part in coronary heart disease (CHD) and causes damage by decreasing oxygen to the heart. Smoking increases BP and heart rate both are bad for the young people; 3 out of 4 deaths of heart diseases are due to smoking.
3. **Skin**—cigarette smoke contains more than 4,000 toxins which are directly absorbed into blood stream and taken into the structures of your skin. It is linked also with early menopause. The most devastating with physical appearance is that of aging effort and likely to develop "smokers face" the skin loses the healthy glow and takes up the yellowish gray cast. The more cigarette smoking the worse ones skin will look it uses vitamin C in body about 35 mg for each cigarette, it is not manufactured in body and the substance that gives skin its plump and youthful appearance. The collage breaks down causing premature wrinkles around the eyes and mouth.
4. **Quitting**—will power and commitment are essential to quit, nicotinic craving experience withdrawal symptoms of irritability, anxiety, difficulty in concentration, restlessness, impatience, tiredness, decreased heart rate and increased appetite and weight gain.
5. **Suggestion**—whenever you have a desire to smoke, take about 15 to 20 deep breaths. Take 2–3 glasses of water after every meal consume at least 12 glasses of water every day to overcome the habit. Chew clove dry, Amla, go for stroll, do 20 minutes exercise, see the money you saved, you yourself realize how stupid you had been in smoking away your money. Practice yoga and meditation regularly.

Stop Smoking Plans—START

1. S = set a quit date
2. T = tell family, friends and co-workers that you plan to quit
3. A = anticipate and plan for the challenge you will face while quitting
4. R = remove cigarettes and other tobacco products from you home, cart or work place
5. T = talk to your doctor about getting help to quit

Six Surprising Reasons to Stop Smoking

1. **Boost your brain power**—Ex-smokers have better reasoning skills and memory than current ones.
2. **Help you look younger**—smoking prematurely ages skin by up to 20 years and makes you four times more likely to go grey.
3. **Increase your fertility**—a study found women smokers reduced their chance of conceiving by a third.
4. **Improve your smile**—the habit is linked to gum diseases, teeth stains and bad breath.
5. **Protect your vision**—it doubles your risk of age-related macular degeneration the main cause of blindness in the UK.
6. **Make your kids happy**—95% of children with a smoking parents wishes that they had quit.
7. **The stress smokers**—you can happily survive without cigarettes until you have a problem at work or a terrible day with the kinds. Smoke to ease tension get moving.
8. **The nicotinic junkle**—upon waking, your first thought is 'cigarette' and you smoke regularly throughout the

day, feeling jittery if you miss one. The chemical addiction feels particularly strong. Try out some nicotinic replacement therapy.

9. **The social smoker**—you forget about cigarettes when alone, but as soon as you are with other smokers you succumb get a quit buddy.
10. **The habitual smokers**—it has been part of the rhythm of your day for years, from your morning tea break to winding down in front of the TV at night the serial quitter-you have tried giving up many times-sheer will power.

Counseling

1. Encourage smoking cessation-although much damage has been done to the lungs and blood vessels by many years of smoking elderly persons can still benefit from smoking cessation by increasing quality of life.
2. Encourage physical activity to promote fitness.
3. Identify alcohol abuse and recognize signs and symptoms like difficult gait and balance, acute change in cognition, frequent falls and accidents, changing in drinking pattern, poor nutritional intake, poor hygiene and self-care, look for social isolation.
4. Evaluate and counsel on dental health.

Tobacco Habit

Adverse health effects of smoking—

1. Lung cancer, COPD, increased severity to asthma and various respiratory infections.
2. Coronary heart diseases, angina pectoris, heart attack
3. Peripheral vascular diseases.
4. Earlier wrinkles, finger nail discoloration, psoriasis.
5. Esophageal, oral, bladder, kidney, stomach, pancreatic, cervical cancer and many other places developing cancers.
6. Disc degeneration, osteoporosis, osteoarthritis, delayed fracture healing, less successful back surgery, musculoskeletal injury.
7. Infertility, impotence, decreased sperm motility and density, miscarriage, earlier menopause.
8. Fetal growth retardation, prematurely, still birth, birth defects, intellectual impairments, sudden infant death syndrome.
9. Brain attack, stroke.
10. Cataract, macular degeneration, snoring, stomach ulcers, impaired immunity.

About 3 million deaths attributed to tobacco consumption in different forms. Thirty percent of cancer deaths among them. Tobacco related diseases young people who take up smoking have been shown to experience an early onset of cough, phlegm production and shortness of breath on exertion.

The harm from maternal smoking can extend beyond pregnancy, affecting the child's growth and development.

People tend to misjudge the hazards of the tobacco. When an young adult begin it to smoke, they do not witness the high morbidity and mortality associated with their behaviour until they reach middle age.

At present, about 1070 million male and 230 million females in the world smoke. The withdrawal symptoms include irritability, anxiety, craving sleep problems, headache, tremors and lethargy. Withdrawal symptoms continue for 4 to 6 weeks and craving may continue for months.

Stop smoking at home, it makes your children more prone to ear infections, pneumonia, bronchitis and coughs.

Keywords

The scary picture, oral health-cardiovascular health-skin, quitting-suggestion, stop smoking plans-START, six surprising reasons to stop smoking, counseling- adverse health effects of smoking.

CHAPTER

11

Tuberculosis

Abstract

Tuberculosis is a worldwide public health problem. TB (tuberculosis) is an infectious disease, which primarily affects the lung parenchyma. It may be also be transmitted to other parts of the body, including the meanings, kidneys, bones, and lymph nodes. TB is closely associated with poverty, malnutrition, overcrowding, sub standard housing and inadequate health care. There are also other factors such as increased immigration, the HIV epidemic, multi-drug-resistant strains of TB, etc. if client develop low grade fever, fatigue, anorexia, weight loss, night sweats, chest pain, persistent cough, get medical advice instantly.

INTRODUCTION

Tuberculosis is a chronic and stigmatizing diseases yet if properly counseled and motivated the patient and family and if patient takes regular and complete course of treatment it becomes more easy and acceptable to patient and he gets completely cured.

Tuberculosis is leading communicable disease in India today.1.6 people per 1,000 populations have bacteriologically confirmed disease. 8.5 million cases of pulmonary TB cases estimated in India. 3.8 million are sputum positive, death quoted as 0. 37 million each year, about 0.8 million cases of pulmonary TB are added every year.

Tuberculosis is a community infection. Tuberculosis is a specific infectious diseases caused by *M. tuberculosis*. It affects lungs in pulmonary TB, it also can affect intestine, meanings, born and joints, lumpy glands, skin and other tissues of the body.

Tuberculosis is a world wide public health problem despite causative organism discovered more than 100 years ago and highly effective drugs and vaccines are available.

Tuberculosis is a curable and preventable disease. It has been estimated that 12–20 million cases world wide and 4–5 million new cases and 3 million death every year "infectious pool"; to make global situation worse tuberculosis combined with HIV is added threat to the world together with incomplete and inappropriate treatment. WHO no single country has succeeded in reaching the point of control.

India continuous to be major health problem. In Asia drug resistant remains high, poverty and economic recession and malnutrition make population more vulnerable to tuberculosis, increased human migration has mixed infected with uninfected, improvement in standards of living and quality of life is absolute.

Disease—on this earth has been present ever since the birth of living beings. It has been problem to human beings. To animals, it is the instincts that make them eat herbs for cure. Man has been able to find out causes for diseases and their cure through research, which has been in oration even today and will continue to be in action in times to come. As the civilization made progress, the theories also changed. The bacteriological era gave rise and new avenues to modern concepts. The root cause of diseases was the core factor for research.

- Age group: 15–49, 95% in developing countries; 45–54 male
- Agent: *Mycobacterium tuberculosis* the bovine strain affects cattle and other animals
- Source of infection—human and bovine. Human sputum is positive for tuberculin bacilli and bovine usually infected milk and milk products
- Sex—more in males than in females
- Rural and urban cases equal
- Social factors likely in persons who are malnourished, overcrowded area living, poor hygiene and poverty
- Transmitted by droplet infection, and inhalation of infected dust
- Period of infectivity—as long as bacilli are excreted in the sputum by the human host. This may be from several months to a few years. If the case is not adequately treated
- Incubation period—weeks to months
- Rural and urban occurrence of tuberculosis is equal
- Mode of transmission droplet infection by an infectious case coughing generates largest number of droplets.
- Other ways—inhalator infected dust
- Early case finding
- Sputum examination—by direct microscopy examination of sputum of patients who has symptoms like cough lasting more than two weeks, continuous fever, haemoptysis.
- Chemotherapy has completely revolutionaries the treatment of pulmonary TB (DOTS).

Clinical Features

- Chronic cough
- Continuous low-grade fever
- Chest pain
- Hemoptysis

- Anorexia
- Loss of weight.

Nursing Care

- Admission to hospital of some cases be considered, those who develop reaction to drug needs nursing care
- Isolation, barrier nursing
- Disinfection of materials and spread disinfection

Multidrug-resistant TB—in resent years, clusters of multidrug-resistant TB (MDR-TB) cases have occurred in several parts of India. Poor compliance or incomplete therapy regimens are factors leading to resistance in an individual. The resistant organisms can then be spread to others, whose initial therapy my not be effective against the resistant organism. The reservoir of resistant organisms grows in such a setting.

India is saddled with the highest burden of TB with nearly 2 million new cases recorded in 2009. out of an estimated 1.3 million people who died of TB in 2008, the nation lone accounted for 2.8 lack lives.

India's case detection was around 67%, while estimated number of TB cases that have become MDR was 99,000 in 2009. Even though the TB mortality rate has fallen by 35%; since 1990, the disease claimed 1.7 million lives has year of which 3.8 lack were women.

According to WHO annual report, global TB control 2010—around 4.700 die to TB daily. An estimated 9.4 million contracted the diseases in 2009.

The big challenge for WHO was an estimated 4.4 lack MDR stains of TB a year which is hard to detect and treat. It was estimated in India that 2009 3.3% of all new TB cases had MDR-TB.

TB mortality rate has drooped from 30 in 1990 to 20 per 100,000 in 2009. 4.4 lack new cases of MDR TB emerging each year and that less than 5% of those cases being properly treated. 5.8 million TB cases were notified through DOTS program.

Control Tuberculosis

Control Measures

1. Case finding
2. Early detection
3. Suspects—sputum examination
4. BCG vaccination
5. Isolation, health supervision
6. Domiciliary treatment
7. Curative and preventive
8. Anti-tuberculosis drugs/chemotherapy
9. DOTS (direct observed treatment)/RNTPC (revised national tuberculosis control program)
10. Nutrition
11. Prevention of cross infection, drug compliance
12. Rehabilitation
13. Research
14. Tuberculin testing (Mantoux test)
15. Health education.

Tuberculosis Over the Years

1. In mid-90s multi-drug resistant TB was first reported
2. In 2006, extensively drug resistant TB (XDR) emerged
3. In 2008, two cases were reported from Italy that had resistant to both first and second line treatment
4. In 2009 15 TB clients in Iran were reported to be resistant to all anti TB drug tested prompting resistance, to coin new term "extremely drug resistant" (X XDR TB) and totally drug resistant TB (TDR-TB)
5. In January 2012, four clients in India were described subsequently reported for further 8 such cases
6. In March WHO said insufficient evidence to use term TDR-TB
7. As per WHO nomenclature, MDR-TB is first TB that is resistant to both of the main first line drugs, Isoniazid and Rifampicin
8. WHO says extensively XDR-TB is MDR-TB with additional resistant to any of the indictable (amikacin, kanamycin or capreomycin, plus resistance to any fluoroquinolones) (WHO consensus, do not use TDR-TB label, new drugs are under going clinical trails and could prove effective against drug resistance stains.)

National Tuberculosis Control Program Activities Comprise of—

1. Early detection and domiciliary treatment of TB cases
2. BCG vaccination of infants and children
3. Isolation facilities, especially for those who require surgery or emergency treatment
4. Training and demonstration
5. Rehabilitation
6. Research
7. The objective of this strategy is to achieve at least 85% cure rate of infectious cases through DOTS
8. To detect at least 75% estimated cases through quality sputum microscopy
9. Involvement of NGO in information, education and communication activities.

Keywords

Disease, clinical features, nursing care, control measures, tuberculosis over the year, National Tuberculosis Control Program activities.

CHAPTER 12

Leprosy

Abstract

Leprosy is an infectious disease caused by the bacterium Mycobacterium leprae. Leprosy has a long history of social ostracism. Around 12 million people worldwide are infected with this diseases, the disease shows a world wide variation of clinical presentation. It is a progressively disfiguring diseases, but rarely fatal. The organism is airborne route. By proper hand washing and personal hygiene, equipment care, client education, establishing barriers and precautions can reduce the risk of disease to household members.

Leprosy is chronic disabling disease caused by *Mycobacterium leprae*. Leprosy is widely prevalent in India. Presently all the districts in the country provide free MDT (multi-drug therapy) services; not all the cases are infectious.

Special Features Which are Peculiar to Leprosy

1. The diseases mainly affect the peripheral nerve
2. Loss of sensation
3. It affects the skin, muscles, the eye bones, tests and internal organs
4. Muscular paralysis
5. Deformities
6. Bouts of increased activity generally known as 'reactions'
7. Hypopigmented, presence of thickened nerves, presence of acid fast bacillus in the skin and nasal smear.

Important Factors

1. Leprosy is now controlled with multi-drug therapy
2. It is curable and its deformities are preventable
3. Value of prevention is vitally important
4. Encouragement during illness and readjustment
5. Remove misconceptions
6. Need of empathy
7. Total management of patient
8. Control leprosy case detection of all cases in the community. This may be done by contact survey, group survey and mass survey
9. Care of hands in leprosy—avoid direct skin contact with hot object
10. When walking reducing pressure and injury
11. Gentle massage keeps the finger mobile
12. Exercise, support the hands
13. Care of feet—look for dryness, cracks, swelling, daily self-examination for blister, redness
14. Care of the eyes use drops to prevent dryness
15. Ways to prevent deformities
16. Educating community counseling, campaign against social prejudice, involve community, and propagate facts to dispel misconceptions.

Leprosy is a chronic disabling diseased caused by *Mycobacterium leprae*. Leprosy also called Hansen's diseases, attacks the skin and nerves and causes skin to swell and become lumpy and discolored. The cause of leprosy is a bacillus (rod-shaped bacterium) 0.0064 millimeter long. Leprosy is one of the most feared diseases because it damages a person's appearance. But it seldom causes death.

It may weaken victims; however it makes them more likely to contact other diseases. Leprosy is contagious, but the danger of catching it from another person is very slight.

Less than 10% of the people exposed to the diseases develop it. To get leprosy, a person must have low resistance and live in contact for many years with person whose body contains large number of bacilli.

Leprosy develops in only about 5% of those persons married to leprosy patients. A mild form of leprosy may develop in about 30% of the children whose parents have severe leprosy. But the diseases persists in only about 6% of there children

India accounts about 64% of leprosy cases in the world.

Badly affected states are—Tamil Nadu, Andhra, West Bengal, Bihar and Orissa

Lesser extent the diseases is found in MP, Maharashtra, Karnataka, Kerela, Jammu and Kashmir.

The overall prevalence of leprosy in India is estimated as 3.7 cases per 1,000 population.

Epidemiological Factors

1. **Agent**—the causative agent is *Mycobacterium leprae*. The organism grows in the foot pads of mice and armadillo
2. **Source of infection**—all cases are not infectious. Lepromatous leprosy is highly infectious
3. **Infective materials**—nasal and throat secretions, skin discharges
4. **Age**—infection can occurs at any age. In endemic areas it affect childhood and signs appear many years later
5. **Sex**—common in man than women

6. **Social factors**—poverty, ignorance, illiteracy, over crowding, poor hygiene and poor living conditions are important predisposing factors
7. **Genetic factor**—suspected for individual susceptibility
8. **Mode of transmission**; contact transmission—leprosy is transmitted by contact between an infectious patient to a healthy but susceptible person. The contact may be direct skin to skin or indirect contact by for mites
9. **Droplet infection**—there is evidence that this diseases spreads by droplet infection
10. **Incubation period**—long and variable, commonly 2–5 years.

Classification

1. In terminate types
2. Tuberculosis type
3. Borderline type
4. Lepromatous type
5. Pure neurotics type
6. Cases further divided into
   (a) Multibacillary leprosy—is lepromatous leprosy and the borderline cases, which are infectious case
   (b) Paricibocillary leprosy includes in terminate, tuberculosis and pure neurotic types of leprosy.

Stress these Points

- Leprosy is a curable disease
- It is a preventable disease
- It is like any other diseases
- It is not hereditary
- It is not the result of divine curse
- Early diagnosis and treatment can control the spread of disease.

Leprosy is curable with multi-drug therapy which also prevents disability and deformity.

Early Sings of Leprosy

- Light colored patches on skin which has no feeling
- Thickening of the skin specially face and ears
- Loss of sensation in fingers and toes
- Pain in the nerves.

Clinical Features

- Hypopigmented patches
- Partial or total loss of sensation in the affected areas
- Presence or thickened nerves
- Presence of acid fast bacilli's in the skin and nasal smears.

Diagnosis

1. Look for skin lesions
2. Test for sensory loss.

Any patient showing a positive skin smear, irrespective of the clinical classification, should be treated with the multibacillary regimen.

Numerous other skin diseases which may mimic leprosy and lead to the wrong diagnosis.

Rifampicin is an essential component of the regimens. Ofloxacin and minocycline are other antibiotics which proven action against the leprosy bacillus.

Monthly supervised treatment is given for children below 10 years, dose adjusted, rifampicin 300 mg, depsone 25 mg, and clafazimine 100 mg.

Patients react to treatment extremely well. Nearly all cases it can be diagnosed on clinical signs alone.

Reactions occur the immune system—often damaging the skin, nerves and other tissues, skin lesions becomes swollen, hot, red, painful, and ulcerative. It can occur suddenly, during treatment, or after treatment has finished.

Delayed diagnosis—disability, deformity, and various nerves will be damaged, leading to loss of sensation and muscle power. Deformities are end result of poorly treatment. So it is essential to intensified case detection activities in both family contacts and people in the locality.

Low Hands, Buns, Wrist Drop, Foot Drop, Face Nose Disfigured

- We have to differentiate leprosy from psoriasis, skin TB, pellagra, lympohoma, kapsos, and sarcoma.
- Infective materials—nose and throat secretions, skin discharges and articles used by the patient acquired in childhood. Signs of diseases will appear several years later.
- Poverty, ignorance, overcrowding, poor hygienic living conditions.
- Predisposing factor—genetic factor.
- Skin to skin, direct droplet contact.
- Education is the main tool for changing and modifying the health practices and superstitious beliefs.

Early Case Detection

- Contact survey, group survey, mass survey, examination of household contacts
- BCG vaccination given (unclear)
- Home isolation, keeping utensils separate, clothes, and towels disinfected.

Care of the Skin

Soak oil to prevent dry and cracks, inspect and protect from thorn or stone. Avoid badly fitting shoes. Inspect feet for redness and painful pressure on walking. Wear right kind of shoes.

Eye and eyelids affected the germ settles in the eye causing burning, some people not able to close there eyes, cover the eyeball, dust touches and they are not able to blink get wound.

Control of Leprosy

1. Case detection—the first step in a leprosy control program is early detection of cases in the community. This may be done by contact survey, group survey or mass survey. Contact tracing involves examination of household contacts specially children. They should be kept under observation for 5 years. Mass survey involves examination of the whole population to detect cases. It is done in hyper endemic areas.
2. Chemotherapy—due to resistance of *M. lepra* to dapsone. Multi-drug therapy is started. Government of India recommended the following multi-drug therapy.
3. Multibacillary cases—DDS 100 mg daily plan rifampicin 600 mg daily for initial and weeks then once a month, clofazimine 100 mg on alternate days for 2 years. Children and adults with low weight should receive a lower dose.
4. Paucibacillary cases—DDS 100 mg daily plus for 6 months; rifampicin 600 mg once a month for 6 months.
5. After 6 months only depsone is continued.
6. Follow-up—multibacillary cases needs annual examination of clinical and bacteriological for 5 years after complete therapy.
7. Chemoprophylaxis—dapsone prophylaxis may be given to healthy children living in contact with leprosy patients. The protective value reported is 35% to 40% the WHO has not recommended mass chemoprophylaxis.
8. BCG-vaccination to control leprosy continued.
9. Rehabilitation—all treated cases restored physically, mentally and socially. This is an important aspect of leprosy control.
10. Health education—is an important factor in ant leprosy camp. The patient, family and the community should be educated on the need for regular treatment, protection of children and family planning.

Community Health Nursing

1. Community health nurse should teach the family about the nature of the disease
2. The need for strict home isolation of the patient
3. The need for regular treatment
4. The eating and drinking utensils of the patient kept separate
5. The cloths towels and linen used by patient should be disinfected
6. Follow up patients should be done before, during and after treatment to find out more cases in home visit
7. Children in contact with leprosy patient should be under surveillance. The children should be protected. The leprosy patient should be isolated
8. The nursing care is demonstrated to the family and the community
9. Advice the family on general sanitation, prevention of over crowding and family planning
10. Education of the community that it is curable diseases
11. It is not divine curse, it is not hereditary
12. Early diagnosis and treatment can prevent deformities
13. Patient needs sympathy and understanding
14. To co-operate with the organizations which help patients in controlling the spread of the diseases.

NATIONAL LEPROSY ERADICATION PROGRAM

The main objective of the programme is early detection of cases and their treatment domiciliary with multi drug therapy to control the spread.

There are Two Kinds of Control Unit

1. SET-survey, education, and treatment centers. It is control unit are established in highly endemic areas, in other areas SET centers are established.
2. The SET centers are attached to PHC. A leprosy control unit covers a population of the 4 lakhs.

Keywords

Special features, important factors, epidemiological factors, classification, early sings of leprosy, clinical features, diagnosis, reactions, low hands, buns, wrist drop, foot drop, face nose disfigured, early case detection, care of the skin, control of leprosy, community health nursing, National Leprosy Eradication Program.

CHAPTER

13

Spirituality Everyday

Abstract

Ones spirituality refers to the degree to which one is thoughtful to contemplative about ones existence, accepts challenges in ones life, and seeks and finds answers to personal questions. Spirituality is expressed through ones religion, cultural influences, spiritual values, beliefs and how one reacts to sickness. Illness can be a time of spiritual crisis and place stress on ones internal resources and beliefs.

SPIRITUAL HEALTH

Sickness a moment of grace—illness can lead to anguish, self-absorption, despair and even revolt against God. It can also make a person more mature, helping one to discern in their life what is not essential. So that one can turn towards that which is an illness provokes a search for God and return to him.

SPIRITUALITY AND HEALTH

Religious practices very according to demonstration-sterilization are prohibited and abortions discouraged. Marital faithfulness, accept modern science condem taking lives in any form, anointing of sick, religion influences enhances life, give meaning and purpose of existence, strengthens ones feelings of self-worth and are health giving and life sustaining. Seek support from faith during time of stress, special healing is movement from brokenness to wholeness.

What is the meaning of scuffing? How should we regard the physical body and its function? Is your illness challenging your beliefs or causing you any distress, e.g. my son was whole life have to remain crippled; there is nothing left for me to live for. Inability to accept illness, I got aids and no one comes near me, who can help me, misery even God does not want me, my living or dying matters to no one. Expression of loneliness and powerlessness.

Assure patient that a nurse will be available to support patient in the time of suffering, give faith, hope and meaning and purpose in life. A nurse's supportive presence is underline, her presence communication value and respect, that she is sincerely concerned and committed in helping to meet his needs. A happy heart is good medicines. But a broken spirit drains your strength drives your bones, bad things can happen in life to good people. Prayer evokes deep feelings, the nurse should be prepared to spent time with patient. Prayer has power to heal and all aspects of life are influenced by spirituality. Illness increases spiritual concerns.

1993—February 11th is A World Health Day celebrated every year. It focuses on the author of all healing the divine physician. The spectrum of sickness is vast, and includes all kinds of ailments. Some ailments fall into the category of the 'marginalized' like addiction, alcoholism, etc.

No one of us can escape sickness, aging and death. What sick need is empathy and compassion? To bring solace, comfort and a sense of security to those in need. Sickness is a typical human condition which shows us ours lack of self-sufficiency and our need for others. When healing does not occur and suffering continuous, we can feel over wheeled, isolated and become depressed and feel dehumanized to face sickness in faith. Faith can do what is humanly impossible. When we are sick we need human warmth, in order to bring comfort to a sick person, sincere closeness is more important than words. Sick find safe anchor in faith.

Prayer for healing—in the face of diseases have faith in Gods love. Never before has man been so much broken in spirit, mind and body as today and in so much in need of spiritual, emotional, physical healing. Prayer for healing is therefore, not a magical formula but a faith process of experience of Gods forgiving inner healing and deliverance. It calls for preparing oneself through repentance, forgiveness and renunciation. Healing takes place in an environment of faith. Just as it is both the power and the love of God healer.

You cannot know the meaning of your life until you are connected to the power that created you.

Association between spirituality and health: It is when an individual is able to engage his beliefs in a higher power and sense a source of strength and support. The healing power of prayer may lower blood pressure, reduce stress before surgery, enhance cancer treatment, reduce depression and enhance immune status. Meditation helps in chronic pain, insomnia, anxiety, etc.

There is a link between mind, body and spirit. A person's inner beliefs and convictions can become powerful resources for healing. Nurses needs to support patients and family spiritually self-concept—what an individual thinks and how they feel about themselves affects the way they in which they care for themselves physically and emotionally and the way they are able to care for others. Individual who has poor self-concept not feel in control of situations and may not feel worthy of care, which himself and has perception of their health are closely related.

Self-esteem—an important lesson in life is to value ourselves. If we do, we will walk with confidence and see ourselves and our experience from the right perspective. We cannot avoid people holding us and our achievements in ourselves, our innate goodness and our values as unique being created in God's image and likeness; we will start living from a different paradigm. We will also begin looking another as fellow human beings, all on the path to the divine and shares in this journey of life.

All areas of life are important—looking after ourselves and maintaining ourselves physically keeping our spirits high and in turn with the divine, widening our horizons, keeping ourselves centered and being conscious of the spiritual and divine.

Innate value is something that is independent of the circumstances of our birth, socioeconomic status and the slot we occupy in life. We will find that all the joys of sharing a simple life and humble position have led us to add value in life.

Values are equated with moral values while the most fundamental moral values are almost universal, life does not stop with mortality. Life is also about giving and talking. Accept yourself as you are and be content with what you have so far achieved, and become worthy children of God.

Be in the now—daily we tend to flow with what is gone and what is yet to come, we function one eye on the past and one eye on the future. We agonize about the future as we are conditioned in that way. Time is neither stable nor permanent, it is transient, it is moving. Time is important resources which cannot be stored or accumulated, replaced, purchased, stopped, and stretched.

Many wonder what spirituality is. What is the definition? The dictionary will tell you that it is something deeply religious, something relating to the spirit and sacred matters. The rest is to them for you to find out. You are left with questions: What is religion, is religion the purpose, the goal, or just the means to the spiritual end? What do we mean with the word spirit and what would be sacred? or what of the sacred is of real importance? This topic tries to give clear answers to these questions.

You are surrounded by spirituality everyday. The definition of spirituality is that which relates to or affects the human spirit or soul as opposed to material or physical things. Spirituality touches that part of you that is not dependant on material things or physical comforts. Let's discover how to recognize spirituality in your everyday life. There is a way to bring spirituality back into the forefront of your everyday life. Spirituality is all around you. Spirituality is in everyone you meet and everywhere you go. You are a spiritual being deep down under the trappings of this material world. Now you can rediscover that spirituality in your everyday life.

Be aware of your surroundings, see past the physical, and see the spirit in all things. Think of the things that make you happy. Look at your loved ones, experience the love you feel for them. That love is pure joy and that's spirituality. What makes you smile? That's new age spirituality. The simple sight and sound of a child's laughter, the quiet peaceful sight of a cat napping in the sun, that's spirituality. A quiet walk on a spring day, the gentle breeze, the sound of birds chirping, the smell of flowers and freshly cut grass, it's all the definition of spirituality.

Whatever makes you feel peaceful, joyful and content is spirituality. Notice all the acts of kindness and good you encounter throughout your day, that's spirituality. Devote just a few minutes a day to quietly meditate on all the good things in your life, that's spirituality. Read books that inspire you and touch your heart will help determine your personal definition of spirituality. Listen to spiritually focused teachers. There are many that inspire and teach an everyday approach to spirituality. Take what rings true in your heart and build on that.

Remember to bring awareness to everyday tasks and remind yourself that you were created by spirit with love and joy. You are a spiritual being first and foremost. Spirituality is your birthright and as much a part of you as the air you breathe. Choose to see spirituality in all things by choosing to see the good and joyful side of life. Radiate this joy and spirituality out into the world and come home to your true self your spiritual essence. Learn how to be happy and you will make your world a better place. Living by example is the greatest gift you can give to the humankind.

Inner meaning: Spirituality is one word, which puts a human being on the highest pedestal of life. It is field of Spirituality traveling on which one reaches the last leg of cosmic life nay the form of human being himself. The goal of spirituality is attaining salvation. The phase of life as a human being announces that the life has come full circle. It is only as a human being that one can get enlightened and attain salvation. Reaching the stage of enlightenment is the last step in the field of spirituality. Spirituality is living life as it was meant to be... not as we may have desired or wanted living it. Living a life of choice is not the forte of all human beings. Those on the path of pure spirituality... the true seekers of spirituality are sometimes able to manifest destiny by establishing absolute control over it.

It is a certain fact that only the true seekers of spirituality become the masters of their destiny. Knowingly or unknowingly many people who have a materialistic goal in life travel the path of spirituality and become successful in life. It was not a happening by chance... all was the result of a law which cannot err. These highly acclaimed individuals unknowingly tread the path of pure spirituality and achieved the goal of their life. Spirituality in other terms means that before we ask God the Almighty for material riches to be bestowed upon us... we need to compensate by giving something equivalent or more back to the community. This is the path undertaken by most successful entrepreneurs. In terms of spirituality we are not supposed to get anything unless we promise to do something in return... in the system of God there is fair play all throughout. As we desire... so shall be the corresponding karma we would be required to perform. Mere false promises bring us nothing.

The famous saying, "whatever we want others to do unto us... we should do unto them" forms the core teachings of spirituality. It is not merely a saying. It has to be practiced in reality spirituality definitely helps one take control of destiny. As we proceed on the path of pure spirituality we tend to develop a positive approach towards life. Reeling all the time under a positive attitude of mind... One is able to fine-tune those critical aspects of life which are an absolute must if one needs to become the master of his own destiny. Spirituality makes a perfect man out of a negative thinker. In the field of spirituality there is no place for any negative thinking. One who has fixed a goal in life and always indulges in positive oriented thinking can not be a loser in life. It can never happen! Spirituality imbibes the following virtues in a human being:

Spirituality makes you feel all the time that there is something higher than the mere existence as a human being. Spirituality spells out that God exists within every living being as our soul (the atman within). It is God within us which guides us on the right path whenever we tend to go wrong. Spirituality inculcates in every human being a feeling of positiveness all throughout. Floating on the positive mental plane brings one closer to our goal of life. It is spirituality and spirituality alone which prompts and guides one in the right direction whenever we feel cheated by the senses prevailing upon us. To be able to come out of the clutches of the five senses is what spirituality is all about.

If we desire to know God truly then we need to follow the path of pure spirituality. It is only as a true spiritual seeker shall we realize God one-day. It is a spirituality which cuts short the path and makes the whole world look like a family. In the spiritual domain there is no space for different religions, dogmas or creeds. Our wants and desires cease to exist... the moment spirituality takes complete control over us! Spirituality truly is the essence of life. However materialistic we may be on the earthly plane... there shall come a day when spirituality would completely wipe us clean of all the impurities within us. Without spirituality the life or a human being is like a rudderless boat going round and round in the unfathomable sea of life.

It is spirituality which teaches every human being the real value of life... being spiritual is not being religious alone... Spirituality teaches us the core values of life... the real essence of us! It is only through the medium of spirituality that God is able to guide the mankind towards its destined goal. As many human beings... as many different spiritual paths! Right from day one when we are born and until the last breath... it is spirituality which keeps our heart pumping all through. It is spirituality which clears all doubts that our soul (the atman within the body) is the real master and our body is but to decay and die.

Spirituality clears all doubts related to the concept of God. Whenever in doubt... the wise follow the dictates of the spiritual masters of the era! Every spiritual being merges his identity with the supreme being (the almighty God). Spirituality confirms that life has to go on... it is a journey to be completed in many phases it is spirituality that confirms that the life of a human being is but a trickle in the total life a span of our soul (the atman within). The total life span of the soul being a maximum of 96.4 million earthly years! Spirituality has no relationship whatsoever with religion. Following a religion means following the dictates of a successful spiritual master... one who has already covered the journey and has become capable of guiding the mankind to its logical end.

Religion is meant for living a single span of earthly life. On the contrary spirituality guides every living being to its logical end in the unending cosmic journey undertaken by the soul (our atman within). It is spirituality alone which removes the fear of death from those who have released the pinnacle of spiritual life. Spirituality gives you a commanding position in life. One can work for above 23 hours per day having gained absolute control over sleep. This is not only possible but can be observed by watching the topmost rung of spiritual masters. The presence of spirituality in our lives cannot be done away with for it forms the inner core of our manifested physical life. Behind every success lies the core of spirituality which guides one inherently all throughout the cosmic journey. Spirituality is not to be practiced merely in theory. Spirituality is not contained in the sacred textbooks alone. We simultaneously need to practice pure spirituality and try reaching the end of the cosmic life. Achieving salvation in the present life would be something every human being would desire.

Spiritual medicine begins with a doctor or practitioner becoming more aware of energy fields. Usually this is as a result of spiritual practices such as: meditation, yoga, tai chi, breath work. The practitioner begins to sense his or her energy fields and only then can begin to sense these fields in the patient.

As the majority of other practitioners do not yet have this perceptual awareness and traditional medicine does not yet recognize energy fields, the practitioners undergoing these shifts have few reference points. Each person's awakening is different but these seem to be common elements. Most begin with a desire to be more in silence, often out in nature. Radios are turned off and the person avoids large crowds and noisy bars and restaurants. Music is soft often without words. More and more time is spent in meditation or other spiritual practices. Dietary changes occur away from alcohol, caffeine and red meat as a result of preferences not abstinence. Spinning sensations are felt in different parts of the body as the charkas or energy centers open up. Often neurological symptoms such as tingling, heat or jerking occur spontaneously. Intense emotions including fear, anger and love rise up from within, often with no apparent connection to external reality.

Faith is developed and tested as the person learns to walk "the razor's edge", relying on intuition rather than logic or the advice of others. Families are often alienated as they sense an abrupt change in the person and resent their advice not being followed.

As energy shifts occur the practitioner becomes more aware of their energy body, especially of weak areas. By working in meditation with weak energy centers, many acute illnesses can be avoided. Whereas before the shift, I would suddenly become ill with a viral infection, I now have a chance to work with weak "charkas" or energy systems and often can avoid the cold or flu. As energy centers open up, one develops an ability to sense or feel things intuitively. Other sources of clairvoyant information develop including spiritual hearing or clairaudience and spiritual sight or clairvoyance. And finally, the strongest intuitive information comes through an acute sense of "knowing".

Spiritual medicine acknowledges this and helps the patient see how conflict resolution is crucial in order to get well quickly.

So how do we become ill?

Each of us has a certain amount of "life force" energy. We can measure this energy with devices that measure the aura. Without such devices we have to rely on our intuitive senses. Often we can feel the energy around the person. People with large bright auras make us feel better and people with dark auras drain us.

Each of us is given as "quanta" of energy, to use for "our daily bread". How much we have at the end of the day depends on how we use it. Life force energy can be stimulated by sunlight, exercise, meditation and vital foods. Any creative activity also increases the energy flow into our field. What depletes us?

The two most significant ways to waste energy is through judgment and defending one's sense of self-importance. Certain types of foods, electromagnetic fields, and additions deplete the field. Addictions actually use up a certain amount of etheric or life force energy with each "desire" created. Addictions can be to a wide variety of things—food, drugs, sex, alcohol, body image and materialism. All addictions suppress spiritual growth by depleting life force energy. All are serving the same purpose, to suppress some form of emotional energy that should be allowed to surface and be released.

What can we do to encourage such releases?

Any activity that causes the release of negativity can infuse us with energy. These include forgiveness, gratitude, praise and praying for others. Healing occurs when there is a large release of negativity rather than the suppression of the energy. The healer helps the patient to transmute the energy.

Do not hold onto old relationships. Energy determines relationships so that if a relationship is not working; release it so that the energy can come back into balance. Do not hold onto any particular relationship; allow change to occur without fear. So many illnesses are related to us holding onto that which no longer serves us. Old patterns of behavior, relationships that are not working, and outdated patterns of thought. What causes us to hold on? Fear including fear of loneliness, fear of separation and fear of rejection. The hell we know is better than the hell we don't know.

Healing is transmuting that fear into faith. Faith that creation will provide us with what we really need, not with what we think we need. Fear causes us to breathe shallowly and causes our life force to diminish.

Forgiveness is a vast topic and one that is crucial to healing. The release of negative energy generated by the onset of forgiveness can stimulate the immune system enough to reverse diseases such as cancer.

Human life is full of desires. To be contented and happy with what we have seems very difficult. But contentment can be achieved by spirituality. It is a way of life. Spirituality leads us towards peace, contentment and bliss, teaches positive outlook towards life, remembering good things that one has and find joy in little things. Contentment is a feeling of satisfaction, be content with what you have, you have God, he will take care of your needs.

Keywords

Special features, important factors, epidemiological factors, classification, early sings of leprosy, clinical features, diagnosis, reactions, low hands, buns, wrist drop, foot drop, face nose disfigured, early case detection, care of the skin, control of leprosy, community health nursing, National Leprosy Eradication programme.

CHAPTER 14

Holistic Medicine

Abstract

Holistic medicine is an approach to medical care that emphasizes the study of all aspects to a person's health. Holistic medicine is a term used to describe therapies that attempt to treat the patient as a whole person. That is, instead of treating an illness, as in orthodox allopathic, holistic medicine looks at an individual's overall physical, mental, spiritual, and emotional well-being before recommending treatment.

INTRODUCTION

Holistic medicine uses techniques to stimulate the "field". Chiropractic, acupuncture, traditional Chinese medicine, massage, homeopathy and other holistic methods increase the energy field and thus the immune and endocrine systems. Spiritual medicine adds to this releasing technique of spiritual healing, forgiveness work, past life regression, and hypnotherapy to aid in the areas of weakness of the energy body. Spiritual practices such as meditation, fasting, yoga, Tai Chi, Qi Gong, and breath work help to balance the energy body. Add to this intuitive diagnosis and you really have lost the majority of the medical profession. But as we say at Millennium healthcare—the shift is on, the shift toward more compassionate and effective healthcare. We are on the verge of an awakening. The institutions of medicine, law, and politics will only shift as those within these institutions wake up and start to shake the belief systems. And as with any transformation, there will be much "gnashing of teeth". But, as we move forward into the 21st century, all we can say is "shift happens".

Holistic medicine is a system of health care which fosters a cooperative relationship among all those involved, leading towards optimal attainment of the physical, mental emotional, social and spiritual aspects of health.

It emphasizes the need to look at the whole person, including analysis of physical, nutritional, environmental, emotional, social, and spiritual and lifestyle values. It encompasses all stated modalities of diagnosis and treatment including drugs and surgery if no safe alternative exists. Holistic medicine focuses on education and responsibility for personal efforts to achieve balance and well-being.

Other Terms Associated with Holistic Medicine

Alternative medicine is often used by the general public and some healthcare practitioners to refer to medical techniques which are not known or accepted by the majority "conventional" or "allopathic" medical practitioners such techniques could include non-invasive, non-pharmaceutical techniques such as Medical Herbalism, Acupuncture, Homeopathy, Reiki, and many others. However, the term alternative medicine can also refer to any experimental drug or non-drug technique that is not currently accepted by "conventional" medical practitioners. As non-invasive, non-pharmaceutical techniques become popular and accepted by large number of "conventional" practitioners, these techniques will no longer be considered alternative medicine. The terms holistic healing and holistic medicine are slightly more stable than alternative medicine and are therefore preferable.

Complementary medicine used as a supplement when needed. In many cases, properly chosen techniques plus properly chosen lifestyle changes can completely and safely heal both acute and chronic illnesses.

Natural healing usually refers to the use of non-invasive and non-pharmaceuticals techniques to help heal the patient. When most people use the term natural healing, they are usually referring to physical healing techniques only.

A practitioner with a holistic approach treats the symptoms of illness as well as looking for the underlying cause of the illness. Holistic medicine also attempts to prevent illness by placing a greater emphasis on optimizing health. The body's systems are seen as interdependent parts of the person's whole being. Its natural state is one of health, and an illness or disease is an imbalance in the body's systems. Holistic therapies tend to emphasize proper nutrition and avoidance of substances—such as chemicals—that pollute the body. Their techniques are non-invasive.

Some of the world's health systems that are holistic in nature include homeopathy, and traditional Chinese medicine.

Many alternative or natural therapies have a holistic approach, although that is not always the case. The term complementary medicine is used to refer to the use of naturopathic medicine, both allopathic and holistic treatments. It is more often used in Great Britain, but is gaining acceptance in the United States.

There are no limits to the range of diseases and disorders that can be treated in a holistic way, as the principle of holistic healing is to balance the body, mind, spirit, and emotions so that the person's whole being functions smoothly. When an individual seeks holistic treatment for a particular illness or condition, other health problems improve without direct treatment, due to improvement in the performance of the immune system, which is one of the goals of holistic medicine.

The concept of holistic medicine is not new. In the 4th century BC, Socrates warned that treating one part of the body only would not have good results. Hippocrates considered that many factors contribute to the health or otherwise of a human being, weather, nutrition, emotional factors, and in our time, a host of different sources of pollution can interfere with health. And of course, holistic medicine existed even before ancient Greece in some ancient healing traditions, such as those from India and China, which date back over 5,000 years. However, the term "holistic" only became part of everyday language in the 1970s, when Westerners began seeking an alternative to allopathic medicine.

Interestingly, it was only at the beginning of the twentieth century that the principles of holistic medicine fell out of favor in Western societies, with the advent of major advances in what we now call allopathic medicine. Paradoxically, many discoveries of the twentieth century have only served to confirm many natural medicine theories. In many cases, researchers have set out to debunk holistic medicine, only to find that their research confirms it, as has been the case, for example, with many herbal remedies.

Purpose—Many people are now turning to holistic medicine, often when suffering from chronic ailments that have not been successfully treated by allopathic means. Although many wonderful advances and discoveries have been made in modern medicine, surgery and drugs alone have a very poor record for producing optimal health because they are designed to attack illness. Holistic medicine is particularly helpful in treating chronic illnesses and maintaining health through proper nutrition and stress management.

Description

There are a number of therapies that come under the umbrella of "holistic medicine." They all use basically the same principles, promoting not only physical health, but also mental, emotional, and spiritual health. Most emphasize quality nutrition. Refined foods typically eaten in modern America contain chemical additives and preservatives, are high in fat, cholesterol, and sugars, and promote disease. Alternative nutritionists counter that by recommending whole foods whenever possible and minimizing the amount of meat—especially red meat—that is consumed. Many alternative therapies promote vegetarianism as a method of detoxification.

The aim of holistic medicine is to bring all areas of an individual's life, and most particularly the energy flowing through the body, back into harmony. Ultimately, of course, only the patient can be responsible for this, for no practitioner can make the necessary adjustments to diet and lifestyle to achieve health. The practice of holistic medicine does not rule out the practice of allopathic medicine; the two can complement each other.

A properly balanced holistic health regimen, which takes into consideration all aspects of human health and includes noninvasive and no pharmaceutical healing methods, can often completely eradicate even acute health conditions safely. If a patient is being treated with allopathic medicine, holistic therapies may at least support the body during treatment, and alleviate the symptoms that often come with drug treatments and surgery. In addition, holistic therapies aim at the underlying source of the illness, to prevent recurrence.

Here are some of the major holistic therapies:

1. Herbal medicine
2. Homeopathy
3. Naturopathic medicine
4. Traditional Chinese medicine
5. Ayurvedic medicine
6. Nutritional therapies
7. Stress reduction
8. Psychotherapy
9. Massage.

Because holistic medicine aims to treat the whole person, holistic practitioners sometimes may advise treatment from more than one type of practitioner. This is to ensure that all aspects of health are addressed. Some practitioners also specialize in more than one therapy, and so may be able to offer more comprehensive assistance.

Holistic medicine: An approach to medical care that emphasizes the study of all aspects of a person's health, including psychological, social, and economic influences on health status.

Holistic medicine a comprehensive approach to health care and prevention of disease employing conventional and many of the alternative medicine modalities, including acupuncture, chiropractic, herbal medicine, homeopathy, massage, and physical therapy which integrates the body as a whole, including mind and spirit, rather than separate systems.

Keywords

Alternative medicine, complementary medicine, natural healing, many alternative or natural therapies have a holistic approach. There are no limits to the range of diseases and disorders that can be treated in a holistic way, purpose, description-holistic therapies: holistic medicine aims to treat the whole person, holistic medicine a comprehensive approach to health care.

CHAPTER 15

Alcohol as a Social Evil

Abstract

Alcohol is considered as a drug. After prolonged consuming alcohol, there are number of signs and symptoms presented such as difficulty with gait and balance, acute change in cognition, frequent falls or accidents, poor nutritional intake, social isolation, danger of malnutrition and increased tolerance to anesthetics, slurred speech, in coordination, ataxia, odor of alcohol on breath and clothing , respiratory depression. Sudden withdrawal of intake of alcohol may precipitated by injury and infection. In female there is an impact on the growth, development and well-being of her fetus.

Nurse is an important pillar in providing health education by means of simple use of teaching aids. She can research further new ideas and reach to the vast public with varieties of cultures, variation in geographical factors, climatic changes, different eating habits, clothing, traditions and customs. Where we have many problems to deal like poverty, illiteracy, unemployment, ill health, poor housing, natural calamities, over population, and communicable diseases.

Health education helps in prevention of diseases to promotion of healthy lifestyle. The modification of the individual behavior in social environment where an individual lives. To encourage people and to adopt and sustain health promoting lifestyle and practices. Indicate to the people alternative solutions for solving the health and health related problems. Education will help to improve quality of life and give security and good position in society.

Nurses play vital role in teaching dos and don'ts and eliminating wrong concepts and giving new fresh knowledge. Because all want to live healthy and happy life. It touches there core of being. It will help in living condition, give dignity, remove incidence of ignorance and teach preventive measures.

Any topic that students select should have relevant, up to date knowledge, reliable matter, appropriate method, group participation and ability to control group.

Alcoholism is a social evil, so she can take this topic and connect to the health problems due to alcohol abuse.

Alcohol is a drug and may be classified as a sedative, tranquilizer, hypnotic or anesthetic depending upon the quantity consumed. Of all the drugs, alcohol is the only drug whose self-induced intoxication is socially acceptable. Alcohol is rapidly absorbed from the stomach and small intestine within 2 to 3 minutes of consumption, it can be detected in the blood, the maximum concentration is usually reached about one hour after consumption. The presence of food in the stomach inhibits the absorption of alcohol because of dilution.

Alcohol has a marked effect on CNS. Alcohol is a disease as agent cause acute and chronic intoxication, cirrhosis of the liver, toxic psychosis, gastritis, pancreatitis, cardiomyopathy and peripheral neuropathy.

Evidence related to cancer mouth, pharynx, larynx and esophagus. It is important factor in suicide, automobile and other accidents and injuries and deaths due to violence. Family disorganization, crime and loss of productivity. Alcohol abuse is an universal problem.

ALCOHOL AND ITS EVIL EFFECTS

Many men take to drinking because of physical exhaustion and gives temporary boost in energy, truck drivers, daily laborers indulge in drinking. Many people are drawn to these habits by friends, just start drinking for company and get addicted. Peer pressure and fashion as sign of modeling. Unhealthy environment living with, and surrounded by such addicts. Ignorance that alcohol gives additional strength and vigor and self-confidence.

It is a root cause of family unhappiness, disorganization of family life. Economic life suffers sudden loss of job and frustration. Health get affected and all the system of body gets affects.

Drink of death—about 60 millions (50%) Indians are alcoholics; this equals the population of France. Two-thirds of the alcohol consumed in India is illegal hooch. More than half of all drinkers in India fall in hazardous drinking category. Ninety-five percent of beverages drunk in India are IMEL. Licensed country liquor, and illicit spirits. Official records show alcohol sales have grown 8% in the past 3 years. There figures do not include illegal liquor sales. Government stats show only 21% of adult Indian men and 25 of women drink.

Percentage of drinking population aged less than 21 years up from 2% to more than 14% in 15 years. Average age of initiation dropped from 19 years to 134 years in two decades.

Employers in poor communities somewhere pay wages in alcohol rather than cash, WHO says alcohol related problems account for more than 5th of hospital admissions.

18% psychiatric emergencies, more than 205 of all brain injuries, 60% of all injuries reporting to emergency now certain study shows in many poor households average monthly expenditure on alcohol more then average monthly salary.

Ban on country liquor in Maharashtra saw wifebeating cases drop by 35% in 2010. In Bengal hooch pouch cost id ₹ 10 for ½ liter. Typically hooch poisoning—its symptoms are vomiting, piercing headaches, frothing at the mouth, complains of burning chest and severe stomach pain, spurious liquor can induce coma, blindness and death.

Traditional tribal make drink from dried flower of Mahua tree and is essential during celebrations. Today also palm wine is made from sap of various species of palm tree. Distilled drinks—Goan spirit, made from coconut or rice of cashew apple most respectable among country liquor. Goa has registered a geographical indicators prepared from formatted sap of coconut flowers, sugarcane grain or fruits.

What is illicit liquor?

It is alcohol beverages are made by formatted of sugary and starchy substances, followed by distillation to increase alcohol concentration. The active ingredient in them is ethyl alcohol or ethanol, any liquor made under unlicensed conditions is called illicit liquor. Usually sub-standard to raw materials is used often this is spiked with other chemicals.

What makes it poisonous?

Under unregulated conditions methanol or methyl alcohol can be produced with the desired ethanol. Sometimes, industrial methyl alcohol or denatured spirit added by illicit to save the cost and is mistaken belief that it will increase potency. There has been incidence where chemicals like Organophosphrous components have been added to illicit liquor. Methyl alcohol is extremely toxic, 10 mL can cause blindness and 30 mL can cause death within 10–30 hours. It is like ethyl alcohol in taste and smell.

What are the antidotes?

Ethyl alcohol and Fomepizole are antidotes' inhibiting metabolizing of methyl alcohol, so that it passes through urine. Sodium bicarbonate used for acidosis. Advanced treatment requires hemodialysis to remove toxic substances from blood stream.

Alcoholism and drug addictions are detrimental not only health and welfare of the individual but to the family, community and society at large/it is a state of periodic or chronic intoxication produced by repeated consumption of drug either natural or synthetic.

Alcoholism means the excessive consumption of alcohol and becoming addicted to it. Small moderate quantities used release tension, relaxed mind and sedate the brain especially to painful emotions and promote a sense of pleasure and well-being.

Most people are not able to control the desire to drink and get into excessive, consumption of alcohol on regular basis and their health comes under danger, ones peace of mind gets affected, home life becomes unhappy business jeopardize reputation clouded when drinking becomes routine.

Men often start drinking in order to forget the miseries and problems of life and to escape miseries. Some drink because of physical exhaustion to get temporary boost of energy and lessens fatigue, e.g. truck drivers, manual workers. People just start drinking just for company, friendship, fashion, sign of modernization, unhealthy environment like living in slums, sudden losses and frustration in love, life ambitions fall, and fall of business. In modern world, people have to make new contacts to extend their business or to increase their professional contacts, late night parties is common. Also urbanization modem city life with mechanical ways of life, materialistic values and cut throat competitions all create tensions and conflicts go to escape accept this way of life.

Habitual drinking cause's personality completely disorganized. Its danger signal is when a person starts drinking in the morning. He needs alcohol to push through the day and he feels he cannot face difficult situation without the help of alcohol. Then the time comes that he cannot manage his life and completely becomes dependant and alcohol becomes absolutely necessity and alcohol becomes significant than company of human beings. He becomes alien to the normal world and to society pathological state.

Alcohol has many evil effects therefore individual should keep himself away from it. Prolonged use health gets affects- tremors, unsteady gait, luster eyes, hanged look, and looses efficiency of self-control, poverty, misery, family unhappiness, violent and abusive language, wife beating and children, becomes anti social, shame to family, no moral and ethical values, gambling, prostitutions and other vices he gets entangled.

SUGGESTIONS

1. The working conditions to be improved
2. Mass communication to explain the evils of drinking
3. Recreational facilities to be provided to divert the mind of people and keep them away from bad habits
4. Improve housing facilities where workers can bring their families to the cities. Together living might help people to keep away evil habits
5. The practice of serving drinking at parties be banned
6. Brothels should be away from the residence and industrial areas
7. Women should take anti-drinking movements, because they are worst suffers when men drink and behave irresponsibly.

First evidence of alcohol being carcinogenic—almost 30 years after discovering of a link between alcohol consumption and certain forms of cancer, scientists are reporting the first evidence from research on people explaining how the popular beverage may be carcinogenic.

Silvia Balbo, who led the study, explained that the human body break down or metabolizes the alcohol in beer, wine and hard liquor. One of the substances formed in that break down is acetaldehyde a substance with a chemical backbone that resembles formaldehyde. Formaldehyde is a known human carcinogen. Scientist also have known from laboratory experiments that acetaldehyde can cause DNA damage and trigger chromosomal abnormalities in cell culture' we now have the first evidence from living human volunteers that acetaldehyde formed after alcohol consumption damages DNA dramatically.

She said out that people have a highly effective natural repair mechanism for correcting the damage from DNA adducts. Most people thus are unlikely to develop cancer from social drinking.

IMPORTANT POINTS SUMMARIZED

What is alcoholism?

Alcohol addiction is a compulsive need for an intoxicating liquid that is from fermented grain or fruit. These liquids include beer, wine, and other hard liquors. Person craves for alcohol cannot limit his drinking. He experiences withdrawal symptoms such as nausea, sweating, shaking, or anxiety. Craving is so great that it surpasses their ability to stop drinking. They need assistance to stop and to rebuild there lives. Alcoholic anonymous describes alcoholism as a physical condition associated with mental obsession. It is a chronic dependency; the personality make up of these people is weak ego and super ego. He has low self-esteem and poor impulse control. He has decreased energy, disturbed sleep pattern, impaired judgment, increase anxiety, depression, manipulative behavior, perceptual changes, and marked withdrawal symptoms.

What are the causes and effects of alcoholism?

It deepens on the environment and traumatic experiences in life. These factors include culture, family, friends, peer pressures and the way person lives. It can lead him to serious problems and is physically and mentally destructive. Currently alcohol use is involved in half of all crimes, murders, accidental deaths and suicides. Problems associated many health's such as brain damage, cancer, heart disease, and the diseases of the liver. Life expectancy is reduced to 10–15 years.

- Too much alcohol can destroy brain cells, leading to bran damage.
- It disturbs CNS, hindering the ability to retrieve, consolidate, and process information
- Brain causing a blackout when totally drunk
- It also can inflame the mouth, esophagus and stomach
- Produce irregular heart beats, risk of high BP, heart damage
- Harm vision, damage sexual function, slow circulation, and water retention
- It can also lead to skin and pancreatic disorders, weakening the bones and muscles, thus decreasing immunity
- A large portion of alcohol is broken down in liver. Liver damage can occur leads to cirrhosis of liver.

What to do with alcoholism?

- Have a desire to stop
- Have the initiative to identify the cause of your alcoholic
- Forgiveness and seek counseling to aid in healing
- Recognize and rehabilitation center for treatment
- Get help from family, friends and above all from you.

To help the patient to take medicine regularly

Reduce anxiety and depression. If the patient is found to be in an acute state of intoxication, attend to medical care and maintain vital signs. Provide adequate nutrition and maintain weight, force eating and add vitamins in the diet. Do not leave him alone; give an hot glass of milk. Rub the back and make him comfortable.

The patient may jump out of window due to disorientation, protect him from injury. Irritation, violent behavior, attacks others so observe for it. Pursued him to maintain personal hygiene. Accept him with his problem provide support of relatives and be non-judgmental. Help the patient to identify his manipulative behavior. Enhance self-esteem, learn that he is important. Call him by name. Help him to socialize, to develop sense of support, and try out new relation. Help him to identify his hobbies.

Help him to find pleasure in life without use of alcohol. To regain insight into life to have hope and gain pleasure in life without it. Attend a follow up clinic. The patient stars his routine job and home.

Keywords

Health education, nurses play vital role, alcohol is a drug, alcohol has a marked effect, alcohol and its evil effects, many men take to drinking because, drink of death, traditional tribal make drink from, what makes it poisonous? what are the anti-dots? alcoholism and drug addictions, men often start drinking in order to, habitual drinking cause's, alcohol has many evil effects, suggestions-alcohol being carcinogenic- to help the patient to take medicine regularly, important points summarized.

CHAPTER 16

Counseling I: Parental and Teacher Education and Counseling

Abstract

There are different branches of counseling. Counseling is a communication process that deals with human problems associated with the occurrence and recurrence of disorders which needs to seek expert consultations. Today parenting has become a challenging task. Parents too chases and compare children for excellence and sometimes unknowingly push the kids over the edge. The role of teachers too is vital in guiding and building a rapport with students.

RENEWING THE CHASE FOR EXCELLENCE

Winning is not just everything: If you do not win, everything is in vain. We forget that the winner is not always excellent and excellent does not always ensure a win. The winner too is only remembered till the next season when another winner steps in and grabs the limelight. We forget past winners so easily that they even forget they were once winners. We are forcing winners to lose sight of life, courage, heroism, dignity in defeat, the power to learn from ones mistakes are all yielding way to one thing.

Push your kids, but not over the edge. Have high but reasonable expectations. Be fair, firm, and consistent. Do not push, facilitate. Put failure in perspective, make your kids play. Are we burdening our kids with our obsessive expectations for high exam scores? Parents are confused how to motivate and guide their kids. They need to know that your love is not dependant on their success. At the same time, they do need to realize that your approval is dependant on their effort. Failure in academics does not mean failure in life.

We do not wait for incidence to happen. We try and identify the problems. We look for signs of dysfunction in children and families—identify the signs of stress and try to arrest the problem. Pressure will always be there, little pressure is important for students to make an effort so you do well in life. Talk about problem with family or peer is a good solution. Many of them are scared to talk to the parents and get messed up in emotions and illogical steps. One should think of parents before taking any drastic step. Your life ends, but what about who live with pain and guilt throughout their lives. Parents are best outlet; you can speak to them about your frustration. It all depends on how much you let the pressure affect you. Each individual will have different ways of dealing.

Not everybody is comfortable with talking about his or her problem, especially teenagers. School should have counseling system and not punish or suspend a child for bad behavior. For constructive action, you must put emotional disorder at an early stage.

The school and counselor must supervise the period/ attention deficit disorder (ADD) so that it can be treated; then. It is important to preserve the self-esteem of a child. If he feels rejected, the consequences can be devastating; also, important aspect is do not mistreat students.

Harassment of Students by Teachers

No school under the guise of enforcing discipline should mistreat any student or parents. The school needs to be aware of the sensitivity and impressionable nature of mind of schoolchildren and must endure that all students, irrespective of their differences are dealt with a dignified manner. Sensitive individual should be protected at any cost especially vulnerable group.

Teaching and learning continues—it also includes the philosophy, objectives, climate of the school, environment facilities, availability of teaches personally, attitude, knowledge, experience, communication and assertive skills, ability to handle the students, problematic students, way of displaying technique used to correct the wrong behavior and maintain good interpersonal relationship.

What does teacher do? A teacher begins with an objective and ends with an evaluation and how best she motivates them. In evaluation, desired result not achieved then re-teaching all over again is important. Therefore evaluation helps modify or revise to get optimal results. The aim of nursing education is to prepare the nurses with head, heart and hand. Teachers need to display leadership students can get inspired. We believe that what happens to others will not happen to us. We apply different standards to evaluate our own behavior and that of others in all fields of activity.

Respect for teachers cannot be ordered, it must be earned. The teachers should regard the pupil as his child. The pupil should regard teacher as his parents. Those who educate children well are to be honored more than parents, for parents only give life and teacher teach the art of living well. The grace of the guru is like an ocean. If one comes with a cup, he will only get a cupful. The bigger the vessel the more will be able to carry. Spiritual teacher enjoys up to comprehend by our soul the infinite spirit which is the depth of the moving a changing facts of the world.

Teachers—all of them so different, what they wear, how they speak, their teaching habits, everything is so different, good looking, intelligent, sophisticated and friendly, popular among students, they hold attention, they left a timeless impression and skill evoke a strong feeling of nostalgia in us you are forever cherished. Clothes make the man. The colors you drape yourself in decide the way you perceive yourself and the way others treat you. The way you look and dress affects what people expect from you. It also declares how you feel about yourself. This decides how you will be treated by co-workers and your boss.

Why teachers punish children—too many students in the classrooms becomes difficult to handle the crowd. High stress levels, students and parents do not take work seriously, as there are no exams students taking back, bad habits, teasing, bullying. Students creating disturbances in class, students form poor background and areas using foul language in class. Parents feel counseling is better option than punishment. Polishing a student's personality is a slow and painstaking process. Turn the problem into solutions.

Is **homework** a waste of time? Homework is a short revision on a daily basis to improve the retention power of children. Only it should be interesting and creative for the children to enjoy it, it helps them to keep pace with study and teaching done in class. They should apply their mind and not take it lightly as they just complete it.

Teacher's speck—every teacher wants the best for his student. It is therefore, advisable to trust a teacher. Good and bad people are there in every profession. Being a bookworm does not help much. You end up forgetting everything if you become a bookworm. It's your dedication, concentration and hard work that matters. Importance of time management is vital.

Teacher's tips—do not give up if you fall down—maintain a daily journal, note down situations or incidents that bother you and because you stress, as this will help you identify and pinpoint the problems and help you find solutions for them. Write down the names of the subjects you dislike and try to find out why. Take a regular break and do what you love to do. Short breaks at regular intervals help you cool down, they also help keep the mind focused and fresh, breaking the monotony of long periods of reading and writing. It could be chatting with friends or watching TV. Organize yourself better, wake up.

All about consistency and practice is success mantra. Work hard, work smart, put in that extra effort, and good planning. Stay calm and conquer. One of the key factors to excel in any exam is to stay calm. How can we conquer anxiety and remain composed when exams are approaching/losing sleep over the boards can affect performance in the exams. Make sure you get at least 6 or 7 hours of sleep. If you are not well rested, writing down on your answer paper all that you painstakingly learn will be an impossible task. Eat healthy and sleep well. Sleep is what will give your mind the time it needs to process all the information you have poured into it. Praying also clears the mind and boosts confidence. It calms you down and makes you sharper. Listen to the songs that make you feel good, which makes you feel happy. Music also stimulates the brain, without stressing it out. Eat healthy and not junk food. Spend time with your family, that your family shares your concern and it supportive. Some light chitter chatter will also help ease the tension.

Student and teacher's rapport is key—technology can never replace a teacher. In classroom, teachers get to know the aptitude of students and their level of understanding. Technology can only support this face-to-face between the students and the instructor—online teaching sessions cannot match or even compensate for such live interaction. An increasing use of technology in school hampers development of skills in a child.

Create scope for innovation with interactive whiteboards, content stored in them can be viewed online and facilities like void conferencing and live broadcasting, smart classrooms can boost pupil's interest in studies like never before. Technology dependence makes students in attentive and impair basic skills such a speaking and writing, making technology an asset rather than a liability depends on a teachers skills. Neither success nor failure is final.

Perseverance is the key to success. Focus on your subject and study your subject well, self-belief is biggest key to handle exam stress. Believe in yourself, keep motivating yourself and boost your self-confidence.

Teacher's tips on how to beat stress—how do you handle exam stresses? How do you revise for the board? What is the schedule you need to keep? It is important to stay calm when exam is round the corner.

1. Make sure that you have your entire stationary ready. Read the question paper thoroughly once or twice. Clear your doubts before you start attempting questions.
2. Begin your exam on a positive note. The positive vibrations will help you in keeping your mind relaxed and this will, in turn, help you work on all the questions. It helps in keeping your mind focused.
3. Answer with discipline as per the pattern of the paper. Try not to go haywire, as this will keep you on track.
4. For the writing exercises, prepare a rough draft, stick to the answers required and make them crisp and clear. Do not exaggerate while answering questions, being to the point helps.

Children should—we cram our children's head with facts or educate them for success as human beings? We teach children how to solve problems in mathematics but give them nothing to help them solve the problems they face in their personal lives. We flood them with a tide of facts, and then tell them as we send them out the door with their diploma. The modern age is fascinated, addicted to factual information such information offers no sense of direction, nor any knowledge of where one might go to find inner peace, poise and a sense of life's deeper meaning and joyous possibilities. The children of today will make the India of tomorrow. The way we bring them up will determine the future of the country. Let us win them over with love. Children who learn to concentrate to increase their awareness and to channel negative emotions are able to handle all the factual information they are taught in school for more effectively. True goal of school must be to help prepare us for that life long learning process. When we are children, we seldom think of the future. This innocence leaves us free to enjoy ourselves as few adults can, the day we fret about the future is the day we leave our childhood behind.

Parenting is now a big challenge—with factors like breaking up of joint families and emergence of nuclear families children has no one to turn to. In the race of score more and more marks children are packed off to various tuition classes, littlie children need to be taught patiently which can be done by their parents, parents must find ways to make the learning fun. Economic pressure are forcing both the parents in more homes to go out to work which has positive and negative effects on children's behavior. In today's competitive age, academic success matters a lot. Parenting is also a challenge due to changing lifestyle. Both the parents are well educated yet, it may be difficult for them to find time to mange children's study. It is necessary for parents to get involved in children's academic, they must communicate with them and be aware of their progress and their daily schedule, and give children time. Parents can make kids independent.

Parents should look out for signs of depression in students, if the child speaks about death and dying he is worried about exams, talks about staying away from the house, talks about leaving school, parents and teachers should get alert. Parents and teachers should be supportive when the students performance is below parents also go though performance anxiety these days due to failure. Parents should help them in developing comfort zone where they can share all their problems with them and it should not be one-way communication.

In today's world, success comes to those who are image ready. With increasing competition and globalization in our economy, one must project an image appropriate to ones role and occasion at hand. This creates like ability and confidence in the people you meet. Your clothes, grooming and body language. The truth is, you may carry certain skills, abilities and experiences, but the people you meet often judge you because of what meet the eye, within second they decide in their mind everything about your personality, values, trust, worthiness, intelligence for job. Visual communication is the major part of any communication at a first meeting. Cloths communicate lot about you to others; your clothes have to be appropriate, personal grooming and hygiene plays an important role in life. Body language is technically the biggest form of communication. Today when almost everyone has talents and technical knowledge managing your image provides that extra edge which eventually decides the final winner.

Top 10 Tips

1. Value your time
2. Know your priorities
3. Practice saying no
4. Do not apologies
5. Stop being nice
6. Say no to your boss
7. Try permitting requests
8. Get back to you
9. May be later
10. Its not you, its me.

Parents ask yourself, examine, and see how does your child spend his evening?

Indulging in computer or video gaming is acceptable once in a while, letting it become an addiction spells trouble for children. For attention deficit hyperactivity disorder (ADHD) to developing symptoms of dysphasia which is a motor learning difficulty.

When we analyze their history, in almost 8 out of 10 cases, we found that the children showing signs of aggression, violent temper, poor social skills, all had one thing in common- they spend hours playing computer games and absolutely no playing outdoor games. If children are taken out mostly in malls instead of gardens, has more psychological and physical damage than parents and kids can imagine.

Following problems may result:

1. **Poor social skills**—too much gaming makes children socially isolated. Often the child gets addicted and gaming takes a priority over everything, else including family and studies.
2. **Poor eye sight**—sitting in front of the screen for hours weakens the eyesight and getting spectacles at an early age is not uncommon with children addicted to gaming.

3. **Impaired hearing**—constant exposure to extremely loud music at gaming arcades and listening to the ear phones leads to early loss of hearing.
4. **Movement disorders**—simple activities like running around, playing on the slide, playing catch-n-cook help improve body movement. Coordination that plays very important part in the intellectual growth of children.
5. **Attention problem**—flashing light and constant music at gaming arcades excite children leading to hyperactivity, ADD or ADHD. It becomes difficult to sustain attention for more than a few minutes and aggravates ADHD in them.
6. **Health hazards**—as they do not spend time outdoor, they do not get enough vitamin D, which requires for strengthening the bones, lack of fresh air or oxygen make the child lethargic. They also develop bad postures. Children visiting malls tend to eat unhealthy foods. They do not get enough exercises this leads to obesity.
7. **Psychological disorders**—research has proved that children who play violent video games are more likely to have increased aggressive thoughts, feeling and behavior. Many even teach the kids the wrong values. They also create a false sense of achievement and children are easily confused between reality and fantasy.
8. **Brain power**—brain needs new experiences to become stronger and healthier. Gaming does not exercise kids' imaginative thinking and develops creativity. This affects their performance at school too and there is decline in verbal memory performance as well.
9. **Get some real play**—according to experts, it is very important for children to stay in touch with nature and indulge in bodily contact games to help muscle and brain develop. Playing with friends help children develop interaction and social skills. Sports teach them teamwork and build the self-esteem in fun environment. Children learn to deal with situation without a conscious efforts as computer generating has calming effect on them.

They have to focus and concentrate—to succeed, you need concentration—on every level of mental activity, concentration is the key to success. The student is talking an exam but is distracted by a popular song running through his head is distraction. A business person trying to write an important contract is worried over an argument he had with his wife. The judge is distracted a teenager appearing before him as he resembles his own son. Lack of concentration means inefficiency, such mind often attracts opportunities as he is focused. There is a power in concentration, concentration awakens our powers and channels them, dissolving obstacles on our path. Concentration implies an ability to release ones mental and emotional energies and focus them on single object. Stillness, stability.

Focus and concentrate at the work place. There is too much going on around you as well as inside your mind. One thing at a time- multitasks priories what is most important for you, give 100% focus task, do not switch off, build mental stamina, your mind may be wandering through a hundred random thoughts, so when your mind is far away, see everything around. Mind power meditation increases your ability to handle tasks better. What also greatly aids concentrations, the glucose metabolism in the brain, which is at its peak after breakfast; people who meditate are able to switch attention between tasks more efficiently than people who do not.

Be an arrow of attention—life is a classroom and you never cease to be student knowledge comes to those who have curiosity that is the mother of knowledge. It is the greatest virtue. What do all science, discovery and invention own their origin to? Curiosity so cultivate curiosity, for curiosity cultivates knowledge. Convert everything into curiosity, what is it about, what is it for, how does it work, how does it fit in with life, if you have a curiosity nothing is dull and tough. Start and look at things with curiosity. Attention is the sharp edge of curiosity, be like an arrow set on its aim for that you should not have diversion, have sense of control.

Opt for hard work instead for easy money. It is to opt for a self-made man formula, when you try to live on your own; you are trying to tap your potential. Everyone is born with enormous potential, but potential can be developed only by hard work. That is the key to success in life. If you are not born to life of hardship, it will activate you and this will give you incentive to work, on the other hand, if you are born into life of comfort, it will kill your motivation. When you try to unfold your potential; that is like embarking on journey that is limitless. Favor may give you temporary relief, but hard work is the only way to achieve great success, rely on your own efforts.

Focus on the following things:

1. **Be positive**—there are students who are motivated, have set goal but they lack proper study method, when they do not get expected result they get discouraged, tensed, and face disapproval.
2. **Negative-motivation**—a student who has no aim in life, lack concentration, find studying boring, can not pay attention- distracted, day dreaming, watching TV, movies, playing, and wasting time with friends ends up his life in failure.
3. **Pressure—**from the parents to get high percentage, can not cope with study, get discouraged, loose concentration.
4. **Parents overstrict**—ambitious parents, parents compare them with others, start building low self image affects their study, social and peer interaction.

5. **Having set goal**, determination, will power, commitment, motivation, encouragement, awareness, realization.
6. Should not loose sight of visions, provide children with safe and loving environment to grow, give them ample opportunities to take studies as self and nation building, skills, proficiency, competence and experty.
7. Most children who get involved in crime, emotionally disturbed, and have no outlet to vent their frustration, parents are busy, friends might be ignoring them, no monitoring system at home and children get exposed to disturbing factors, facts and ideas. If the child is aggressive in school, it could be because of atmosphere at home or it could be parents fault. Students need to be counseled ill effects of drug abuse as a preventive measure. Parents should keep the tract on the kids company and what they do, in their leisure time, parents need to be alert violence all around us, recent cases of raging, physical and sexual abuse have shaken us.
8. **Be your own therapist and drive away stress and pain**—make right choices, life looks up, you attract positive people get in touch with your inner self, clear your mind, clutter creates blocks in the flow of energy within you, when these blocks remain for long it spreads all over your body and mind leaving you in forever irritable mood. Be around nature, the earth elements have the capacity to take away negativities. Drive away negative energy and replace it with positive vibes around you. Good sleep, healthy diet and exercise, drink enough water, which gradually fills us with positive energy.
9. Nowadays time passes with great speed, so only being a time conscious will not be enough, planning the use of time also is essential. So that, an activity is planned consciously, success is achieved. Punctuality is one of the yardsticks for measuring people worth; it is a key to success. Rate it as a top most asset and have respect for task; it will mould your character so that you become a person of discipline, quality and integrity.
10. **Often nothing requires**—more courage than the admission of ones fault. Human beings have a double nature, capable of great sacrifice and charity and at the same time capable of committing heinous acts. The instinct to do well and the instinct to bad are intertwined with both positive and negative qualities. We tend to hurt others with our thoughtlessness and selfish inclination; hence we need to be on guard always. Not to harbor resentment, anger or bitterness, not to be selfish, greedy or proud, repentance means new beginning starting all over again, desire to set things right.
11. **Happiness is a context of being alive with the moment.** You remain unhappy because of problems, like the oceans waves, will keep coming. One has to enjoy despite the waves, despite the problems. We are restless with ourselves because the self we know is empty, shallow, void and unhappy. Fact this fact. We try to be busy because we want to avoid-avoid this. Often you are alone to tend to fear, anger, disappointment and insecurity. Learn to heal the inner hurts, handle your greed wisely, manage your inner insecurity all will automatically get transformed. You will be at peace.
12. **Never mind failures,** they are quiet natural; they are the beauty of life. What would be life without them? We failed so we get strengthen, life has meaning only in struggle.
13. **Burn anger before anger burns you**—it is more distractive than fire or earthquakes. When you get angry, certain glands in your body get activated. This leads to an outpouring of adrenaline and other stress hormones, with noticeable physical consequences. Your face reddens, blood pressure increases, voice rises to a higher pitch and breathing becomes faster and deeper, your heart beats harder and your arms and legs muscles tighten, your body becomes tensed. The culmination effect is that it increases risk of coronary heart diseases and other life threatening diseases like stroke, ulcers. When you are calm, peaceful, happy, digestive process in your body work normally. It is not individual or situation that cause anger, it is your own reaction or response to situation, develop the habit to control anger.
14. **Education** without character, science without humanity, commerce without morality is useless and dangerous. The end of education is character, teachers teach with passion and students learn with enthusiasm.
15. **Mind grows in magnitude**—the mind thinks, it discovers and invents newer modes of thinking.

Follow these habits of a highly effective management guru—

1. **Be proactive**—choose your own course. Highly effective people do not dwell on the thing they can not do and are not reactive to outside forces, instead they focus on what they can do and those consequence.
2. **Begin with the end in mind**—determine what your end goal is, including your broader life goals, so you know what you are working toward.
3. **Put first thing first**—parities tasks based on importance, rather than urgently and make sure your plan drives you toward the goals you outlined in habit, once you have prioritized tasks, execute accordingly.

4. **Think win-win**—aim for solution that mutually benefit both parties in a relationship.
5. **Seek first to understand the to be understood,** try to recall, listen to other people and be open to influences which should help them do the same for you in order to help create a more respectful environment an better solve problems.
6. **Synergies**—use teamwork to reach goals unattainable by one person working alone. To get the strongest performance out of team players encourage meaningful contributions and end goals.
7. **Sharpen the saw**—to be more effective over the long hand make sure to keep your body mind and spirit fit an refreshed via exercise, prayer or meditation community service and stimulating reading.
8. Accept the problem and seek help, it won't resolve on its own.
9. Enhance creative abilities.
10. Jot down the disturbing thoughts (as and when it occurs) on a piece of paper and throw it in the dustbin.
11. Connect with positive minded friends and relatives.
12. Do something therapeutic e.g. Observe sun watch child at play.
13. **Tips**—understand and empathetic with a person. Be firm and do not cater to all his demands, do not use abusive language, discuss a solution with family and friends, do not take risk, never mange probe of your own.
14. If you are confident that you are competent and prepared to work hard, you can achieve anything make your child stronger and intelligent find out weather a child has a problem of poor appetite, weakness, other stomached, irritation, poor concentration, poor memory, phobia to resolve these problems need to give proper diet and maintain daily regimen of your child. Prevent diseases by strengthening immune system, improve physical strength and stamina, help the retention of memory power, and protect the child from seasonal diseases and different kind of allergies. For healthy and happy life through early diagnoses, therapy of diseases, testing of heath.

Education—a new hub that is fast track education board, based curriculum and global perspective to equip students the relevant qualification and training that serves as a spring board to a brighter future. Today's education system that is; competitive and encourages young minds to be analytical. Talented students get quality education with an array of specialized courses; students can enjoy a number of choice acclaimed teaching facilities.

Lessons learnt for life from honeybees—

1. **Lesson 1–divide duties**—bees lead a structures life. There roles are well defined, they are genetically programed not to trespass into another's territory. The drones mate with the queen. The queen lays eggs and the workers bees are beasts of burden. The last lot handles every responsibility from scavenging, storing pollen and processing the nectar to feeding the queen bee. There is no conflict of roles and that is the perfect model to develop in any organization.
2. **Lesson 2–cooperation**—the spirit of cooperation is more important to bee then the spirit of competition. It takes a cluster of them to drive honey; they know they can not do it alone. That is possible only because they cooperative. Members of professionals team must bring in their own experience and expertise to a project to help create an effective produced communicating and sharing ideas is crucial.
3. **Lesson 3–be loyal**—loyalty to once community is the key to its long-term survival. If bees are strong pollen and processing nectar from a mango plant, they will not be distracted until the time they are done working on that particular plant, in a very silent way, there is a mutual understanding from the flower and the bee about what they had like to achieve from each other. The flowers trust them because over time bees have established themselves as a loyal species, a loyal employee is one who sticks to guidelines working hours and meets.
4. **Lesson 4–work hard**—ever watched a worker honeybee do her job. She is perpetually on her feet, its work ethic have even inspirited (being busy as a bee) male Drones that is male bees are lazy they do not work. That is why the worker honeybees female end up attacking them. This could happen to you some day. Loyalty is an ethic that is highly valued.
5. **Lesson 5–be punctual**—punctuality is a common ethics that most of us fall short on for bees everything depends on the sun. They start their day soon after the sun rises and they return to their hives around evening keeping time helps them develop optimum results.
6. **Lesson 6–duties comes first right next**—for bees society comes first and then comes self-later. It is a fiercely protective species. In a hive, one worker bee serves as a guard who protects intruders, who try breaking into the hive, if threatened it stings when a bee stings it dies. It sacrifices its own life to protect its community and colleague for bee, it is duty first.

Turn conflicts into challenges—is it true that a mind full of conflict is a diseases mind. When ease is disturbed, it is disease. When in conflict, our peace, ease and serenity are disturbed; conflict is the fire that ravages our well-being. Despite material prosperity, we are bound to be unhappy as long as this fire exists in us. How to put an end to it? The moment you become aware of this fact, put an end to it. Find the cause- you have a choice. Our conflicts go on increasing because we go on fulfilling topical desires only.

To train the mind to analyze rather than memories so that it may distinguish truth from error to strengthen the will, that it may have the power to practice virtue and reject vice, to stimulate ambition to disregard mediocrity and develop leadership, to maintain high academic standards and to present the current and complex problems of modern life.

Illuminating them with varied information give quality education to the young, shape minds, the core value of quality honesty, integrity, team work, excellence learning, sharing and respect for individual.

Measurement of intelligence—William Stern, the German psychologist introduced the concept of IQ. 100 (to avoid decimals) obtain IQ when the mental age (MA) is divided by the chronological age (CA) which is the actual age of the person in years and multiple.

It is inborn all round mental efficiency and also as mental energy capable of being transferred from one activity to another. It is a innate mental ability, we grow with are from infancy to maturity gradually the perceptions become accurate and keen. Child is able to concentrate on all sorts of tasks and his memory improves. Intelligence enables us to understand things to see the relationship between the things.

Many devices are used to show the results or scores of an intelligence test that is call IQ intelligent Quotient. IQ provides information about the relative brightness or dullness of the individual. It is obtained by—

$$\frac{IQ = MA}{CA \times 100}$$

If a persons, CA is 10 and his MA is 12, his IQ will be how much find out.

Levels of Intelligence

Near genius/genius are in range of 141 or over.

Levels	*IQ*
Idiot	0–25
Imbecile	26–50
Moron	51–70
Borderline	71–80
Low normal	81–90
Normal	91–110
Superior	110–120
Very superior	121–140

Mentally Retarded Level IQ Ranges

Mild	50–70
Moderate	35–50
Severe	20–35
Profound	<20

As intelligence tests employed to measure IQ generally, have an error of measurement of about 5 points. For example, 50 IQ means an IQ of 50 + 5, depending on the adaptive behavior. He causes of mental retardation is chromosomal abnormities, inborn errors of metabolism, single gene disorder, prenatal causes, e.g. infection of rubella, syphilis, birth trauma, hypoxia, intrauterine growth retardation, psychiatric disorders.

Understanding problems—(observe the students in your class if any child facing below mention problems—advised counseling and note you do not make it known to others in the class and do no discuss in the class about a child facing any problem, keep it confidential).

1. **Academic**—poor performance, clever but not scoring good marks, clever but lazy, not writing, slow in understanding, low grasping power.
2. **Hyper active**—very difficult to sit at one place, not paying attention, involved in different activities.
3. **Behavioral**—misbehaving especially with girls, fighting, disturbing the class, unnecessary arguments with minors as well as teachers, passing comments, giving indecent remarks.
4. **Indiscipline**—does not care for teachers, takes everything granted, often going out of the class, bunking class and school, does not follow rules and regulations.
5. **Adjustment**—no adequate peer interaction, feeling lonely, not speaking much, not having friends.
6. **Emotional**—involved in any relationship and friendship, feeling hurt easily, crying easily, looking disturbed, looking like lost.
7. **Suicidal tendency**—attempted committing suicide, self-harm, irregular and interrupted sleep and food intake, keeping self-aloof from others, keeping distance from close friends, looking disturbed, losing interest in life, talking to friends about committing suicide.
8. **Single parent,** step parent, adopted child-by divorce, separation by law or death of a spouse (be alert regarding these point, do not ask child directly or indirectly, you may come to know through the parents or through any other source of information).

Can you deal with emotions? Your emotional Quotient is valued as much as your intelligence Quotient, at work and in classroom. Why is it that kids who excelled in school often turn into average professional as adults? It could be because a lot of what happens in classrooms is related to intelligence quotient (IQ). IQ at work he will express his emotions a healthy way, and understand those of his colleagues, thus enhancing professional relationships and performance.

Improve your IQ; make an effort to reflect on what emotions you are feeling at various times. Once you start reflecting, you will understand them and their immediate causes better. An important part of improving your IQ is being able to spot stress triggers, and bring yourself back to feeling calm and relaxed. Be open to experiencing various emotions, even negative ones. Once you experience then without resistance you can accept them easily. Learn to come up with healthier options for dealing with negative emotions, yes, you are upset, but that does not mean you stop talking to people. Observe non verbal cues of those around you. They are an insight into what they may be feeling. Be pen to criticism, and analyze if the criticism holds any merit. Be goal oriented; chalk out short and long term plans.

Ask These Questions

1. I am able to understand what makes me angry, upset or frustrated
2. I give up easily
3. I can sense what others are feeling without any verbal cues from them
4. I generally respond to a situation based on the first option that comes to my mind
5. I have goals for my future and assess them from time to time
6. I believe getting work done is a important than talking care of feeling of others
7. When faced with difficult situation, It can motivate others
8. One cannot tolerate people who are slow in their work
9. I am able to share even my intense feelings with someone
10. People can share their opinions, thoughts and feelings with me without fear
11. I am aware of my strengths and weakness
12. I get stressed when things do not go as I had planned
13. I believe expressing my emotions makes me weak
14. I have interests and hobbies that help me improve my mood.

The career dilemma, students have no idea sometimes so as to what career they should take up in future. What are the career choices that are there, there are architecture, journalism, design, art, science and so many more? It is confusion, they have to know which field they have to pursue and what colleges they want to go. Know your talents and interest; make sure what you do not want to do, do something you are passionate about, what you enjoy. Go on adding more knowledge along the way, winners never quit, inculcate basic values in young minds at there early stage of education.

What is your career choice? With the responsibility and accountability that go hand in hand with freedom, today students have the liberty to choose a career of their choice. They are under no pressure to support the family or do something in order to earn quick bucks, experts speaks that students come up with the basic query, I want to be rich, I want success and all the luxuries in life by the age of 25 hence what is the career that would suit me. The counselor asserts that there are no good or bad career options; if a student puts his mind into something he can always make a positive. An open mind is what student need to adapt to any situation. Engineering still ranks among the favorites followed by advertising and other fields in mass media. There is considerable drop in the field of reaching and doctors; the legacy that my parents were doctors so I want to do the same is change. It is largely because the amount of efforts and time you invest while the returns are slow. The expert says that it is the attitude and the application of mind in a job that will do wonders, irrespective of its nature. It is the mind that needs to be mentored. There is increasing trend for psychology, now every organization needs a councilor. So if you put your heart and soul into a profession you can turn it to your advantage, which is when a good or bad job is not a matter of concern. Do not prepare future for your students but prepare your students for the future.

Do our schools prepare our students for future endeavors? As grooming ground for treasures of tomorrow, it's a school that facilitates the harmonious development of all power, potential and capacity. The second home provides the best ambience to nurture physical, mental and spiritual growth and conducive environment to embark on a life long learning. Importantly it teaches us the art of living. The seed of greatness is sown into impressionable young minds. The tiny tots, who enter school, emerge as creative, confident and competitive citizens of the future. School ignites the passion to progress with perfection. A school is not worth a great deal if it teaches young people how to make a living but does not teach them how to make a life. It is a place where many students of diverse cultures and attitudes coverage. One recognizes ones strength and weakness. It teaches the pre-requisites of life—the meaning of tolerance, team work and how to handle life without much trouble it teaches. By mixing and socializing in school, one learns to fit into society and live according to its norms. The ability and skill one acquires in school enables one to make a respectable and decent living. Life itself is a school and experience, individual aptitude, attitude and the indomitable will to succeed prepares one for life. Compulsive education in schools could at times be outdated and far removed from practicality tending to appear bookish or mundane. Originally the uniqueness seem to be lost in the mass manufacturing to literature, meant doing out of heaped spoonfuls of education in schools will not equip anyone to face the dynamic realities of life. In olden days Sundays and holidays used to ring bells of fun and joy for the children. All the fun has lost its meaning as students are busy doing homework and preparing for the tests. This has become the part of their daily routine. Good grades are helpful only in getting a good job, but they are a completely unfair indication of how a person will perform under the pressures of the real world. With the spate of competitive examination, children are suffering from a high level of stress. The aim of education should be to equip students for the tough battle of life. At a time when moral values are getting eroded.

How to manage the time—today money can buy almost everything, except time. Since the tine in person's life is constant and irreversible, nothing can be substituted for time. Worse it, it is wasted, it can never be regained. Today people have numerous demands on their limited time, so time needs to be effectively managed for gain.

Change is inevitable, it is the truth each one needs to understand and accept completely. Some changes are welcome, some are not, accept them compassionately. Change is the only thing that matters in life. Life without change is not possible. Change keeps things rolling. Change is exciting and something challenging but it always keeps up refreshed. We develop new perspectives to old problems. Change is necessary; else, we would all die of sheer boredom. Variety is the spice of life, we all love to have change weather in school or home.

Going against the clock? Sleep well—good sleep is not a waste of time but a guarantee for better work performance. The mismatch between the body's internal clock and our daily schedules increases discrepancy between the daily timing of the psychological clock and social clock as a result of this social jet lag people are chronically sleep deprived. Each of us has a biological clock; we can not set those clocks according to our whims like watches.

Effort is input and outcome is the output. If the effort invested is enough and in the right direction, then the outcome ought to be positive. Input parameters are more in ones control, only assessing effort without focusing on outcome would also not be right. Its only when we correlate our effort to the results achieved are we able to give feedback

Seeing with inner eye—good and bad nature in everyone's life, good hears the inner voice of consciousness and bad discourages it and focuses on materialistic ambitions for power and wealth. They lack spiritual vision. Person's inner world is weak. The eye is the lamp of the body, if your special eye is sound, your whole body will be full light

The original source of all tension is becoming. One is always trying to be something; no one is at ease with himself as he is. The being is not accepted the being is denied, and something else is taken as an ideal to become. So the basic tension is always between that which you are and that which you long to become.

If the problem can be solved why worry? If the problem cannot be solved, worrying will do you no good.

Love for mobile devices may trigger personality disorder—our obsession with latest tech like smart phone, tablet to laptop may cause not only distraction, but it can change out personality. Our brains are not developed to be constantly engaged like this.

Dear parents, listen to your children. There are many stories that need to be heard. direct, easy, fearless speech is the first sign of empowerment in your child.

Balancing the brain—your child may be left or right brainier, but its best to use both sides. The behavior of different sides of the brain was discovered in 1981 by Roger Sperry, who initiated the study of the relationship between the brain right and left hemispheres. Left half tends to function by processing information in an analytical, rational, sequential way. The right half tends to function by recognizing relationships, integrating and synthesizing and aiming at intuitive insets. The left side brain deals with the problem or situation by collecting date making analysis and using rationales thinking to reach a logical conclusion. The right side approaches the same problem by making intuitive leap to answers based on insight and perception. The left brain tends to break down information for analysis while the patient tends to put up information together to create whole picture.

The human brain begins developing early in prenatal life—3 weeks after conception-but in many ways, brain development is a lifelong project. Brain also responsible for the strong information, and the; new skills and memories throughout life. Children absorb variety of information, developing skills and honing unique learning styles he/she might display the predominance of either left or right side of the brain at different times. It is only at a mature age that abilities and style get stabilized and can therefore be identified

Right-brained child finds it tough to remember, facts and figures may not fare well. Parents should use tools that force both sides to interact. Expose your child to toys within the sense of sight. Both the sides of the brain must be used equally for fuller developing. Make a thorough analysis of the child's strengths and behavior. An equal emphasis is essential for enhancing capabilities related to academic, arts, creativity and language related to both sides of the brain.

To find out left or right ask the following questions

1. Which hand do you write normally?
2. Which hand do you use to eat?
3. Take a step, which foot did you use?
4. Which hand do you use when brushing?
5. Which hand do you sue to open cola?

If you answer left you are right brained, if you answer right you are left brained and if mixed result you could be more whole brain.

Examples of becoming a youngest MD Dr Sho Yano who is also person both MD and a PhD in (PhD molecular genetics and cell biology) he wanted to become physician as he felt that people come to the doctor when they are in highest need for help. They share their secretes as he will keep them confidential, and they share some of their private moment with him. Doctors does not have an option to walk away from patient, no matter what the disease is, they have to cure it. Yano reportedly was reading by two, writing by three, playing classic music on the piano at age of four, and composing at age of five. He then entered the Pritzker school of medicine at the University of Chicago which designed for MD and PhD. Becoming youngest person to graduate and awarded master's degree at 21, he was awarded PhD at the age of 18 years old. So you can see that there is no limit to what you can do. Sky is also not a limit and one life is not enough to learn.

No one saves us but we ourselves must walk the way. What we think we become. Discover everything for a joyful life, right around you.

Piano man in the making—Ethan Bortnick, 11, the youngest solo piano artist making headlines through his concrete tours, he started playing piano when he was three years old. He uses to listen to the music on TV and recreate it on a toy keyboard. He practice 40–50 minutes and composed new music. He feels honored as thousands of people come to see his program. He performs classical, jazz, rock, and roll written and composed by him. He invites people on the stage, ask them to play ring tone from the cell phone then compose a brand new musical piece on the sport.

Therefore, you see each one is unique and is blessed with plenty of talents and potentials just discover your own uniqueness.

Counseling in mental health—nurses or the health personnel play an important role. She provides counseling services to the patient, family members, community people regarding various issues related to stressful life events. She also provides crisis counseling for the victims. She also counsels regarding health promotion, health maintenance and good health habits and good lifestyle. She gives counseling to the individual regarding drug abuse, alcohol abuse. She conducts counseling sessions to deal with stressful situations in life, which can contribute in occurrence of mental illness. She gives guidance to the parents of mentally retarded children regarding the care, toilet training and acceptance of child in the family. Gives counseling to couples regarding genetic disorders, refers to the psychiatrics.

Qualities a counselor should have to guide students are—

1. Should have a good ear for listening
2. Non-judgmental
3. Warm
4. Approachable
5. Genuine
6. Mature
7. Confidential
8. Objective, sense of humor
9. Make time
10. Creative
11. Perceptional
12. Notice non verbal expression and pain
13. Good pacing
14. Confront appropriately
15. Calm
16. Knowledgeable
17. Supportive, pleasing eye contact
18. Has resources
19. Will refer if and when appropriate
20. Dresses appropriately
21. Shows interest in client
22. Able to speak about upsetting things
23. Can deal with panic and anxiety, stress, tension and worries
24. Has liking for people
25. Caring attitude
26. Well-maintained and records
27. Punctual for appointment and therapeutic.

Be a leader; show the way, a leader is one who knows the way, goes the way and shows the way is as per found role of a leader who shows the right direction, he influences behavior and work towards achievement of specified goal. Leadership and management go hand in hand and they are linked everything falls and rises ion leadership and every school should develop the art of leadership.

Conclusion—counseling is a method that helps the client to use a problem solving process to recognize and manage stress and that facilitates interpersonal relationships among client, family and health care team. It develops a set of goals for future behavior of an individuality is an helping relationship in that someone seeking help, someone willing to give help that is capable or trained help in a setting that permits help to be given and received. It is not giving advice, not giving information, and it is not interviewing. It is a professionally trained person who can assist a person who seeks help. To help the client to accept actual changes that is resulting from stress. To encourage and develop abilities and right attitudes, and help a client to grow, explore in the period of confusion or turmoil and establish proper identity. Counseling varies from situation to situation. Counselor assists the client to accept reality and provides information on all the aspects to problem. Here the students develop an attitude of self-acceptance and attain social harmony.

Keywords

Push your kids, but not over the edge, harassment of students by teachers: Teaching and learning continues, what does teacher do? Why teachers punish children, homework? Teacher's speck-teacher's tips-do not give up if you fall down, student and teacher's rapport is key, perseverance is the key to success, tips on how to beat stress, children should, parenting is now a big challenge-parents should, tips, parents ask yourself, examine, and see how does your child spend his evening? Focus and concentrate, be an arrow of attention- opt for hard work, effective management guru-lessons learnt for life from honey bees-turn conflicts into challenges-train the mind to analyze, understanding problems—deal with emotions, be a leader; conclusion—all about consistency and practice is success mantra. Work hard, work smart, put in extra-effort, and good planning, improve your iq; career dilemma, future endeavors, change is inevitable, balancing the brain-counseling in mental health.

CHAPTER 17

Counseling II: Stress/Suicide/Juvenile Crime—Understanding Student Psychology and Disorders

Abstract

Stress is a change in the environment that is perceived as a threat, challenge, or harm to the person's dynamic equilibrium. A limited amount of stress can be a positive motivator to take an action. Excessive or prolonged stress can cause emotional discomfort, anxiety, possible panic and illness.

Family is the building block of society—its significance cannot be ignored. Teaching of values at home as it is the child's first school of life. Counselor is often faced with dilemma dealing with ill-mannered children. The generation is not taught to be polite. You adopt it as a way of life by watching parents what they do. The child will pick up the traits automatically with a challenging job, long hours at work and unpredictable schedules, couples from double income homes have little time or patience to get their kids to do as I say and as I do. Environment can also pay a role in moulding behavior patterns. When left unconnected rudeness can manifest itself in various aspect of behavior with positive reinforcement encouraging and supportive parenting, negative behavior can be easily, older. Most parents today complain about there children being so preoccupied with there phone, ipads and laptops, that they have no time or inclination to what someone is saying. The true character of a person is reveal in interaction with people less powerful than themselves. Give your child your time; be aware of what is happening in their life. Understand their emotions, let them express their feelings and thoughts freely and respect their views. Do not be judgmental; do not compare your child with other siblings. Set an example, be a good role model, do not be abusive in front of a child. Listen like a friend, but be assertive as a parent.

Today youngsters are a stressed lot. Be it studies, peer pressure, parental demands or societal expectations. They are pressured from all sides. Home is the only place where the child can be himself. Parents need to support their children; instead, they are usually the ones who pressure them the most. Society itself is judgments in terms of what achievements means. Constantly monitor your own thoughts. Handling pressure can be turned into an enjoyable task. Handling pressure could one of the biggest lessons in life. Stress is an inherent part of human life. Right from the planning to it's conceiving. Birth marks the first pressure that a human being faces, beginning an unending series of events, each of which bring in varying amounts of stress of pressure. Stress is perceived by the mind as positive and negative and according to it comes response either adrenaline release (positive) or corticosteroid release (negative) children need to be conditioned to perceive any event as a challenge, rather than overwhelming if you kick a stone in anger, you will hurt your own foot.

By the end of adolescence the individuals intellectual structures are nearly completely developed, although learning and intellectual growth go on throughout the life span of individual.

Stress—the original source of all tension becomes something, for that no one is at ease with himself as he is. The being is not accepted, the being is denied and something else is taken as an ideal to become. It is not the situation that is causing you stress, it is your thoughts, that you can change that right here and now. The greatest weapon against stress is our ability to choose one thought over another.

Obsession—childhood trauma may lead to obsessive tendencies. How to handle it? Obsession can be dealt with if tackled with patience, thrive reinforcement is the first step. The object of obsession should be desensitize, they should gradually distance from the obsessed person. A voice keeps telling them, I am not good enough, we make them realize that this is a distressed thoughts and relate it with childhood memories. We reprocess past disturbing memories.

In the heat of the sun, grass withers, flower fades and wax melts but an oak tree does not wither. In the slightest wind needs are shaken, grass bends but the mountain do not move, however strong the it may blow. A man who has no control on his will is like a ship.

Insomnia in children—it might be the food they eat, or the mounting pressure of the studies, bed not right, its not dark enough, wrong food, they are too tired. Be around when they go to sleep, pray with them, do not let them watch TV or play computers games before bedtime. Try to keep consistent bedtime.

What drives an individual to take his own life?

What is life and what sustains it? The physical frame is sustained and supported by air, food and water. However, at psychological level it is hope, the exception of self-worth and moral strength that affirms the will to live. Hope is the springboard of all activity, a new house, a new dawn; a new year all holds hopes.

A fractured mind, like broken mirror does not reflect reality. It leads to misconceptions and creates confusion, leading one to jump to conclusion. A united mind is the key to peace, happiness and fullness.

Water from many rivers continually flows into the ocean but the ocean never over flows. Be content with what you have, rejoice in the way things are.

Never give up in life—always live on the edge. Never get complacent. Train as hard as you can; but always remain calm, it pays off. Desire to achieve motivated me. Leadership is not attained in a day's time, the qualities are innate, once you are motivated in right way you can become good leader as it is within you.

What is self-esteem? Self-esteem is rating ones worth because of external factors like physical looks, wealth, achievements, acquisition, and success. Thus, we are encouraged to achieve and acquire and to measure ourselves according, this posses a problem, since we are bound to fall, grow old, fluctuate in weight and suffer financial setbacks from time to time. You are not being nice to yourself if you define your worth by your achievements. Eventually, you turn into a less balanced human and more a pendulum; you will be insecure with every achievement, because you have based your worth on it. Your survival begins to depend on things which are not essential to survival at all. What you need to do is forgo the trouble and accept yourself, you are what you are, stop rating yourself, you are responsible for your action, but you can change them. Non-achievements will bring disadvantage. This will help you to embraced change and stabilize a sense of worth

Get rid of mental stress—wake up, brush, have breakfast, commute, attend school, eat lunch, study, go for tuitions, commute, eat dinner, sleep. This is the lifestyle of almost every youngsters today which; leads to mental stress.

Never ending deadlines, house chores etc stress builds up in our lives. While little stress can be helpful, but too much of it can have a severe effects on you.

Practice These Techniques

Breathe when you feel too stressed out; take 10–15 slow deep breaths. Inhale slowly from your nose and exhale through your mouth, which will help you to relax and give you a good frame of mind.

Be assertive and say no, respect your own boundaries, helping people is great but you have to think about yourself, always agreeing with everything will create havoc for yourself.

Avoid negative people—if you are in company of pessimistic people, you will never be able to live positively, be with constant optimistic people, which matters.

Exercise helps to reduce tension and increase blood flow to the brain.

Listen to music, which is medicine for your heart and mind, it is soothing.

Stop cribbing, accept what you can't change, things that bothering you, take it up as a challenge and face it.

Cry it out let your tears come out, it is natural way of releasing toxin from your body and easing stress.

Take a break will improve your performance and elevate stress.

Be a child they think about present without bothering about the future or the past.

Laugh, laughing is a great way to kill stress.

Spiritual activity.

Balance diet, healthy eating will help you stay focused and feel less stressed in your daily life.

Suicidal attempts among schoolchildren—the suicide of a loved one throws bereaved families into a wilderness of silent, relentless torture. There is so much stigma and lack of understanding surrounding suicide in addition to their intense grief; families have to handle the prejudice and unqualified opinion of others, who cannot even bring to comprehend what it is like to feel such despair. More than one lakh lives are lost every year in our country; in the last two decades it has increased.

Suicidal tendencies in students—What pushes students over edge?

Deadly cocktail

1. Depression - 23.7%
2. Stress - 14.51%
3. Parental pressure - 20.1%.

Counseled

1. Lonely/aloof - 27.3%
2. Quiet - 20.95%
3. Behavioral change - 19.7%
4. Anger - 4%.

To prevent suicide, teachers should

1. Consult counselor - 25.9%
2. Talk to child - 21.25%
3. Talk to parents - 20.06%
4. Inspire them - 6.26%.

Teachers believe that talking to a child and talking to counselor is one of the most effective means to control suicide.

Students idolize teachers and often look up to them for more than they look up to their parents. Teachers are in very good position to help prevent student's suicides. It is important that they use their positions responsibly. Today teacher's suicidal tendencies.

Any change in behavioral in child should be view as a sign of depression.

- It is important to recognize anger.
- Note sentences- I will not come to school tomorrow.
- I am a burden to my family.
- I am useless.

Counseling in its intense form is only a decade old in the city. The need to be equipped with the necessary emotional first aid for crisis should be given importance. Be sensitive to lonely children, isolated, aloof or quiet children.

Risk factors are family history, academic challenges, socio-cultural factors, biological factors, mental health/ psychological factors, environmental factors. There are attempted suicide, completed suicide and self-harm suicide.

Common symptoms like frequent sadness, anxiety and restlessness, mood swings, continued sleep disturbances, confusion and irritability, decreased interest in daily activities, self-injuring behavior, loss of self-confidence and self-esteem, not able to enjoy usual things, avoid close friends, finding it hard to function at school.

Prevention: Deal with social and emotional problems, identify emotional level and feelings, assess intensity of such feelings; manage, control, reduce and know the difference between feelings and actions. Develop positive attitude towards life, implement positive lifestyle, educate and counsel the parents. Teach parents methods of strengthening child development. Identify risk factors for violence among children. Explain clearly and directly, listen carefully and answer truthfully. Teach to handle problems, encourage sharing their grief, and help to let out by crying. Have a positive attitude towards your children. Parents are responsible to give honest and correct information to the school counselor. Sometimes parents hide essential information that can cause harm to the child.

Understanding Student Psychology; Developmental Disorders and Parent-Teacher Education and Importance of Counseling

Parental education and counseling is important for proper management of the following difficulties and disorders in children.

The various mental disorders in childhood are behavioral and emotional. There are specific developmental disorders of speech, habit disorders, etc. dyslexia is a developmental reading disorder. The child delay in learning to read, write and spelling are also impaired. The problem may include failure to understand simple mathematical concepts, failure to recognize signs and symptoms and mathematical tables.

Articulation errors, distorted words like wabbit for rabbit, ca for car, bu for blue, etc. restricted vocabulary, difficulty in selecting appropriate words, and immature grammatical usage, below par understanding of language failure to respond to simple instructions. Poor coordination of daily activities of life, inability to perform fine motor tasks.

In autism child there is absent of social smile, lack of eye contact, lack of awareness of others existence feelings, treats people as furniture, lack of attachment to parents and absence of separation anxiety, prefers solitary, absence of fear in presence of danger, etc.

There are children who have lack of verbal or facial response to sound or voices might be thought or deaf initially. Abstract thinking is impaired, stereotyped behavior like head banging, body spinning, hand flicking, and resistance to slightest change in the environment. Children should be given behavior therapy, help in regular routine with few changes, structured classroom teaching, maintenance of acquired learning, teach self-care skill, give speech therapy.

Attention deficit disorder—a common disorder occurs in about 3% of school age children. The onset occurs before the age of 7 years and the symptoms seen at the age of 4 years. In ADD hyperactivity where child has poor attention span with distractibility, fails to finish the things started, shift from one uncomplicated activity to another, does not seem to listen easily distracted by external stimuli and often loses things, child finds difficulty in sitting still at one place for long, moves about here and there, talks excessively, interferes in other peoples activities. Acts before thinking spontaneously. Difficult in wait for turn at work, and play.

The diagnosis can be made because of teachers' school report. Parents reports, clinical examinations, counseling and behavior modification, behavioral education.

In conduct disorders characterized by frequent lying, stealing or robbery, running away for home and school, physical violence like rape, assault, use of weapons, cruelty towards other people and animals.

In Tic disorder, (rocky mountain spotted fever, Lyme diseases takes place by Tic bite) children have eye-blinking, grimes, strugglers of shoulders, tongue protrusion, facial gestures, stamping, jumping, hitting self, squatting, twirling, coughing, barking, throat clearing, sniffing, clicking, repetition of heard phrases and words.

In habit disorder child may have thumb-sucking, nail biting, pulling out of hair, head banging, teeth grinding, masturbation pricking of nose, biting parts of the body, skin scratching, body rocking, and breath holding and swallowing of air.

Other disorders like—separation anxiety disorders, phobia anxiety disorders, social anxiety disorders, sibling rivalry, mixed disorders of conduct and emotions and reactive attachment disorders of childhood.

Give play facility, encourage to develop there skills, explain discipline, control emotions and motivational factors in early children's life, change perception by new experience, give factual knowledge, make them aware of problem, seek reliable help from advisor, identify source of problem which will help to understand, recognize and accept individual differences. Help they live in the world of reality. Give them personal worth and dignity. Give your child a chance to become a knowledge explorer for life.

Juvenile delinquency—Violence committed by a person below the age of 18 years. Offences committed like theft, sexual assault murder, burgling or inflicting injury, running away from home, fire setting. This habit may be developed due to poverty where child is deprived of want of things, lack toys and play facilities, broken family, neglected child's needs, lack of affection, lack of security, children may develop bad habits in bad company.

Juvenile crime went up by 13%. A big worry—murder, attempt to murder, robbery, molestation, sexual harassment. It is a dangerous reflection of the temperament of the city teenagers who resort to such mindless bloodshed on a provocation, which is most cases, is absolutely trivial.

Criminals in the age group of 7 to 18 years, are dealt with more humanly under the Juvenile Justice Act, 2000. Their cases are taken before a juvenile law stipulated that the maximum penalty for a minor. Even for murder. It is 3 years of reformatting.

The law in the other countries—United State depending on the gravity of the crime and if the accused is a habitual criminal, a juvenile as young as 14 can be tried as an adult in some states. America is one of the few countries where juveniles do not have bail as a right and can get life imprisonment without parole.

In United Kingdom a juvenile charged can face trial in an adult court. Canada youths aged 14 to 17 may be tried and sentenced as adults in conditions including murder, attempted murder or aggravated sexual assault.

The juvenile justice act—special unit-under the juvenile justice (care and protection of children's) amendment act, as soon as a juvenile is apprehended by police he has to be put in charge of the special juvenile police unit or designated police officer. He has to be placed before the board within 24 hours.

Claim and juvenility—if an accused, not perceived to be a juvenile, is sent to court and claims to be a minor, the court has to make an inquiry. A claim of juvenility will be recognized at any state even after final disposal of the case

Maximum punishment—a juvenile can be sent to a special home for a maximum of 3 years.

Identify protected—no visual media shall disclose any particulars that could identify the juvenile.

Over 51% of all the 804 juvenile arrest in 2011 in Mumbai were crimes in pursuit of material gain like robbery of theft and 40% in violent crimes like murder.

A cop invoke new child abuse law talking a tough stand the protection of children from sexual offense act victim friendly, gender neutral and defines a child as any person aged below 18 new anti-child abuse law.

Prevent violence for adolescents

1. If angry, irritable or hostile, talk to a friend about what is troubling you or call toll free helpline number 18602662345.
2. When there is an emotional assault within or friends suggest, revenge, wait for a day and think it over.
3. How parents can help—seek help from relatives and friends when elders other than parents, advise the child he/she is more receptive to making behavioral changes.
4. Talk to a counselor if the child becomes too violent.

Common primary prevention factors—improve in social economic condition, eliminate malnutrition, prematurely and prenatal factors improvement, education on removal of misconception, good prenatal medical care to prevent infection, trauma, obstetric complication prevention, immunization, genetic counseling. In secondary prevention-early detection and action, early remedial measures for correctable disorders, early recognition as delay in diagnosis, many cause unfortunate help child to integrate with normal individual in society and no kind of segregation or discrimination should be avoided, help them to reach their own full potential. In tertiary prevention can be applied behavioral modification, positive and negative reinforcement, parental counseling to lessen the levels of stress.

What has happen to our value system? Why don't we think before inflicting pain on another? Why has the manifestation of violence in our behavior reached such dangerous levels? Can we start the re-operation process today in our own little ways? Be the change you wish to see in the world. If one wants to transform our society, we have to begin with ourselves. At an individual level, we have to learn the art of situation management. We can do this by responding positively to negative situation. We can stop the vicious cycle of violence from continuing. Social evil do not erupt all of a sudden they germinate, grow over a period, sometimes assuming monstrous proposes. One practical way to begin the process of humanizing society is to make motivational education accessible to all. Family is the building block of society; its significance cannot be ignored. Teaching the values at home, the child's first school of life, only then can society starts developing on positive note. You need to concentrate on updating yourself, pay attention to how you convey your thought to make a positive impact. Develop language skill, basic grammar, pronunciation and effective expression and pay attention to voice modulation. In exam set goals, e.g. if your child is scoring 65%, set a target for 70%. It is achievable and succeeding at it will help boost his confidence.

Internet kids—may turn into isolated adults. The increase tried of youngsters being addicted to the internet and their dependence on the virtual world for emotional support worries that these wired youths may grow up into adults who will find it difficult to adjust to their real surrounding. They are so attached to the friend in the virtual world than these surrounding them. In long run, they may face extreme isolation and insecurity. We find many children with face book addiction syndrome, where they feel helpless, if they do not check their accounts regularly and virtually chart with their online friends. The internet addiction has robbed them of interpersonal contact in real world spending so many hours on net point at addiction. Parents fail to see that children can fall in bad company online as well. Moreover, this affects the development of a child. Most of the kids depend on social networking sites to express love, anger and grievances. Many lie to their parents abut the time they spend online, also many parents were unaware of what their children do online which is a serious issue, locking themselves in room hours. Internet addiction is how hitting children at an early are. Eighty-seven percent use social web sites to express feelings since they do not want to share personal life with the parents. Sixty-eight percent chat more when they are sad and 54% feel good as uploading a nice picture on social site, 13% kid's parents have discussion on ill effects of excessive internet use, 2% know about cyber laws. Possible implications of over dependence on virtual world may be due to rise in teen depending extreme isolation, reduced support system in real world increase impulsive behavior, loss of verbal skills both expressive and receptive.

Access to other humans has reduced for children with both parents become breadwinner and families become nuclear. This ahs lack to most children depending on the online world for emotional stability, parents need to set time limits for internet usage and spend more hours with their children.

Preventive measures—parents must bone up on tech and warn children about web misuse. Set norms for social media and internet use. Limit the time a child can spend online or on a computer. Put computer in a common room, not in child's bedroom. Keep an eye on profile and activities; discourage chatting with stranger's online and sharing personal information. Educate child not to share password.

To minimize exposure to violence curb tech overuse and develop a social life where they ca actively participate. Cut down TV hours, limit time spent playing video or online games, most of which show violence and blood shed. Monitor child's cell phone, most devices come with net and social media access, encourage habit of sitting together and having family conversation.

Debate of Juvenile Crime

Should the law be amended to allow minors who commit heinous offences to be criminally prosecuted like adult?

Different opinions and reflections and reactions

1. There assailants cannot be labeled "juveniles". If they can resort to murder, they are murderous and should not be shown any leniency. If they are sent to juvenile homes, they are bound to corrupt the inmates there.
2. They are not juveniles, they are sadists, and they derive pleasure from harassing helpless women. They prey on the vulnerability of the weak.
3. These guys are not normal human beings; they are the hyenas and the wild dogs of the city. Time has come to take responsibility of our own safety and learn to fight back.
4. Strict action needs to be taken against every eve teaser-how can they forget that they have their mom or sis in their family. If someone misbehaviors with them, how would they feel?
5. Eve-teasers should be punished so that the girls can walk freely.
6. The culprit are not human, there are people with a criminal mindset, when they go to jail they will learn new techniques for crimes rather than reforming. When these criminals know people can hit back they will lose the pleasure they derive from teasing people.
7. This is kaliyuga. Parents are unable to control the present day youth.
8. The guys need to be off the streets permanently, maximum sentence should be given.
9. Why were photos of these criminals not published? To protect their privacy or because they are minors and it would impact their future I not a reason. They did not care for the privacy of the girl or the life of a fellow human being. Their photos and crime details should be published and the government should fast track the case and put them behind bars for a very long time.
10. Our future goons, if allowed to get away, will grow up to break the law time and again.

11. It is ridiculous law that threat such people as "minors" it needs to be amended speedily.
12. Age limit to the juvenile must be fixed at 12 or so. The criminals of today are all aged 15–16 up ward and walk free as they are minors.
13. Today 16 and 17 years olds should not be considered minors. They have all the dirty knowledge this would requires, they know how to pass lewd comments, kill a person. Severe penalty like death can be a solution. The maturity levels of today are something one needs to see, rather than age a 2-year-old can operate a tablet computer, etc. The exposure is high, kids learn very fast.
14. Such criminals should be hanged for their crime of killing an innocent person. Unfortunately the Indian courts may take a lenient view as the criminal happen to be minors. The us carries out death sentence even if the accused happen to be a minor at the time of the crime. Just wait for the criminals to turn 18 and hang them.

The only way out is within—do you feel well? If you are feeling joyful, content, grateful, alert your system is faring well. If not plug the leak, face fear, banish worry and practice forgiveness then your energy system will begin to recover, as you continue to detoxify yourself, your self-awareness increases. What you focused on expands breath, medicate, cut cord, and steal joy.

If you have no right values, success could lead to downfall. Work hard, study hard, nothing comes easy, there are no short cuts, no matter how menial the job is. The important thing is to do well. Tell the truth always for lies destroys you. Test of status and power can disregard ethics in getting things done. God does give another chance for those who are willing to repeat and re-order their lives based on moral and ethical standards. Power could do much good if used for the benefit of common good.

Keywords

Family is the building block of society - youngsters are a stressed, obsession-never give up in life, what is self-esteem? get rid of mental stress- practice these techniques- suicidal attempts among school children, what pushes students over edge? juvenile crime, prevent violence- for adolescents, value system, internet kids- preventive measures - debate of juvenile crime- the only way out is within.

CHAPTER

18

Counseling III: Who Needs Counseling? Why They Need It, Let Us Follow

Abstract

Need for counseling varies according to the problem faced such as parents of a child with birth defect, mental retardation, or possible genetic disorders, and condition tends to run in family. Each needs to be recognized, screened, and tested for risk.

New media is where the future is—your place is the right at the top, start your climb now. Challenges make us grow bigger and deeper, therefore dare to challenge.

The boom of new media in the recent years has fostered the emergency of new career opportunities realizing the value of technology and wiring in. The dynamic nature of technology that is still developing, Corporate houses are increasingly realizing the value additions to their brands through digital platforms, weather it is creation of full-fledged online sales channel; everyone is jumping on, so the digital bandwagon, creation of specialized content for new media is increasingly the need of the hour. Now media requires a combination of technical skills and conceptual creativity. Creativity allows you to think of how the medium can be harnessed the technical skills which allows you to actually do it. There are constant innovations in the real of new media and those working in this field need constant updates.

Invest in the future—our children hold the key to our collective good. A growing child can aspire to be an astronaut sending rockets into space, a cricket battling legend, a government ministers, a bollywood film star or a teacher set to inspire a new generation of children. There are no secrets to success. It is the result of preparation, hard work and learning from failure.

Be positive—we live in a holistic world where all of us have a constant need to be accepted, loved and admired. Our fears, dislikes and our bursts are mostly mere manifestations of our negative thoughts. Out positive thoughts can change your attitudes. Recognize negative thoughts as they arise and bury them before they take roots. Do not let emotion take the better of you. When you surround yourself with people who are delight to be around, you will start behaving like them too.

Champions are made from something they have deep inside them—a desire, a dream, a vision. They have to have late, minute stamina, they have to be a little faster, and they have to have the skill and the will. But the will must be stronger then skill. They keep playing until they get it right.

They are not supernatural, they just fight one more second when everyone else quits, sometimes one second of effort gives you the victory, fight till the end.

Face failure, never mind failures, they are quiet natural; they are the beauty of life. What would be life without them? It would not be worth having if it were not for struggles. Why do we fail? Is it because we are unlucky? Is it because we have not worked very hard? It is for different reasons that we experience failure.

It is strengthening our consciousness that God grants us defeat. Life has meaning only in struggle. Triumph or defeat is in the hands of God, so there are suffering and defeats in life and no one can avoid them. Happiness is contact of being alive with the moment. Even a problem can make us alive, problems like an ocean waves, will keep coming, one has to live despite the waves. We are restless with ourselves because the self we know is empty, shallow, void and unhappy. Face this fact. We try to be busy because we want to avoid this void. Once you learn to manage your life wisely, you will receive peace. It is important how you frame your experience that matters, learn from the mistakes of others, and that is your challenge. Nature has its own way of punishing and rewarding. Forgiveness is like taking a psychological bath that keeps you fresh. Success depends on one's ability to make the most of every opportunity.

Willpower—Are there ways to build up willpower?

Willpower is a component of self-control. Self-control is setting goal, willpower is taking you wherever you want to go. Some people are born with greater will power then the other but all can develop conscious effort. Willpower is somewhat like muscle. It can get fatigued if overused.

If you want to have perfect willpower, you should have perfect mastering over your body control over the body influences the mind and the mind determines the will.

Put your career top of the gear, a happy employee is a productive employee. Happy people achieve better results. To open to new thoughts and ideas exercise your creative instinct.

To succeed in the career you opt for planning it right is crucial. Taking the right step in the right direction, after a careful analysis of your strength, weakness and ambitions becomes vital.

How will you deal with a grumpy coworker?

1. Do not be defensive—respect them and make sure they respect you too. They are whom they claim to be, so be content with that. Some people have issues with life which are portrayed to others by their temperament, and the mere you understand that, the better you will deal with it.
2. Get the right boundaries—cerate healthy boundaries whenever you have to cross paths with them. You do not want to be unfair to them just because of the way they are. At time, they just might say things without giving it a second thought. Do not take everything personally.
3. Do not be gossipmonger. At times, your coworker might get to know that you have been gossiping about them behind their back. That might be the reason why they are bitter to you.
4. Keep a check on yourself; make sure you do not react while approaching the person. Keep calm and make sure not to upset a person.
5. Ask if you can be of help. Try taking it out with person and do not pester them, just let them be.

Dealing with this requires conscious efforts towards living in the present open to accept the reality, attend to priorities in life, rather than being perfect, take 'do it yourself' approach. When faced with set backs, does not retreat into a shell, sharing problems with others lightens our load and creates possibilities for new solutions to emerge. Favorable and unfavorable events come and go in our life with the regularity of our seasons. Life is a journey of experience, create positive beliefs around our setbacks, we feel more empowered and experience greater equanimity.

Show more understanding—we sometimes become righteous about our own beliefs and our own goodness and look down upon others. Who is good and who is bad? No matter how bad we think someone is. We believe God provides for everyone, even to an unbeliever too he provides food. There are people who cheat, who deceive others, and who slander others. There are people who hurt others, even kill others; it takes all type to make the world. Yet God provides life to each of them. No one is without fault we should be kind and amicable towards all, each one of us is different, so show understanding towards all.

In matter of communication, a lot of what we give and receive depends on our vibes, body language, facial expression, speech, tone, speech speed and eye contact. Though it comes from your upbringing and your past experiences, it can be changed by conscious effort, with regular practice. Give positive vibes and believe in it, you can decide how to respond to the request. In arrogance, vibes relax, soften your facial muscles and work on the eye and direction of the nose. Tell yourself I am clam and cool flash a warm smile.

Orientation/motivation—dealing with ups and downs in life is a matter of having the right attitude and right thinking in life. Living up to your expectations in life is a biggest challenge. Sometimes we feel insecure when things are not in our control, then we are under fear, insecurity runs higher. At that moment overcomes that fear and insecurity is the most important to live healthy and peaceful life. At that, moment faith in God helps overcoming fears and insecurity. When after doing everything there are moments you feel things are not in your control then leave that completely on God, allow Him to take control of your life, and do not give up, continue your work, it will make you stronger to face the challenges of life. Sometime when you look back, you will laugh at yourself things for which you lost sleep are of not importance. Be true to yourself and your feelings and actions are clean at heart. Let head and heart work independently, head thinks and heart feels and we need both.

Many things you cannot change. It determines the types of family into which you are born your race and the type of body in which you are born. You might wish to change the shape of your nose or increase your height by a few centimeter where changes seems impossible, you always have the choice within your power.

In today's scenario, we require persons who care, who are sensitive enough to provide succour to the wounded, the hurt, the ailing, together for humanity.

Love is the best fuel—life is a journey and the human being is the vehicle and best fuel is love. To make the journey smooth add love or else you make frequent breakdown, love is available in plenty and it does not get depleted. Every human being is the source of this fuel. Love appeals to true being or soul. It constantly seeks peace, stillness and stability. The universe is waiting and longing to fill us with love but it needs only to take a small step first, believe in the power of giving first. The language of power—what is power? Power is exercised in the way we relate to one another—knowledge is power.

'Me' represents our self-centered instincts to take things personally. We are quick to judge our successes and failures, compliments and critique and take them personally. Every untoward incident raises the question of why is it happening to me? Actually, nothing is happening uniquely to us, every one has their share of challenges; it is how we react to them makes the real difference.

Why are we not born equal? All are created equal. You are the architect of your own destiny. The good and bad affect us, and remains with us until we balance them out.

The harmony between our dreams and reality that is which keeps us going day after day. The pinnacle of success is to recognize yesterday is hard work and a great zeal to strive for the bright new future. No path leading to success is easy without painstaking. If we pursue our goal with energy determination, persistence and definitive desire noting can stop us in our achieving our goal in serving through excellence.

Change is unpredictable, the unexpected creates stress. It is human nature to resent new and shifting demands. It is also a human nature to bloom and thrive rather than shield away from the more you accept change as a constant the more prepared you are. Resistance generates stress and inflexibility. You develop new strengths when you focus and work to welcome change. Your confidence in your skills grows, that means that you invest your effort and energies where your power lies.

Be positive—developing positive self is important way to reduce stress in your hectic and monotonous work life. Try avoiding negative talk, negative energy as this could cause you additional stress. Maintain a positive frame of mind, do not let others around affect you with their comments about yourself, try imbibing all the good points and forget all the other remarks as they come.

There are also simple things to keep in mind at home for a clear mind. Clean home gives positive energy, breath in fresh air, brings in positive flow of energy, listen inspirational music which brings smile on face.

Being desk bound can erode physical mental health, long hours daily desk bound is bad for health and can affect your mental well being.

A positive state of mind is not merely good for you, it benefits everyone with whom you come into contact, literally changing the world. Think positively and master life fully with confidence and faith and life will become more secure. Keeps your thoughts positive because they become your words, keep your words positive they become your behavior, keep your behavior positive, it becomes your habits, keep your habits positive, they become your values, keep your values positive, they become your destiny.

Power begets power; the most dangerous are those who are powerful and corrupt as well as intelligent. Intellect is a double-edged sword it can cut either way. It can even justify a wrongdoing and untruth appears like truth. Find like minded people who have respect for truth and ethical values.

True realization of the actual nature of this material world, its perishable, transitory and illusionary aspects best dawns on a person in suffering.

Motivation—do not be a bird in a cage when you can fly high free yourself of all block, created by none but you.

Being honest—helps keep unnecessary stress away. There are no internal stress, there are no internal conflicts for the individual. People who are dishonest often live in the fear of being caught, rights fear keeps them on hooks of anxiety, which affects there mental health negatively. Honesty makes you feel confident and fearless, feels positively in all aspects of his life. Honesty is the main ingredient of recovery and without it no progression. Self-development makes us accountable which in turn enables us to set an agenda for our lives.

Imprisoned by our own thoughts—the state of your life is nothing more than a reflection of your state of mind. We do feel a sense of internal imprisonment, the feeling of restriction of a lack of space and freedom, all comes because of our thoughts the mind, which creates this thought from childhood to this day. It generates worries, anxiety, fears, jealousies, greed, anger, these thoughts and emotions imprison us and often leave us powerless, throw useless thoughts away leading ourselves to break free of imprisonment.

Shaking Off the Past

A moral with message–A wise man was telling a joke to a group of people. All those present were highly amused and appreciated the humor. After a while; the man narrated the same joke again, for the second time, then again at third time. When he tried to repeat for the 4th time, a member of the group burst out, why are you repeating a joke so many times? I am not amused, it is irritating, then the wise man responded, if repeating a joke ceases to amuse after a few times, then how do we carry on with repeated remembrance of past painful stories. Moving on life with often an unsavory incident requires one to view it as just one among many events and incidents in ones life. Most people try and strive to up root the weeds of unpleasant memories. The past should never be empowered to affect the present. Every event is the outcome of a host of complex factors; most of them are not predictable or controllable wake up to dream about the wonderful future that beckons us.

Some easy lessons for you–do not dwell in the past or worry about the future. Do not have expectations. Indulging in thoughts of making vast sums of money, receiving abundant love, getting recognition and honor for a lifetime of work, etc. if you think you will be happy when some of these dreams come true, you are chasing a mirage. Be happy as you are now and enjoy peace. Cultivate patience, do not give importance to a change of place, you are not lying on a bed of nails here. Therefore, experience joy wherever you are now. Do not get attached to a place. Do not long for an extraordinary experience. This disturbs the mind. Do not crave for gadgets like ask what the need for these things is for me. Do not think of illogical obstacles and difficulties. Moreover, evaluate every task in terms of spiritual values. Do not get addicted to work, enjoy work, the increase desire to excel itself leads to frustration, raising the bar constantly gives rise to tension which robs you of peace of mind and contentment.

Keep your thoughts positive because your thoughts become your words, keep your words positive because your words become your behavior, keep your behavior positive because your behavior becomes your habits, habits positive becomes values and values positive becomes your destiny.

Spiritual—will you change the way you will look at people you cannot get along with and look at them with the eyes of love? Spend time with a sick housebound person. Do others have to lose in order for me to win? Reconciliation is even more important than offering worship and sacrifice. There are dimension to life vital to fulfillment and happiness that are not satisfied by financial security or material wealth, what are those in your life? Do to others, as you would have them do to you. Today there are many subtle forms of 'possession', which are more dangerous than external positions, consumerism, selfishness, ignorance and better the thou attitude-we need to ask the lord to exorcise these demons from our lives. We expect to be forgiven by others when we do them harm after we have said sorry, and sometimes, if they forgiver us, we get upset with them even more. We need to apply the same verdicts to ourselves when others ask for forgiveness from us. Better let people hear not what we say but what we do. If the Lord were to visit the temple of your life, what would he find there?

How can one balance one's spiritual quest with living in the world?

Maintain works as medicines. Doctors send patients to meditate to overcome physical sickness and psychosomatic diseases. Some come because of psychological, emotional reasons. Therefore, you can use meditation as medicine therapy, psychological exercise to increase memory and brain actively. You can use it as a microscope or a telescope, to see your; life clearly, or to understand the world. You can meditate to develop spiritual qualities like joy, peacefulness, compassion, while meditating we might achieve peace and equanimity.

Peel off your longings one by one like an onion. Nourish the heart—the happier we feel, the happier ourselves and the more harmoniously we function, nourishing our emotional health can be challenging in a modern world in hectic lives. You can choose your attitude of each day, love yourself, mix with positive people, see the funny side of life, think big, think positive and stay happy always.

All of us have faced situations in life where we feel terribly helpless completely at wits end. No amount of thinking or talking seems to bring any solution. We feel boxed in from all sides, without any obvious escape or relief from the situation. This can be very stressful and can play havoc with our minds and bodies.

The feeling of helplessness comes when we are faced with circumstances where we can neither run away, nor fight. We find ourselves extreme stressed and strained such situations are extremely frustrating and the pressure that build up within start damaging our body and mind. We arte surrounded all directions, only path open are up or down. God has to show the right way. For example, investors are stuck with investments which they can nether redeem nor hold on, employees on job they can not leave nor continue with it, teenager cannot leave with or without their parents, one who suffers with chronic disease where treatment is as bad if not worse then the diseases itself. Do I value my personal freedom more or do I want harmony, what price am I willing to pay for my choice?

A man, who realizes the potential of his mind by means of introspection and contemplation, does not lack self-confidence. He has control over his mind and he is able to realize its full potential. Be a lamp for yourself. Be your own refuge, all things must pass, strive on diligently, do not give up, with the realization of ones own potential and self-confidence in ones ability, one can build a better world. It is confidence in our bodies, minds and spirits that allows us to keep looking for new adventures, new directions to grow in and new lessons to learn which is what life is all about. Your chances of success in any undertaking can always be measured by your belief in yourself.

We are peaceful, if we are happy, we can smile and blossom like a flower and everyone in our family our entire society will benefit from our peace. Power love will replace the love of power. Then will our world know the blessings of peace.

Every individual has to work to survive but earning a living becomes the exclusive focus and priority of ones life, problems can arise when we live to earn rather than earn to live. Check for unchecked greed which can bring unnecessary problems, the inner wealth is our mind, our consciousness; mind is like a wish fulfilling jewel. The most important kind of knowledge is one that makes a kind person a decent person, a person worthy of respect.

Every chance you get, you have to give it your all. You can not give anything less than your best because there are a thousand people standing in line just behind you.

Breath is life; breathing is such an accepted reality of life that we do not give much significance to it until we are deprived of it. Ask an asthma patient the agony and distress of walking up in the middle of the night, with a feeling of suffocation, shirt ineffectual cough, labored breathing and wheezing.

To live a meaningful life we need to balance our thoughts words and actions. Both we think too much or too little in either cases our actions are gravely affected for those who think too much action is wanting and for they thoughtless life turns out to be a causality. Although harmonizing thoughts and actions is desirable for acting wisely unless thoughts, words and actions are in vision you cannot strike a balance. Mind is the seat of our thoughts words and actions, cultivation of mind is of paramount important where is the mind when the body is here, the kind of auto reminder help to keep body and mind together.

Attachment—most of us suffer in life because of confusion between love and attachment. Love is a positive quality but attachment is getting tied to person—it causes bond age as well as disappointment and ultimately makes us sad. We all have strong attachment to money, name, and fame—most time it creates bondage and bind us in the process, so you suffer the more you are attached, the more you expect something out of that relationship when there expectations are not met it causes misery. Too much attachment or identification to possession is harmful. Blind attachment to children, you will fail to take objective stand while dealing, attachment leads to clinging.

Organize and execute around priorities—how to do the best, some work urgent some are not so urgent, goal setting, time tracking to be aware to know where your time actually gets spent, self-monitoring make adjustment. Concentrate on doing on task at a time, throw unneeded things way, know when to stop a task, ensure time is set aside to accomplished high priority task.

Travel light on your journey in life. Your desires and expectations are heavy baggage, which slow you down thwart your progress, let them go. We live in a wonderful world that is full of beauty, charm and adventures. We can have if only we seek them with our eyes open.

Get started, winners never wait for tomorrow, because tomorrow never comes. So never, leave until tomorrow that you can do today. Success is reserved only for those who dare to venture into the unknown territories. Winners always do in time and that is why they never lose. Smile today, tomorrow could be worse.

It has been scientifically proved that laughter releases that feel good endorphins in the brain that helps reduce stress. It keeps mind fresh and happy despite the work stress. The right kind of humor allows people to be more open to different ideas and helps them think out of the box. It keeps employees and colleague happy, creative and productive. Laughter is the best medicine.

How do you manage your anger?

Anger management—anger is an abnormal state that varies in intensity from mild irritation to intense fury and rage. Like other emotions, it is accompanied by both external and biological changes. When one gets angry; the heart rate and BP goes up, and the levels of adrenaline and non-adrenaline too changes. Anger is a natural adaptive response feeling and behavior, which allows us to fight and defend ourselves when we are attacked. Expressing ones anger is an assertive, non-aggressive manner is the healthiest easy to express anger. It can b supported. One holds the anger and stops thinking about it a focuses on something positive. The aim is to convert it into a more constructive behavior. Unexpected anger can create other problems. The goal of managing anger is to reduce both the emotional feelings and the physiological arousal reaction. Some people are really hot headed, than others; they get angry more easily and more intensely than the average person does. There are also those who do not show their anger in loud spectacular ways, but arte chronically irritable and grumpy. Some have low tolerance to frustration.

Angry people cannot take things in stride; they are infuriated being corrected for minor mistakes. It is not okay to vent your anger out, letting it rip with anger actually escalates anger and aggression and does nothing to help you resolve the situation. It is best to find out what it is that triggers ones anger and managing with relaxation tools. Changing the way in thinks when one is anger, once thinking can get much exaggerated and overly dramatic and makes you feel worse. Angry people tend to jump to conclusion, which can be inaccurate. Do not say the first thing that comes into your head but slow down and think carefully about what you want to say at the same time listen carefully to what the other person is saying and get your times before answering. It is natural to get defensive when you are criticized. Do not fight back but listen to underlying message. Maintaining your cool can keep the situation from becoming disastrous one. So do not allow it to get out, control, and turn it destruction. First empty your mind, only then you can make room for wisdom to come into attain wisdom, we must purify the mind by making it free of all impure thought.

Life is beautiful inside and outside—how should you live? You do not have you possess something to enjoy it. Look at the butterfly, its lifespan is so short, yet it enjoys itself thoroughly. It goes from flower to flower, the most beautiful creation of nature. It sucks nectar the sweetest thing in nature. It chooses best honey, speak only sweetly, think and live beautifully and enjoy life. Sweetness is the secret of a beautiful life. This should become our nature. Life than becomes easy, weightless, otherwise the mind is full of problems and we are always ready to fight. Let not external world disturb your mind. Everything divine is within you and around you. To find happiness you have to find divine in everyone.

Keywords

New media is where the future is, Invest in the future- be positive- face failure, willpower—show more understanding, in matter of communication, orientation/motivation—love is the best fuel—the harmony between our dreams and reality, change is unpredictable, a positive state of mind, motivation—the feeling of helplessness, realizes the potential, to live a meaningful life, organize and execute around priorities- get started, winners never wait for tomorrow, because tomorrow never comes, life is beautiful inside and outside.

CHAPTER 19

Stress Adaptation in Nursing

Abstract

Stress management can help clients control illness, improve self-esteem, gain control and enjoy life more fully. Stress involves clients education, finances, job, family, habits and positive and negative coping of a person. Identify stress, make more time for yourself, and say no to responsibilities that you do not have time for.

Stress a word taken from the term "distress" is a part of life. Everyone feels stress at one time or the other. Stress is balanced for obesity, drugs, alcohol use, divorce, child abuse and feeling "stressed" out: in common and talking stress breaks to do physical exercise is recommended in many work settings. With stress such a part of everyday life, it is easy to see that an additional health problem, such as an illness as injury can increase the physical and psychological effects of stress.

Stress is a disease of the 21st century. Every one seems to be in stress from a child to a retiree. The only time you are free from stress is when you are inactive, activity brings mental agitation. What disturbs the mind, bad boss, nagging spouse, which cause mental turbulence caused by unusual and unfulfilled desires, when desires fulfilled you want more desires leads to delusion, all these creates lot of misery and tension. Persons who are obsessed for money never enjoy the money, he has all the best he can bye money but he has so stressed that he does not enjoy any of it. More desires unsettles the mind, the mind lingers in past and future, unable to concentrate in the present. This leads to failure. The way out is manages your desires with intellect. From stress go to destress.

Basic Concept of Stress and Adaptation

1. Stress
2. Stressors
3. Adaptation
4. Homeostasis

1. **Stress**—is a condition in which the human systems respond to changes in its normal balanced state. Stress results from a change in the environment that is perceived as a challenge, a threat, or a danger. The major source of stress in an society arise from interpersonal relationship and performance demands rather them from actual physical threat. Stress affects the whole person in the entire human dimension (physical, emotional, intellectual, social, and spiritual) positively and negatively.
2. **Stressors**—is anything that is perceived as challenging, threatening or demanding. Stressors may be internal, e.g. an illness, a hormonal change or fear or external, e.g. loud noise, or cold temperature.
3. **Adaptation**—when a person is in a threatening situation, immediately response occur. These response which are often involuntary, are called coping responses. The change that takes place as a result of the response to a situation to a stressor is adaptation.
4. **Homeostasis**—the environment includes the external environment which strained our bodies, and the informal includes mechanisms that regulate body and the surrounding body cells. To maintain health, the body's internal environment must remain in a balanced state. Various physiologic mechanisms within the body respond to internal changes to maintain relative constancy in the internal environment which is called homeostasis. Maintenance of physiologic and psychological homeostasis—the effects of physiologic and psychological are interrelated, are the mechanism that are consciously or unconsciously used to maintain its response to stress. The autonomic nervous system and the endocrine system primarily control its mechanisms.

Local adaptation syndrome (LAS)—is a localized response of the body to the stress. It involves any specific body part such as a tissue or organ instead of the whole body. The stress precipitating the LAS may be traumatic or pathologic.

1. **Autoimmune disorders**—hypothyroidism, rheumatoid arthritis, ulcerative colitis, psoriasis, myasthenia gravis.
2. **Cardiovascular disorders**—hyperextension, coronary arterial diseases.
3. **Respiratory disorders**—asthma.
4. **Gastrointestinal disorder**—esophagus reflux, constipation, diarrhea, ulcerative colitis.

Threat—(increased blood pressure, peripheral vasoconstriction, increased metabolism, water retention, dilated pupils)

↓

Fight or response—(state of resistance, coping and defense mechanism)

↓

Recovery (stage of exhaustion, vasodilatation, increased pulse and blood pressure, panic, crisis, rest and recovery or death)

Physiologic indicators of stress—backache, constipation or diarrhea, dilated pupils, dry mouth, headache, increased urination, increased pulse, BP and respiration, nausea, sleep disturbances, stiff neck, increased perspiration, chest pain, weight gain or weight loss, decreased sex drive.

Types of Anxiety

1. **Anxiety** is a vague, uneasy feeling of discomfort or dread from an often unknown source.
2. **Mild anxiety** increases alertness and perceptual fields e.g. vision and hearing and motivates learning and growth.
3. **Moderate anxiety** is manifested by a tremors, increased muscle tension, butter flies in the stomach and slight increased in vitals.
4. **Severe anxiety** is characterized by extreme fear of a danger that is not real by emotional distress that interferes with everyday life and by avoiding situations that cause anxiety. It is manifested by difficulty verbally communicating increased motor activity, a fearful and facial expression, headache, nausea, dizziness, tachycardia, and hyperventilation.

Panic causes the person to lose control and experience dread and terror. Panic is manifested by difficulty communicating verbally, agitation, trembling, poor motor control, sensory changes, sweating, tachycardia, hyperventilation, dyspnea, palpitation, chocking sensation, sensation of chest pain or pressure. The person is unable to learn, concentrate, experiences a feeling of doom. This level of anxiety can lead to exhaustion and death.

Coping mechanism—anxiety often is managed without conscious thought by coping mechanism, which are behavior used to decreased stress and anxiety. Typical coping behavior include crying, laughing, sleeping, physical activity, exercise, smoking, drinking, lack of eye contact, withdrawal, limiting relationships, withdrawal behavior involves physical withdrawal from the threat or emotional reactions such as becoming apathy or feeling guilty and isolated. Compromise behavior is usually constructive, often involving the substitutions of goals or negotiation to partially fulfill ones needs.

Stress and basic human needs—stress is common to all people. Adaptations to stress require energy and motivate behavior. Stress in a healthy person may promote health, e.g. the fear of developing lung cancer may motivate a person to stop smoking. Stress in health also facilitate normal growth an development, provide the stimulus for learning constructive adaptive behavior, provide problem solving abilities, encourage social relationships and help develop spiritual social relationships and help develop spiritual strength. The effects of stress on a sick or injured person are in contrast, usually negative, stress can cause illness and illness causes stress.

Effects of Stress on Basic Human Needs

1. **Physiologic**—change in appetite, activity or sleep; change in elimination pattern, increased pulse, respiration and blood pressure.
2. **Safety/security**—feels threatened or nervous, uses ineffective coping.
3. **Love/belonging**—is withdrawn and isolated, blames others for own faults, demonstrated aggressive behavior, becomes overly dependent on others.
4. **Self-esteem**—becomes a workaholic, exhibits attention seeking behavior.
5. **Self-actualization**—refuses to accept reality, centers own problems, demonstrates lack of control.

Caring for a family member at home for long period can also cause prolonged stress which response in chronic fatigue, sleep problem, and increased incidence of stress related illness.

Crisis—is a disturbance caused by a precipitating event, such as a perceived loss, a threat of less or a challenge that is perceived as a threat to self.

1. **Maturational crisis** occur during developmental a teenager moves into adulthood.
2. **Situational crisis** occurs earn a life event disturbs a persons psychological equilibrium such as loss of a job or death of a loved family members.

Commonly Occurring Defense Mechanism

1. **Compensation**—a person attempts to overcome a perceived weakness by emphasizing a more desirable trait or over achieving, e.g. a student who has difficulty with a academic may excel in sports.
2. **Denial**—a person refuses to acknowledge the presence of a condition that is disturbing, e.g. despite fining a lump in the breast a women does not seek medication help.
3. **Displacement**—a person displaces an emotional reaction from object or person to another object and person, e.g. an employee who is angrier kicks chair.
4. **Introjections**—a person incorporate qualities or values of another person into his own ego structure. This mechanism is important in the formation of conscience during childhood, e.g. preschool sister not to talk to strangers, experiencing his parents values to his younger sister.
5. **Projection**—a persons thoughts to impulses are attributed to someone else, e.g. a person who a person who ends any sexual feelings for a coworker accuses him of sexual harassment.
6. **Rationalization**—a person tries to give a logical or socially acceptable explanation for questionable behavior, e.g. a patient who forgot to keep an appointment says, if patient did not have to wait three

months to get an appointment they would not have forgotten.

7. **Reaction formation**—a person develop conscious attitude and behavior patterns that are opposite to what she likes rally to do, e.g. a married woman is attached to her husbands best friend but constantly rude to him.
8. **Regression**—a person returns to an earlier method of behaving, e.g. children often regress to soiling diapers or damaging or bottle where they are ill.
9. **Repression**—a person voluntarily excludes an anxiety providing event from conscious awareness, e.g. a father may not remember shouting his crying baby.
10. **Sublimation**—a person substitutes a socially accepted goal for one whose normal channel of expression is blocked, e.g. an individual who is aggressive toward others may become a star football player.
11. **Undoing**—an act or communication used to negate a previous act or communication, e.g. a husband who was physically abusive to his wife may bring her an expensive present the next day.

Physiologic stressors—it has both a specific effect and general effect. The specific effect is an alternation of normal body structure and function. The general effect is the stress response. Primary physiologic stressors include chemical agents (drugs, poisons) physical agents (heat, cold, and trauma) infectious agents (viruses, bacteria) nutritional imbalances, hypoxia, genetic and immune disorders.

1. For example, accidents cause stress for the victim, the person who caused the accident and the families of both.
2. Stressful or traumatic experiences of family members and friends.
3. Horrors of history such as zazo con, camps, the dropping of the atomic bombs on Hiroshima, terrorist attacks.
4. Fear of aggression or mutilation, such as muggings, rape, murder and terrarium.
5. Events of history that are brought into our homes through television such as wars, earthquakes, violence in schools.
6. Rapid changes in our world and the way we live, including changes in economic and political structures and rapid advances in technology.

Psychological stressors—include both real and perceived threats. The person's responses are continuous and include individualized coping mechanisms for responding to anxiety, guilt, fear, frustration and loss. The mechanisms serve to maintain psychological homeostasis.

Personal factors—ones physiologic reserve and genetic inheritance are important in maintaining homeostasis and adapting to stressors. The ability to adapt is decreased in the very young, the very old and these with alter physical to mental health, which do not have the necessary physiologic reserve to cope with physical changes such as dehydration or fluid excess. Adequate nutrition and sleep are necessary for enzyme for immune responses; wound healing and energy production and restoration, malnutrition, dietary deficits or excess sleep deprivation all impair ones ability to adapt to stress. Social factors and life events are also implicated in adaptation to stress, with people who have strong support systems and relationship better able to adapt to stress and remain healthy.

Stress and adaptation in nursing-activities identified as highly stressful include the following—

1. Assuming response for which are not prepared
2. Working with unqualified personnel
3. Working in an event in which supervisors and administrations are not supportive
4. Caring for a patient during a cardiac arrest or for a patient who is dying
5. Experiencing conflict with peer.

Student nurses also experience stress and may have difficulty adapting to the request and response of caring for others. Factors causing stress in student nurses include the following—

a. Fear of failing the classroom and clinical lab components of each course
b. Fear of failing the licensure examination after graduation
c. The demands of the nursing program
d. Fear of injuring patient
e. The need to meet financial and family response
f. The complex of behavior is called burnout. Burnout can be compared with the exhaustion stage of anxiety and is characterized by a wide range of behavior. Some nurses try to become "superior nurses" expecting perfection in themselves and others. Some withdraw and do only minimal work; still others resort to drugs or alcohol. Many nurses who cannot handle the stress have the profession.

The following diagnosis in nursing may be made when stress is the cause of the problem

i. Anxiety related to conflict about values and goals in life threats to self-concept, threat of death, threat of or change in health status, threat or change in environment or role situation maturational crisis or unmet needs.
ii. Stress overload related to single parenthood, inadequate economic resources and chronic illness.
iii. Moral distress related to cultural conflicts, and of life decisions, conflicting information about ethical decision making or prescribed decisions.
iv. Defensive coping related to loss of job and economic security.
v. Ineffective denial related to continued smoking behavior.

vi. Decisional conflict related to placement of parent in nursing home.
vii. Disabled family coping related to lack of knowledge about home care of child on ventilators.

Teaching healthy activities of daily living—a person's normal lifestyle greatly influences his/her perceptions of and reactions to stressors.

1. **Stress reduction through exercise**—regular exercise helps maintain physical and emotional health. The benefits of exercise include an improved musculoskeletal system, more effective cardiovascular. Exercise improves the general sense of well-being, relieves tension, and enables coping with day-to-day stressors. The type of exercise depends on what the person enjoys, e.g. walking, jogging, bicycling, swimming or sports such as golf or tennis.
2. **Rest and sleep**—help the body maintain homeostasis and restore energy levels. Adequate rest can provide "insulation" against stress, but stress may interfere with ones ability to sleep.
3. **Nutrition**—plays an active role in marinating the body's homeostatic mechanisms in increased resistance to stress. Reduce intake of salt, refined sugar, animal fats and cholesterol. Eat more fruit, vegetables and whole grains. Eat less red meat and more fish and poultry.
4. **Encouraging use of support system**—it provides emotional support that helps a person identify and verbalize feelings associated with stress.
5. **Encouraging use of stress management techniques**—stress created emotional distress that often produces physical sign and symptoms. One person may have tension headaches, another becomes irritated, another clenches his fists. Many people take legal or illegal drugs drink or smoke to excuses or eat compulsively. These behavior can be modified by adoptive mechanisms.
6. **Relaxation**—techniques are useful in many situations such as child-birth, pain, anxiety, sleeplessness, illness of anger, and other uses are being discovered. Relaxation promotes a body reaction opposite to that of the fight or flight response. Relaxation can be taught to individuals or groups. Various techniques like rhythmic breathing alter state of consciousness. The positive technique of this relation is it improves quality of sleep, reduces fatigue, improves ability to tolerate pain, increased confidence and improves coping mechanism.
7. **Meditation**—in quiet surrounding, comfortable position, mental image on which to focus with closed eyes, relaxes the major muscles.
8. **Anticipatory guidance**—focus on psychologically preparing a person for an unfamiliar or painful event.
9. **Using cutaneous stimulation,** message, application of heat or cold or both intermittently, acupressure, hypnosis, administrating angelic.
10. **Therapeutic effects of laughter** which increases levels of epinephrine the stress hormone; activates the immune system; elevates the threshold for pain and can minimize the pain sensation; promotes spiritual and psychological coping; helps one to face difficult or unpleasant procedure, deepens respirations, and causes muscles to contract.

Keywords

Stress is a disease of the 21st century. Basic concept of stress and adaptation- types of anxiety, local adaptation syndrome-coping mechanism-stress and basic human needs, crisis-psychological stressors-personal factors- common occurring defense mechanism- stress and adaptation in nursing- teaching healthy activities of daily living.

CHAPTER 20

Importance of Time

Abstract

Time is an important factor in human being. Life moves around the clock. From morning to evening time controls human being. Every second is vital and purposeful. People who management time make a great success in life.

The value of time is very important factor in student's life. Once passed from life it will never come back. Time is the strongest force of nature that surely rules both nature and humankind. Time has 3 important impressions of its nature, past, present and future. It ruled past that's why we call it history, it rules present and we call it development and it's always prepared to rule future, so we call it vision. Every person has different ways. To relate and value time. We often forget to understand its importance, some power packed words defining time and its control on our lives is perfect to remind us constantly, what a beautiful gift, and life has given us, in the form of time. Some great quotations or words of expressions are just the reflections of our state of mind, how we feel and relate with life. To make us understand the value and power of time. Remember, lost time is never found again.

Time is precious—time is free but it's priceless. You can't own it but you can use it. You can't keep it, but you can spend it. Once you're lost it you can never get it back. Time is more valuable than money. You can get more money, but you cannot get more time. We are all obsessed with doing that we have no time and no imagination left for being. As a result, men are valued not for what they are but for what they do or what they have for their usefulness. Time is really the only capital that any human being has an the only thin he can't afford to lose.

Time explains its value—time is most precious thing in our lives—although we can't keep control on it, but if we manage it in a constructive way, it often serves us with the most memorable and successful experiences of our lives. To realize that value of one year, as a student who failed a grade. To realize the value of one month, ask a mother who gave birth to a premature baby. To realize the value of one week, ask the editor of a weekly newspaper. To realize the value of one hour, ask the lovers who are waiting to meet. To realize the value of one minute, ask a person who missed the train. To realize the value of one second ask a person who just avoided an accident. A minute now is better than a minute later. Therefore, treasure every moment. Yesterday is history, tomorrow is mystery, and today is a gift, that's why it's called the present.

Time is a great reminder—clock is a machine of great moral value to man, allaying his concern for the future by reminding him what a lot of time remains to him. For a long time it had seemed to me that life was about to begin-real life. But there was always some obstacle in the way, something to be gotten through first, some unfinished business, time still to be served, or debt to be paid. Then life would begin. At last it dawned on me that those obstacles were my life. We all have our time machine, some take us back, they're called memories, some take us forward, and they're called dreams. You may delay, but time will not.

Time guides our plan—there is a time for departure even when there is no certain place to go. Time is too slow for those who wait, too swift for those who fear, too long for those who give too short for these who rejoice, but for those who love, time is eternity. We make plans, but time guides them. No matter how much we try or put efforts, to materialize the according to out will, our plans, actions, words, everything is guided by time. It is the most important factor that rules our lives. To achieve great things, two things are needed, a plan, and not quiet enough time.

Make the most of each day—a bank credits your account each morning; it carries over no balance to tomorrow. Every evening you lose the balance you failed to use during the day what would you do? Draw out every cent, of course, each of us has such a bank, its name is time. Every morning, it credits you with 86,400 seconds. Every night it writes off what you have failed to invest, if you fail to use the days deposits, the loss is your. There is no going back. Invest it so as to improve get from it the utmost in health, happiness, and success. The clock is running, make the most of life today, a minute now is better than a minute later.

Time is a fantastic healer—every moment brings different situations in life—sometimes success, sometimes failures, sometimes happiness and sometimes sadness. But with every situation it brings along a positive source that teaches us to react to the situation we come across in life. I think and think for moment and years. Ninety-nine times the conclusion is false, the hundredth time I am right/our greatest glory is in never falling, but in rising every time we fall. Until you value yourself, you won't value your time. Until you value your time, you will not do anything.

Time brings revolution—time flies over us, but leaves its shadow behind. History has witnessed many big revolutions in the world, as whenever the time has influenced; to change things around it. No revolution can be values as much, as the time covered in bringing the revolution into practice. It is the time that rules and provokes the situation to develop such as impact as to define it as revolution in the world. So the strongest of all warriors as these two—time and patience. More than any other time in history, mankind faces crossroads. One path leads to despair and utter hopelessness. The other, to total extinction, let us pray to have the wisdom to choose correctly. So, just remember how to use your time, tomorrow you might bring a revolution.

Have patience with time—the only reason for time is so that everything doesn't happen at once. Life takes its own sweet time to offer us what we want, but we have to be very patient with time because there is no control on time. Things will happen when time allows, so all you have to so is let things happen on its own, according time. A sense of value of time—that is of the best way to divided one's time into ones various activities is an essential preliminary to efficient work, it is the only methods of avoiding hurry. If something anticipated arrives too late it finds us numb, wrung out from waiting, and we feel nothing at all. The best things arrive on time; it is a mistake to look too far ahead. Only one link in the chain of destiny can be handled at a time.

Time is a great teacher—there is no great teacher then time, it teaches us every day, every moment, about value of life and our living. Our experiences are time's certificate to us, for passing life's tests and learning the value of time. Reality is a question of perspective, the future you get from the past, the more concrete and plausible it seems, but as you approach the present, it inevitable seems incredible. Time is the only comforter for the loss of a mother. The finest workers in stone are not copper or steel tools, but the gentle touches of air and water working at their leisure with a liberal allowance of time.

Time management is important—yesterday is a cancelled check, tomorrow is a promissory note, today is the only cash you have- so spend it wisely. Time management is very important to lead an organize life, both personally and professionally. It also helps us in achieving our goals without wasting time. Good time management knowledge is our ability to recognize and solve many problems in life. With good time management skills you are in control of your time and your life, of your stress and energy levels. You make progress at work. You are able to maintain balance between you work. Personal and family lives. You have enough flexibility to respond to surprises or new opportunities, remember lost time is never found again.

Keywords

Time is precious—time explains its value time is a great reminder, time guides our plan—make the most of each day, time is a fantastic healer—time brings revolution—have patience with time—time is a great teacher- time management is important.

CHAPTER 21

Information Technology and Nursing Education

Abstract

Experienced nurses have to prepare students for leadership role. Tomorrow belongs to the nurses who prepare for it today. Nurse contributes to the professional development of peers, colleagues and others. Her decision and action on behalf of patient are determined in an ethical manner. To be most effective, a health care system must do more than provide equipment, supplies, facilities and manpower. It must guarantee universal access to an assured standard of care. It must use health resources effectively and efficiently—balancing efforts to promote health with capacity to cure disease.

Fill the gap between theory and practice. Theory without practice is of no use. The clinical facilities for nursing practice are quite insufficient. This affects the performances as well as the job satisfaction. Boosting the opportunity for higher education for nurses faulting needs to be made available.

INTRODUCTION

Impact of social changes and challenges—The change in nursing is quite slow and not keeping the pace with other countries. We have to take the momentum, and have to expand our horizons. Comprehensively, the nursing profession is expanded quantitatively and qualitatively, as there are more nurses who are willing to take responsibilities, and are willing to be active in the process of change.

Public is now far more informed and desires to be involved as educated partners in health care. Today patients are demanding improved access to services, many of which are expensive.

Nursing practice should focus on area of specialization and seize the opportunity for creating innovative new roles within the current system. Nurses, as strong and vital professionals, should have advanced skills and creativity. As they provide individualized, holistic care, integrate research into practice.

Nurses must be valued for their unique contribution to the system and recognized for their ability to adopt and adapt to change not only in patient population but also in health care delivery. Technology and telecommunication advances allow for instant local, global linkages with cost-effective information transfer and intelligent gathering. Nurses have to access to these technologies and equipped with necessary knowledge and skills to use these devices for optimum impact. Accountability, collaboration, competence, effectiveness, efficiency, affordability, public participation, self-regulation, transparency and universality to improve and reinforce professional regulation are the principles of nursing.

The nursing profession struggling to keep pace with rapid development in medical science and technology. Nowadays people are better informed, they have more health awareness and there are more demands for improved health care facilities. In order to meet the increased health needs, nurses will have to be better informed and highly skilled. They need creation of specialized nursing posts in different areas to give quality nursing care where they can increase their confidence and result in better services. However, we have to admit that there are many positive changes in nursing profession.

Shaping the future of India—innovation essentially means good, new ideas that lead to socioeconomic benefits for a society as a whole. Internet and web too of the greatest innovation of out time. Great innovation such as batteries, birth control pills, penicillin, DNA, forensics, computers, the MRI scan to name them a few, all originated and flown into the market. Not just rocket science for progress, India must motivate scientists.

Stress among Nursing Professionals

Stress amongst care professionals is currently a major concern in health policy. A certain level of stress is normal to help one complete the work and deal with the challenges of life.

There are 2 types of stress:

1. Good stress
2. Bad stress/distress. Too much of it causes the body to expand in unpleasant ways and adversely affects efficiency of nurses in providing care to the patients.

Stress is a subjective phenomenon based on individual perceptions, producing positive and negative perspectives. There responsibilities of a nurse are manifold and so are the reasons of stress.

Overburden, underemployment and underpayment of nurses along with their own personal reasons leads to stress.

Sources of Stress

1. **Workload**—they have to look after the patient 24 hours round the clock in different shifts. It requires devotion to patient and their relatives. Requires understanding, carry out doctor's instructions on medication, food, clinical tests. They have non nursing activities like answering phone calls, supervising stock of dugs; housekeeping may be due to inadequacy of nursing staffs. High work load takes a toll on their mental as well as physical health and results in out burn.
2. **Shift work**—particularly night shifts, can have effect on personal and social life. Prolonged shift work has health risk, long-term night shift working has even been suggested to increase the risk of cardiovascular disease.
3. **Lack of reward**—not paid to the proportion to their qualifications.
4. **Workplace stress**—requires high level of skill, team working in variety of situation. They have to listen to their seniors, adjust to the colleagues, administrative department, coping with patient and relative, deal aggression and violence, emotional needs of families of poor, death and dying at times takes a toll on the mental health of nurses.
5. **Hectic time schedule** not only at work but at home, time pressure leads to various symptoms of stress.
6. **Leadership style**—poor control, poor group cohesions, lack of adequate supervisions support, lack of clarity about task, personal clashes, harassment.
7. **Professional conflict**—detect mistakes and corrective action, inter professional conflict, disagreements.
8. **Traveling**—far from hospital stay requires long hours of traveling.
9. **Social status**.
10. **Family stress**.
11. Pleasing one and all.
12. **Acting strong**—due to controlling of emotions at times person is stressed out.
13. **Increased expectations and desires**—any person today expects good food, best children, beauty, great body, perfect homemaker. Tensions is aroused due to kids not studying, husband very busy has no time to listen to wife.
14. **Unnecessary worries**—some being emotional and sensitive take more tension.

All of this above leads to a burnout which has to be controlled, otherwise it gives following symptoms:

Psychological Symptoms

1. Get irritable, short temper, increased level of arousal, and mental acuity
2. Get out of control and forgetful
3. Anxiety, apprehension
4. Fatigue and lethargy
5. Unnecessary augmentation
6. Inability to concentrate
7. Feeling gloomy, boredom
8. Depression
9. Negative attitude
10. Poor decision making skills
11. Burn out that is emotional exhaustion, deceased personal accomplishment.

Physiological Symptoms

1. Increased arterial BP and clinical hypertension
2. Headache, neck aches, back ache, joint ache
3. Cardiovascular problem—increase in palpitation and coronary heat disease
4. Restlessness
5. Tremors
6. Stress induced diabetes
7. Indigestion and ulcers
8. Atherosclerosis
9. Insomnia or poor sleep
10. Weakened immune system
11. Constipation or diarrhea
12. Weight gain or loss of appetite
13. Gastric disorders
14. Menstrual problem
15. Asthma attack.

Are Nurses for Export?

Developing counties now treat nurses as an export commodity that can earn vital over seas currency. India reported to have trained 8 million nurses compared with just 3.8 million 10 years ago.

Proper selection of nursing students needs to be considered other wise resources are wasted.

School libraries, sitting accommodation, independent study and wide reading.

Right kind of teaching staff; capable of inspiring students to approach learning in right spirit to be strengthened. Examination conducted in language familiar to the learner. Student must have high ability in English so as to compete in national and international job market.

The aim has to be providing a platform to all health care professionals and advanced high tech environment. Promote higher values and effects in all segment of nursing profession that is health-care education administration and research. It will definitely get excellence in areas to meet the expectation of people.

Do what you can with what you have, where you are?

Our trouble is not ignorance, but inaction. The action of today becomes the destiny of tomorrow.

Chronic stress causes depression—do not let stress get you down. When knocked down in life or work, talk about your feelings. Be aware of difficult thought and sensations in your body, observe it and let it go. Take an emotional audit with help of friend's counselor. Yoga and Vipasana helps calm the mind. Disconnection from friends, family and peer could cause depression. Once in while talk about your feelings with someone you trust. Any thought about death should be examined for its intensity. Basic neurochemical equation, daily stress could over time cause a build up of harmful chemicals in the body, which in turn could lead to chronic anxiety which can end up in depression.

Heaven and God are not high above us far away, they are deep within us. Heaven is not a distant country where there are trees and houses and other objects. It is a plane of consciousness within us seekers of eternal truth will realize their eternal heaven within their aspiring hearts. At every moment we are creating heaven or hell within us. When we cherish a divine thought an expanding fulfilling thought we create heaven in us. When we cherish ugly, obscure, impure thoughts we are just entering into our inner hell.

Forensic digital is the science of gathering digital evidence to solve crime and for investigation purpose. It is the discovery, analysis and reconstruction of evidence extracted from computer system, computer networks, computer media and computer press pherals that allow investigations to solve the crime. In today's cyber age, digital formats like e-mail, charts, documents, digital pictures, pen drive, mobile phone, etc. the imaging recovery and analysis of such information is called digital forensic. Technology is ever evolving and with new devices soft ware and encryptions being introduced everyday, specialized software and hardware produced at rapid pace.

WWW—World Wide Web—the internet which is network that connects other networks. WWW refers to the complex links among web pages or websites across through URLS that is called universal resources locators.

- com—for commercial sites.
- ors—for organizations.
- edu—is for educational institutions.
- gov—for government sites.

Consumers can access websites from computer in their homes, public libraries, school, cyber cafes, etc. computer access is rapidly increasing they have become standard instructional tools and computer assisted instruction allows students to proceed at their own speed, provides immediate feed backs and allows dissemination of information to remote areas. It enhances academic information age. It is a challenge to keep abreast of the information on any subject; on our abilities and updates. WWW and internet both classic and the most current information can be found on any topic. Computer revolution in the form of computer assisted instruction.

Most new educational buildings are wired to accommodate technology wireless technology, plug in laptop for network or internet access. Projectors liquid crystal display panel that allow computer screen to be displayed to the entire classroom.

Distance learning education where students at satellite sites participate in educational experience. There are many models for distance learning. The computer is ideal for conducting certain types of learning educations like survey can be completed on line.

It is data warehousing—the accumulation of large amounts of data that are stored over time. Computer in nursing administration are well suited to assist the nurse in these functions. Computer-based patient record CPRs or EMRs (electronic medical records) permit electronic patient data retrieval by care givers. DSM—diagnostic an statistical manual of mental disorders. MMDS the nursing minimum data set.

MIS—a management information system.

HIS—a hospital information system.

Nursing on internet—for the health care profession the internet provides a variable treasure chest of information, but mixed in with the nuggets of gold is a vast amount of irrelevant or useless data. Many hours can be wasted searching for the precise information you require, so the trick is to learn to navigate the internet. Various articles and information like published facts about diseases, data on drugs, news services, educational materials, etc. if you know where to find it information then almost any topic is available. Valuable site with an extensive complication of links to online nursing sites and journals, colleges and universities, higher degree nursing education program, an index of the nursing health development agency, health professionals, national electronic library for health national health services.

Gluing chips for faster computers—companies 3-M and IBM announced that they plan to jointly develop the first adhesive that can be used to package semiconductors into densely stacked semiconductors onto densely stacked silicon "towers" they are aiming to create a new class of materials which will make it possible to build for the first time, commercial micro-processors composed of layers of up to 100 separate chips.

Such stack in would allow for dramatically higher levels of integration for information technology and consumer electronics applications.

Processor could be tightly packed with memory and new working, e.g. into a "brick" of silicon that would create a computer chip 1,000 times faster than today's fastest micro processor enabling more powerful smart phones, tablets, computers and gaming devices.

For example, new types of adhesives are needed that can efficiently conduct heat through a densely packed stack of chips and away from heat sensitive components such as logic circuits.

Today's chips, including those containing 3-dimensional transistors, are in fact 2D chips that are still very flat structures.

Our scientist are aiming to develop materials that will allow us to package tremendous amounts of compact power into a new form factor a silicon 'skyscraper'.

Information therapy as important as prescribing medications—how convenient it would be to get patient specific information. Information therapy is an important a part of treatment as prescribing medications. Today patients and doctors are waking up to information therapy across the globe. It gives right information to the right person at right time to make better health decision. The information can be directly from the treating doctor form any form of technology or books and pamphlets is educating to the patient

For web users, even blink is a long wait, wait a second, no which is too long. When you wait a few seconds for a computer to respond to a click on a website or a tap on a key bund subconsciously, you do not like to wait. Google and other tech companies are on to make fast go faster. The reason is that data hungry smart phones and tablets are creating frustrating digital traffic jams, as people download maps, videos clips of spots highlights, new updates or recommended. The competition to be quicker is fierce. People will visit a website less often if it is slower than a close competitor. A person will be more patient waiting for a video clip to load than for a search results. Four out of 5 online users will click away if a video stalls while loading.

Search for truth is called research. Computer is in research—this 21st century is known as computer age. When it was invented, it was so big that for installation it required whole room. Today it is become small and smaller and the size is reduced yet the strength, power, capacity is increased tremendously.

Application of Computer in Medical Field

- Application of computer in community and public health managed.
- Application of computer in the hospital and nursing homes, clinic.
- Helps to increase efficiency and better care services to the patients by computerized methods of diagnosis. Saves time our non-clinical work like record keeping, billing, accounts, etc.

Internet—we can access libraries in the world, converse with professionals in a fraction of a second. It is possible because of high-speed internet connection and is joined to WWW dynamic adding new sights every day, thousands of computed added daily to these net works and with that comes thousands of opportunity at our door steps for information exchange.

Advantages of net—electronic mail or e-mail, remote file access, information retrieval, medical information, patient care. There is innumerable source of information available on the WWW.

Services like Yahoo, Google, Jocose, Magellan provide easy interfaces to the web and its contents. These search engines gather information about sites located on web by sending out 'spider' or 'crawlers' that query each site they encounter on the content they find. This information then classified and entered into a database.

In built computer technology plays a great role in imparting latest knowledge available in medically field due to which world is shrinking faster in communication.

Due to changing techniques in the care of patients and their treatments the nursing activities are also changing very fast.

Way Forward

India seems to be on the brink of massive digital environment, since digital technology is now affordable; the systems are expected to penetrate the smaller towns and rural areas. Life science research and drug discovery and development.

A new dimension of electrocardiography (color touch screen long rhythm recording up to 5 minutes) health care is a growing sector in India and there is lot of potential for growth and demand for medical electronics, consumers are demanding cost effective monitoring and health management products that can use at their homes, e.g. blood glucose meter, blood pressure machines, heart rate monitor, digital thermometer and pulse Oximeter. This has fueled the need for portable and miniature health care solution.

Era of ultra high performance—the evolution of technology—the digitalization of the Cath laboratory images was one major leap in terms of technology the latest trend in the Cath laboratory is the introduction of newer interventional tools that enable quick and confident diagnosis and assist in making the therapy precise with better clinical outcomes. A revolutionary technology that improves the visibility of the deployed Stent in the coronary arterial disease during interventions with Stents becoming increasingly thinner is very challenge.

Network—computers connected to the network are used to transfer the documents at a very low cost as compared to telegrams, mailing, etc. it makes all programs, data and peripheral devices available to authorized user or nodes on the network. It helps in reduction of costs being spent on nodes attached to the severe computers as all necessary hardware components are attached to server instead of nodes. Nodes can access required information from severe. The data supplied for one computer to other computer is of high reliability. You can make more than one copies of all files, on one or more computer, so that if any file gets damaged due to hardware failure or due to some reason, the other copies could be used.

Types

Local area network, wide area network, metropolitan area network, peer to peer network.

Internet—it is world wide network of networks. It is the common way whereby dissimilar computers with various operating systems are able to communicate with each other, using a set of protocols connection to the internet open the door to a vast world of information and communication that resides in files on host computers, including computers that follow the TCP/IP protocol.

Finding a file on the internet is similar to finding the location of an individual in a city, for this the user needs the files add. Add are the key for receiving and sending information on the internet.

Internet requires a dial-up telephone line, an internet access account with an internet service provider, communication software, a modem, a computer with either a serial port for an external modem or an expansion slot for an internet modem.

All computers within an given network are connected to each other with help of a cables.

Internet services—electronic mail (e-mail) provides a on to one and one to many communication mechanism to send and receive textual messages. An email program is used to compose and send the mails to the recipient add. This mail then goes to the local mail server, which forwards the mail further to other mail servers until it reaches the recipients mail box. For example, e-mail program are Yahoo mail, G-mail, Rediffmail, etc.

Attachment with e-mail—over a period of time, people felt the need for sending various other types of information like images, software, spreadsheets, etc. along with the textual message through e-mail. MIME was designed to enable different types of information to be attached with e-mail message.

File transfer protocol—allows web user on one host to access and copy files to and from another host over the internet. The file transfers protocol service is used to exchange relatively large information. This information can be any file format. The commands allow the user to list directions, change directions, get file, etc.

WWW—is a highly graphical collection of multimedia documents which use simple hypertext-based navigation.

Web servers—is to host a variety of information. There are many web servers on the internet. This number of web serves increasing every day. An organization can have one more web servers. This web serves usually hosts information pertaining to a company and its product. The information store on web server is in HTML format.

Internet relay chat—is the services on the internet that allows people to communicate over the internet in real time. IRC allows one to one meeting as well as many too many real time charts. IRC services hosts different channels.

Patient management computers are used for planning and controlling purpose by health professionals. Computer equipments are used to maintain pulse rate, BP, vitals. The loads to convert and fast diagnosis hospital used for clinical application which helps the doctors in his professional practice, administration, financial accounting, billing, inventory, control, both are related to each other. A powerful computer can do several tasks. You can net worked large hospital so that information about each patient would be available throughout the hospital. In hospital there should be separate software which are related to medical treatment. It is an integral and essential part of hospital tasks. If it gets any damage then whole work will be stopped.

Password restrictions are necessary for every software; so that unauthorized persons cannot use the system. Patients records, operation list, bill generation, lab test, treatment card, IPP, reports becomes easy manage routine documents, follow up patients internet medicine, ECG, analysis, etc. are done by computer program.

Computer is a machine that handles data. Data can be raw facts or figure facts that are gathered and entered in to the commuter. It stores, retrieves, sends and analysis and synthesizes that data to produce information.

When two blades of scissors act together the scissors does its job. You cannot cut a piece of cloth with just one blade of the scissors. Therefore, fate and free will both necessary for action.

What is the role of technology in development?

Technologies rapidly transforming the way we live work and spend our leisure time. It has extended to spread of knowledge immensely and made its sharing easy, promising almost near universal empowerment of the people, provided we make innovative uses of these new technologies. As a result, winds of change now sweeping across much of the world are paving way for an open world. Today's advances made by man are fundamentally transforming the organized human life—dawn of a new era—the information age.

Today events talking place in any corner of the planet becomes known the world over almost in no time. Change talking place rapidly and on such a vast scale that globalization is become reality.

Information age—today IT media has assumed significance, which they never had before, media has become a mechanism to govern our lives. It has become a way of life itself. Many of the societies are already changing from being advanced industrial societies to "information societies" their network and other enhanced forms are major force. US engaged more than 46% of the workforce, which earns over 55% of the labor income.

Companies are in process of building a vast web of electronic network, information super highways of fiber optics and computers. This network will deliver an abundance of goods and services at your office and homes. Video images, phone calls, enormous amount of data on various required fields by a user or customer. They promise to change the way people think, work, live and use their leisure time.

In the last few years break through in satellite and high speed computing have given leading users an over whelming economic advantages over those who have not kept pace.

The "pull" for the "lasts" and the "best", there have been revolutionary changes in IT, which both provides challenges and opportunities. IT increase the efficiency in terms of speed, spread.

Amazing times acquired new meanings. What used to be distant is no more that far away, what used to be local has become global.

Telephone, TV, commuters are getting inter-twined with each other holding out promises of a world in which innovation and human dynamism would be main driving force.

In the seamless world of tomorrow mind would matter. The wireless web further facilitates connectivity. The quality of images and the speed of downloads will improve significantly multimedia mobile message will be the next rival of e-mail.

Today, there is greater access to mass media and internet in India and other developing countries.

India gas developed a niche for itself in the area of computer software development and as a service provider. IT is a powerful force.

IT means a whole range of technologies like computers, telephone, TV, internet, etc. that facilitates human communications in terms of quality, quantity and speed. Technology is the means by which goods are manufactured in an economy. Due to that goods are made cheaper, faster and more efficient. A balance is required therefore so that both technology and living condition of the people improve.

Digital divide—Digital divide between the developed and developing countries. It changes informative environment in the new millennium.

Other features of the present day situation which is microprocessors and the "chips" have not only made possible in physical terms, but economic terms, its technologies and computer is transforming business operations, broadcasting, telephone system and human interaction. We are on threshold of having a high resolution two-way video and personal computers tied to net works, so that sitting at home or office, one can receive information from and to anywhere in the world and engage in a two-way video conversation across the world.

Rural Innovative

1. For example, public call offices (PCOs)—In around 600,000 villages provided PCOs in India have been provided phone connections.
2. For example, automatic milk collection system (AMCS, Amul).
   - Major information centers are connected through internet. Each such center is computer connected by a phone line; the villagers come to the center get information of nominal rates of their product in different markets in order to negotiate better deals. The benefited of Gyandoot reach over half a million people in more than 600 villages.
   - VKS—village knowledge center set up Chennai, for empowerment of tribal and rural women who are barely literate. The process helps the women in creating a relevant database ad sharing with other

leading to awareness, behavior change and action to improve their economic well being an life itself
- SEWA—Self-employed Woman's Association in Gujarat using a satellite communication to train women both urban and rural.

21st century—our communication-wireless, our dresses topless, our phone cordless, our cooking fireless, our youth jobless, out food fatless, out labor effortless, our conduct worthless, our relation loveless, our attitude careless, our feeling heartless, our politics shameless, our education valueless, our arguments baseless, our job thankless, our salary very less.

Wake up its time for your vertical growth, so gear up, life is too short, sheer determination, dedication, desire and optimism we can achieve goals.

Nursing has under gone rapid change in its move towards full professedly. It has rapidly expanded nursing on the brink of advancement of full professional states. When mind and body are together at the same time, at the same place, there begins the awareness of the self.

Internet vs human mind—over-usage of the internet and search engines made us over dependent, because we do not think, today people do not apply logic and reasoning simply because they do not have the time. Now who has the time to open an encyclopedia or read books, we simply go to the net, our brains now rely on the internet for memory, we just refer to it. The search engine is acting like a remote control of our brain, which gives you desired information and it saves time. But we need to brainstorm as well. Try to read books and find answers, efforts should be made to inculcate creative thinking. Go to library, put on your thinking cap and search for answers, read books and you will see the difference. Spending hours in face book, surfing, and music download, emails send, etc.

Mobile users hear imaginary ring—people hear imaginary ringing of their mobiles in pocket due to misinterpretation of sensory signals in the brain, ringing in the head because people are often anticipating a call, they interpret unrelated stimuli, so they feel that their mobile is ringing when it is not. The imaginary phone vibrations experienced.

Present scenario-digital divide—In the US, 56% of adults access online services, whereas in the developing countries, 2–3% or even less have access to the internet. The whole of Africa has just 14 million phone lines that is less than what they have in New York or Tokyo.

A third of the world's people have never made a phone call in their lifetime. One-fifth of the world population lives on just a dollar a day. Such inequalities themselves as rural areas become more isolated and fall further behind. That is where IT globalization and poor stand. In addition, why we need AV aids in India and in nursing schools to teach the people in simple manner. After the introduction and our present stand of education, let us turn to the educational aids. Its importance in health care practice; and why are they relevant today.

Telephone, TV, computers are getting inter-twined with each other holding out promises of a world in which innovation and human dynamism would be main driving force.

Today, there is greater access to mass media and internet in India and other developing countries.

India has developed a niche for itself in the area of computer software development and as a service provider. IT is a powerful force. An internet user has access to a wide variety of services, electronic mail, file transfer, vast information resources, interest group membership, interactive collaboration, multimedia displays, real-time broadcasting, shopping opportunities, and much more.

The internet consists primarily of a variety of access protocols. Many of these protocols feature programs that allow users to search for and retrieve material made available by the protocol. Almost every protocol type available on the internet is accessible on the Web.

IT means a whole range of technologies like computers, telephone, TV, internet, etc. that facilitates human communications in terms of quality, quantity and speed. Technology is the means by which goods are manufacture in an economy. Due to that, goods are made cheaper, faster and more efficient. A balance is required therefore so that both technology and living condition of the people improve.

Shrinking the globe, binding India together, conquering distances, breaking boundaries, bringing people closer together, making cultures interact, opening up opportunities, giving wings to dreams, making the world one market, driving the economy, pushing the wheels of the progress, talking the country to the sky.

The gold of human dignity that lies hidden in every living soul waiting to shine through, only we will give it a chance.

Education is something, which makes an individual self-reliant and selfless. By education can bring out all round drawing out and the best in the child and man and body, man and spirit. Education is the manifestation and divine per formation already existing in man. Education means enabling the mind to find out the ultimate truth making truth its own and giving expression to it.

Disadvantage the Indian nurses have against their foreign counterpart is the lack of quest for knowledge, research and excellence. They are satisfied with status quo; foreign nurses are deeply interested in updating their knowledge and their careers.

Computer influence in every sphere of human activity brings many changes in education, health care, scientific research, social science, law, music and painting. Uses of computer save the time, economizes energy and help the nurses to provide quality nursing care. You just keep getting better every day. Your best is always the next one. Learning and assimilation what is learnt what remains and becomes basis for future growth and enters into personality. Reconstruct ideas and enlarge interest. Human being has the upper hand on technology. The media can now illustrate, discuss, analyze, form concepts. How attention is gained, how meaning is transferred, how opinions and attitudes are created or modified, exchange of ideas, knowledge.

Animation in Medical Education

- Shifting of a passive teaching to active learning
- Transmission of biomedical knowledge to development of professional skills and attitude
- Verbal media to audiovisual media
- Computer technologies to the extent of making self-learning modules
- Computer based 3D interactive program
- Computer with multimedia capacity added with sound animation and 3D videos
- Digital drawings are made on a computer screen, the computers calculates the details like movement, color, light, etc.

Advantages—in the movie field, TV educational programs, medical education, for health-care professional, for health care education of patients regarding various procedures, mass media health education program, medical website design and development.

Medical animation in macromedia flash format—flash media is available in most of the computer systems, the file size is very small, it opens quickly, it can be made interactive. They are available to demonstrate human anatomy, physiology, principles of various investigations and interpretations of results. It has unique value of grasping, it makes unseen visible, making the abstract thoughts concrete, very close to the real appearance like the blood cells flowing in the circulation. It has the motion features is shown step, by step. It attracts audience giving rich expression; the whole thing can be reproduced at any time any place, its attractiveness arousing attention and perception makes the learning so effective. All topic cannot be taught with this, it is time consuming and tedious. However, the medical animations are having its wide use in medication profession.

Microteaching is a system of controlled practice that makes it possible to concentrate on specific teaching behavior and to practice teaching under controlled condition. It's characteristic that is reduce the complexity of the teaching situations and reduces the teaching skill and size of the topic.

Its basic principles—enforcement, practice and drill, continuity, microscopic supervision.

- Its steps are defining a specific skill, demonstration of skill, micro lesson plans, teaching a small group, fed backs, re-planning, re-teaching and re-evaluation.
- Its five "R" are recording, reviewing, responding, refining, and re-doing.
- It is a time consuming.
- Man gets cultured and civilized through education.
- Education as the power by which man is able to control his environment and fulfill his possibilities.
- An all round drawing out of the best in child and man body mind and spirit.
- Aim of education is complete living harmonious, mental, social, moral, physical, and character, culture, individual, self-knowledge developed.
- The method should suit and adapt to the capacity of the students. Review knowledge, do rehearsal, use handouts, pictures after demonstration, pace the steps.

Audiovisual materials are devices by which helps to clarify, establish and correlate accurate concepts and facilitates understanding of spoken words. It stimulates and reinforces learning an makes learning dynamic and concrete, effective, interesting, inspirational and vivid experience, helps better assimilation, retains, recall thinking and reasoning, can get direct experience of situation, enables to look listen and learn, quicken the phase of learning, active participation.

It must be easy to see and understand, simple and different, easy to handle and transport, emphasis key points, accurate, encourages viewers to eye your ideas, attract the vision of others, neat, clear, easy to bold, attractive colors and clear.

Arrange AV aids in sequence and have them within easy reach, present right moment in proper sequence.

Supportive supervision plan is the first ever large-scale initiative for nurses in India—what is supportive supervision? It is "monitoring" guidance and feedback on professional and educational matters to promote enhance patients care. It deals with technical issues, e.g. skill and knowledge.

It is aimed at motivating and supporting health-care providers to improve their work performances. Supportive supervision is a process that promotes quality at all levels of the health system, focusing on the identification and resolution of problems, and helping to optimize the allocation of resources. It is a key element in continuing education; it focuses on problem solving on the spot with the joint participation of the supervised and supervisor. It combines three elements like impact, support, and motivation. It worked with health staff to establish goals, monitors performance, identities and correct problems there by improve the quality of health service. Identify and address weakness on the spot, thus preventing poor practices from becoming routine. Supervisory visits are also an opportunity to recognize good practices and help health workers to maintain their high level of performance.

Keywords

Sources of stress difficulties faced by nurses—the nursing profession, shaping the future of india, stress among nursing professionals. There are 2 types of stress, psychological symptoms-physiological symptoms-chronic stress, forensic digital, distance learning, nursing on internet- gluing chips for faster computers-web users, application of commuter in medical field, way forward-internet services-rural innovative-21st century-our communication-internet vs human mind- mobile users hear imaginary ring- present scenario-digital divide, animation in medical education, medical animation in macromedia flash format.

CHAPTER 22

Nursing Care Plan

Abstract

During nursing education, a nurse has to take up different clients for case study and prepare the nursing care plan for the client. Here some case study examples are given just for her to get an idea how to do nursing care plan to meet patient's needs.

A nurse has to do nursing care plan in clinical areas as well as in the community field, so she has to change her shift to the area of work and keep the principles of nursing care plan the same with all the steps. Few examples of it will help her understand this concept better.

Characteristics of a Profession—Case Study

1. Intellectual—carrying with high responsibility
2. Learned in nature based on body of knowledge
3. Practical rather than theoretical
4. Technique can be taught through educational discipline
5. Well organized internally
6. Motivated by altruism/selfless service.

Case Study—Meeting Urinary Needs

Client's reports of loss of urine while standing, urgency, dribbling with coughing and frequency every hour.

- Thirty years' old female well-nourished.
- T 98.4° F, P 76, R 18, B/P 116/78.
- Skin warm, dry and intact, pale pink in color.
- Abdomen soft, non-tender, non distention, bowel sounds audible in all four quadram.
- No bladder distention.
- Voiding frequencies in small amounts—clear yellow urine
- Pedal pulses palpable, no pedal edema.
- **Nursing diagnosis**—stress incontinence, weak pelvic muscle.
- **Planning**—expected outcome—states kegal exercise have helped increase ability to retain urine. Reports less dribbling with coughing and no loss of urine with standing.
- **Implementation**—nursing intervention—describes Kegel exercise to the client and encourages client to practice exercise 10 times/day.
- **Evaluation**—client states that with exercise she is experiencing no loss of urine while standing and only dribbling slightly while coughing.
- Why evaluate?
  To measure attainment of client goals re-direct plan of nursing care.
- How to evaluate?
  Develop evaluative criteria collect data and compare it to standards. Summarizing findings and make interpretations. Identify courses of actions. Take corrective action based on findings.
- Types of evaluation—determination of the clients findings of goal achievement, review the nursing process. Participation in quality assurance program.
- What do they want to know—what interventions are most successful in achieving desired outcome.

Case Study—Meeting Respiratory Needs

Client complains of a 'cold' fatigue, loss of appetite, increased shortness of breath, fever.

- Obtain sputum for culture and sensitivity
- Oxygen at 2 L/minute via nasal cannula
- Postural drainage and chest percussion
- complains of 'shortness of breath'
- T 100.6° F, B/P 120/76, P 98, R 26 and labored
- Breath sounds audible bilaterally- decreased in left base Rhonchi present, left greater than right
- Arterial blood gas results—Paoz 56 mm Hg, $PaCO_2$ 52 mm Hg.

Nursing diagnosis—ineffective airway clearance, excessive secretions and ineffective coughing.

Planning-expected outcome—demonstrates improved airway clearance. AFB effective coughing techniques and breath sounds clear to auscultation.

Nursing intervention—encourage client to maintain adequate hydration by drinking 8–10 glasses of fluid/day. Teach and supportive effective coughing—technique perform chest physical therapy encourage position charged every 2 hours. Assess breath sounds before and after coughing episodes.

Evaluation—respiration are 20/minute and slightly labored, breath sounds are clear bilaterally in the upper lobes and left lobes are slightly decreased, coughing is productive of a moderate amount of thick, yellowish secretions.

Case Study—NCP Administering Medications

Client came in emergency room—has developed severe itching and rash

- T 98.4°F, P 60, R 20, B/P 120/70.
- Many areas of raised reddened spots on forearms and lower legs with evidence of inflammation.
- States intense itching and cannot help scratching.
- No known allergies.
- No talking any medications at present.
- Has not eaten any new foods recently.
- Immunization completed.
- Physician ordered Benadryl 25 mg PO start and q4h pm for itching.
- Apply calamine lotion at affected areas
- Return to dermatology clinic.
- Report any symptoms further spread of the rash.
- **Nursing diagnosis**—high risk for impaired skin integrity.
- **Planning**—skin will be intact.
- **Nursing interventions**—explain the Benadryl will help relieve the itching. Administer Benadrly as order. Explain effects and purpose of taking drug. Demonstrate how to apply calamine lotion to affected areas to decrease itching. Teach him to keep nails short and clean, not to scratch his skin, keep his towel and clothes separate from other family linens, and wash his hands before and after applying lotion.

Evaluate—inspection of skin of arms and legs shows no more rash and no breaks in the skin.

NCP-IV Therapy

Client with gallbladder diseases—70 years old cholecystectomy surgery performed.

- He is still receiving IV therapy and talking ice chips occasionally by mouth
- IV of 5% dextrose in 0.9% saline
- Ambulate in room
- Discontinue Foley
- May have clear liquid post nausea.

Nursing diagnosis—high-risk for injury, presence of IV needle in right arm.

Planning—exhibit no edema or pain at IV site. IV line patent and infusion running at ordered flow rate.

Nursing intervention—support arm with IV infusion on pillow. Teach client to be careful when moving arm. Check that needle and tubing are securely taped. Monitor IV flow rate every hour to see whether it is on schedule. Assess client on orientation/hour. Check tubing for kinking/hour.

Evaluation—assessment of IV site reveals no edema. Client states he has no pain at sight. A tourniquet placed above the IV site stops infusion.

Case Study—NCP Person with Wound

Patient with hysterectomy for excessive menstrual cycle bleeding is due to multiple fibroid tumors. No known health problems. She has a mid-line abdomen incision from below the umbilicus to the symphysis pubis. She complains of discomfort at the incision site when she moves and has not other problems.

- Regular diet as tolerated
- Vital signs/4 hours for 24 hours, then routine
- Routine postoperative dressing change with 4 × 4s and abdominal pads daily
- Voiding without difficulty
- Ambulates to bathroom without assistance
- Vital sings within normal limits TPR, BP of 1 degree.
- Complaining of abdomen discomfort at incision site
- Midline abdomen incision, 8-cm long extending from umbilicus to symphysis pubis
- Sutures intact, black silk interrupted sutures
- No wound odor
- Minimal swelling along suture line
- Small amount of crusted blood along incision.

Nursing Diagnosis

Impaired tissue integrity, mechanical disruption of surgery abdomen hysterectomy, 8" lower midline abdomen incision with interrupted silk suture in place minimal amount of serosanguineous drainage on dressing.

Planning expected outcome—shows wound healing without complication. No wound drainage continued decrease in swelling along incision line no infection, confined decrease in incision discomfort. Appropriate stage of healing for 72 hours after surgery.

- Implementation: Nursing interventions—wash hands before after dressing change.
- Remove dressing and note type and amount of drainage and inspect wound each day. Don sterile gloves, cleans wound incision with sterile isotonic saline.
- Reapply sterile dry dressing.
- Check patient TPR at regular intervals as determined by hospital policy.
- Instruct patient on importance of splint wound with small pillow when she coughs or changes position.
- Instruct patient about the need for a dietary intake for wound healthy with adequate protein, vitamin, iron. Assist patient to choose meals.

Evaluation

- 0.5 cm amount of serosanguineous drainage on dressing.
- No evidence of wound infection wound margins appear cleans no redness minimal swelling around suture noted. Wound edges approximated with crusted serosanguinous drainage along incision line.

- No evidence of wound dehiscence, wound at appropriate stage of healing.

Case Study—NCP

Patient in emergency department with acute abdomen pain, which is intermittent in the mid-epigastric area and radiates to right shoulder.

- Nausea and vomiting, no diarrhea
- A diagnosis of acute cholecystitis with chelelithiasis
- Midepigastic pain 24 hours duration
- Nausea and vomiting 12 hours duration
- Skin and sclera slightly jaundiced, skin dry, flakey, intact
- T 38.2°C, B/P 135/80, P 100, R 40
- Pupils dilated bilaterally.
- Abnormal lab values. Total Billruia 2.4 WBC 15,000
- States no known allergies.

Nursing Diagnosis

- Fear of hospitalization, surgery and anesthesia.
- Expected outcome/planning; fear related to impending surgery and anesthesia.
- Nursing intervention: Use therapeutic communication skills to encourage expression of subjective feelings, perception of coping ability provide explanation of surgical procedure sequence of surgical events, initiate teaching and return demonstration of coughing deep breathing and leg exercises, pain, wound care, home self-care.
- Offer comfort measures, observe status of fear.
- Risk of infection: Ensure operating room cleanliness establish sterile field, use aseptic technique. Ensure proper surgical hand scrubs technique and hand washing, ensure proper skin preparation of operative site, proper gowning, glove and draping technique, implement corrective action for any breaks in aseptic technique.

Evaluation

Verbalize fear of anesthesia provide return demonstration and acknowledge, transported to preoperative holding area via stretcher, check vitals.

- Operative site clean and dry to prevent infection.
- Wound edges closed, adhesive strips in place.
- T tube secure minimal drainage around tubing, states no tenderness at operative site.
- Vital signs—TPR, BP.

Purpose of NCP

1. For patient provide quality care, monitor progress, and ensure consistency/continuity.
2. For nurse—communicate information, organize care and evaluate care.
3. For clinical unit—make assignments, organize time related activities, direct shift report and evaluate nurse's performance.
4. For administration—secure resources, distribute resources and evaluate nursing practice.
5. For nursing—educate practitioner, develop professionalism, define nursing parameter, test and develop theory and research.

Case Study—NCP Psychological Needs

Lupus

Is an inflammatory disease that can cause deterioration of the connective tissues of muscles and bones in various parts of the body.

Law self-esteem and sadness reluctance to joint friends, difficulty in making decision, slightly over weight not accepting self/calls.

All developmental milestones of infancy and childhood reached successfully.

Diagnosis of Lupus

Nursing Diagnosis: Situational low self-esteem perceived loss of friend's secondary of illness lupus.

Planning: Expected outcome—initiating contact with friends.

Implementation: Nursing interventions: hypothesize about what her friends think and feel when she refuses their calls. Show confidence in patient ability to make change.

Evaluation

- Vicious pattern broken
- She initiated a call to a friend
- She visited with friend in hospital
- She accepted invitation to a party and engaged in activities to enhance her self-esteem.

Diagnosing is the interpretation and analysis of patient data to identify patient's strength and health problems that independent nursing intervention can prevent or resolve. Nursing diagnosis may change from day-to-day as the patient responses to health illness change.

Case Study—NCP Meeting Perceptual Needs

Patient with multiple injuries—clavicle, left femur; the chest X-ray showed a pneumothorax:

- Bed rest.
- 20 lbs skeletal traction to left leg
- Immobilize left arm in a figure of – 8 bandages.
- Left chest tube to 20 cm of suction
- Foley catheter to dependent drainage
- IV – D5 ½ NS at 125 cc/hr
- Demerol 50–75 mg IMQ 3–4 hours

- T 36.5° C, B/P 132/78, P 72, R 18
- Oriented
- Agitated restless, and combative
- Pulling at IV, Foley catheter and chest tube
- Foley to dependent drainage
- Radial and brachial pultes - 2 + bilaterally
- Capillary refill brisk
- Movement and sensation intact in left lower extremity
- States she has pain in the ribs and left leg
- Nursing diagnosis—Sensory/perceptual alterations to an unfamiliarly environment and an insufficient amount of meaningful stimuli
- Expected outcome/planning: answers questions demonstrating that she is oriented to person, place, time and patient role responsibilities
- Interacts with family, friends and hospital personnel
- Nursing interventions—orient patient, teach environmental stimuli, place calendar in view of patient, speak slowly, make frequent meaningful content with patient, bring personal items from home, provide communication board with pictures to facilitate interaction.

Evaluation

Patient is oriented to person, place and time, patient not pulling at IV, Foley or chest tubes. Patient is able to interact and communicate her needs.

NCP

Altered Nutrition

Less than body requirements inability to ingest sufficient nutrition.

- Discuss food preferences with patient
- Teach types of foods needed to meet daily requirements of a minimum of 1200 calories
- Allow patient to select eating times and food to be eaten
- Closely observe and record caloric intake at and between meals
- Promote conservation of energy to prevent loss of calories through excess activities that raise metabolic rate
- Assess of water and electrolyte imbalances.

Fluid Volume Deficit

Excess fluid loss, decreased fluid intake secondary to nausea vomiting and diarrhea.

Nursing Intervention: Asses for presence of thirst/8 hours

- Offer small amount of clear fluids.
- Assist with oral hygiene 18 hours.
- Lubricate lips with lanolin or petroleum jelly
- Record I/O
- Monitor IV fluids
- Record characteristics of vomits and stool.

Planning

The nurse and patient work together to develop patient's goals and identify the nursing interventions most likely to assist the patient to meet the goals.

It is important for the plan of care to be consistent with nursing standards, congruent wit other planned therapies and realistic in terms of the patient and nurse abilities or resources.

Computerized NCP

Will allow nurse to address patient care problems at the nurse's station.

These program are set up so that reference texts are edited and individualized before the care plan is saved on the disc and printed—one such program describes the patient's medical symptoms, nursing diagnosis, patient's goals, measurable outcomes and nursing interventions. There is also documenting the care given.

Benefits of Computerized NCP

- Expanded knowledge base
- Documentation of direct care and independent nursing intervention like teaching emotional support
- Improved record keeping and audit and quality assurance
- Documentation of all members of the health care team with print outs for the patient's record for change of shift report
- Reduction of time spent on paper work.

To search comprised literature: 5 items are needed: a telephone line, a communication card, a modem, a cable to connect the modem and the serial card and communication software. To access the desired data base the user needs to obtain a password and an account number.

Examples of nursing process—heart failure

1. **Assessment**—for observing the effectiveness of therapy. Any sign and symptoms of pulmonary fluid overload. Patients emotional response to diagnosis, sign and symptoms of dyspnea, shortness of breath, fatigue and edema, sleep disturbances (sleep suddenly interrupted by shortness of breath) number of pillows, needed for sleep, altered mental status, the rate and depth of respiration increased blood volume fills the ventricle with each beat, level of consciousness.
2. **Diagnosis**—based on assessment data—activity intolerance and fatigue, breathlessness from inadequate oxygenation, anxiety, ineffective therapeutic regimen management related to lack of knowledge.
3. **Planning**—promoting activity and reducing fatigue, relieving fluid overload symptoms, decreasing anxiety or increasing patients ability to manage anxiety teaching the patient about the self-care program.

4. **Interventions**—prolonged bed rest, pressure ulcer venous thrombosis and pulmonary embolism, exercise, managing fluid volume, controlling anxiety, monitoring and managing potential complications, teaching patient self-care.
5. **Evaluation**—maintains heart rate, bp, respiratory rate and pulse oximetery within the targeted rang, maintains fluid balance, isles anxious, sleeps comfortably at night, takes medicines as prescribed, performs and record daily weight.

Examples of nursing process—leg ulcers

1. **Assessment**—careful nursing history, the extent and type of pain, appearance, temperature of skin, quality of peripheral pulses, edema, vascular insufficiency, nutritional status is assessed.
2. **Diagnosis**—impaired skin integrity related to vascular insufficiency, impaired physical mobility, imbalanced nutrition (increased need for nutrition that promotes wound healing) infection, gangrene.
3. **Planning**—restoration of skin integrity, improve physical mobility, adequate nutrition and absence of complication.
4. **Intervention**—restoring skin integrity keep the area clean, poison the leg, elevate extremity, avoid trauma, provide protection, bed rest, relieve pressure, use bed cradle, avoid heating pads, not water bottle, hot baths, heating pad may produce injury burn, improving physical mobility (when infection resolves for promoting arterial flow and venous return).

Keywords

Characteristics of a profession, meeting respiratory needs, administering medications, IV therapy, person with wound, nursing diagnosis: examples of nursing process–heart failure, fluid volume deficit, etc.

CHAPTER

23

Nurse's Notes

Abstract

A nurse has to maintain daily diary book where she has to collect patient's data, perform physical examination, keep nurse's notes and nursing care plan as per format.

NURSE'S RECORD AND DOCUMENTATION GUIDELINES

Nurse's notes are an important part of the documentation. As soon as the nurse receives the patient, she has to document in nurse's notes the observation of the patient that she has seen and are present at that moment when she takes the handover.

How do you know that you exist?

Because you breathe, you eat and you speak, etc.

Therefore, besides your assignments, you must know also other details of the patients in the ward too.

Do not limit your abilities, but constantly grow in knowledge.

Find fine balance. You have to improve on education side as well as service side.

Constant review, open discussions, it is a joint effort.

How do you know that the client brought on bed is oriented/ not oriented?

By asking questions and collecting following observations.

What is the meaning of nurse's notes and how are they maintain?

What are the important points the nurse keeps in mind while documenting nurse's notes?

There are following points to keep in mind:

1. Each nursing notes depends on the diseases condition of the patient.
2. Each patient observed independently, e.g. surgical, ICU, orthopedic, neurological, etc.
3. Keep in mind that changes can be rapid and dramatic or slow and subtle.
4. Patient needs frequent testing, eye sign, motor and sensory nerves, ICP, vitals, headaches and vomiting.
5. Your assertive self, your attitude at work is of importance.
6. Keeping your mind in what you do.
7. Be alert, be observant, be vibrant and be vigilant.
8. Maintaining the quality care and your dignity upholding.
9. When patient arrives in ward, causality, check the consciousness of patient and his ability to follow instructions, check the abilities and limitations.
10. When patient is transferred to the ward was the condition stable, was he drowsy unconscious, ex-tuba Ted, transported on trolley, stretcher, accompanied by whom.
11. Handing over patient to other staff find out any fresh complains,
12. New developments if any, observation of improvement/ worsens condition.
13. Patient received with other illness like DM/HT/IHD/ MI/asthma/allergy.
14. Patient received on bed with vein-flow, peripheral IV, RT, Foleys, ET, CVP, ART line, dialysis catheterization, drain.
15. Patient had episodes of vomiting/loose motion/rigors and medications given as per doctors order.
16. Morning/evening/night—hourly given/not given/pending/ reason.
17. Investigation name them like HIV, HBsAg done and reports attached, or awaited, or informed consultant about laboratory finding.
18. Vitals BP, TPR, noted, no change, there is a change.
19. Patient is for Sx/surgery preoperative orders carried pout/kept NB till noon, skin preparation, shaving, explained sequence of surgery/procedure, obtained consent, special needs meat, taught deep breathing and coughing exercises, active passive exercises. Send to OT, time.
20. Patient received from OT after surgery v/s checked, had breathing difficulties, abdominal girth checked, operation site no bleeding, oral fluids taken, NG aspiration till peristalsis reappear, frequent change of position, continuous monitoring, IV fluids types and amount, frequent mouth care, surgical incision is clean and dry.
21. Postoperative sutures removed, allergic reaction to procedures, medications prompt information to surgeon/physician.
22. BT given, blood group or blood on wait, storage 1–6 celsius, complication of BT.

23. Patient slept well/not slept well/restless/awake.
24. Diet plan-liquid diet, inability to take food, not able to tolerate food, had normal diet, clear fluids, pt took nutritious balanced diet.
25. Input/Output chart maintained he had 1000 mL of liquid containing tea, coffee, coconut water, kanji, fruit juice etc intake by mouth-item and amount, by IV, urine out put, vomit us, drainage, bowel any other, volume of urine output is in balance with fluid intake.
26. Bowel and elimination open, normal, urine and bowel elimination are re-established.
27. Instructions given to patient, family, relative about the psychological supports given.
28. Doctor visited and new orders of medication ordered, old orders remain cancelled/changed.
29. Dressing done with dry, wet, there was pain, fluid and discharge at wound site, contractures, necrosis, dead tissues, sensation absent, abscess, healed, cleansing medication use, applied medication, antiseptics, non-antiseptic dressings, pressure dressing, swelling, numbness, tingling reduced/increased, applied bandage, adhesive tape.
30. Drainage tubes-fluid, color or secretions drain purulent, pale, watery, clear watery, shortening of drainage, doctors purpose achieved.
31. Nebulization, steam inhalation.
32. Oz 4l/min by nasal catheter 8 hours.
33. Prepared patient for scopies, diagnostic test, test results, significance of test.
34. RBS, urine sugar, AG.
35. Regular medication, drug added.
36. Maintenance of ventilation-deep breathing and coughing, exercise, patient moves in bed, or physiotherapy advised.
37. Patient is free from pain and discomfort, good sleep, no complains, no manifestation of complications present, or patient weak and easily fatigued.
38. Fluid intake and electrolytes are normal.
39. The circulating fluid volume: arterial blood pressure is within the CVP and the pulmonary artery pressure.
40. The serum electrolytes (sodium, chloride, potassium, calcium, phosphate, magnesium, glucose) within normal range.
41. The heart rate is, the heart rhythm is regular, lungs are free of crackles/wheezes on auscultation.
42. Acid base balanced restored, blood urea and cretinin levels are normal, patient is alert and conscious, eyes opens spontaneously, verbal response shows orientated to time, place and person, motor response are coordinated and appropriate to command, the skin is warm, dry and normal in color, the limbs are free of contractures.
43. Respirations are effortless.
44. Patient is able to perform activities of daily living, good hygiene maintained.
45. Serum electrolytes and pH are within normal range.
46. No bed sore, weight stable, peripheral edema absent.
47. Progressive and duration of complains.
48. Report and investigation arrange chronologically.
49. Every continuation sheet attached to IPD main case paper, put serial number, so any page detached, missed will know.
50. The event of complaint that the patient was not seen or neglected this entry becomes useful.
51. If the patient is referred to other specialist, observation and advice must be entered if computerized, necessary standard format issue of certificate prepared by doctor also.
52. ICU treatment sheet—high risk consent, BT, parental nutrition, laboratory requisition, critical care flow sheet, OPD case paper, IPD case paper, history sheet, provisional diagnosis, treatment sheet, nurses notes, IV fluid sheet, RBS reading, I/O by mouth/IV anesthetic record, pre-operative check list, e.g. vitals, consent, NBM, allergies, investigations, shaving, general hygiene, dentures, loose teeth, nail polish, contact lenses, jewelry, intraoperative nurses notes, postoperative notes by RMO, billing chart, etc.
53. Aim of documentation should be accurate, concise, current, factual and organized data to be entered with your professional responsibilities.
54. Record patients observation of behavior, record nursing intervention and the patients response.
55. Chart precautions or prevention measures used, document in legally prudent manner.
56. Charting for the purpose to give concise information pertinent to the patient during hospital stay.
57. The day of admission is counted as 1st day of disease, marked "S" surgery "E" enema, 'D' delivery. "T" for telephone, TPR graph marked with firm dots in proper column so that straight connecting lines can be drawn.
58. Record date on each new page on top.
59. Diet is charted as medication.
60. Summarize significance observation.
61. Order of charting during hospitalization-BP, I/O, diabetic record, graphic sheet, doctors orders, physicians order, history and physical examination, laboratory report, X-ray report, consultation record, request for ECG, other special examination, operation report, nurses notes, summarizing sheet.
62. Concise record of all current orders, when an order is discontinued, draw a line through it and write at the right side the date it is discontinued, if a medication or treatment is omitted circle the hour.

63. Admission chart all pertinent information including time of admission, how admitted, apparent symptoms and complaint in nurses notes.
64. All elevated temperature to be taken 4 hourly unit; normal temperature above 101 report.
65. Chart type of examination, specimen sent to laboratory, examining doctor.
66. Morning care—offer bedpan/urinal, brush teeth, bath face, ears, neck and hands. Straighten bedding, keep unit clean and neat, observer any change, offer fresh water, check drainage and empty/record, give breakfast, give bed bath with back care, change bed linen, comb hair, adjust side rails.
67. Afternoon care—loosen bed linen, change position, observe any change, offer fluids, message back.
68. Evening care—put extra blanket if needed, give special instruction for laboratory and X-ray, surgery, etc. to be done, next morning record care given, general condition and observation.
69. Transferring patient—complete charting up to time of transfer, time and mode of transfer, room and ward to which patient is being transferred, transferred out and time. Nurses receiving patient any untoward reactions caused by transfer, write transfer in and time.
70. What ever information you enter must be complete, concise which is your professional responsibility.
71. Record as mentioned above patients observations and behavior, and note problems in orderly sequential manner and chart precautions and preventive measures used.
72. Record all medical visits and consultations for the other nurses to be aware for better client care.
73. Chart in time and indicate each entry and date, your interventions all this is crucial in notes.
74. When more seriously ill patient come your responsibility of recording becomes significant.
75. Update admission, transfer, discharged, procedure performed, and change in patients status.
76. Fluid administered (to correct electroplate imbalance).
77. Measured neurological status.
78. Monitored vital signs and neurological status/hour.
79. Patient is kept NBM/on NPO.
80. Assessed Glasgow Coma Scale.
81. Provided emotional support.
82. Monitored for ICP/15 minutes.
83. Head elevated to reduce venous pressure.
84. Assessed peristaltic waves and bowel sounds.
85. Tube clamped.
86. Medical management and diet modification explained.
87. Color of urine noted and documented.
88. Air mattress/water mattress used to prevent ulcer of the skin.
89. ECG taken.
90. Oz administered as prescribed/checked oz saturation.
91. Warm compression given.
92. Dressing inspected.
93. Audiometric done.
94. Notified physician of patients condition.
95. Test blood glucose and test urine for ketones 3–4 hourly done.
96. Monitored transfusion reactions (temperature, chills, dyspnea).
97. Physicians orders reviewed.
98. Sigmoidoscope/proctoscopy done.
99. Cleansing enema given.
100. Patient to be sent for MRI test.
101. Patient is put on assisted ventilation.
102. Given oral hygiene 4 hourly.
103. Blood and urine samples obtained.
104. Applied ice pack.
105. Rectal tube inserted for flatus.
106. Foley's catheter inserted as prescribed.
107. Skin, mouth and eye care provided.
108. Monitored gag reflex and ability to swallow.
109. Administered stool softness.
110. Provided gait training.
111. Insulin administered.
112. Health education and psychological support given to patient and family.

Every patient has right to know the nature of his illness, its prognosis, its treatment, its preventive, enhancing and rehabilitative aspects. In addition, the health problems that he may have to face in the future for that the relatives also should be aware of these facts in order to help the patient.

Patient's responsibility—a long life is a gift–if it is a healthy one. Learn how to live better and how to manage the condition that creep up on your body interne, computer too can guide you how to go about. Dialogue with your doctor and ask him to explain the diagnosis and the course of treatment. If you do not get convincing answers, do some research in the internet about the illness, and be armed with information so that you can have a meaningful dialogue with your doctor.

Your health is too important to be left to the experts. Detection of illness is critically important in effective cures. Do research on internet on health issues. Getting older does not interfere with your ability to use a computer. You can enter the world of technology at an awkward age too. New technologies and economic opportunities are influencing the essence and quality of life. Fast changing lifestyle, western culture influence, and electronic media is urgent need.

Better late than never, where hope grows, miracles blossom, fear ends, faith begins. Awareness is power.

Students, anyone looking at you will say what type of nurse you will be in future. If you build up confidence in skill, you will stand up even everything goes against you.

How nurses must respond to the patient—patient in the hospital is considered as a paying guest; he expects medical attention, efficient nursing care, physical comfort and protection. He is sick and dependent, sensitive and emotional. He expects kindness and support. He has anxiety during illness, financial stress; it affects his wellness to accept treatment. Confined to bed affects and interrupts his job. He is dependent on others for his physical need so he gets irritated. Insecurity due to strange place, no privacy, multiple beds, strange people attending to him. She to be kind and understanding and make him relaxed comfortable, explain to him routine, his treatment plan, see patient facial expression, emotional reaction to pain, fatigue, maintain therapeutic environment and attain patients need immediately. Never leave seriously ill patient along.

Conclusion—when a patient is brought to the hospital, he/she is initially taken to the causality, where on duty doctor does primary check up, determines the seriousness and nature of illness. History of illness collected, all past investigations and summary collected, and in accordance with the nature of illness the medical doctor on duty recommends a particular specialist under whose care the patient will be treated. The relatives will choose the class of the bed where the charges for operations. Investigations and all other services may depend on it. The hospital diet, preparation of case paper, advanced money and med claim if any all the details collected. When the patient is taken to the ward, the nurse will explain the further details and all the orientation of the place. After receiving the patient, the nurse will have to keep nurses notes as per her observation.

Keywords

Nurse's notes, documentation, ICU treatment sheet, Order of charting, care, patient's rights, patient's responsibility.

CHAPTER

24

Bag Technique

Abstract

Community health nursing is the back-bone of rural villages. Bag technique is an important aspect of community health.

During the nursing training students, have educational visits to the urban and rural community. They have to go to the field and live and work with the people in actual situation and experience.

The customs, cultures, health habits, lifestyle, pattern of living, pattern of food, rituals, etc. They also have to conduct deliveries, check up antenatal mothers, visit schools and help in ICDS, Anganwadi programme and get all the information relevant to their study.

They do survey, prepare family folders, family welfare services, prepare nursing care plans, give individual and community health education.

Visit the PHC, and sub-centers daily and know the functioning, staffing pattern, attain OPD, and do procedures IPD and help the staff.

They also take part in the visiting families' daily; take part in camps, and mid-day meal programme.

Through different AV aids and skits, role-play, songs and dances teach the people and give health related and social issues related such as alcoholism, smoking, tobacco chewing advice and its ill effects on health.

All together, it is very tiring, hectic field experience, where they feel hungry, thirsty, hot sun and dust walking and walking sometimes miles where they in practical level practice their skills. They get deep and rich experience and get to know the India that lives in urban slums and rural villages.

This experience becomes a stepping stone in their life where they remember and relish it later on. It teaches them the value of life and the value of abundance and the unfortunate people who live day in and day out. They also get to know why people are sick, and what background people come to the hospital, so that they can show the extra solidarity towards the poor fellow men of ours who live in same India that we live. So it is also a value education.

There we have to practice certain procedure with bag, which contains all the necessary articles. The bag is light and easily carryable and washable. Community nurse is recognized by her bag. She carries it door to door to visit people, and in emergency she has enough articles where she can attain the basic first aid needs of the people. So here I have developed certain training skills that are demonstrated and re-demonstrated by the students in the actual field.

How the bag should be?

The bag should be made of canvas, leather or light metal. It should not be very heavy, it should be such that bag can be carried by the hand or on the shoulder. It should contain only essential equipments. No home visit should be made without bag. The bag is like a small dispensary. It is very handy and useful in the field area. I myself have found it very useful and was able to attain small emergency in school, Anganwadi, slums and in villages at their door step. People get benefited by it at their home. Once in a week bag and its contents must be fully checked, cleaned and refilled. Empty the bag completely and boil all the articles, sock other equipments in antiseptic or soap water. Do not handle the contents of the bag without first having washed your hands well. Always put the bag on a stool, cot or box after placing a clean paper and not directly on the ground.

How the bag technique is done?

1. First as you enter the village or urban area and go for home visit, ask the family first permission to enter the house. If there is a patient of fever, eye infection, any minor dressing or any minor illness you can carry out the procedure.
2. Look around and see a clean surface that is away from the animals and children
3. First spread the newspaper and keep the bag on it
4. You can unbutton the bag and keep half open
5. Ask the family to give you a bucket of water and mug where in an area where you can wash your hands. That is keep the water ready
6. Then you can open the outer pocket and take hand washing articles
7. Go and do community social hand washing
8. Wash hands with soap and water
9. Come back to the area of bag and now you can take a newspaper and spread one for you to sit, one for preparing sterile field, and one for the patient as shown in the figure
10. Take the plastic sheet our and put on a newspaper as shown in the figure

11. To carry out the procedure you take the spirit bottle, cotton balls and make the sterile field
12. Now remove what is need for particular procedure the articles.
13. Wash hands and replace the articles in the bag
14. Used articles place them in separate extra plastic bag
15. Fold the used newspaper with used side inside and keep it in the outer pocket.
16. Burn the soiled dressings and wash all the instruments and send for sterilization to use on the next day for another procedure. Once the articles are sterilized it is ready for the next use. As it can prevent cross infection by carrying contaminated articles from house to house.
17. Do not unnecessarily open the bag. Take once and for all the needed articles. Does not misuse the bag by keep personal articles in it?
18. Follow the strict aseptic technique
19. Follow the steps of each procedures
20. What ever you do, do it keeping the scientific principles and abide by it scrupulously
21. The bag will have rubber goods, thermometer, bottles, cord ligature, eye antiseptic, instruments, dressing materials, strict aseptic technique it is disinfected each articles. Once this is completed, close the bag and place on clean newspaper, so that it will be ready for next use for any procedure open bag, wash hands, remove articles required, close the bag
22. Bag technique remains the same for all procedure, only different procedures need different articles and following its steps and principles. The basic remains the same for all procedure.

Example in procedure of eye care the student is instructed and taught how to clean the eye from inner canthus to outer canthus using a separate swab at each stroke. For crusted secretion place a wet warm gauze piece until the crust becomes soft. If the eye is infected and there is more pus formation use separate swab each time until the eye is fully cleansed. She has to follow the instruction of opening, closing and taking out articles and replacing back the articles with step by step keeping the scientific principles which are remain the same in field and in hospital. Nurse opens a sterile set for eye care and dressing procedure open top most part of the covering wrapper away from him. This leaves sterile equipment and supplies well covered and are not contaminated. Then she opens the second layer of the wrapper, it still leaves sterile equipment and supplies covered with the last layer of the wrapper. As the last step nurse opens final layer of the wrapper towards herself/himself. Now the wrapper becomes the sterile field. As shown in the figures. Pouring sterile solutions liquids on a sterile dressing bowl. The outer surface of the cap are un-sterile so do not allow the inner surface touch an un-sterile area. Same the sterile forceps should not touch the edge of sterile wrapper a outer are considered un-sterile. Follow the basic principle that only an sterile object can touch another sterile objects.

Examples of some procedure given below that are done through the home visit bag technique-

1. Example in procedure of care of nose and ear
2. Example in procedure of testing for urine foe sugar, albumin. Hot and cold test
3. Example in procedure of for steam inhalation
4. Example in procedure of hot and cold application
5. Example in procedure of physical assessment
6. Example in procedure of pediculosis treatment and its advice
7. Example in procedure of minor small dressings
8. Example in procedure of talking vitals and temperature
9. Example in procedure of blood pressure
10. Example in procedure of baby bath
11. Example in procedure of domiciliary delivery
12. Example in procedure of cord care
13. Collecting blood for peripheral smear (obtaining a small sample of blood by skin puncture) to detect malarial parasites and to detect blood cell abnormalities. The thin smear you can put a drop of fresh blood on the middle of the slide and use another slide to spread the blood drop along the slide. Then leave the film to dry. For thick smear put 3 drops of fresh blood on the left hand quarter of the slide and with the corner of another slide mix the blood and smear 1 cm in diameter.

Giving a **baby bath/tube bath** to clean the skin of the baby and for promoting hygiene and comfort in the home setting

Giving a **lap/leg bath**—bathing a baby by placing him/her on the legs in a home setting which is the traditional method used in bathing a baby at home in rural communities

Oil bath—premature babies oil is applied all over body and is wiped off with cotton balls or rag pieces. When baby is covered with vernix caseasa, an oil bath is given to remove it.

Home Visits

Go to the people, learn from them, live with them, start with what they know, build with what they have.

Home visiting is the back born of MCH services. The home visits will provide an opportunity to observe the environmental and social conditions at home and also an opportunity to give prenatal care. The **purpose** is to carry out simple nursing care in the home which helps in prevention of diseases and promotion of health of the members of the family. Home visit needs proper planning, follow up, evaluation. It follows certain principles such as it should be made according to the needs of the people. In home visits we need to collect background information of the family to identify heath problems. (Students can get all the information through survey and preparing family folders.) It has advantages and disadvantages too. Caring for the sick at home has become a highly specialized area of health care and major component of comprehensive health care. Nurse must demonstrate respect in their personal surroundings and arrive fully prepared and equipped with objective for home visit use of domestic articles in home nursing. Use of earthen pot instead of bedpan, using a piece of clean cloth or sari in place of bandage using a glass bottle instead of hot water bag, use disposable items in home nursing teach then to drink safe water, boil milk, eat hot cooked foods, properly wash, use personal towel, get immunized, use mosquito nets, get rid of rats, wear shoos, stay away from sick people, burn sputum, etc. four things you must keep clean, i.e. body, cloths, house, surrounding.

Procedure of hot compresses—heat has soothing effect on the body. Heat reduces the muscle tension, relieves pain, and speeds up the healing. Heat dilates the blood vessels and reduces congestion. Hot compress is effective way of applying heat to the body.

Procedure—folds a towel four fold, soak it in hot water and wring it out. Apply to the affected area. Replace when it becomes cool. Keep the hot water covered with lid, check that hot water is not too hot, otherwise it will cause burns.

Hot water bottle serves the same purpose. Moreover, it remains hot for a longer time and does not require to be changed frequently.

Procedure cold compresses—it is used to stop bleeding, to reduce bruising and swelling and to relieve pain. It contracts the blood vessels and enhances to stop the bleeding. It can reduce swelling after the sprain.

Procedure—takes a small towel and four fold it. Soak the towel in ice-cold water and wring it out, apply it to the affected area. Replace it when it becomes warm. An ice bag has the same effect which remains cold for longer time and does not need to change frequently

Explanation—Outline of the figures that will follow in the chapter is given below. This will explain all the figures in the chapter:

1. The figures show the home visits in the field area where students are trained to visit door to door and give medical first aid and attain the emergency as well give individual and group education. They also can see people as they are, where they are, which makes people comfortable, approachable, cooperative and student friendly as they spend time with them. So it becomes easy to reach them at their level in the actual radical situation.
2. Students in the figures showing the community hand washing and teach the simple techniques of checking the urine sugar at home
3. Showing them how to take care of the eyes when any infection comes
4. How to do the simple dressing and prevent infection
5. The people too are rich in their customs, they taught the students there ways of giving traditional leg bath
6. Lap bath
7. Oil bath, which you can see in the figures
8. Tub bath
9. Government runs many programs for children by Balwadi and mid mid-day meal, teaching and educating, etc. Students enhanced and took active part with the teachers and helped them and taught them the value of education, cleanliness and how in simple way them can be healthy
10. In the field itself they have to visit near by social institutions where they had educational visit and displayed there talents by bringing moments of joy and happiness on the faces of inmates.

Through the community bag a students performs number of procedures. It is like small dispensary where she has to use bag technique as per need of situation. Therefore, lots of pictures are given where she works and does her procedures in actual field of urban and rural area of her posting.

Keywords

Bag, bag technique, procedures, Eye care, blood smear, home visit, hot and cold compression.

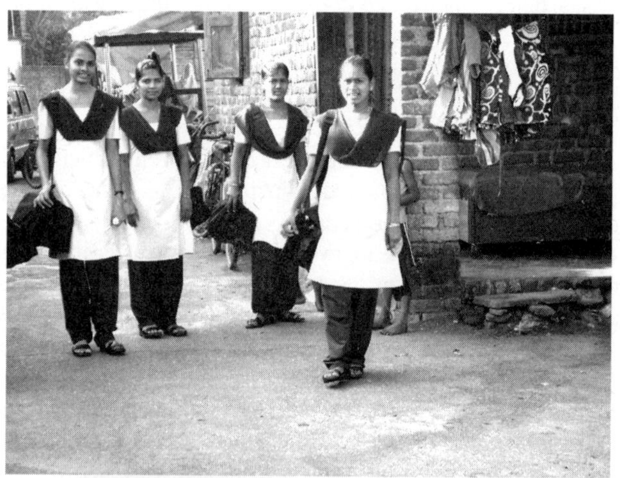

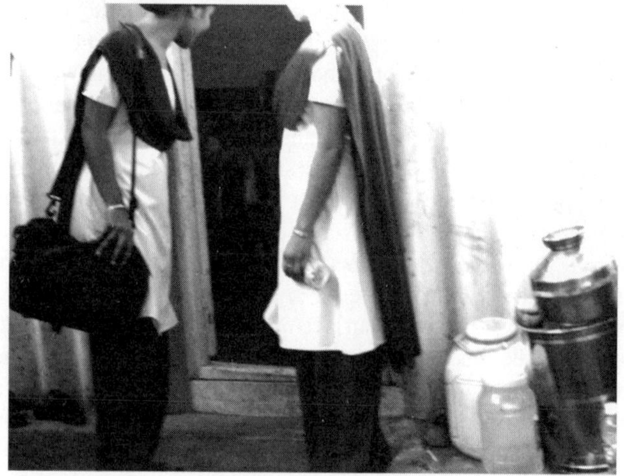

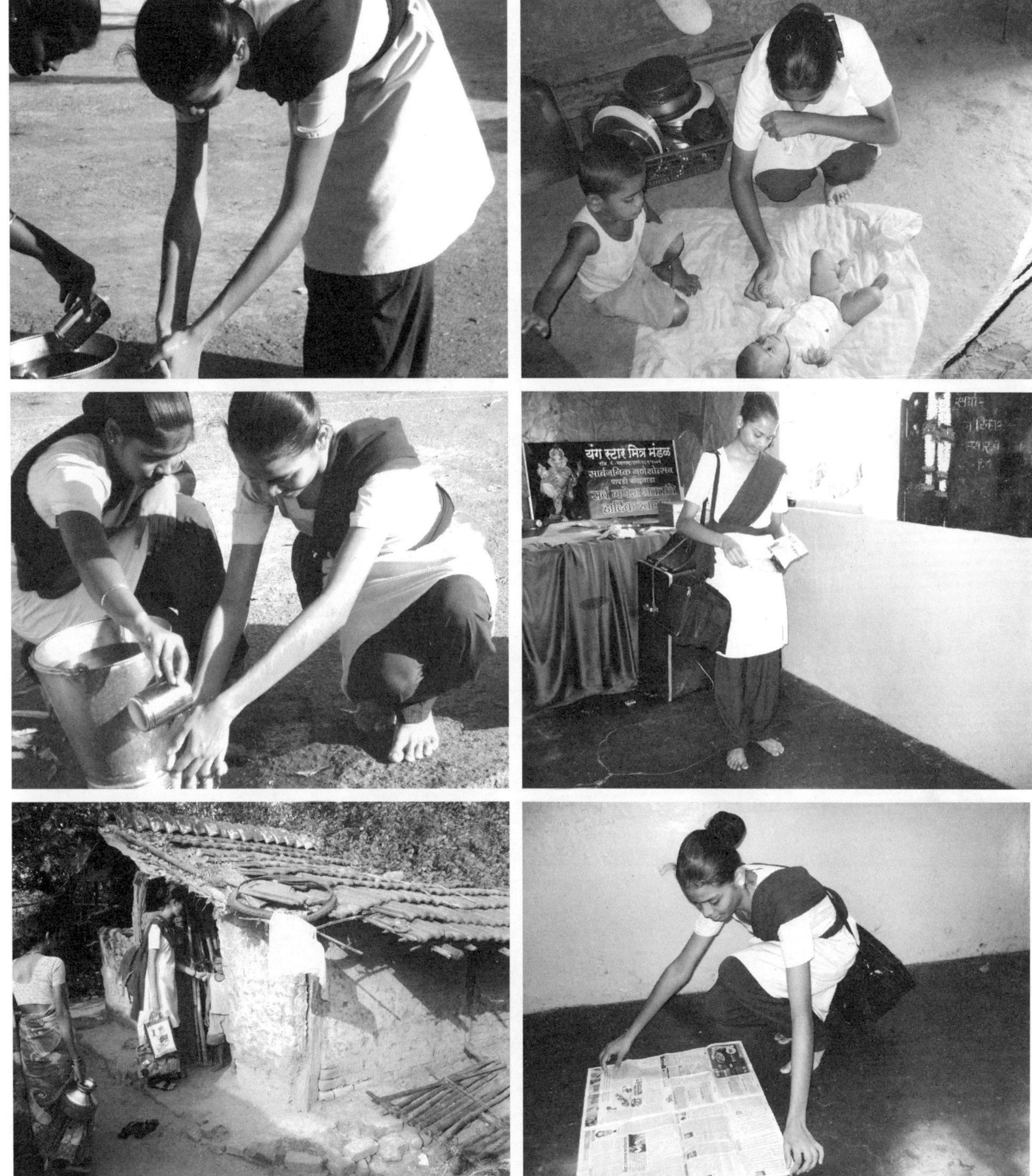
यंग स्टार मित्र मंडळ

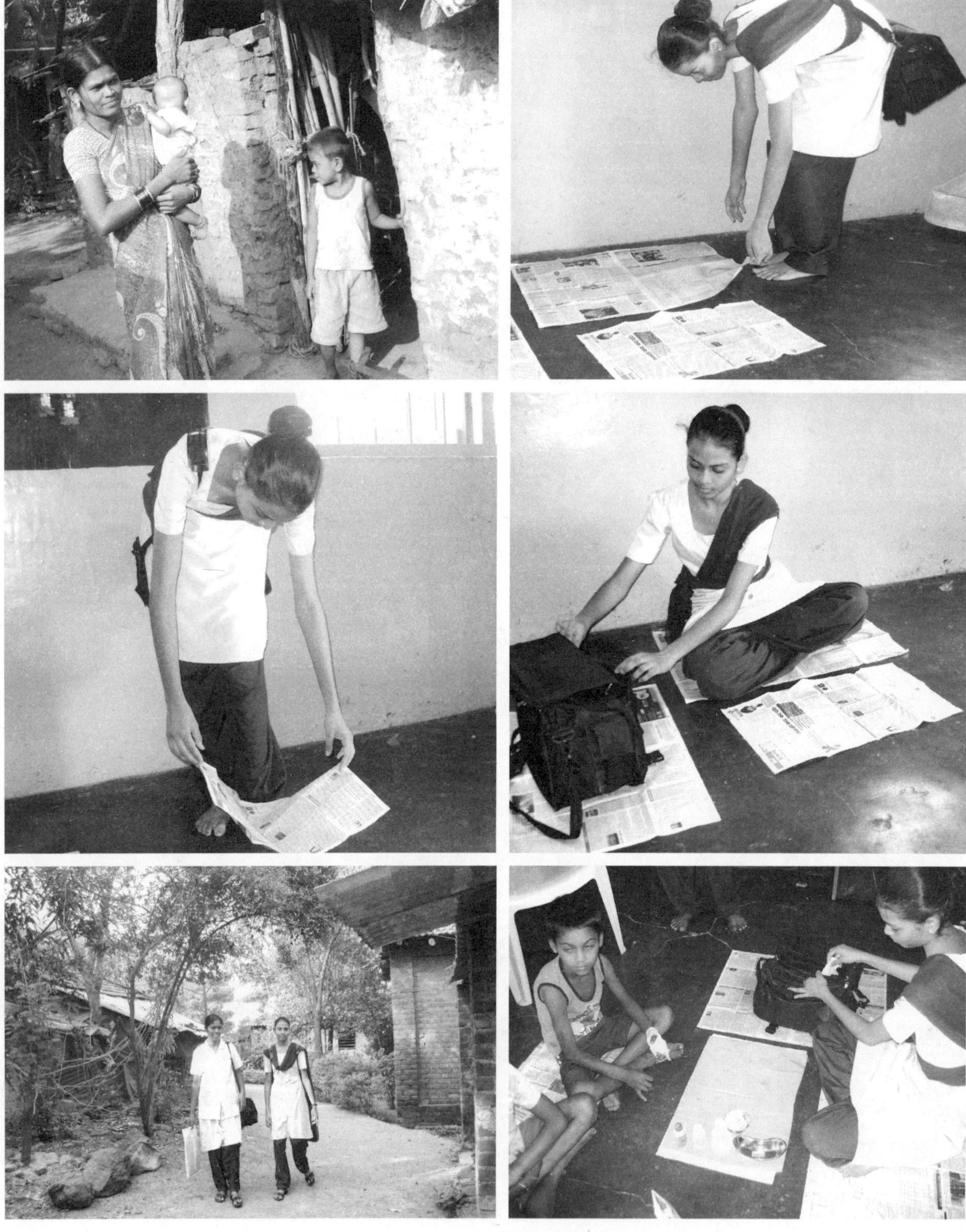

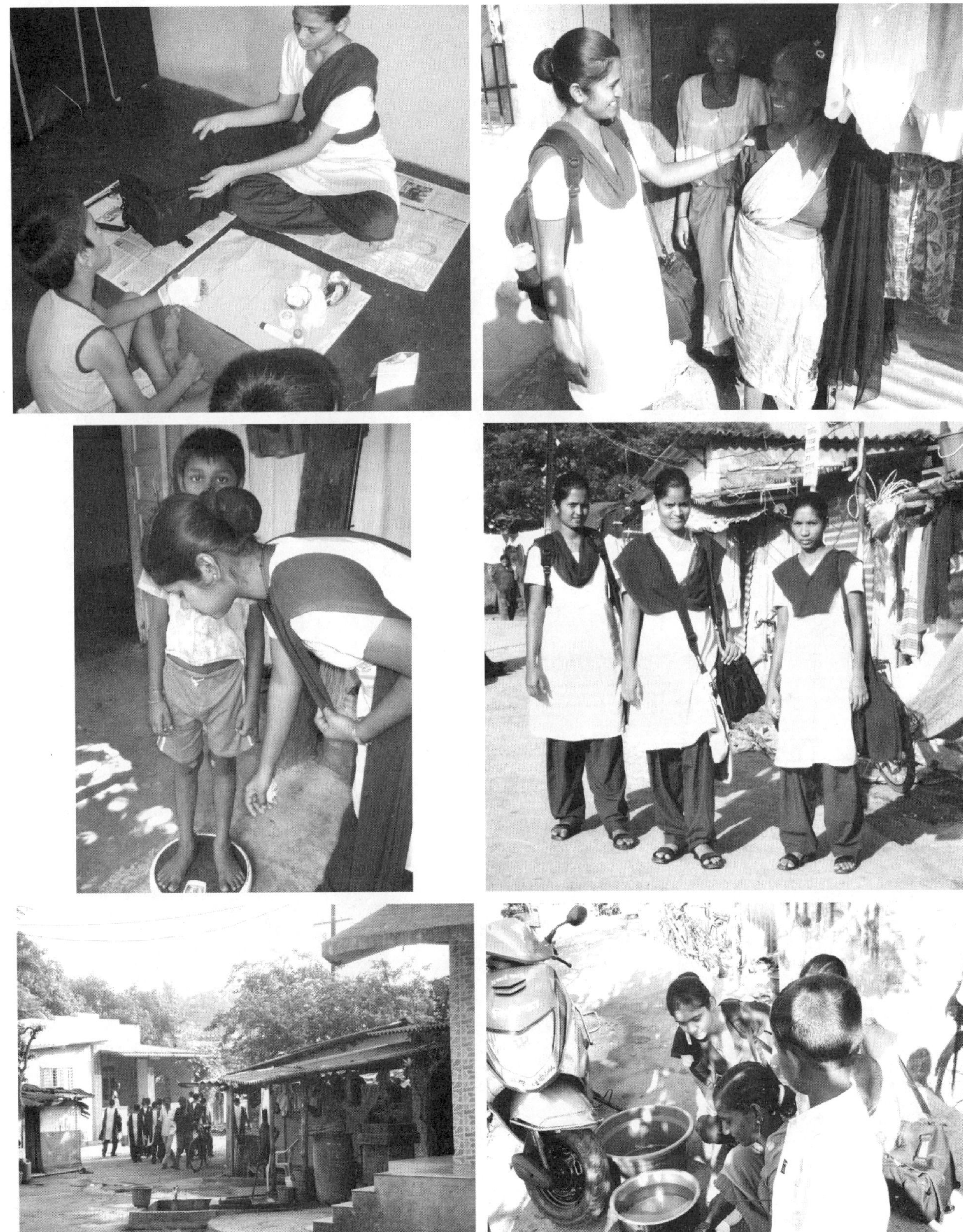

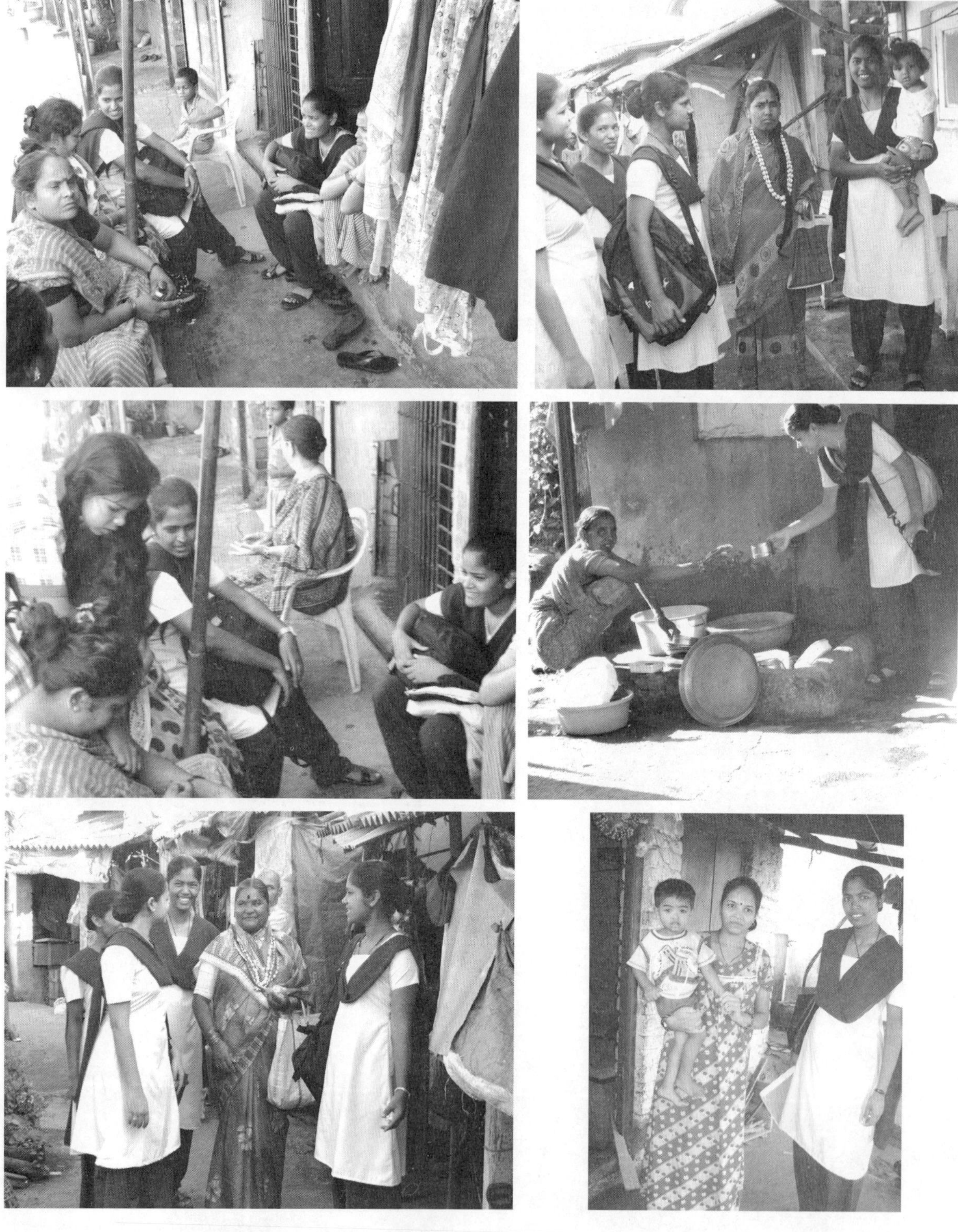

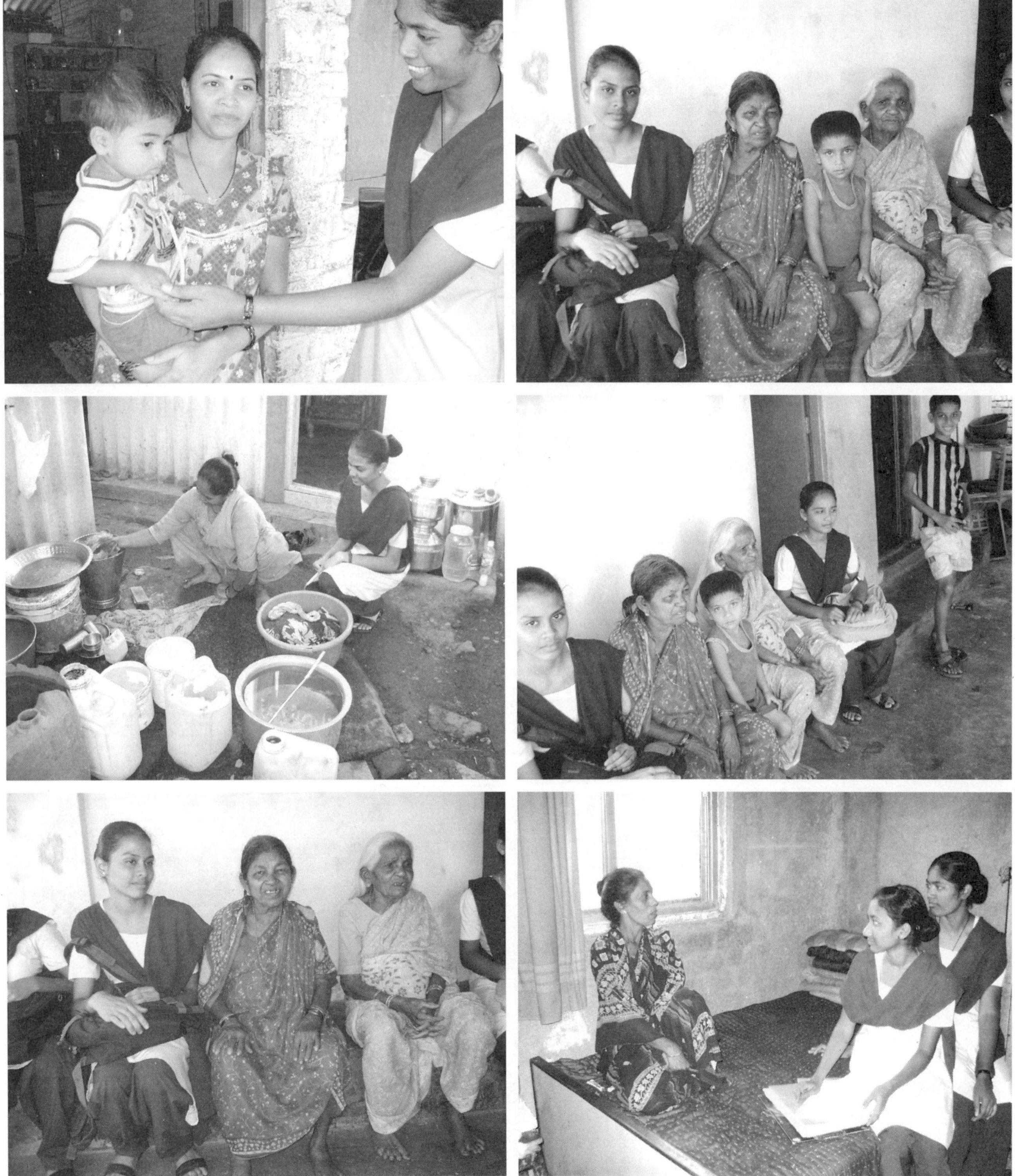

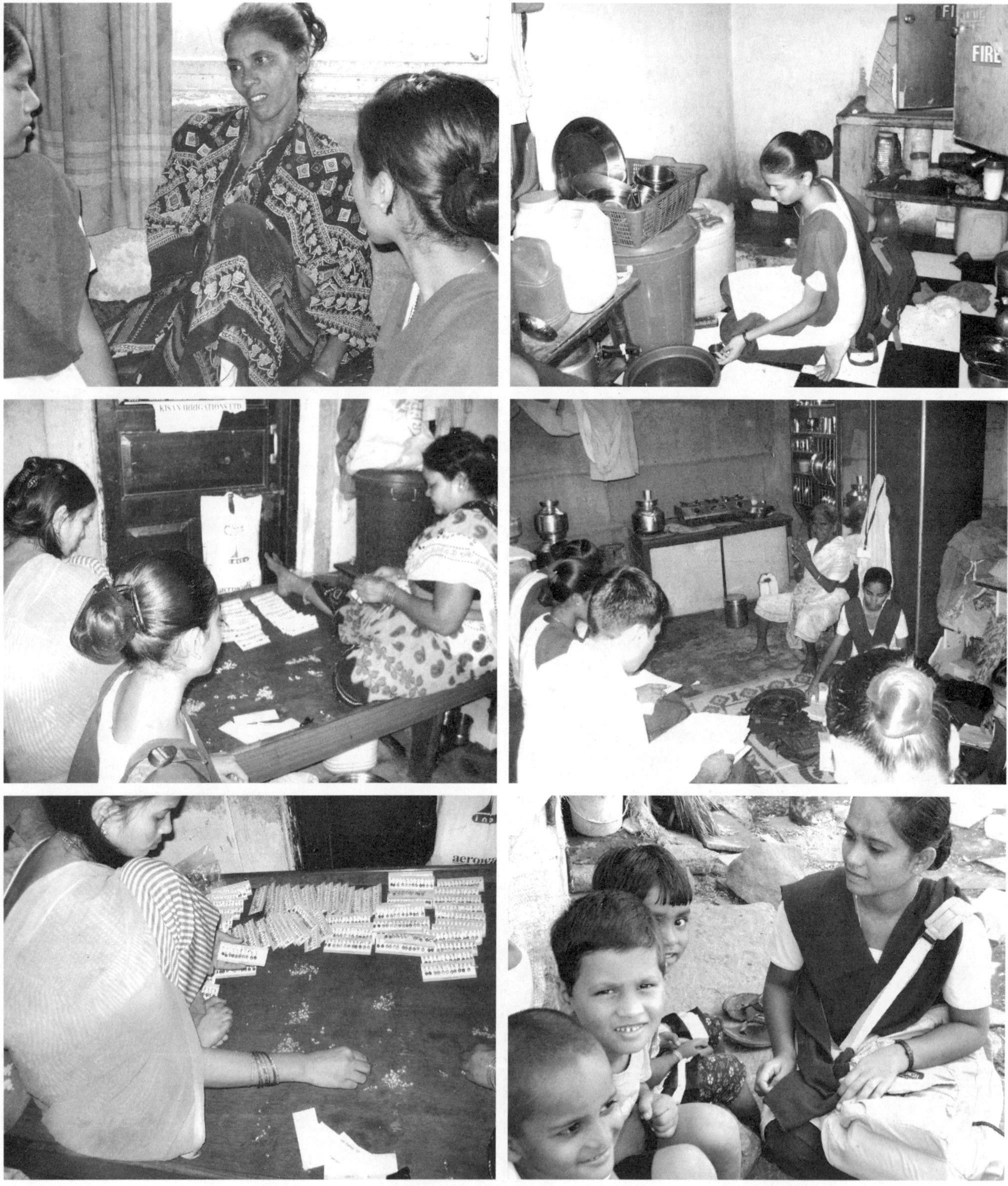
FIRE

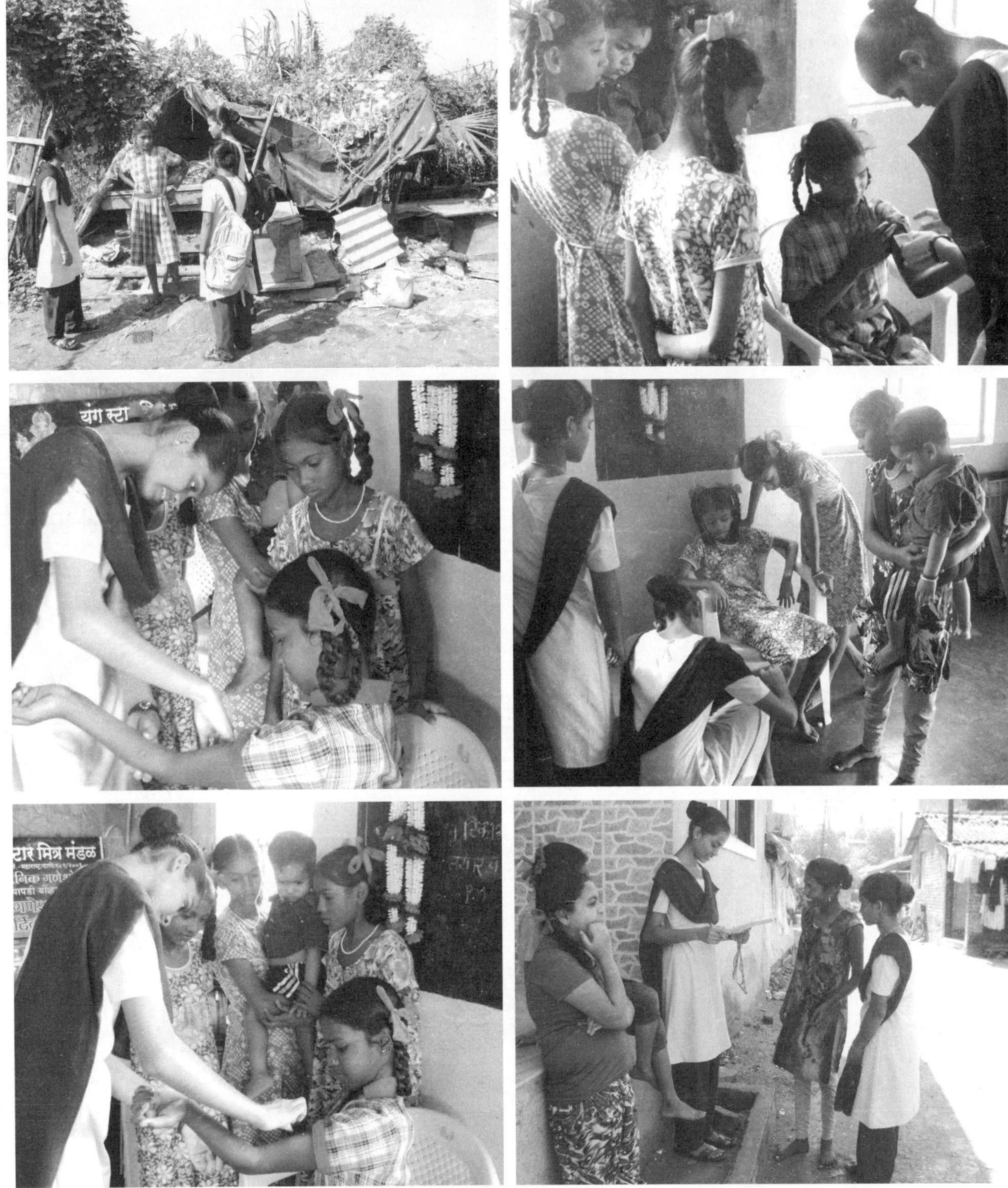
मित्र मंडळ

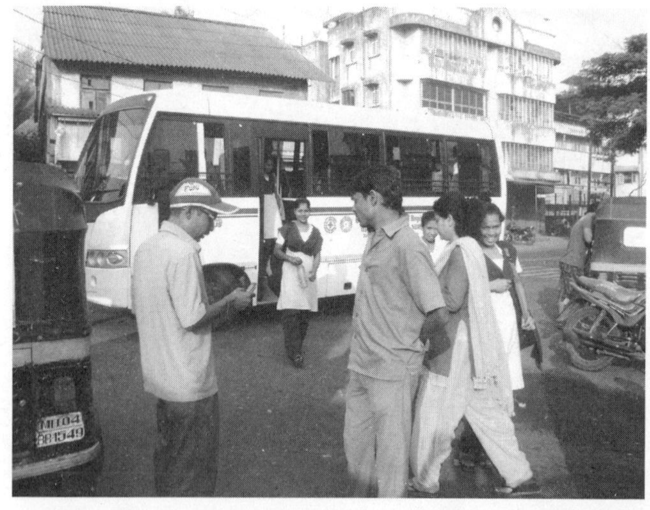

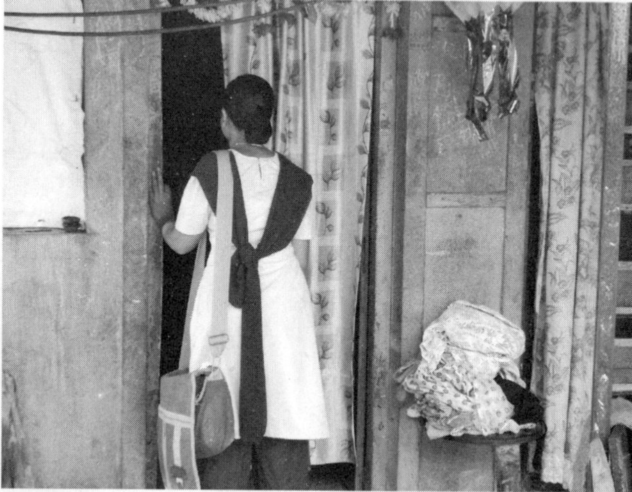

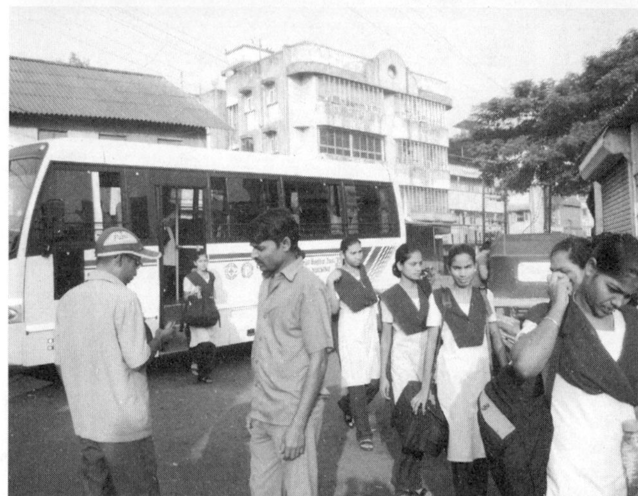

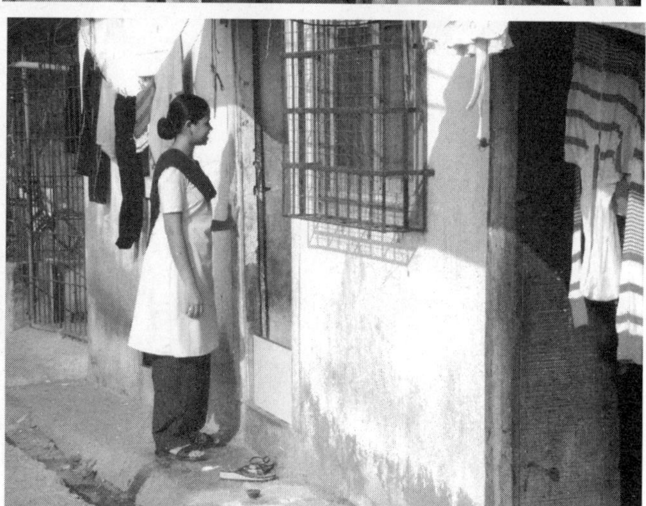

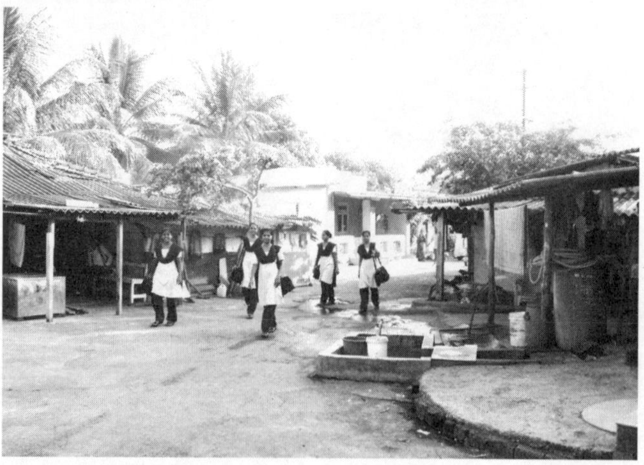

Hand Washing and Urine Sugar

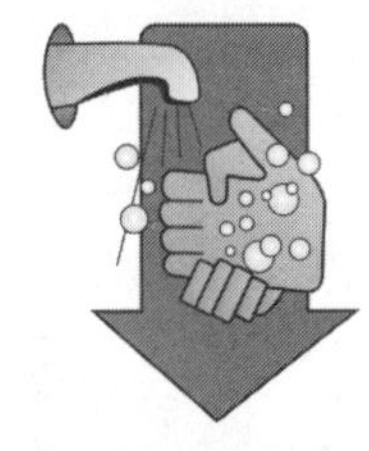
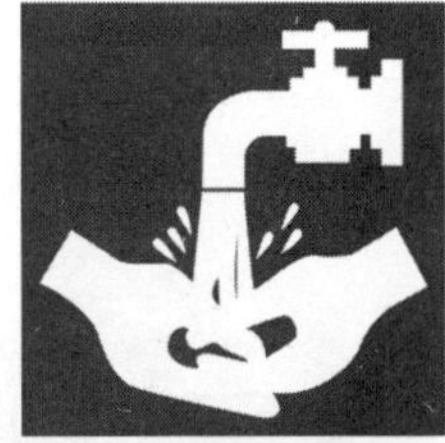
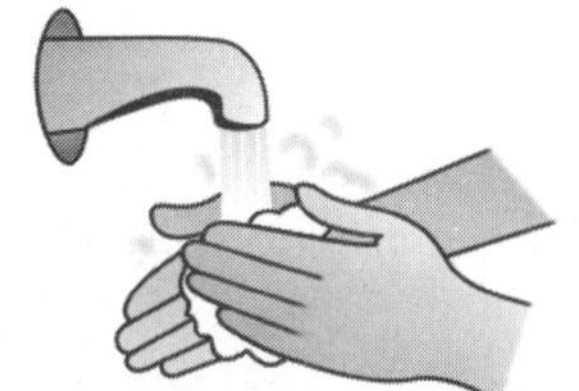
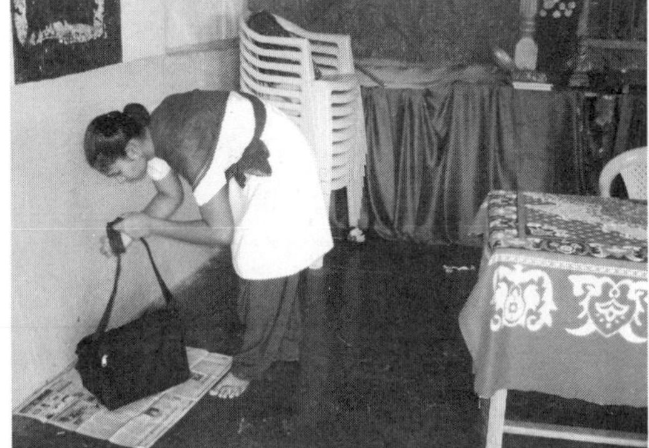
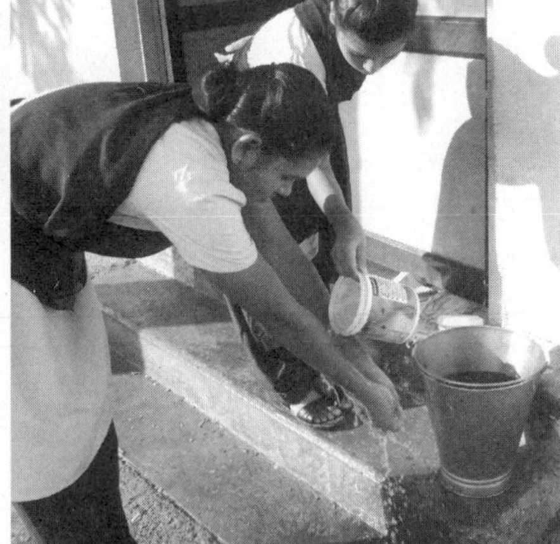
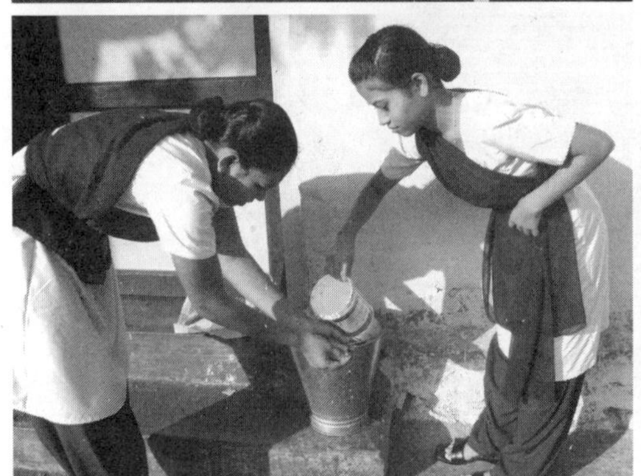
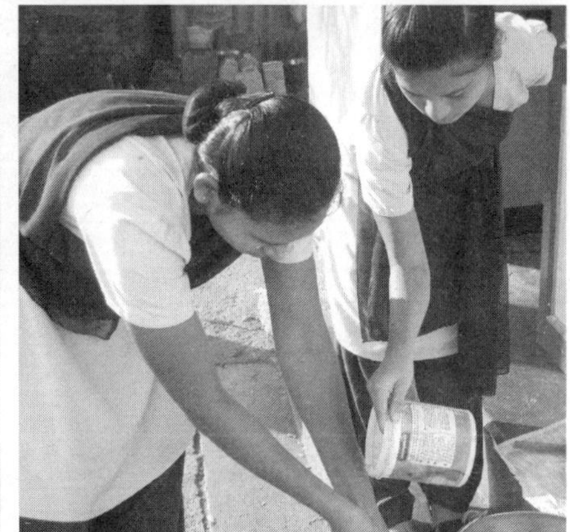
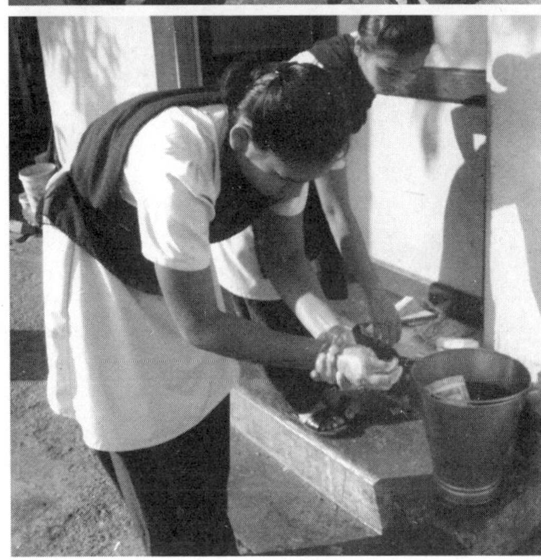
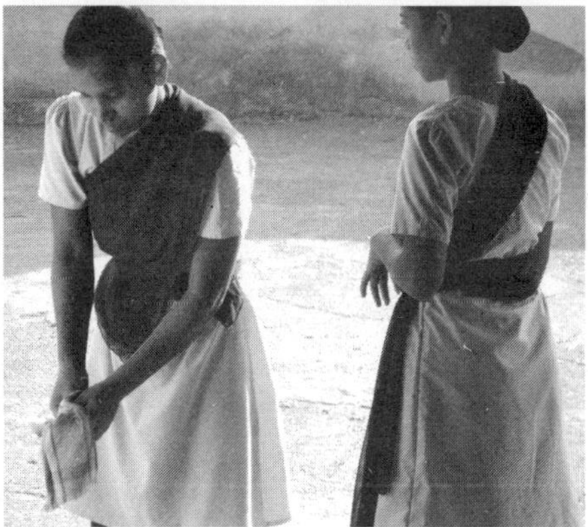

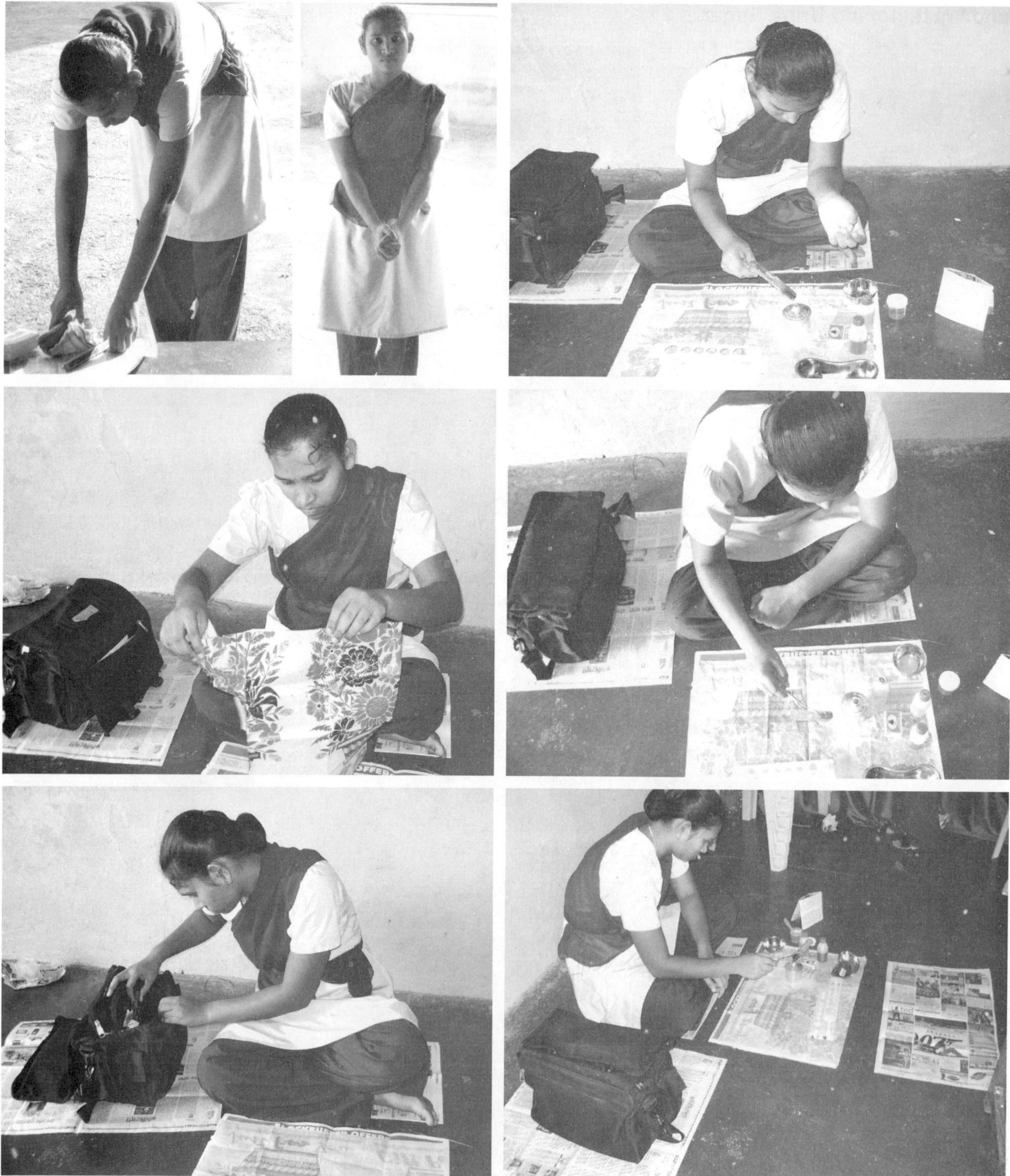

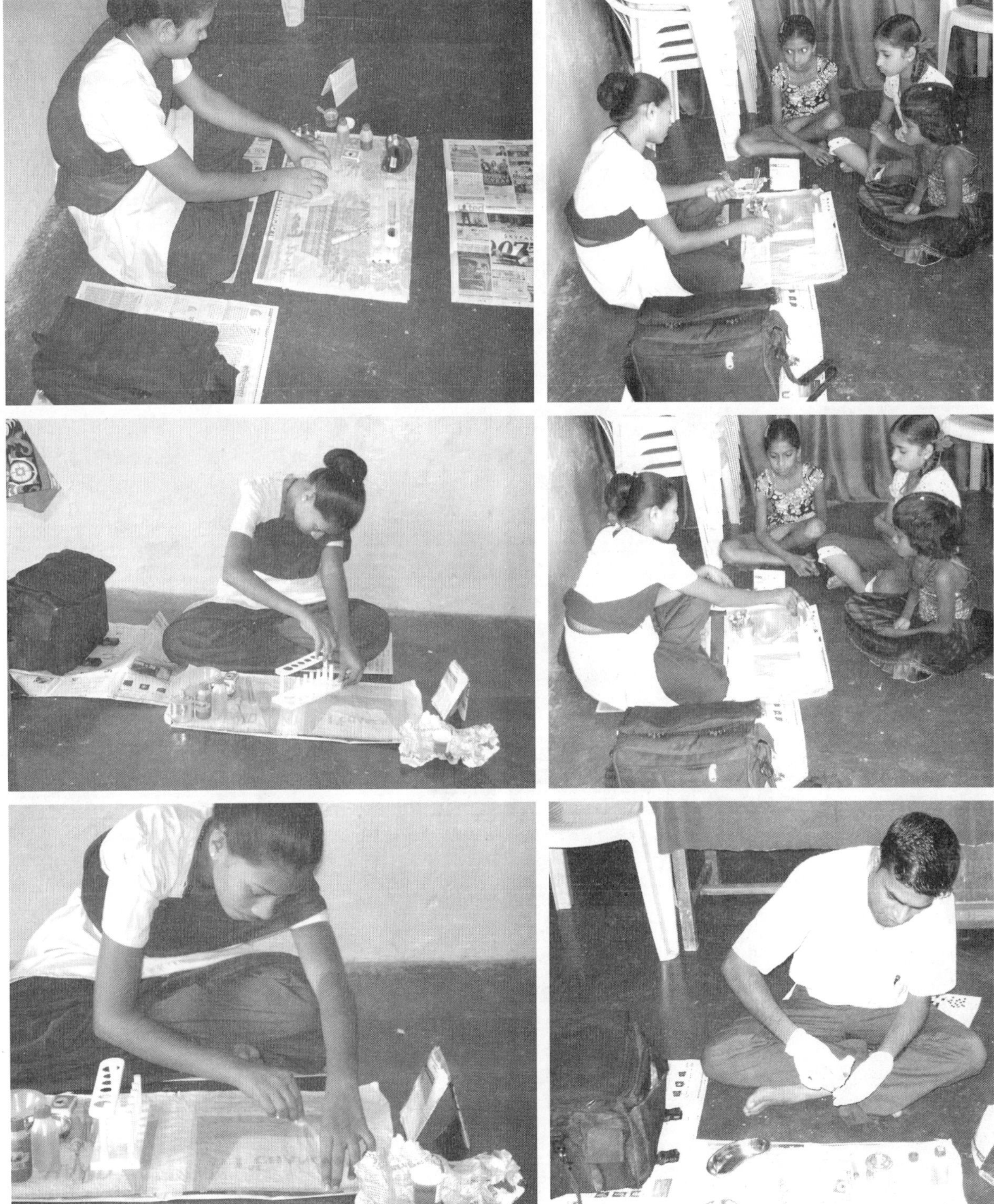

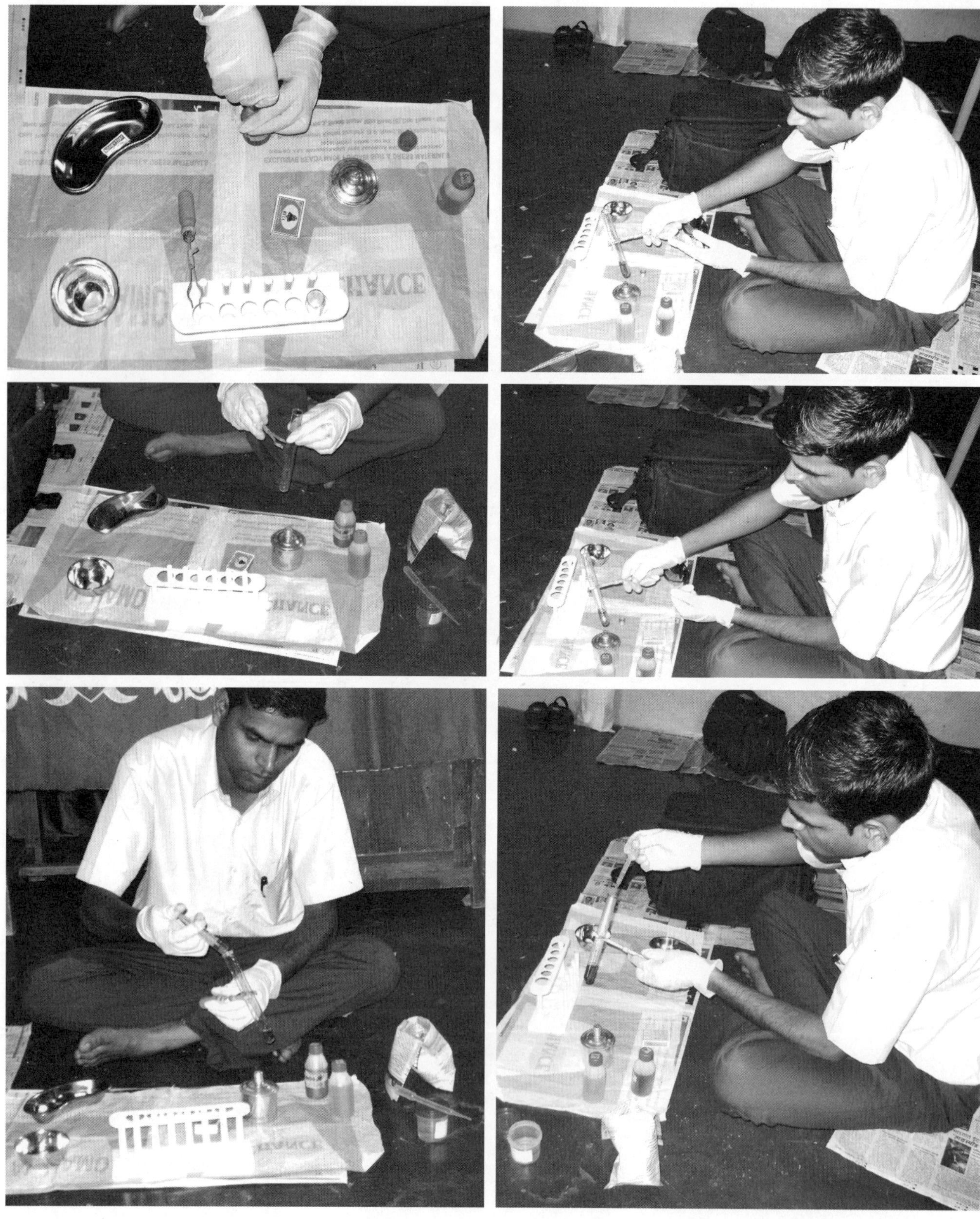

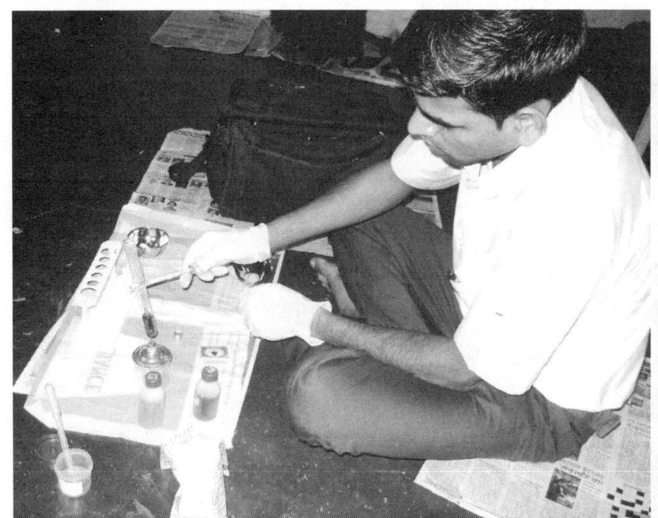

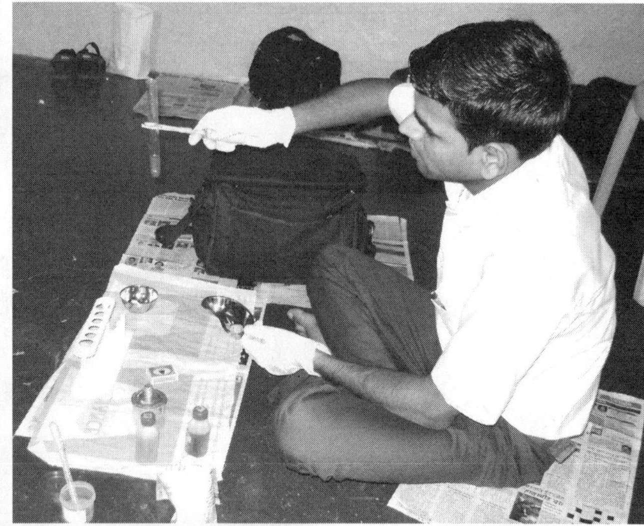

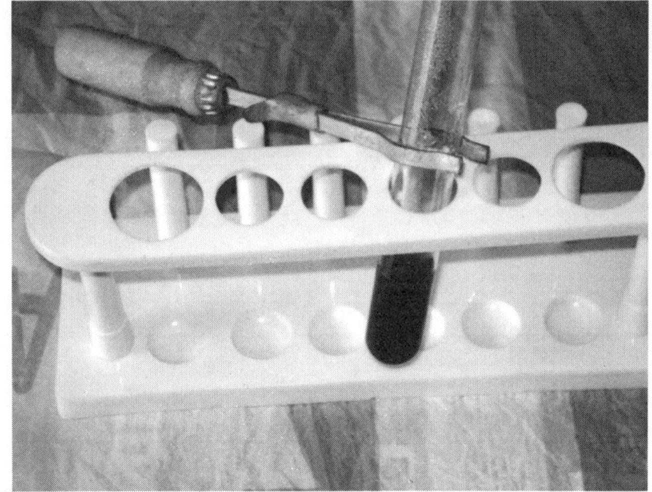

Dressing

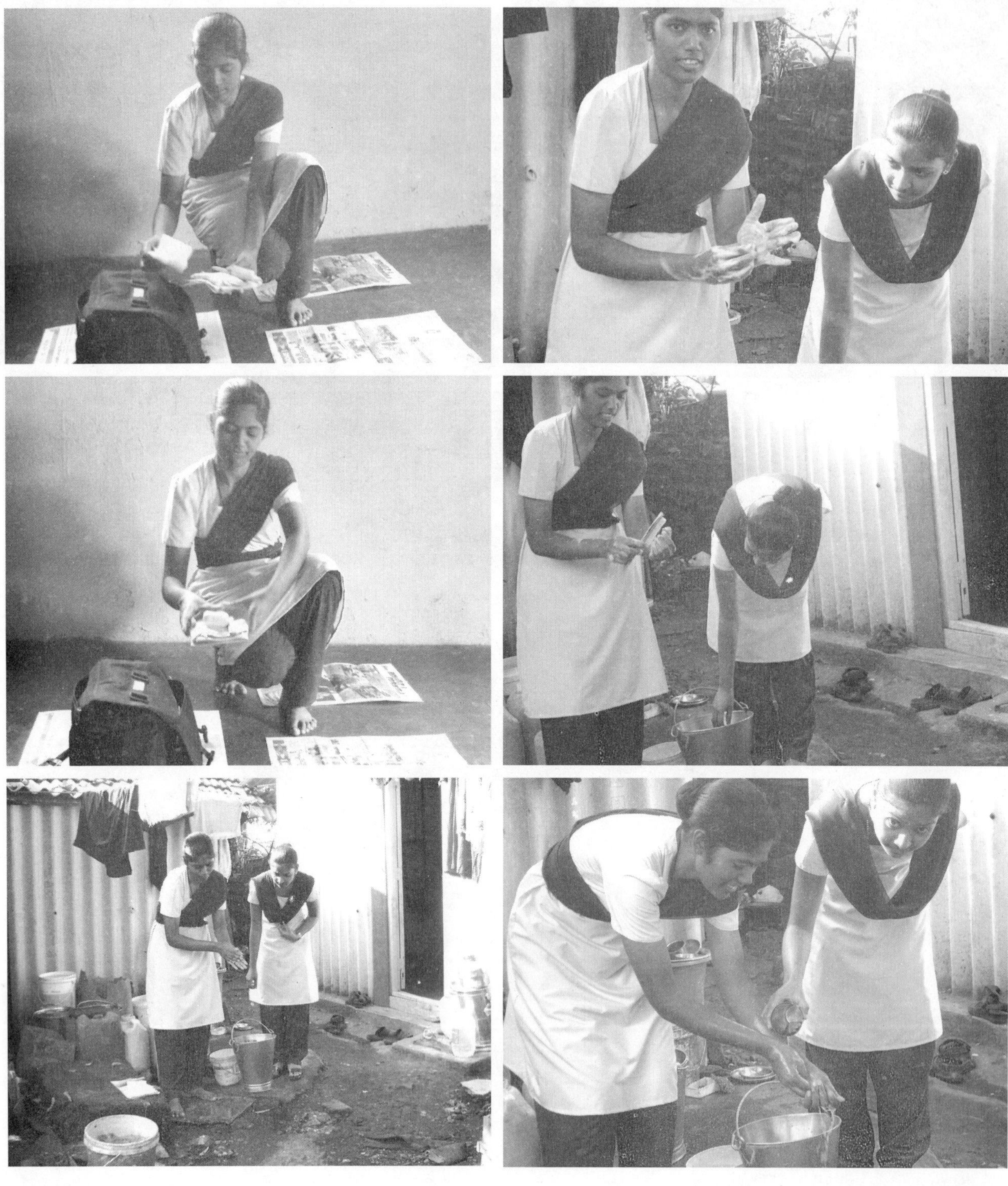

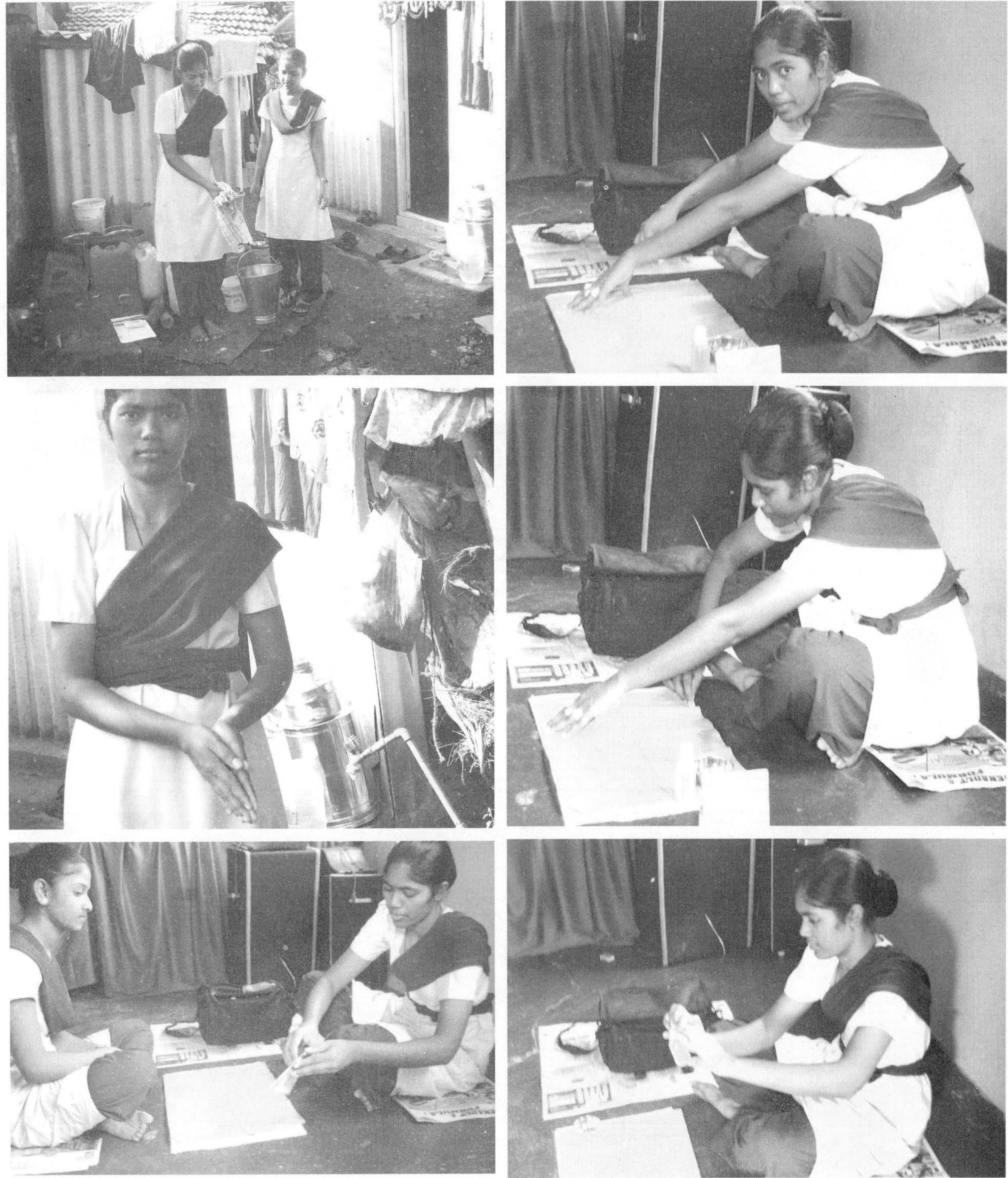

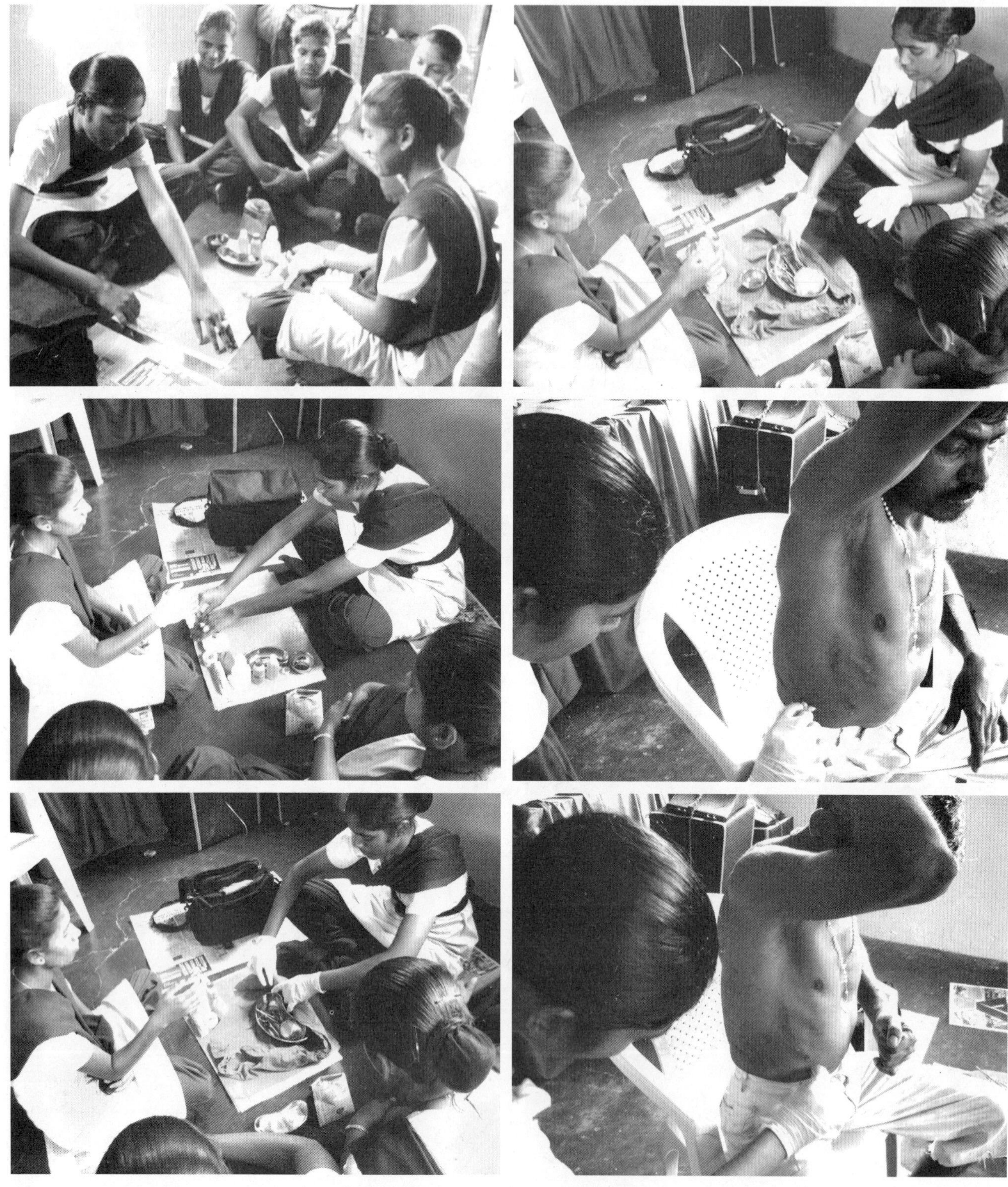

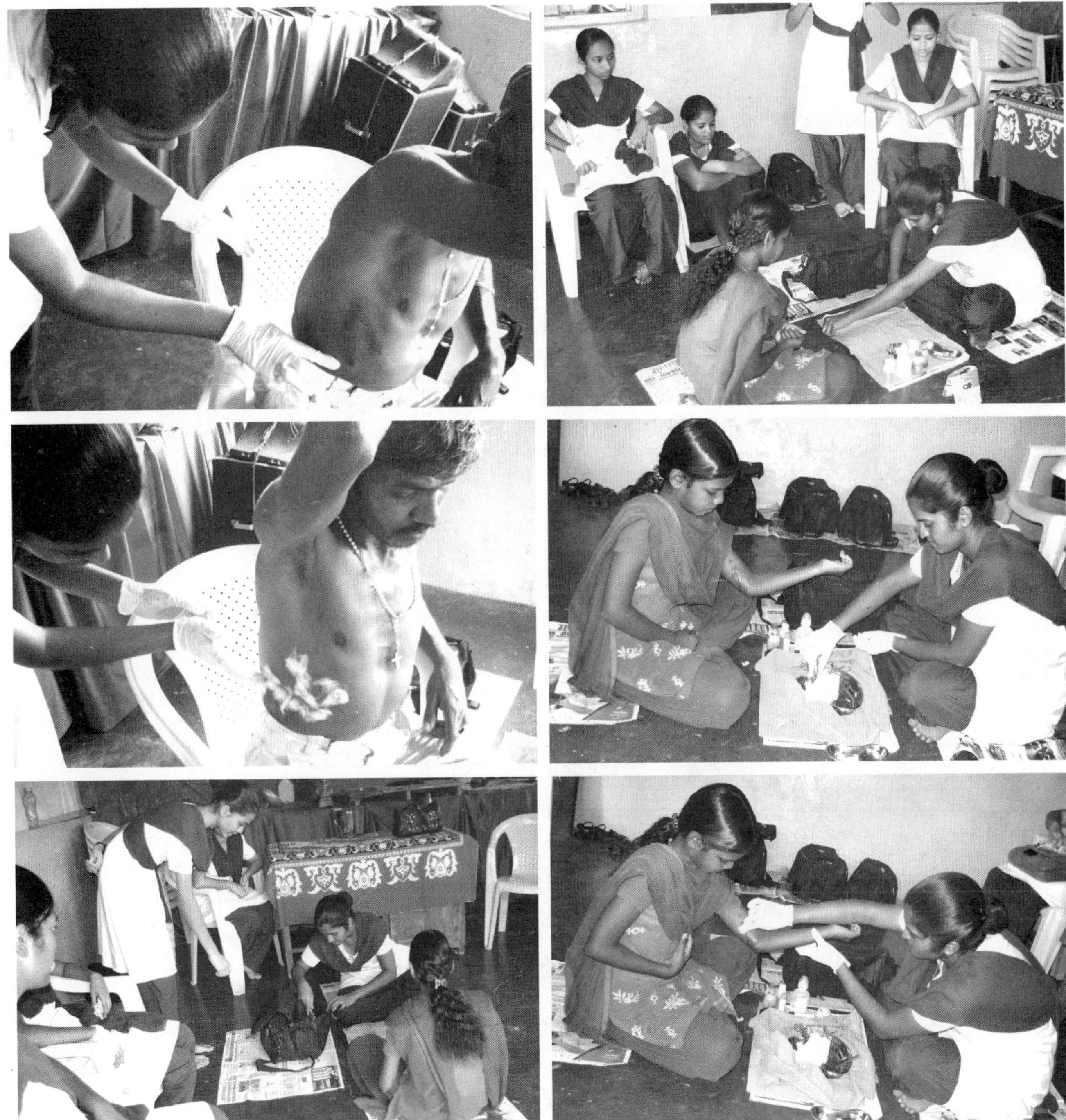

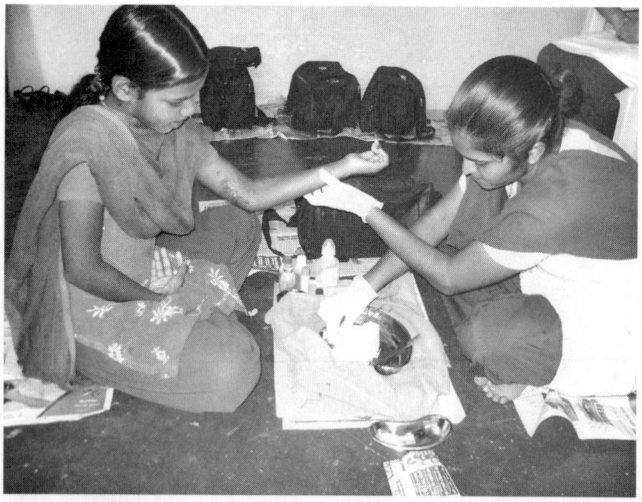

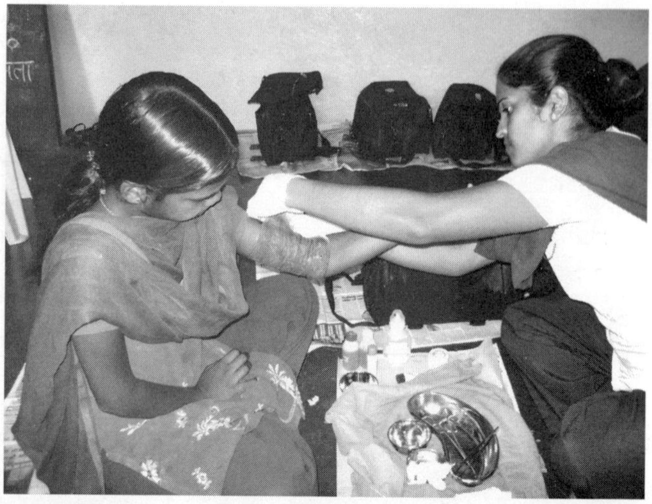

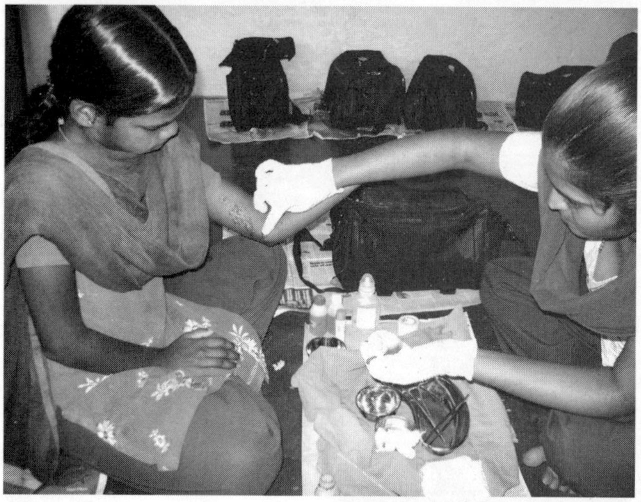

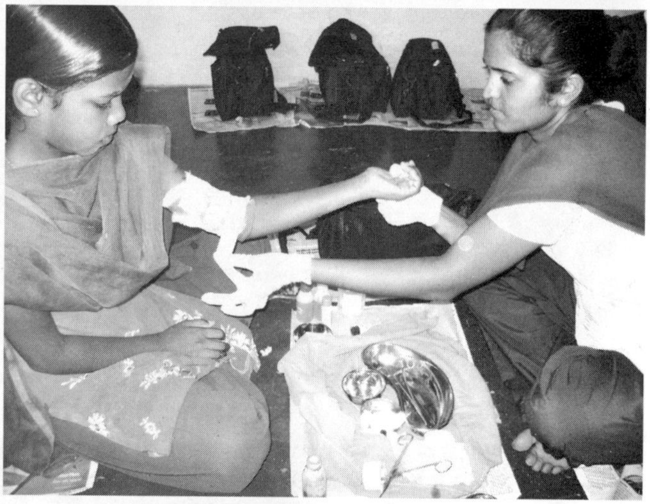

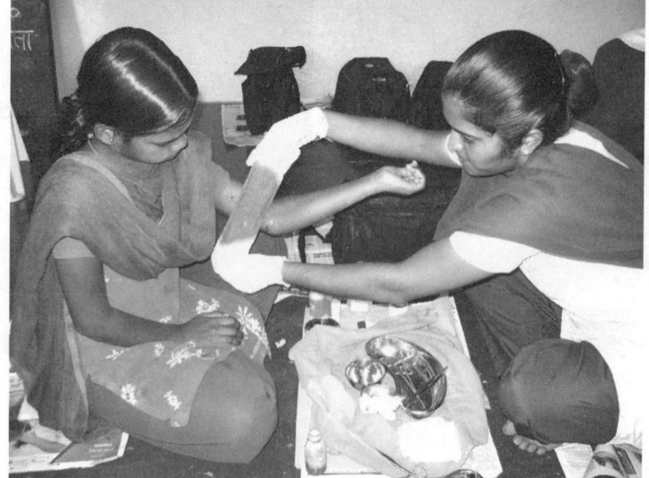

Eye Care

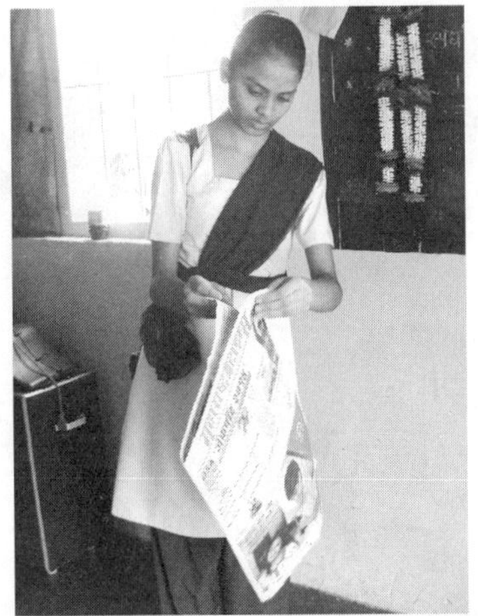

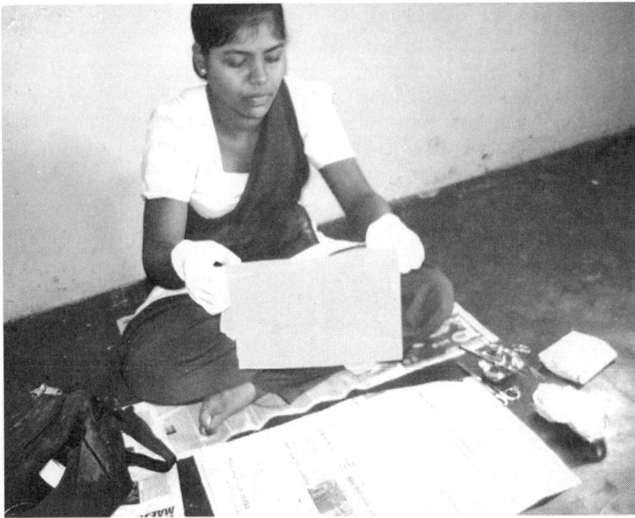

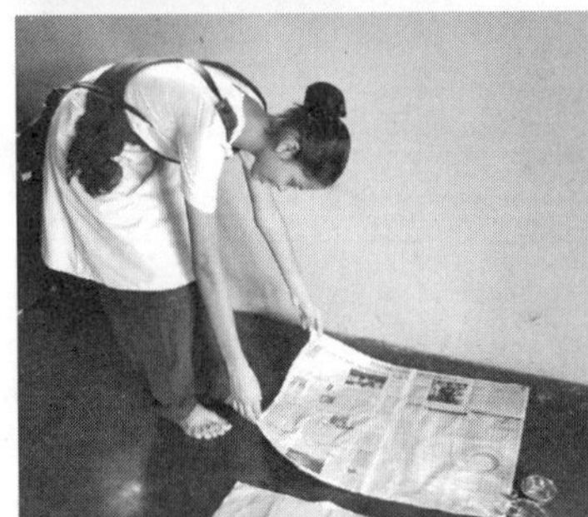

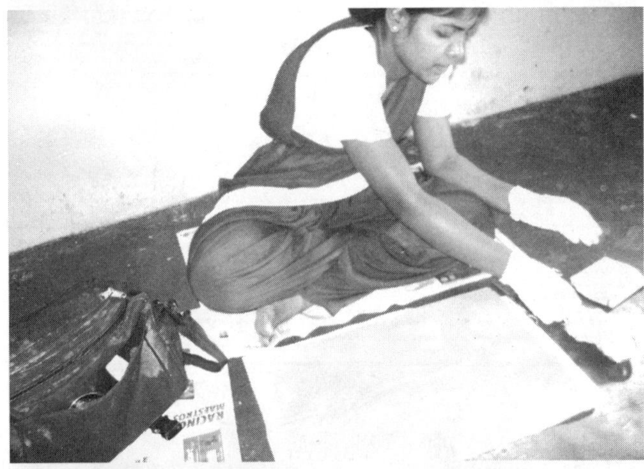

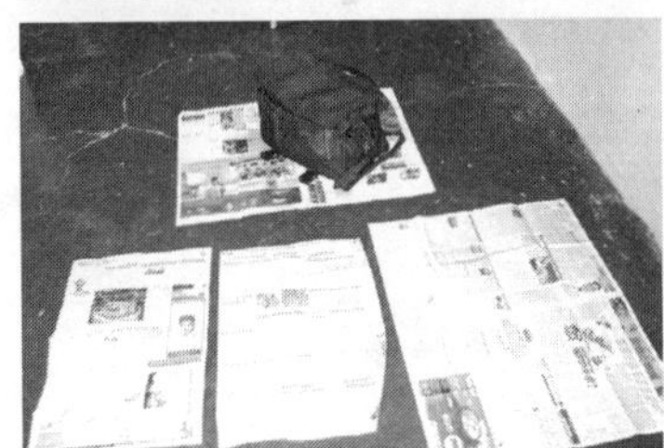

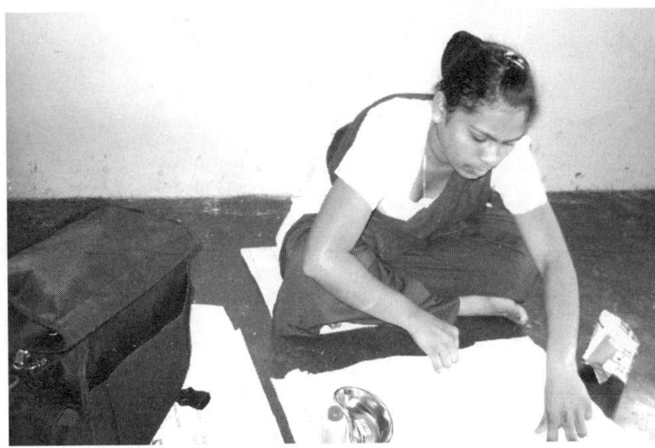

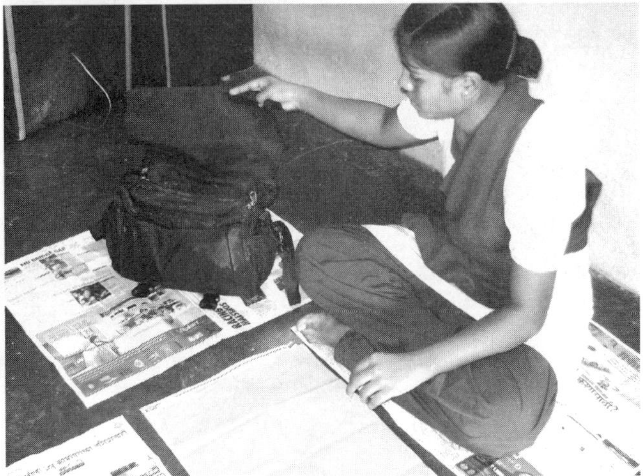

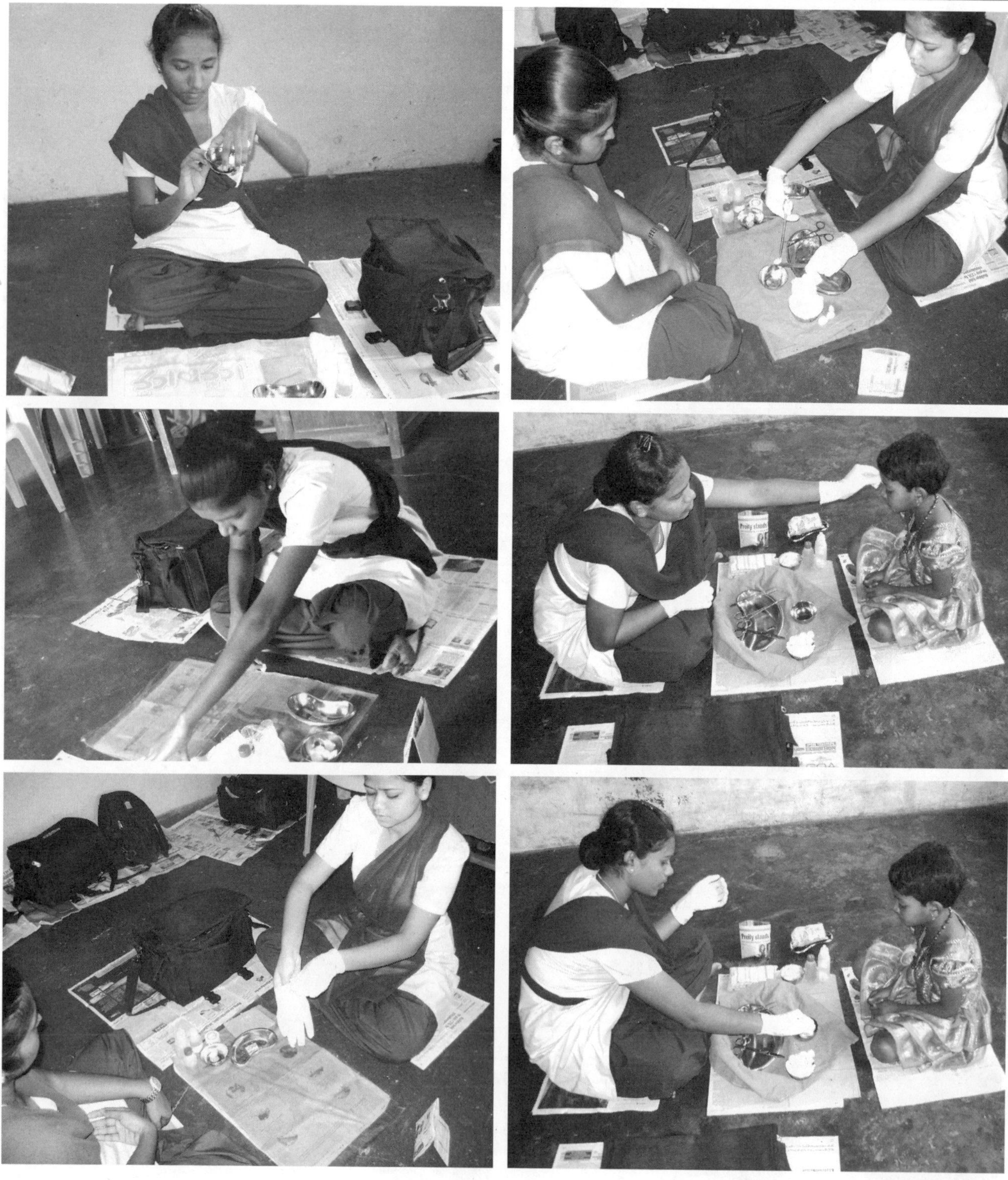

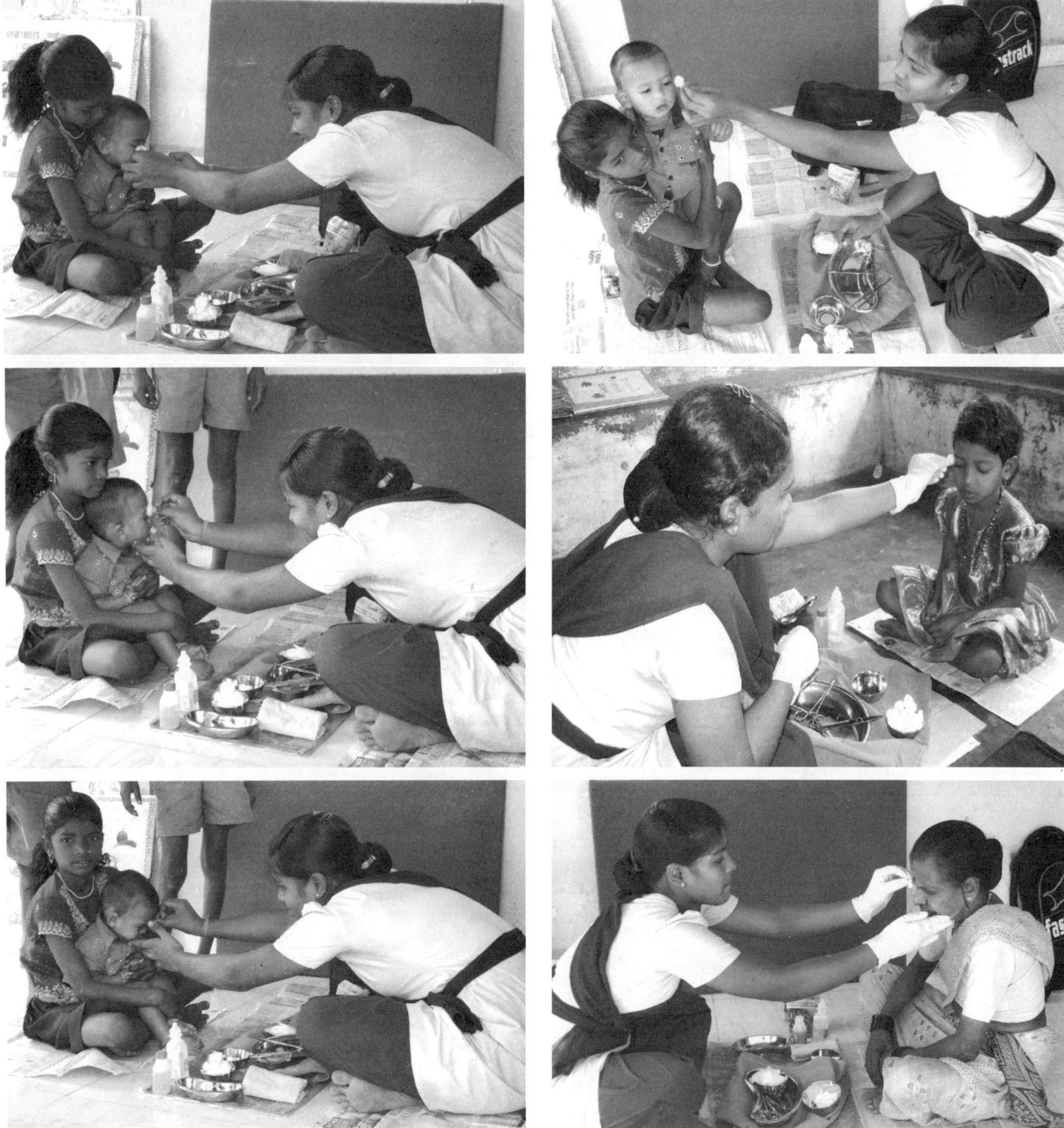

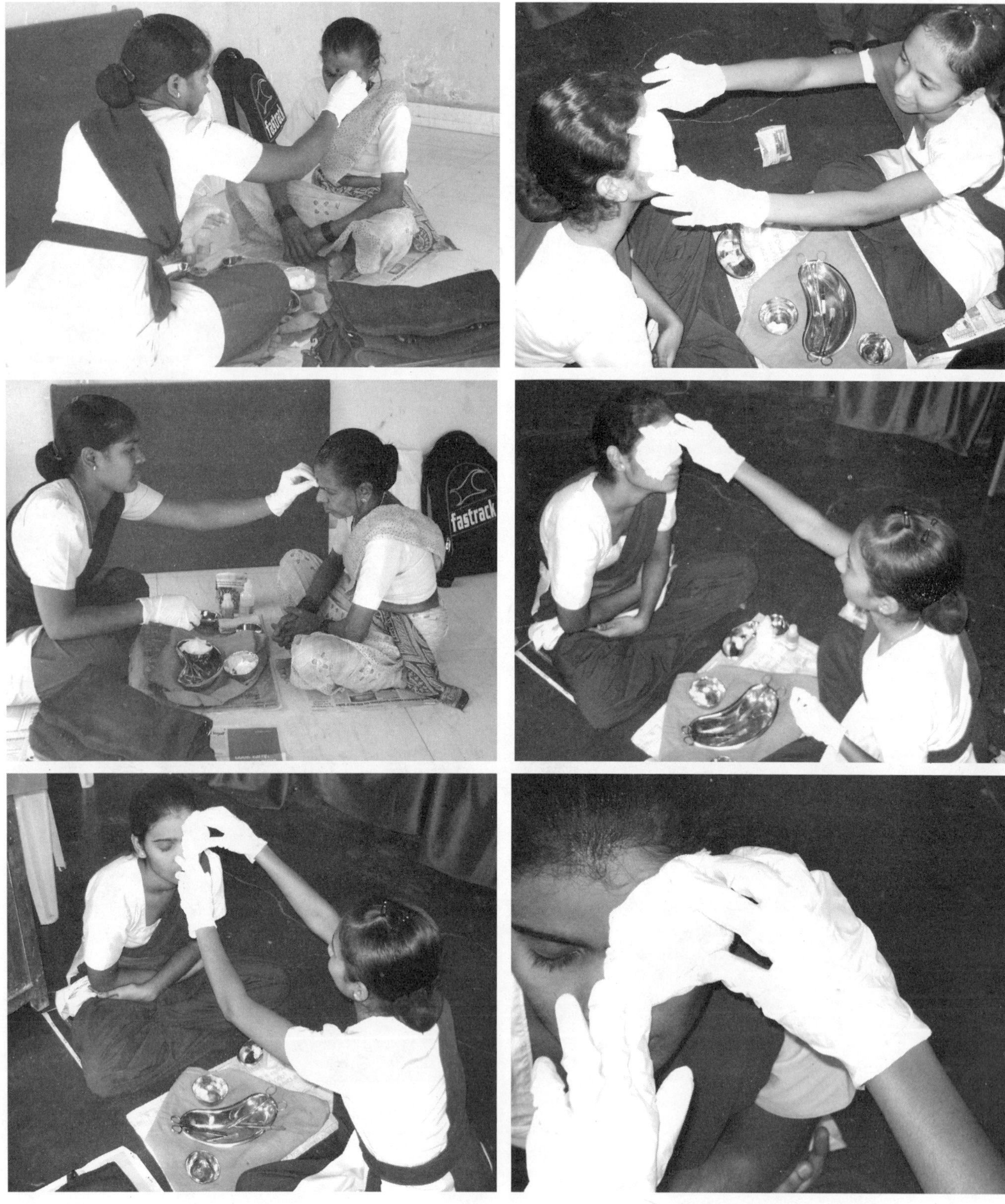
fastrack
fastrack

Bag Technique with TPR

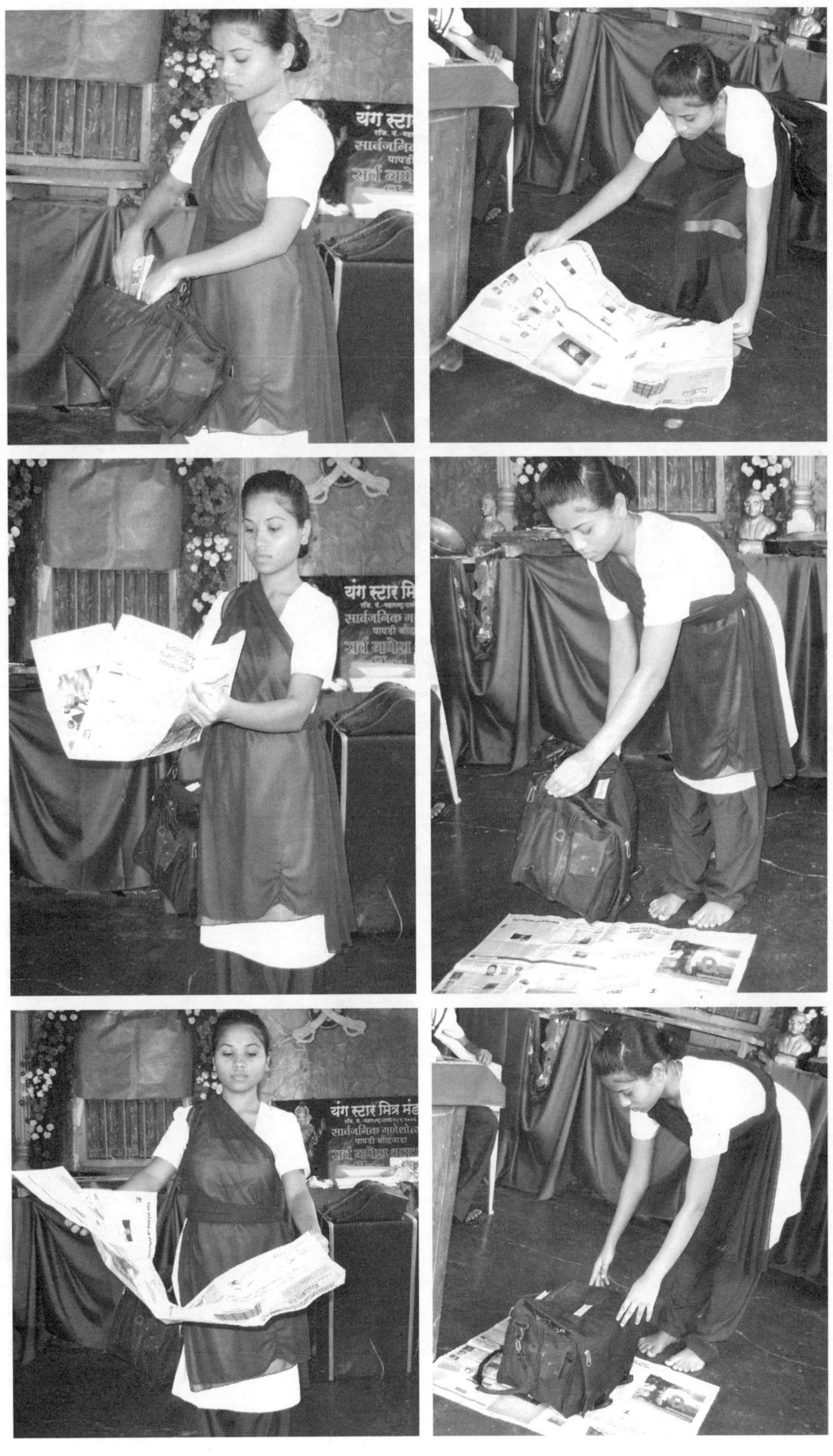

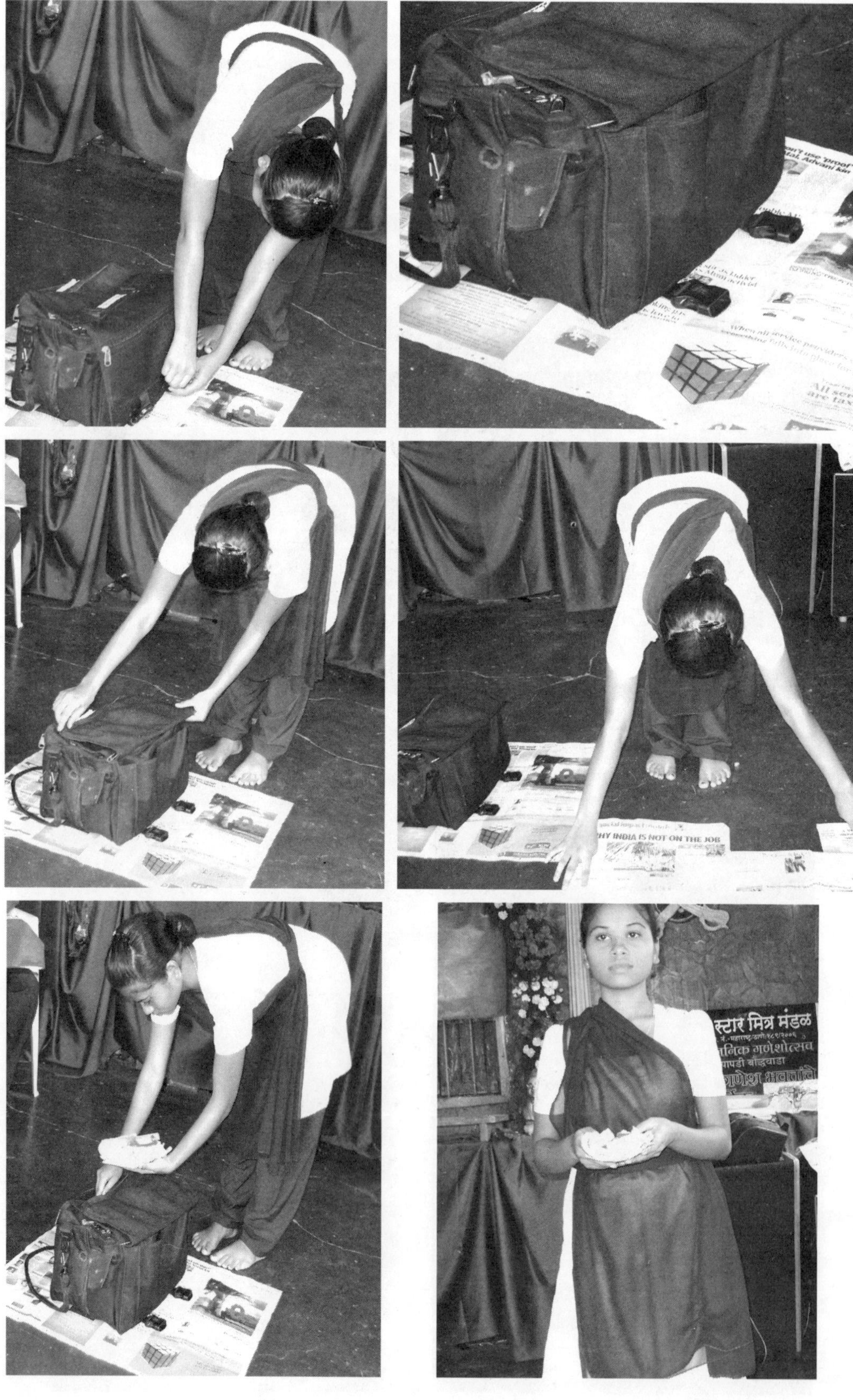
HY INDIA IS NOT ON THE JOB
स्टार मित्र मंडळ

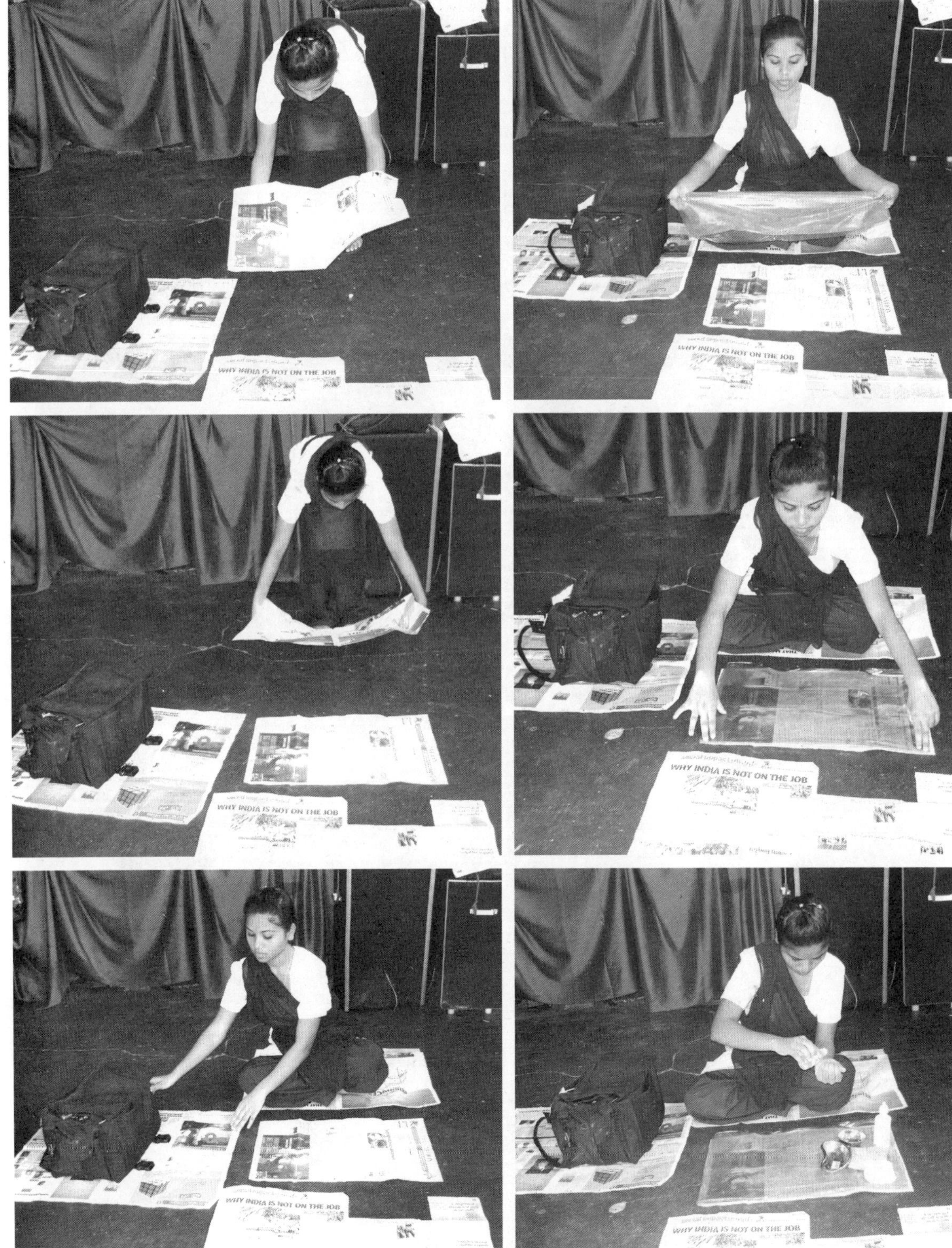
WHY INDIA IS NOT ON THE JOB

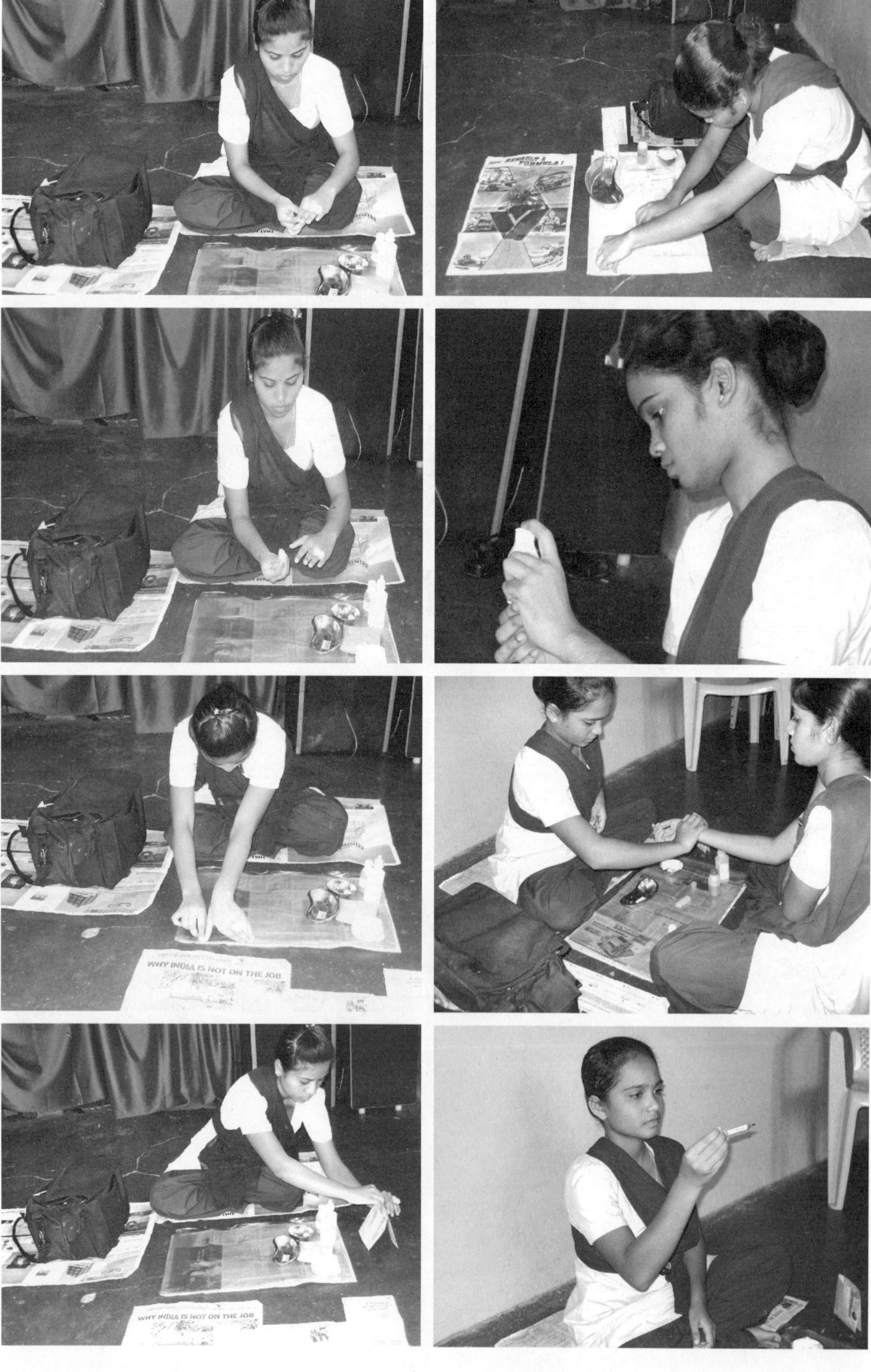
WHY INDIA IS NOT ON THE JOB
WHY INDIA IS NOT ON THE JOB

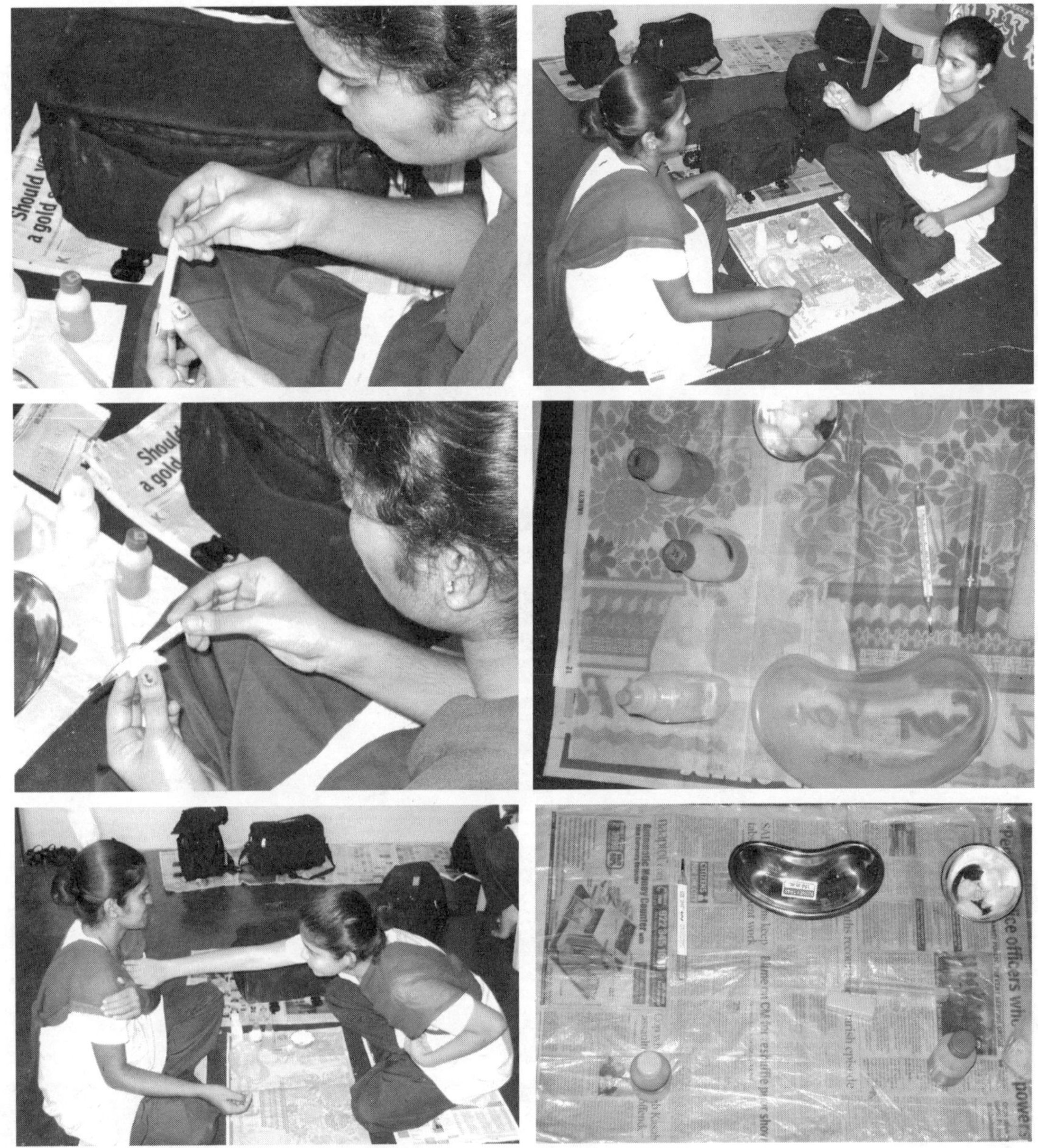

Baby—Oil Bath

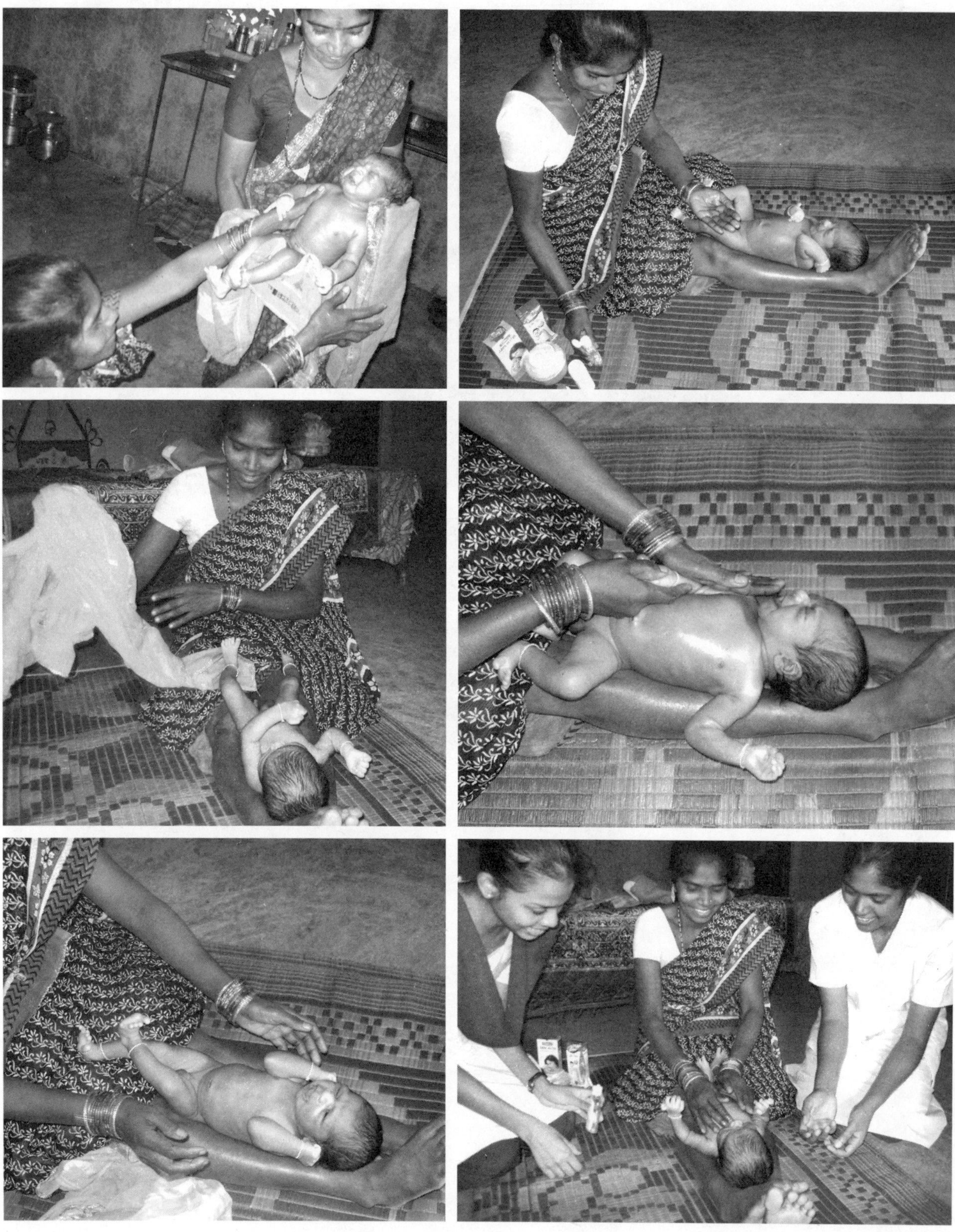

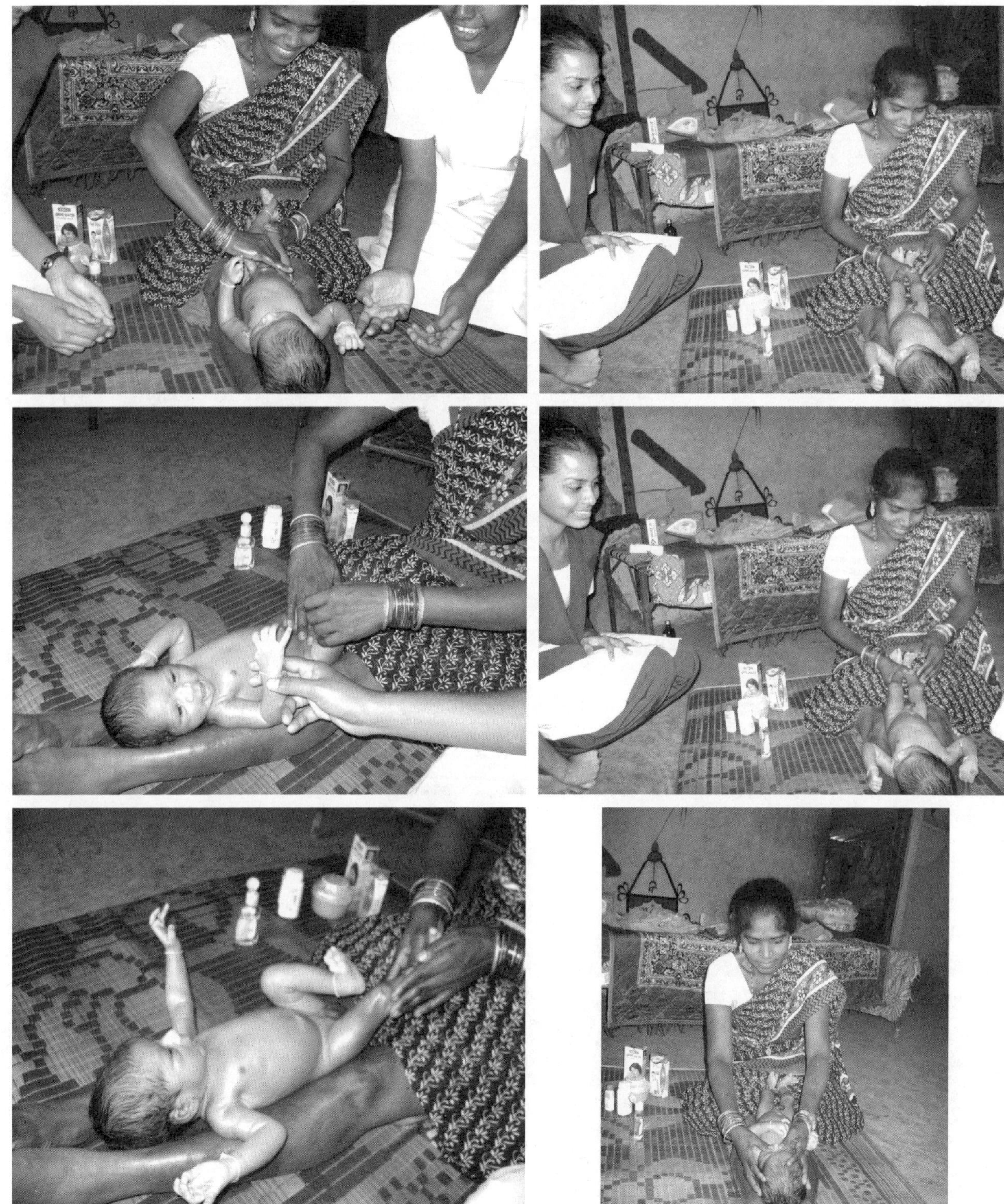

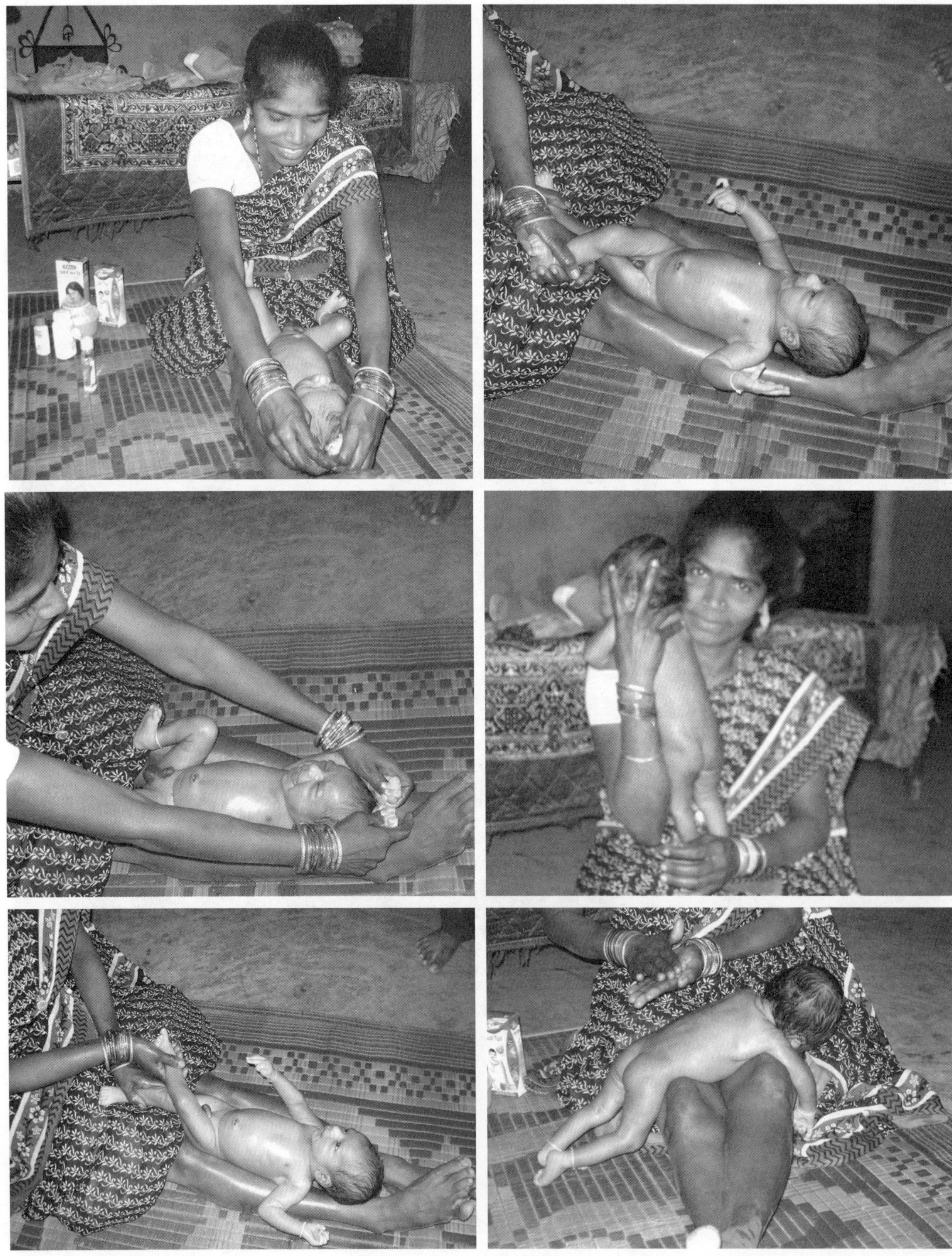

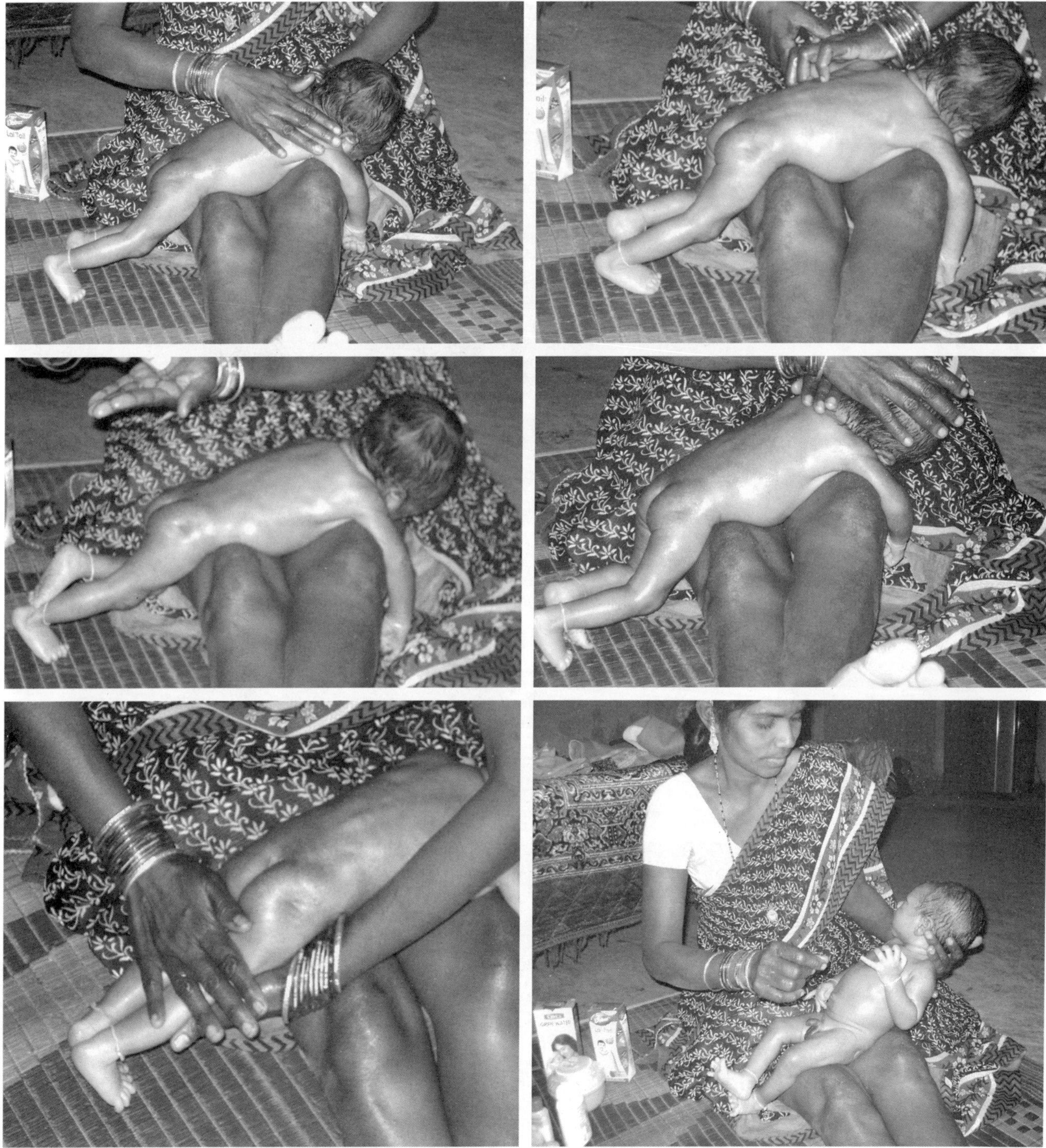

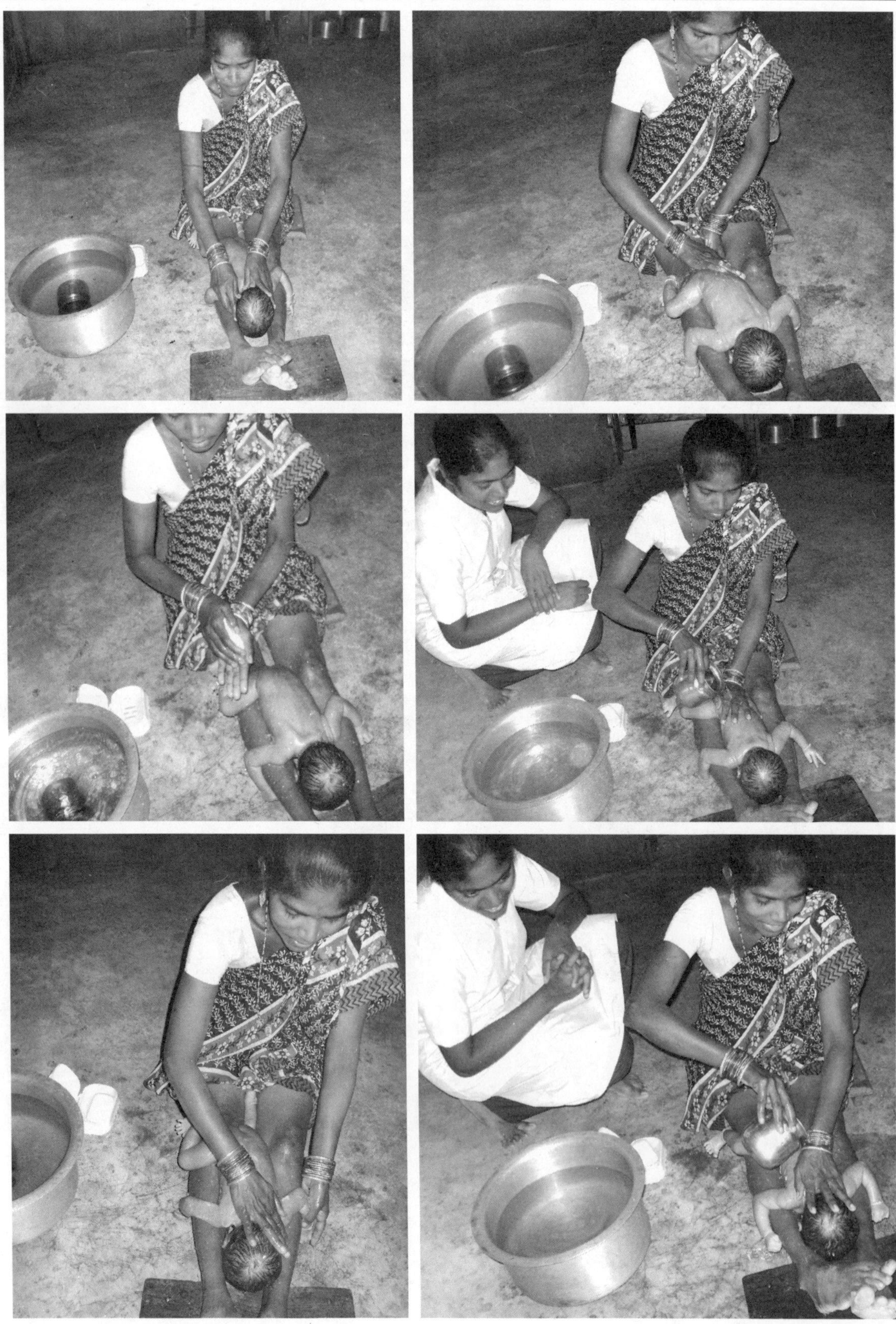

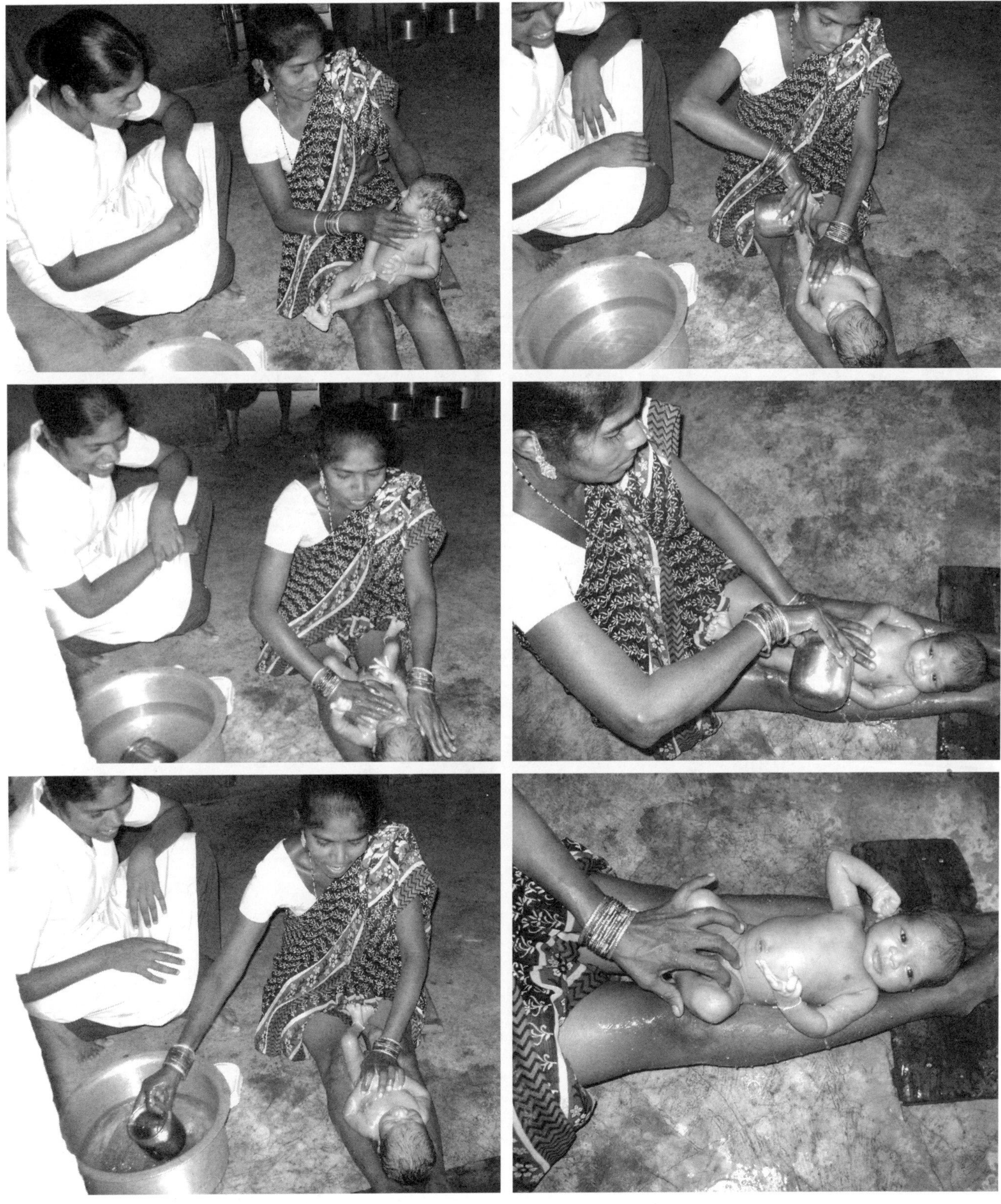

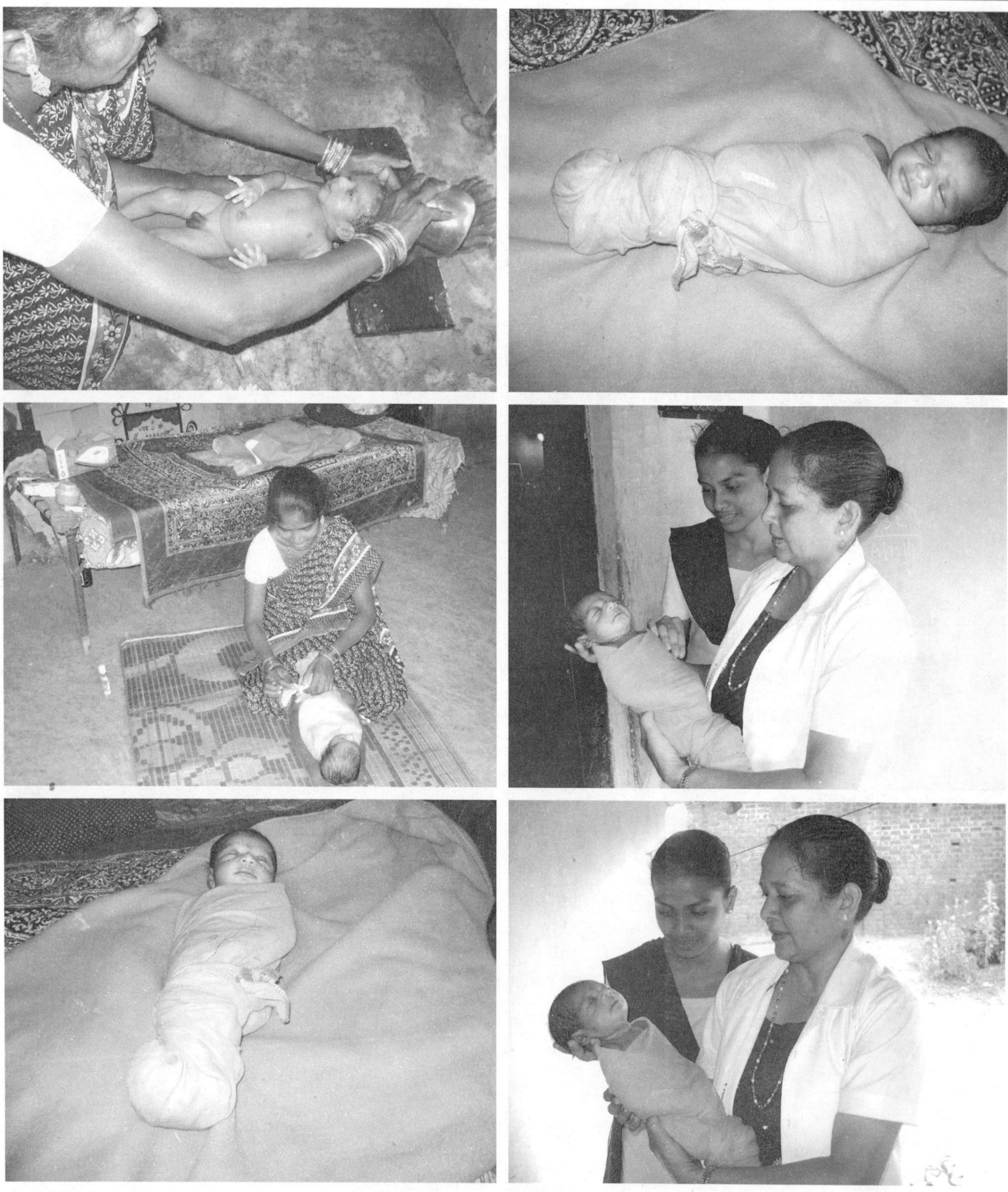

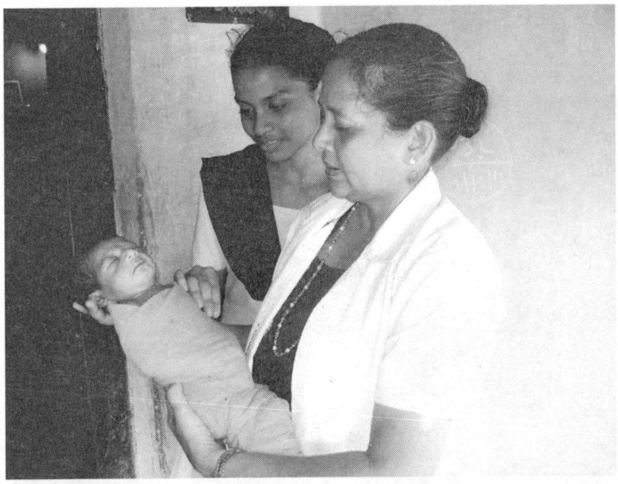

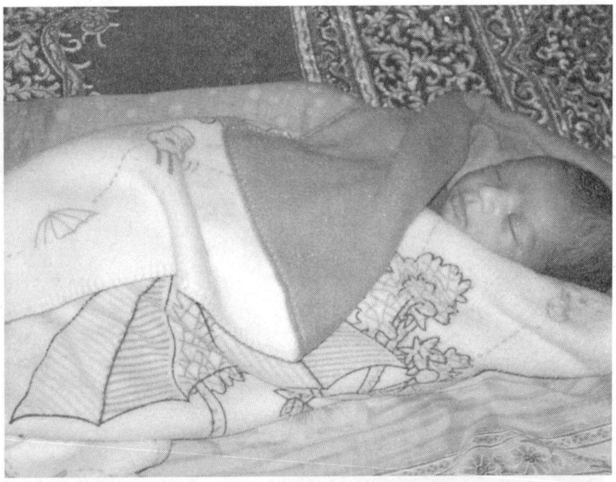

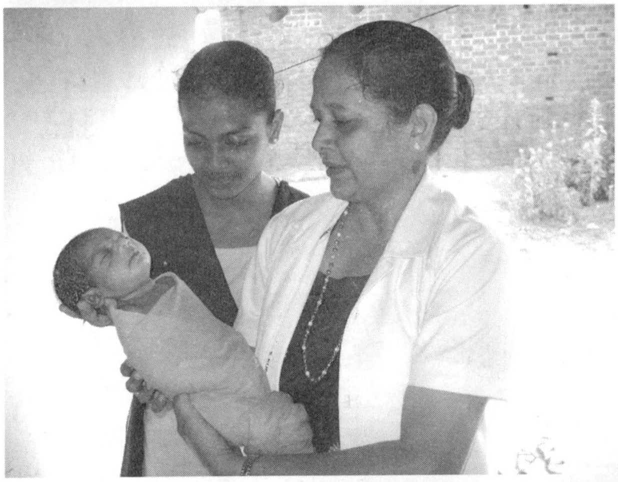

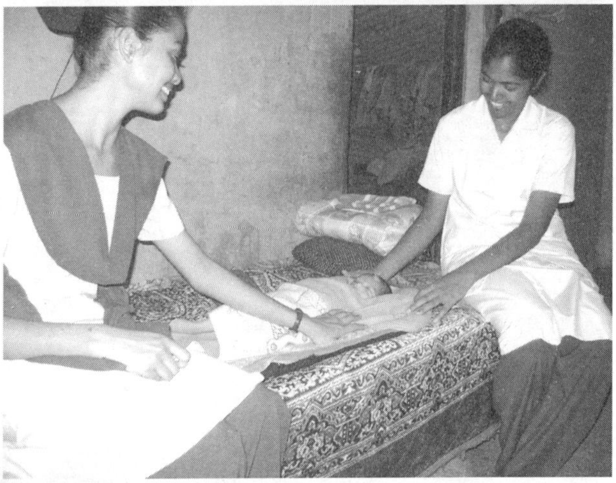

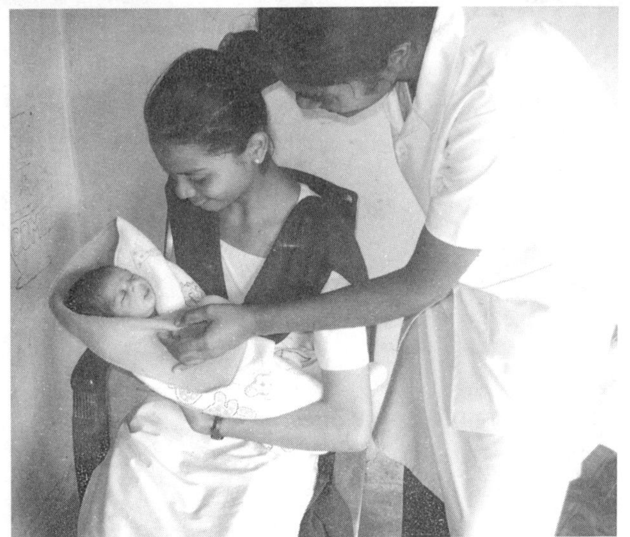

Baby—Leg Bath

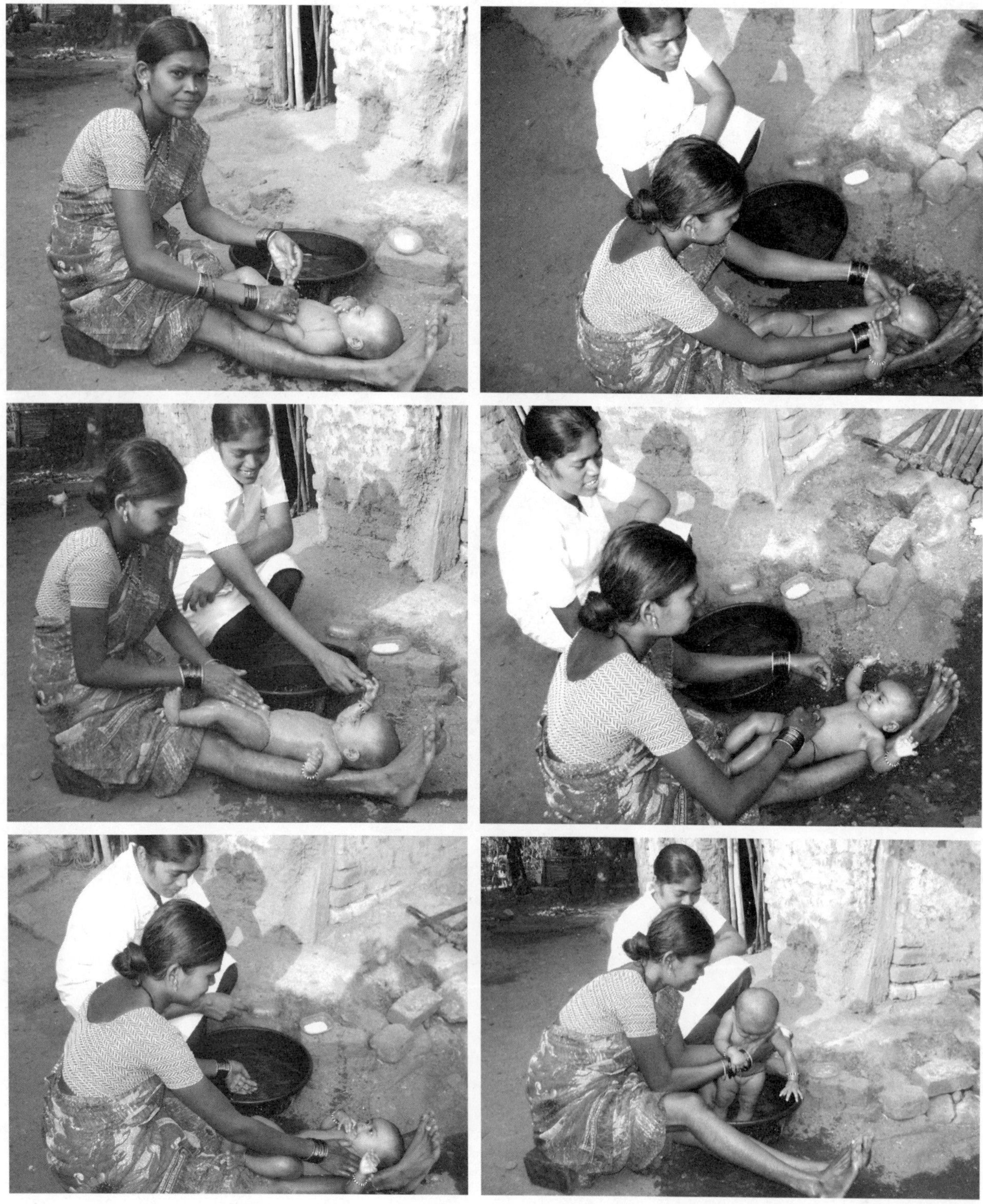

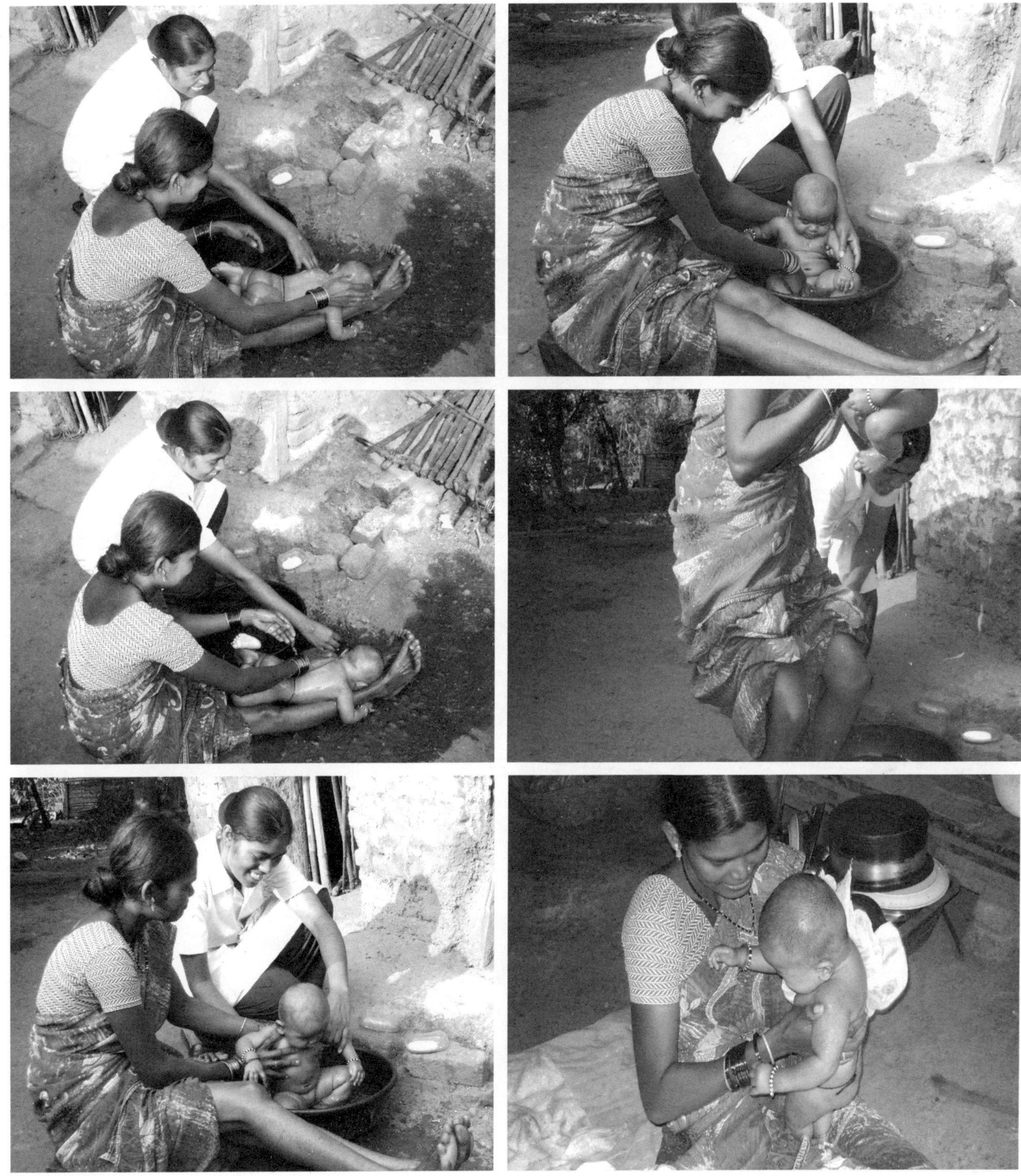

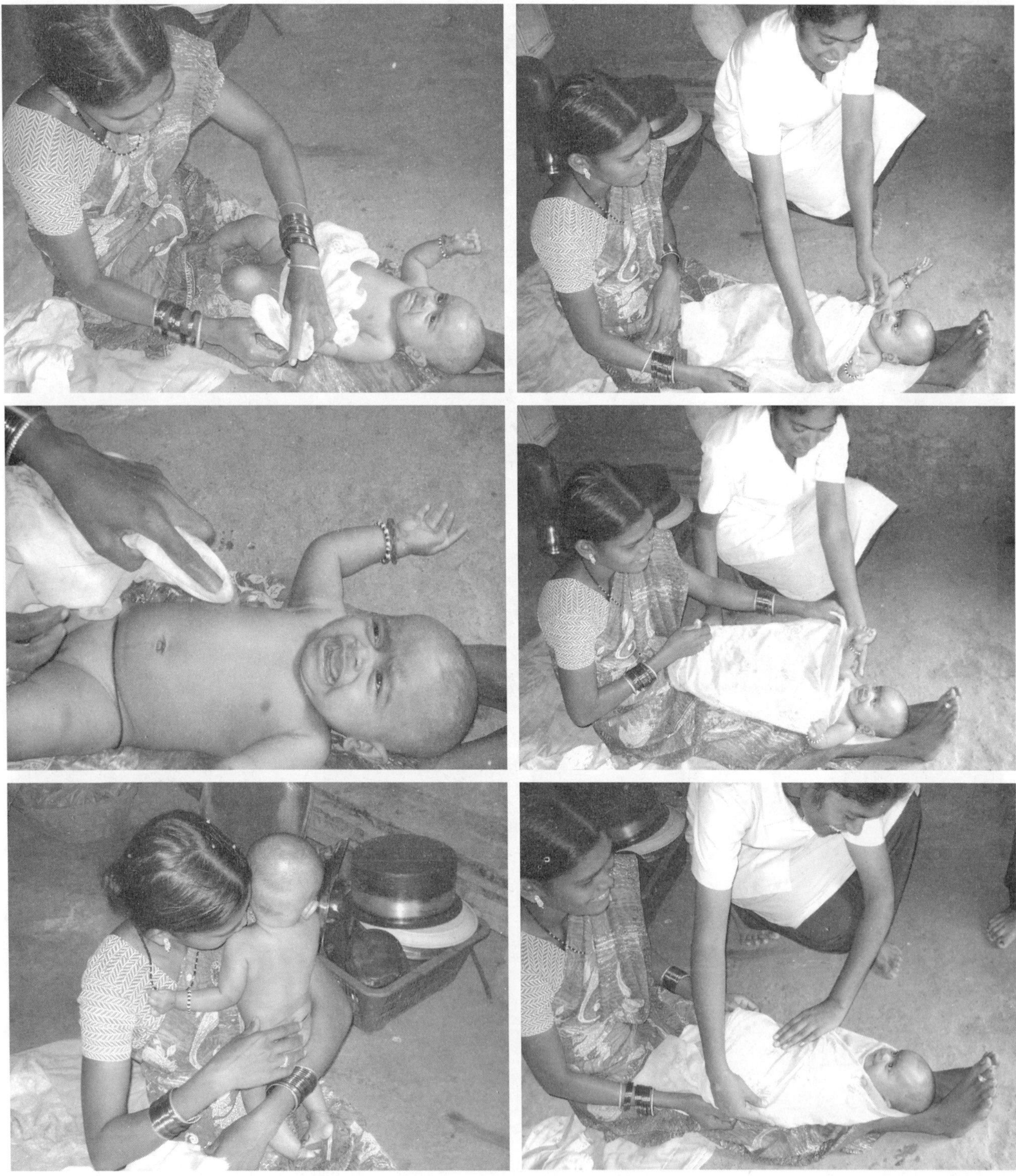

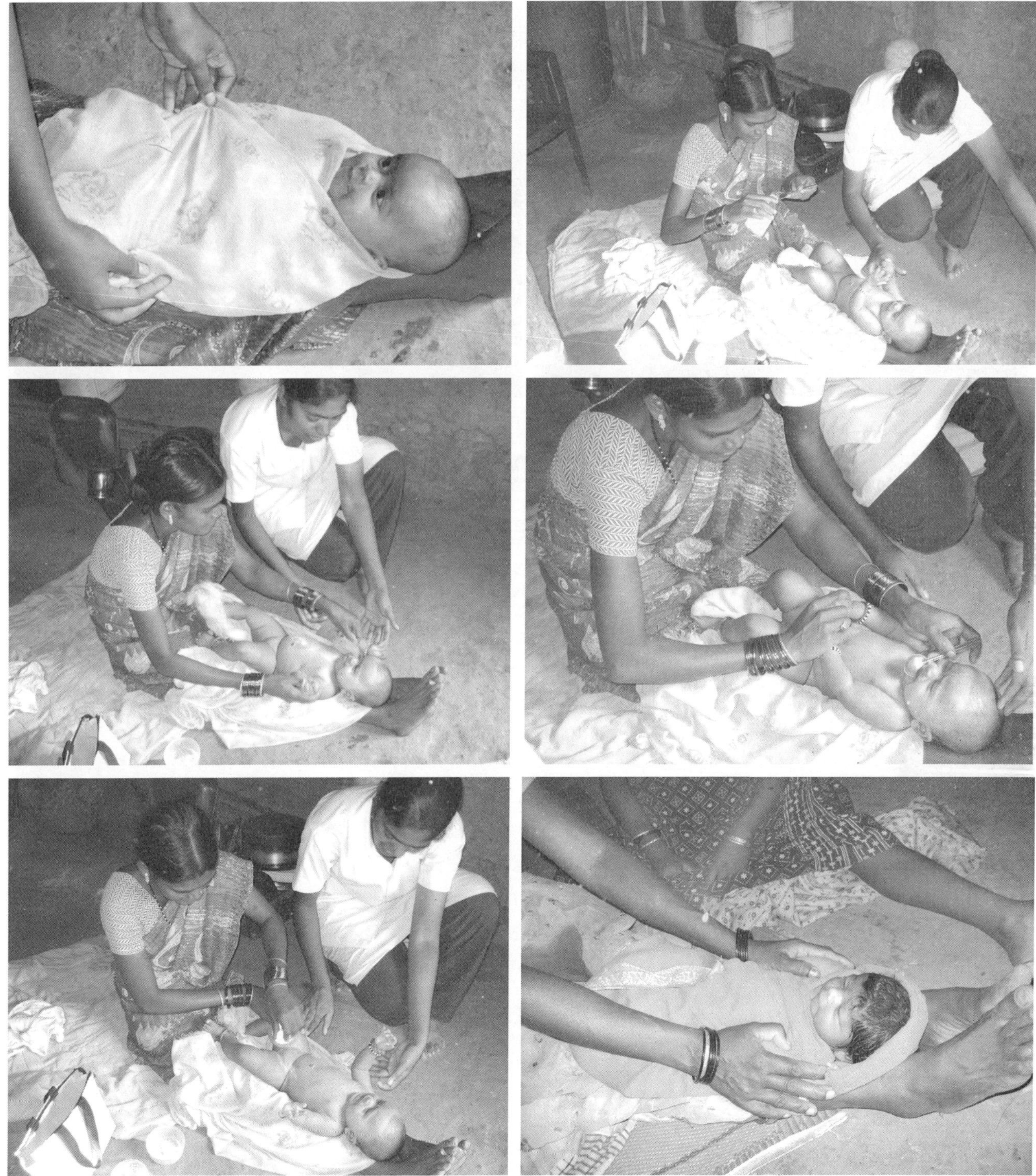

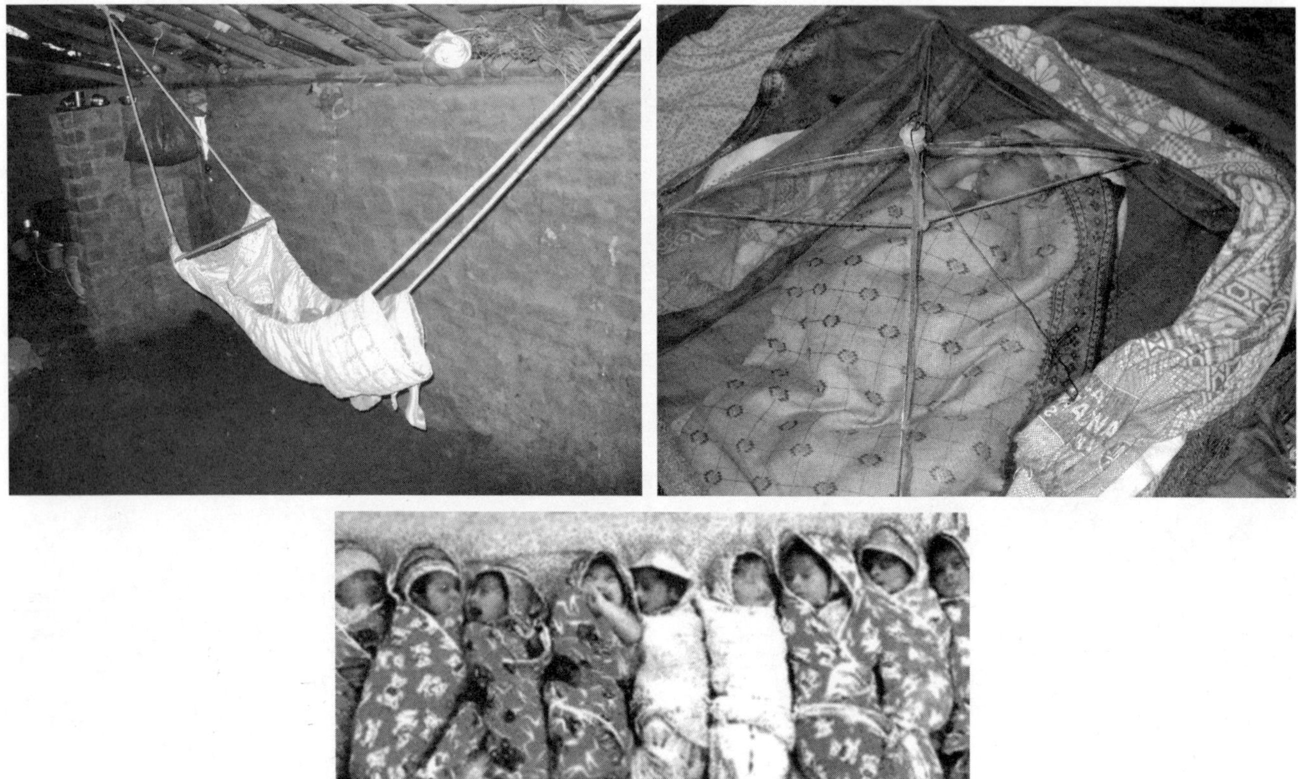

Baby—Tub Bath

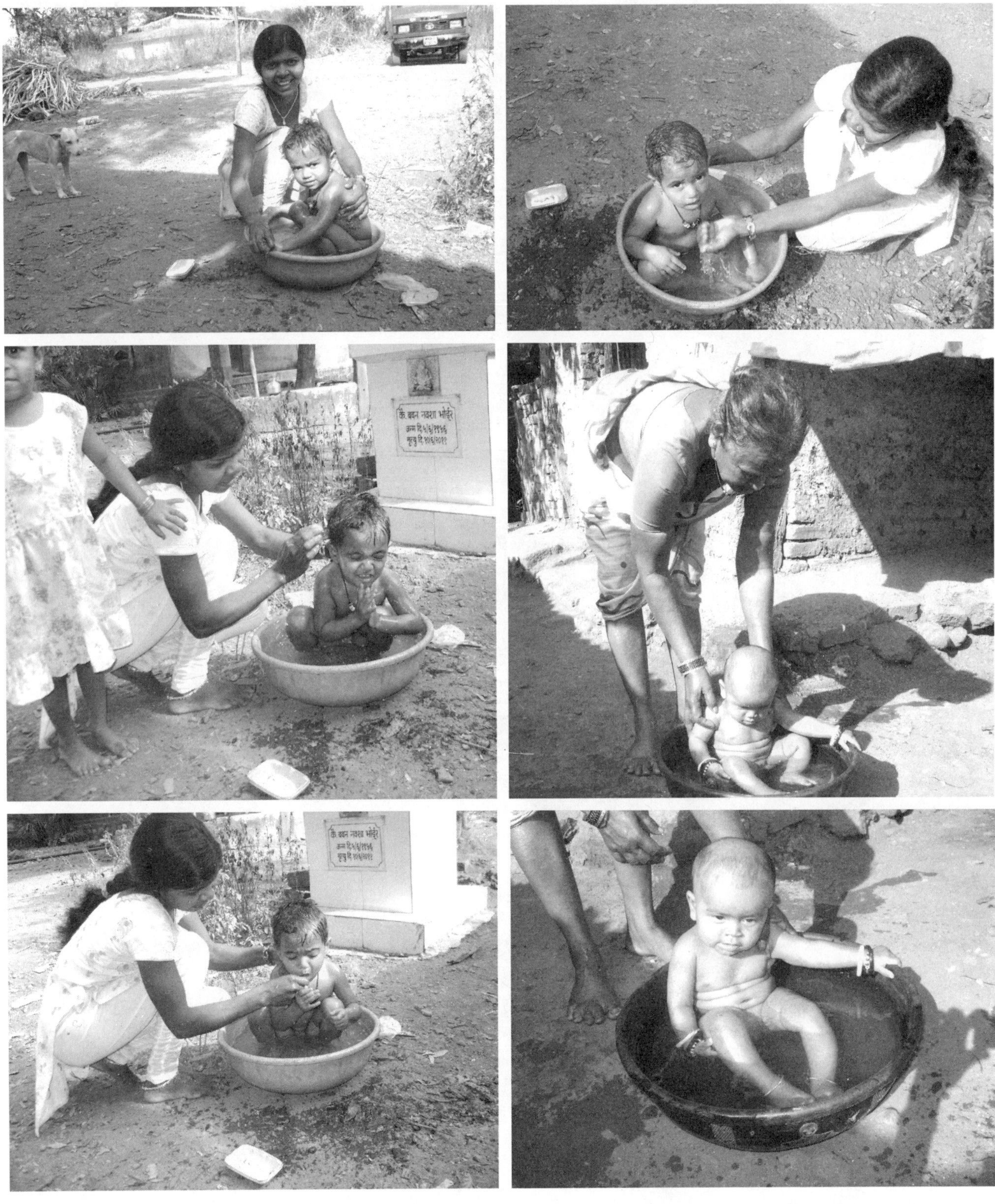

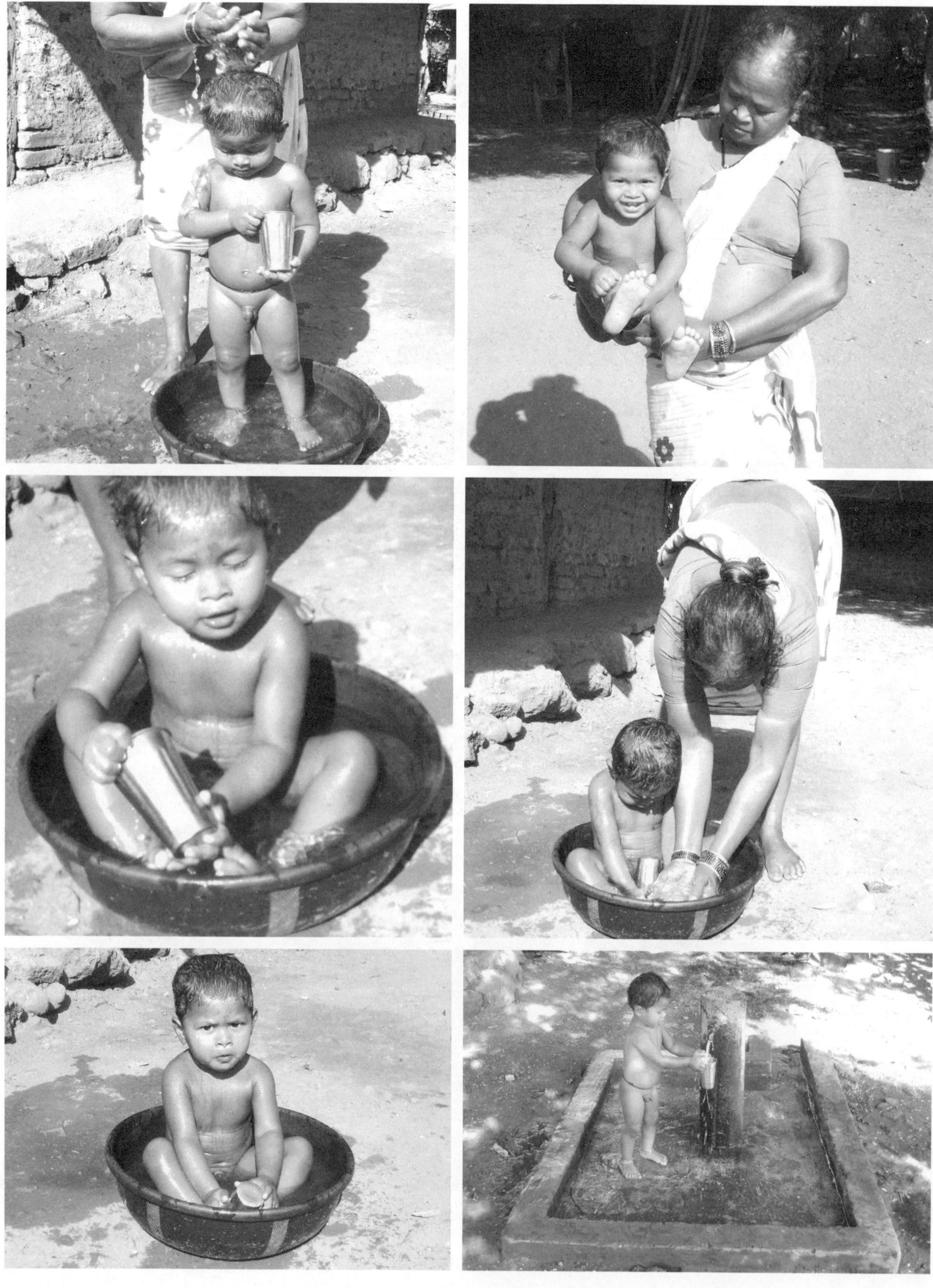

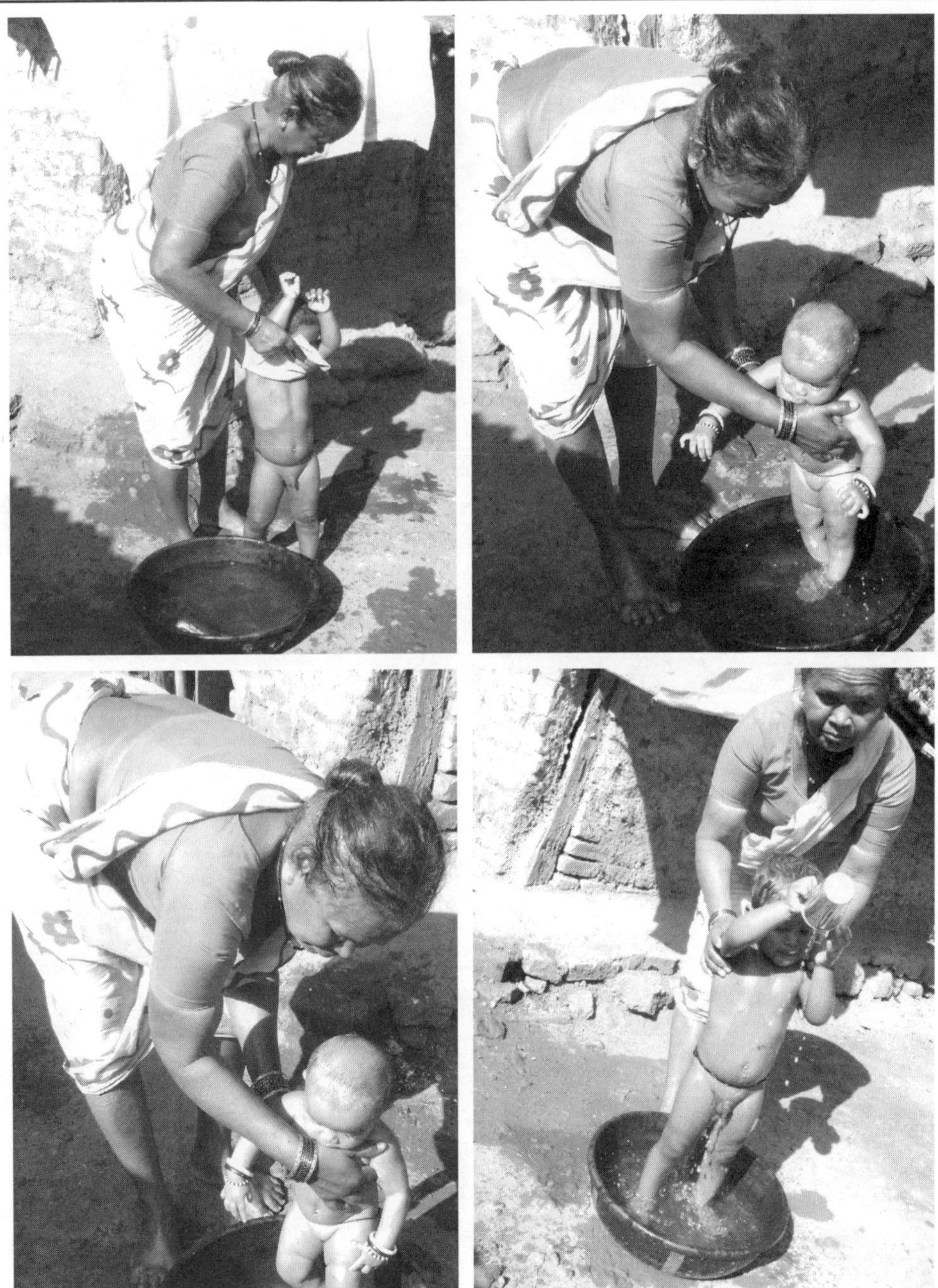

ICDS

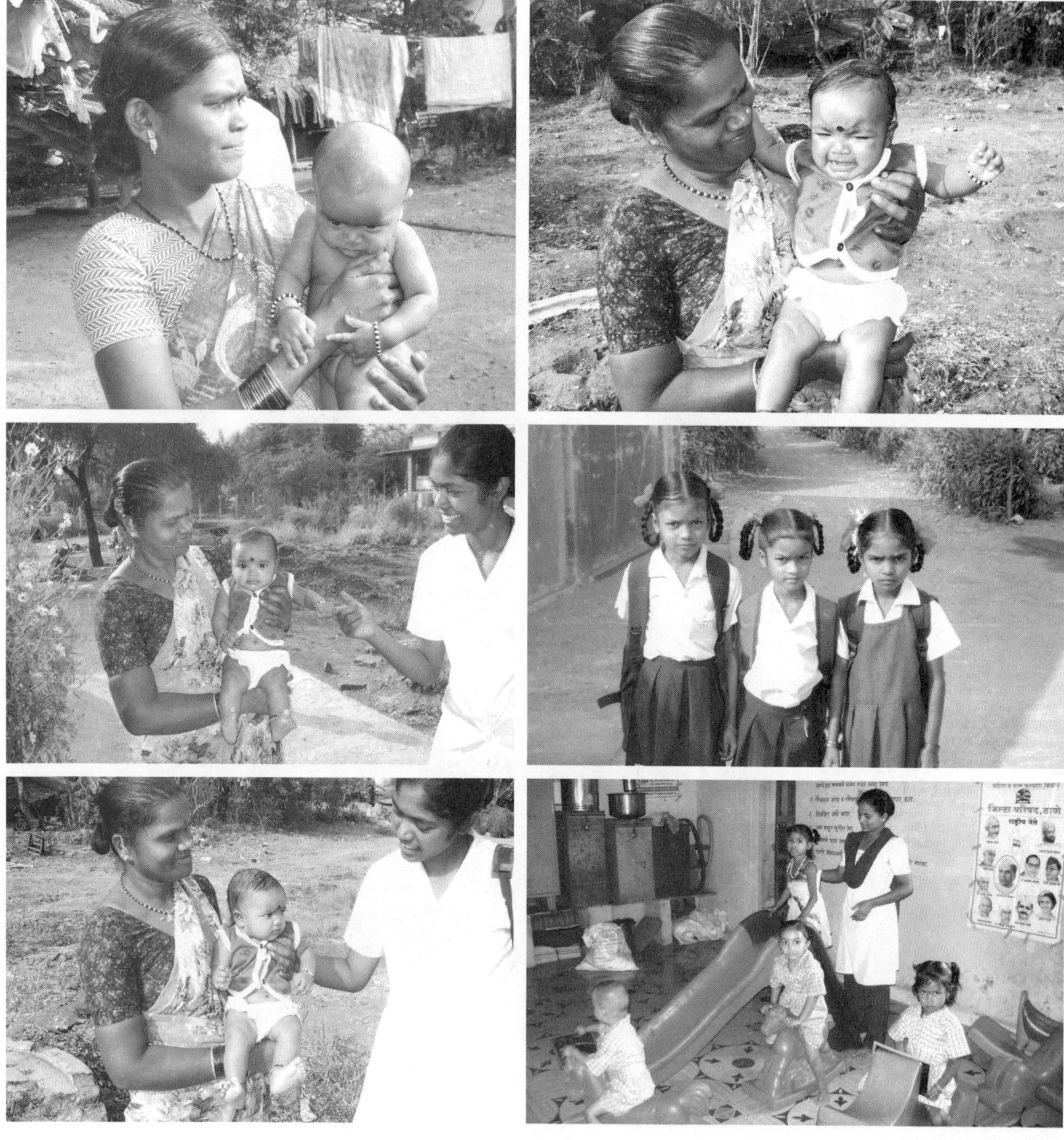

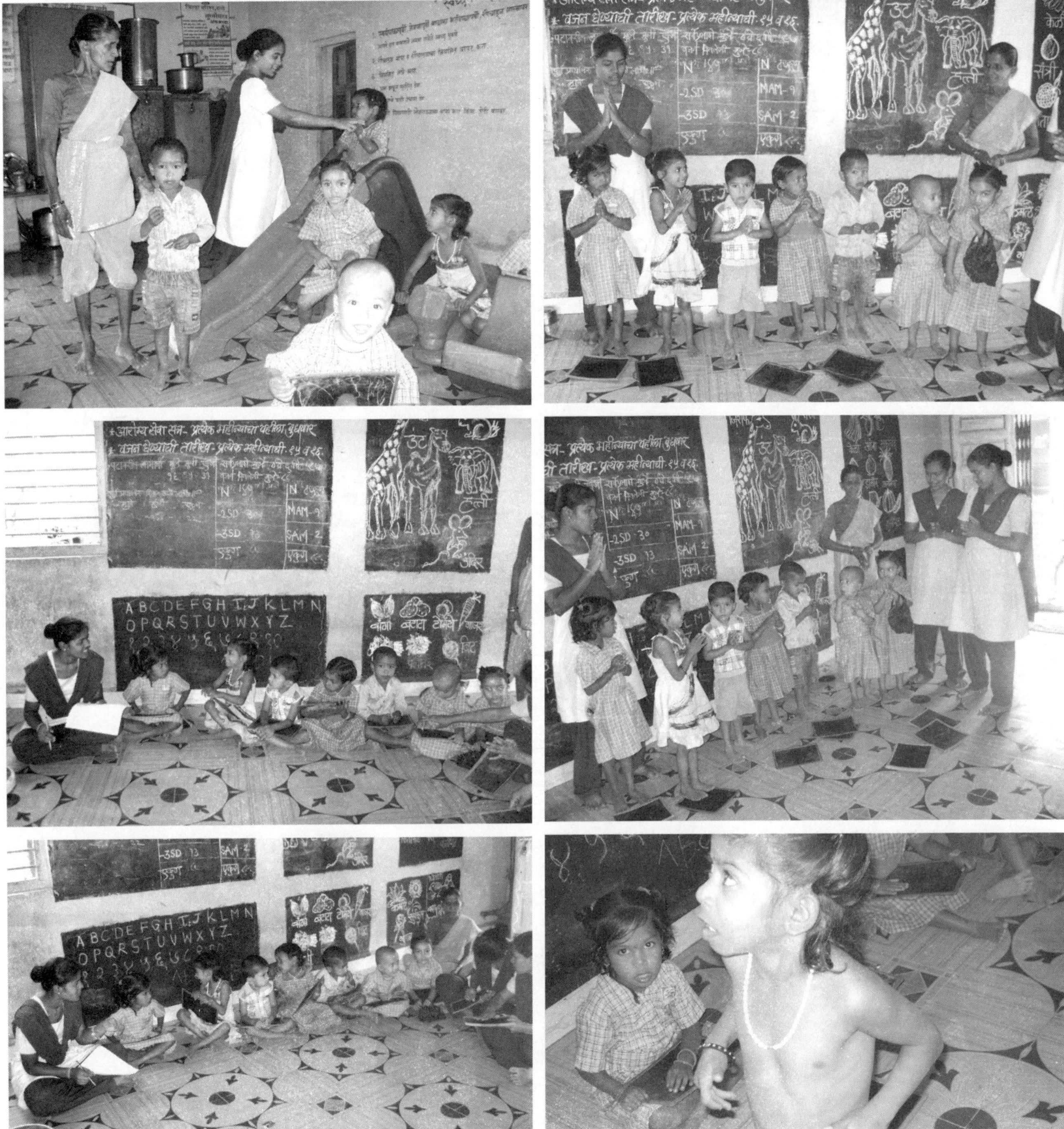
A B C D E F G H I J K L M N
O P Q R S T U V W X Y Z
-2SD 30
-3SD 13
MAM-1
SAM 2

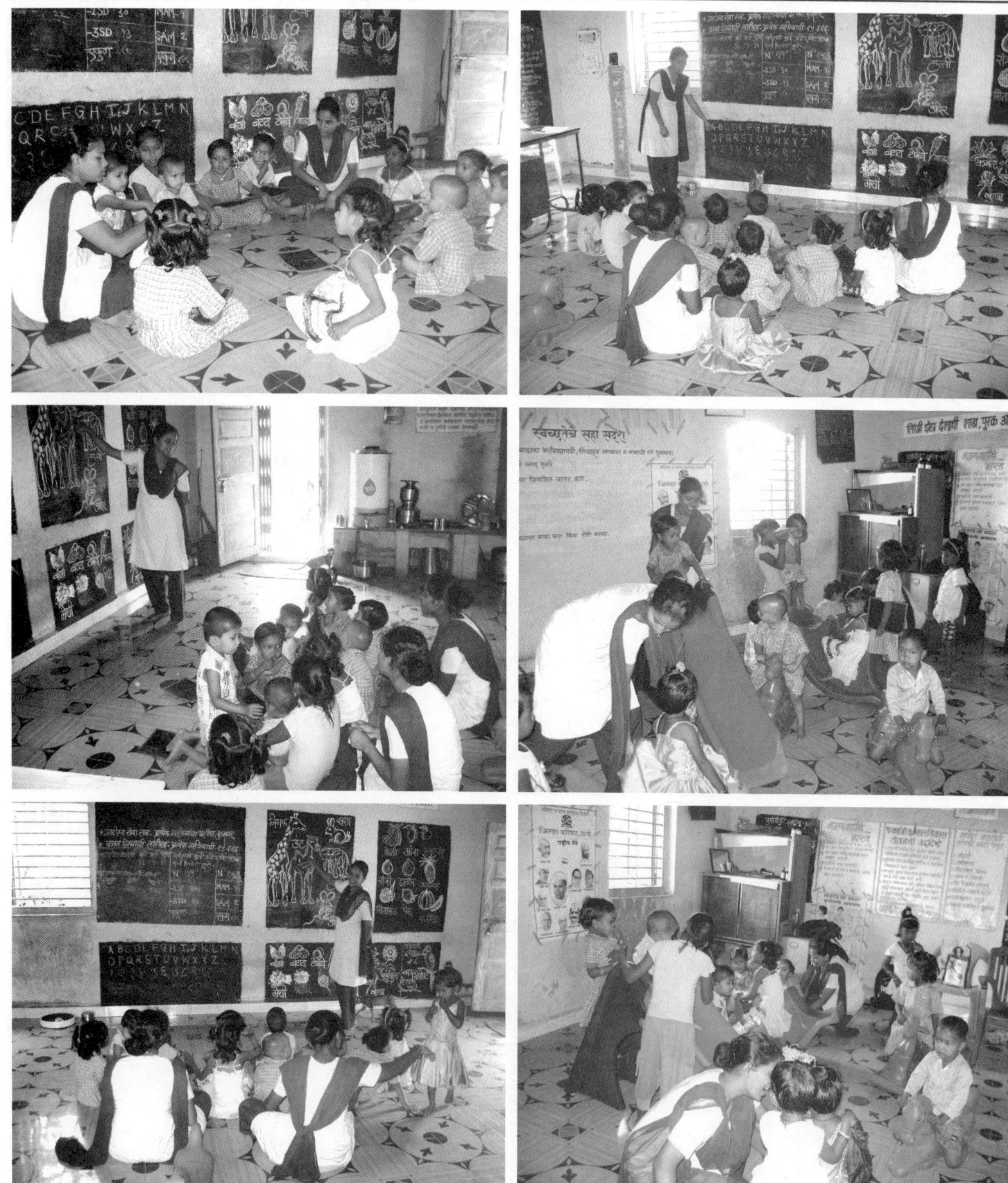
ABCDEFGHIJKLMN
OPQRSTUVWXYZ
स्वच्छतेचे सहा संदेश

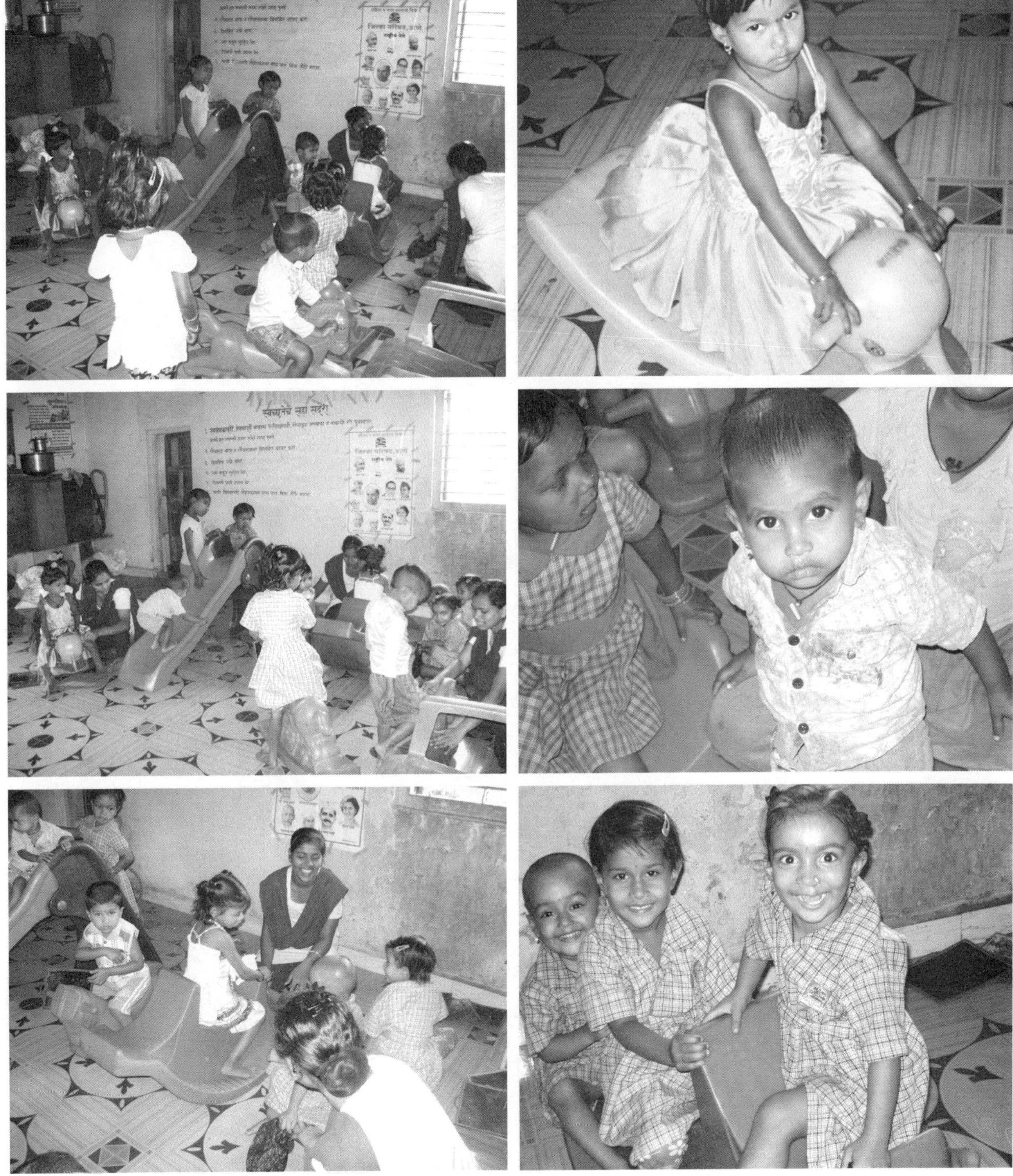

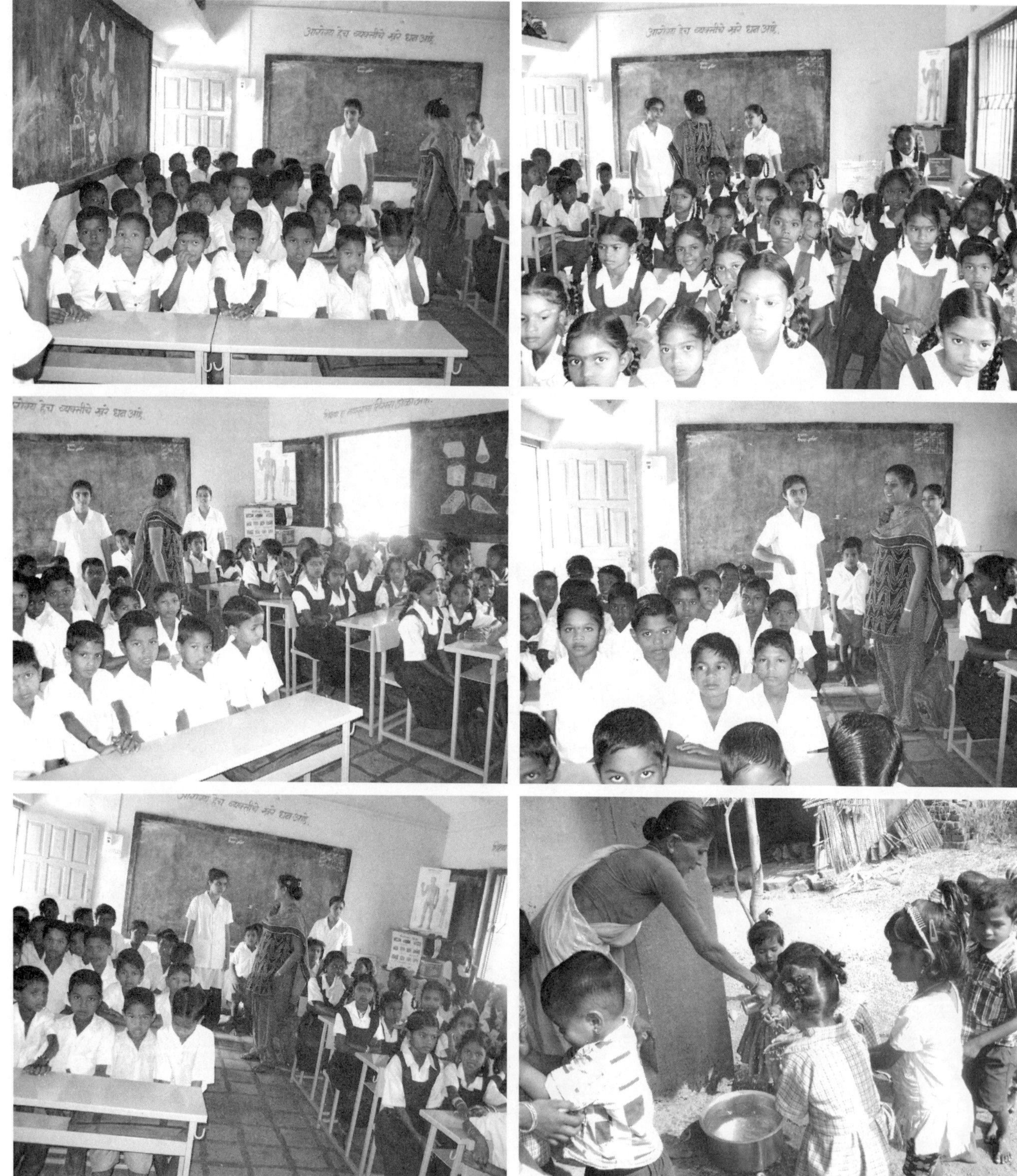

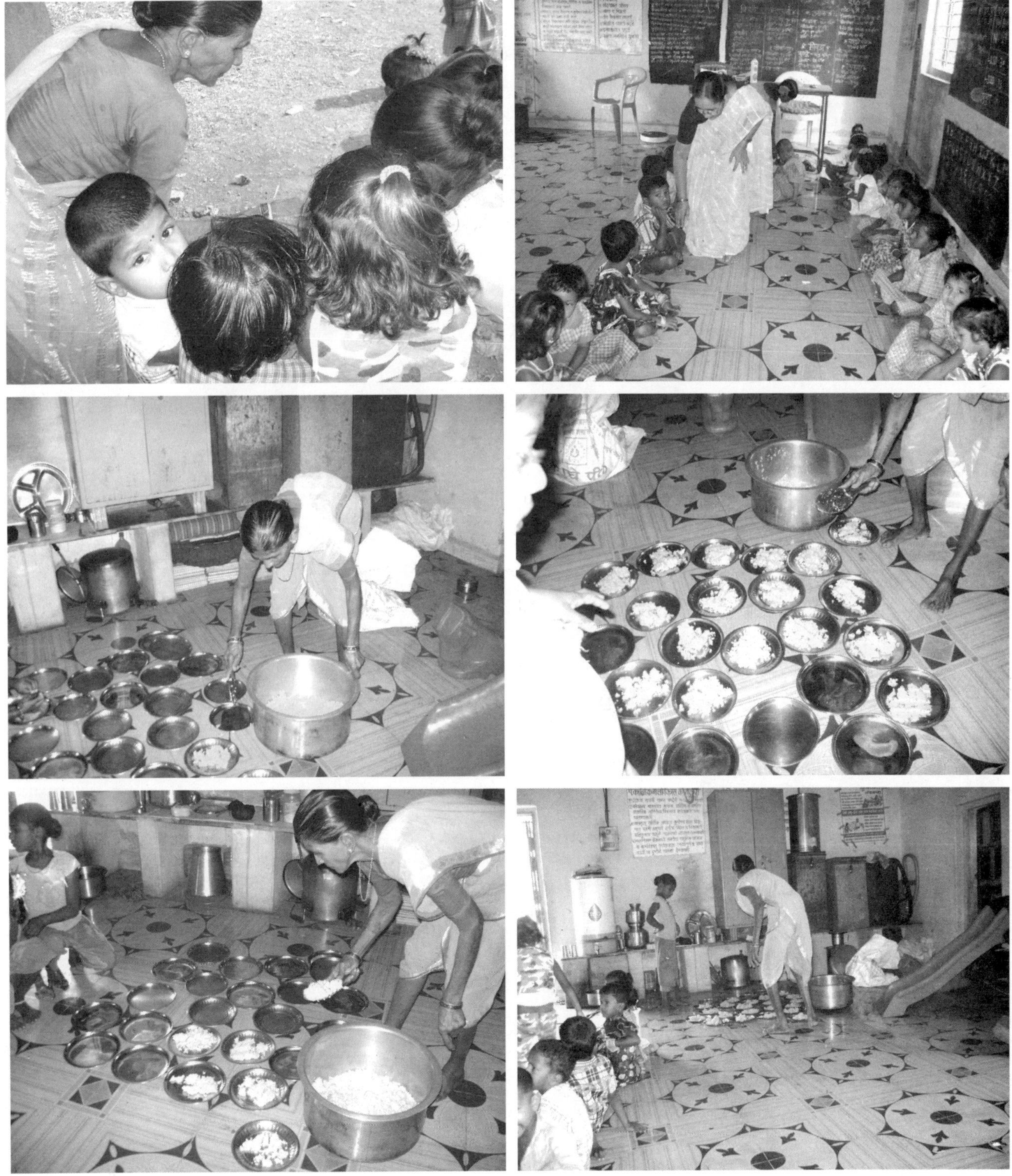

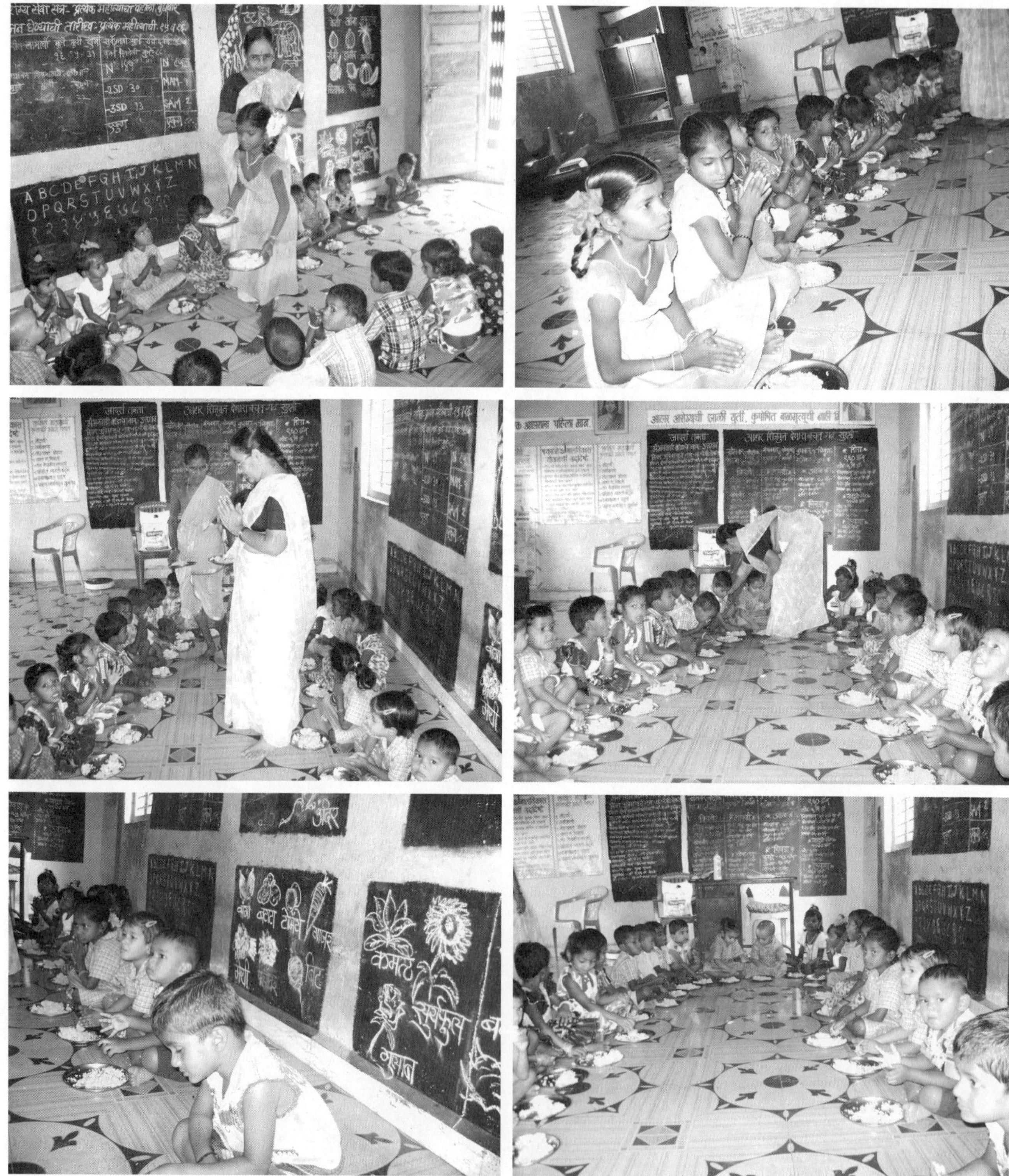
A B C D E F G H I J K L M N
O P Q R S T U V W X Y Z
सूर्यफूल
गुलाब

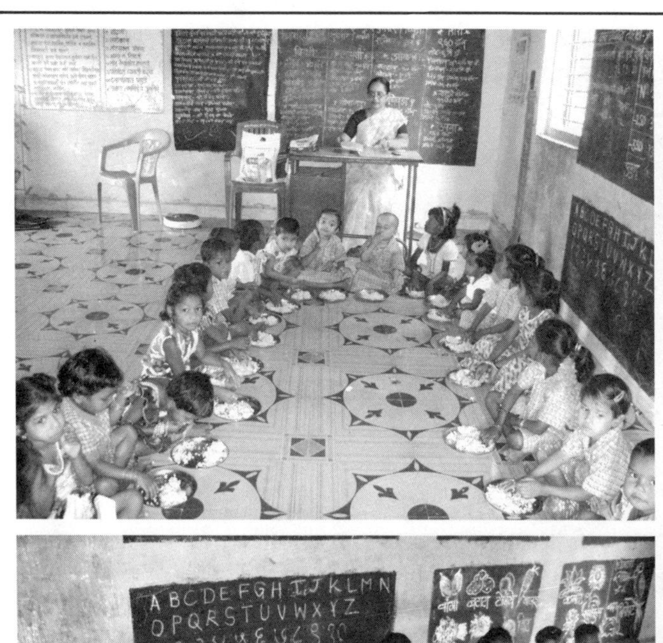

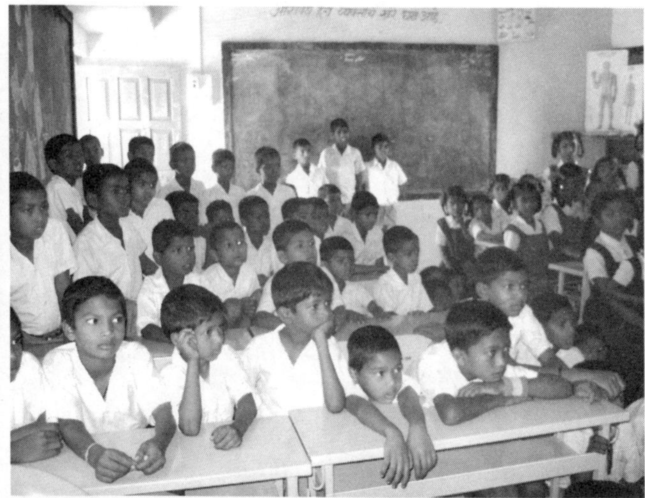

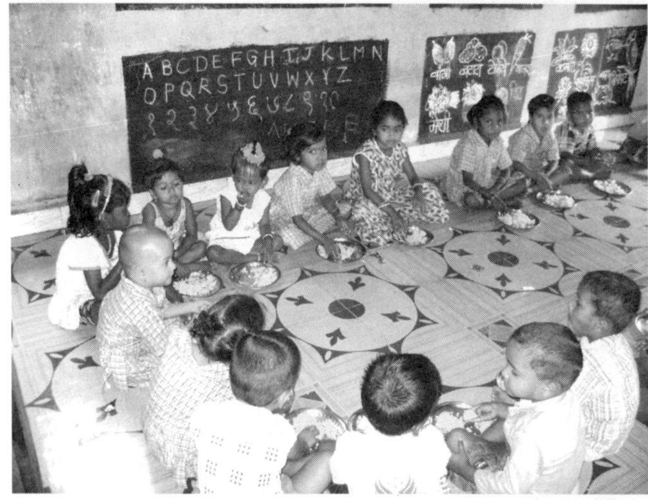
A B C D E F G H I J K L M N
O P Q R S T U V W X Y Z

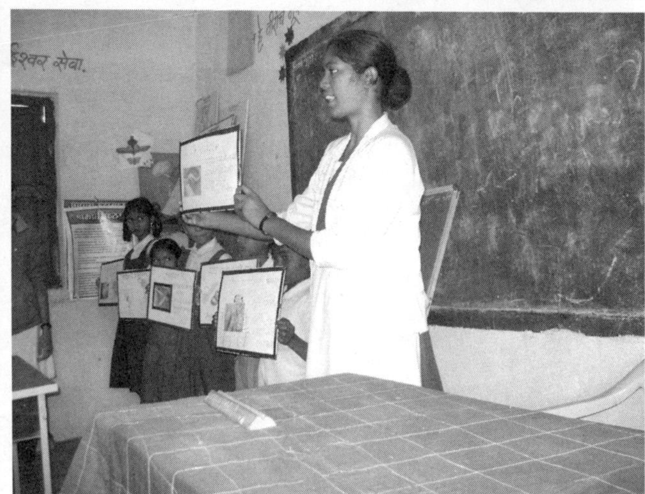

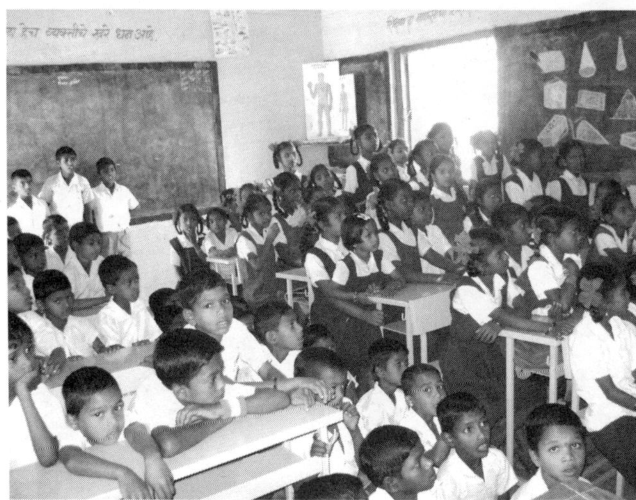

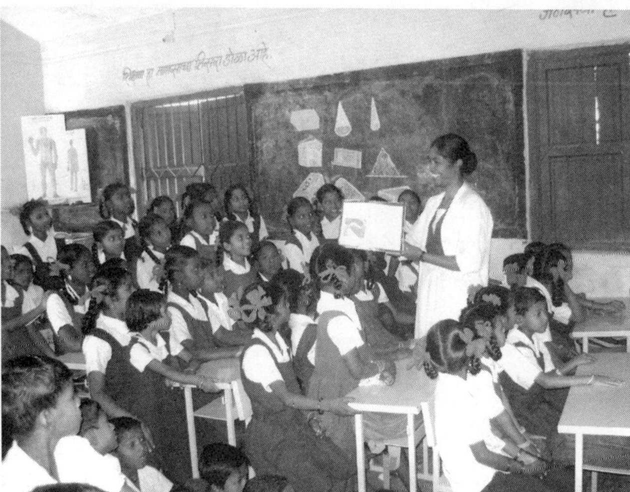

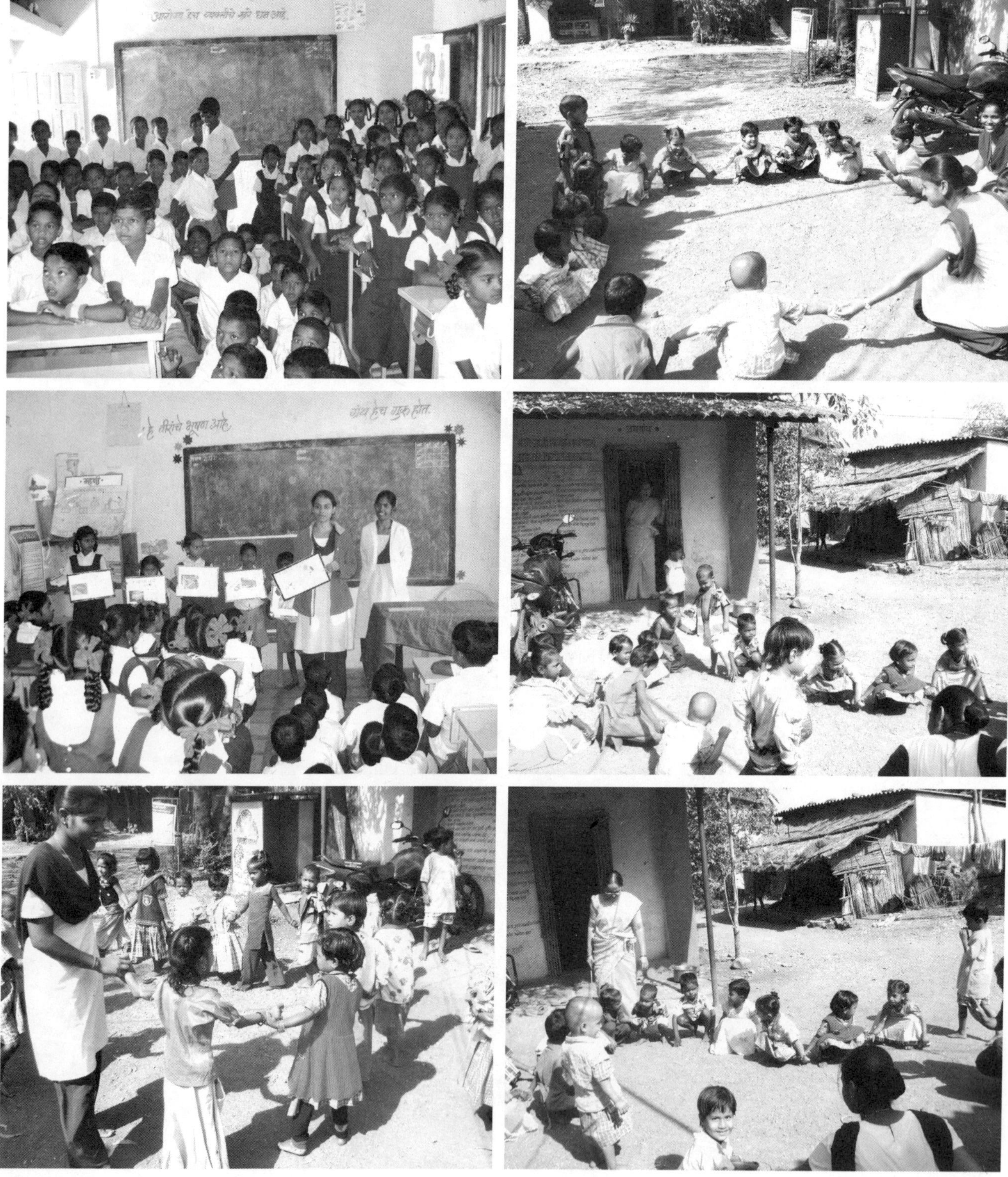

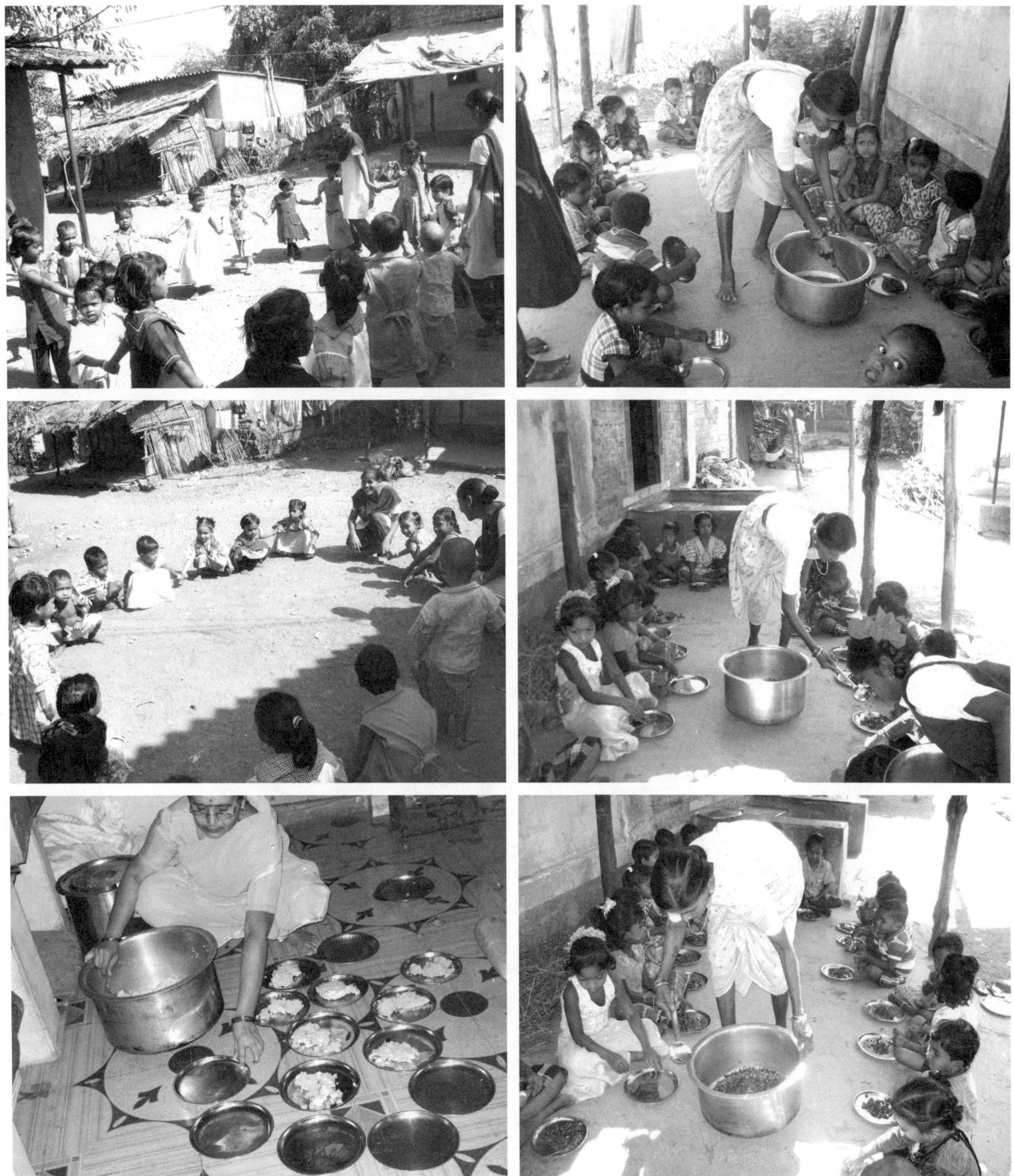

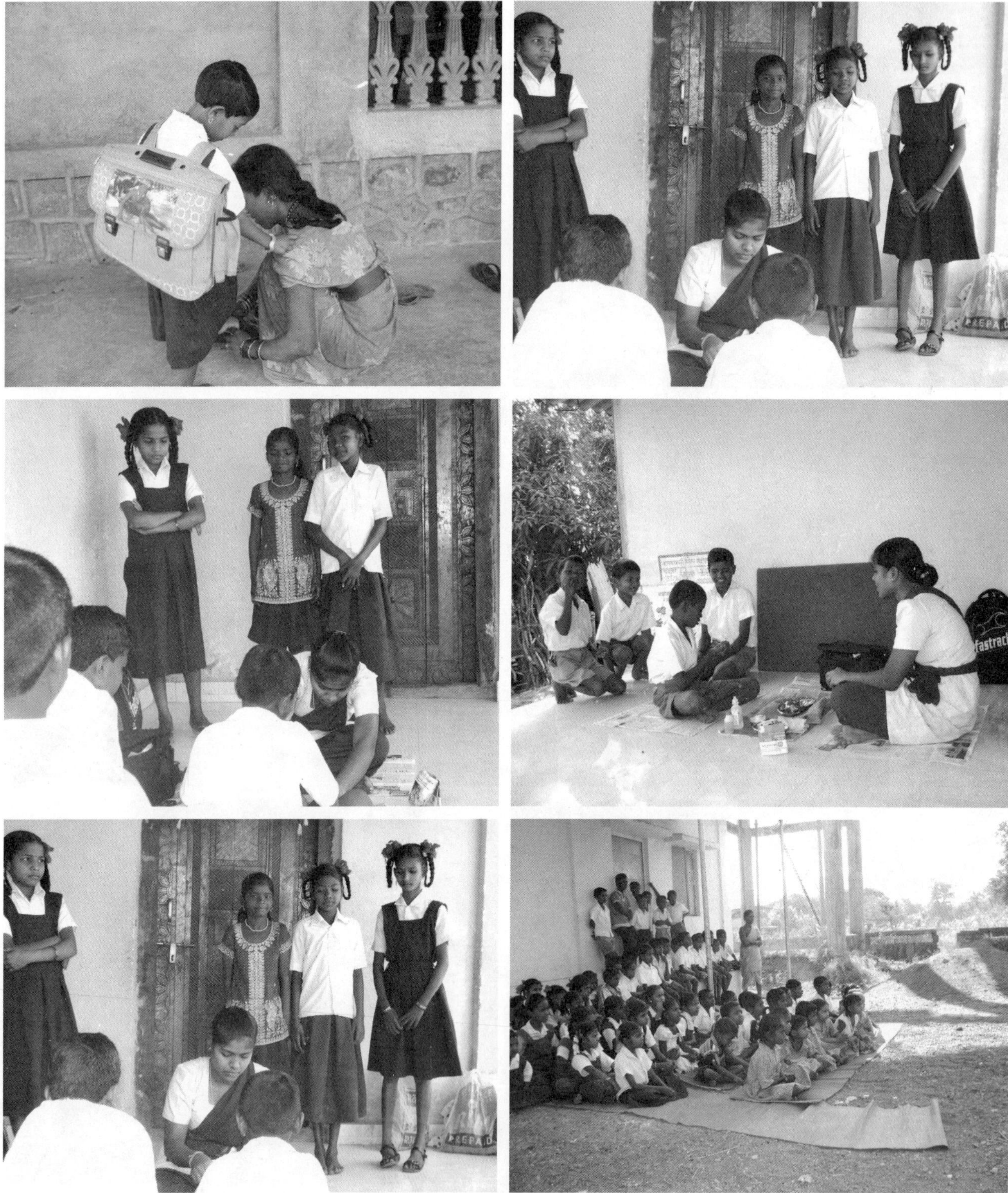
fastrack

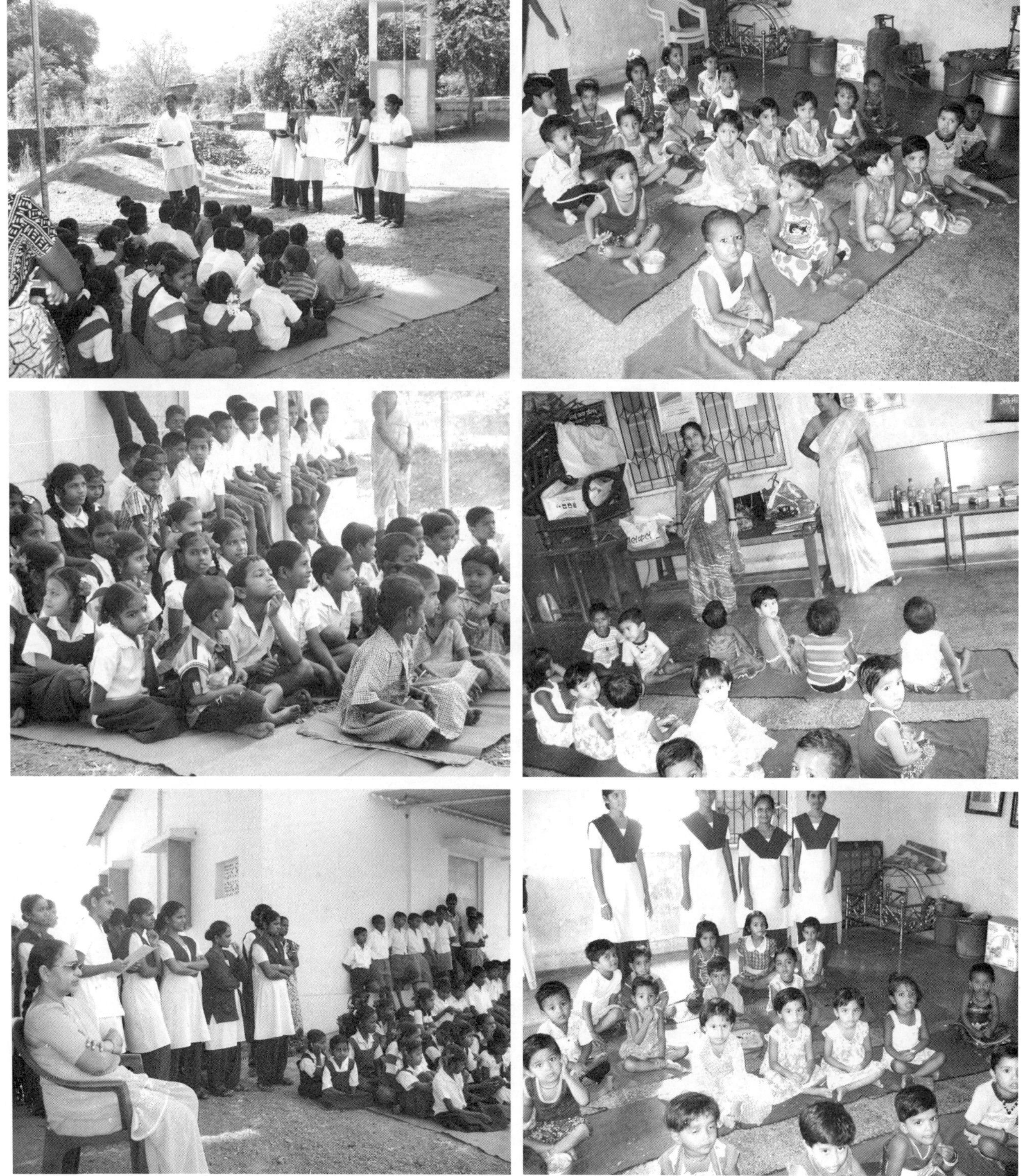

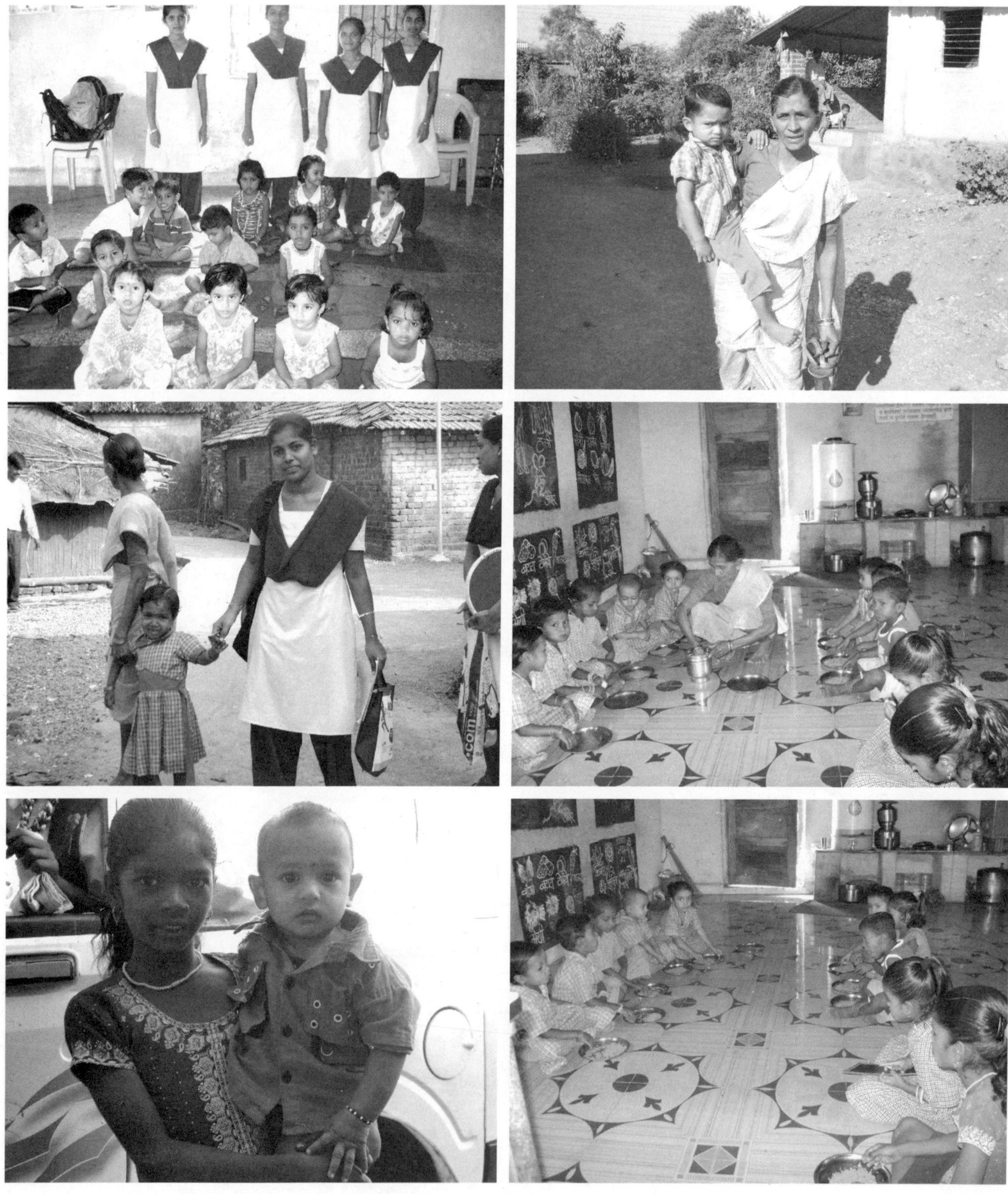

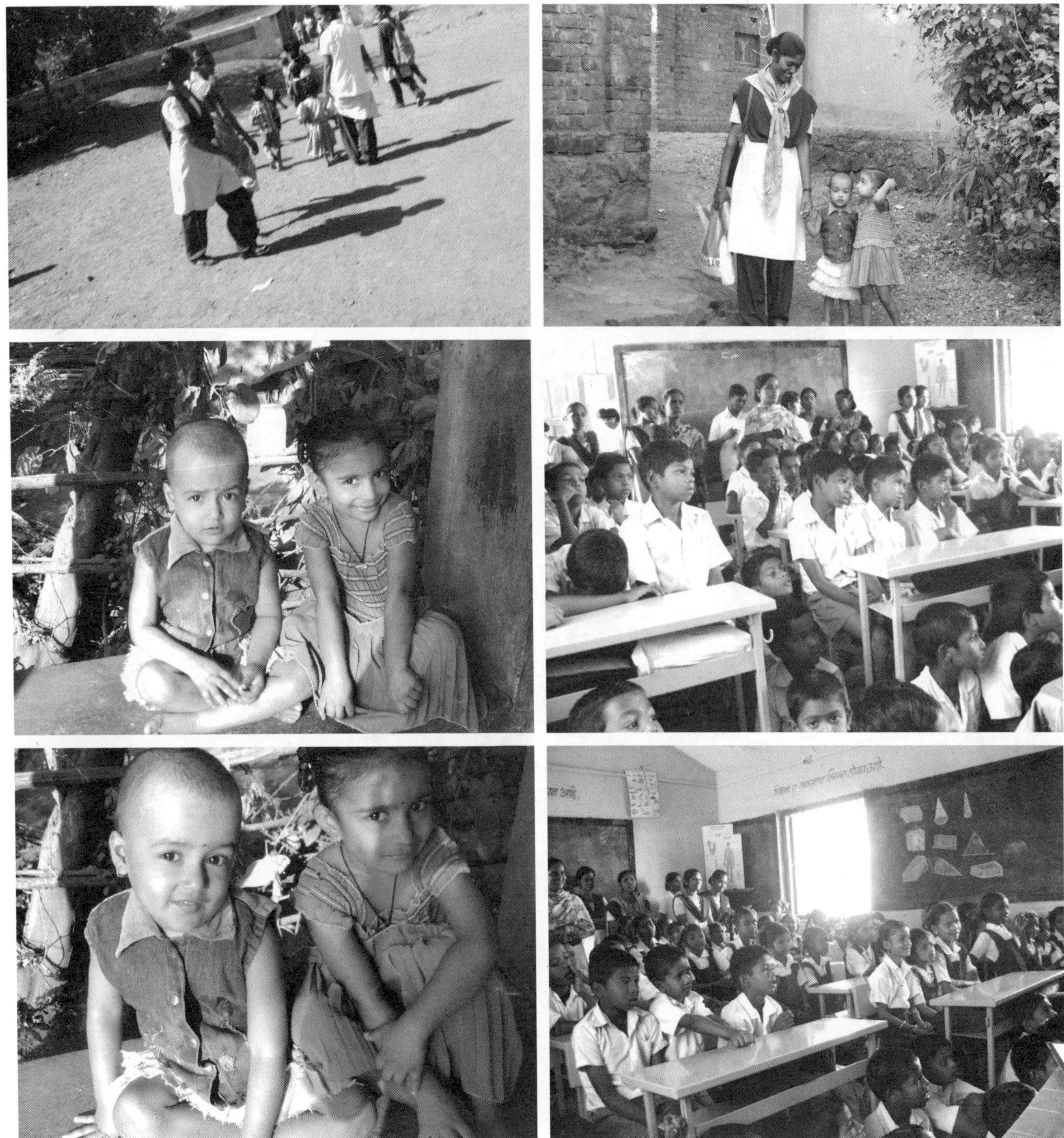

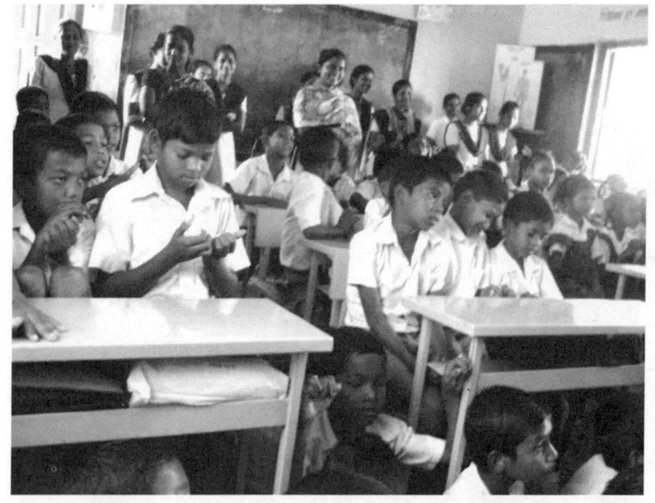

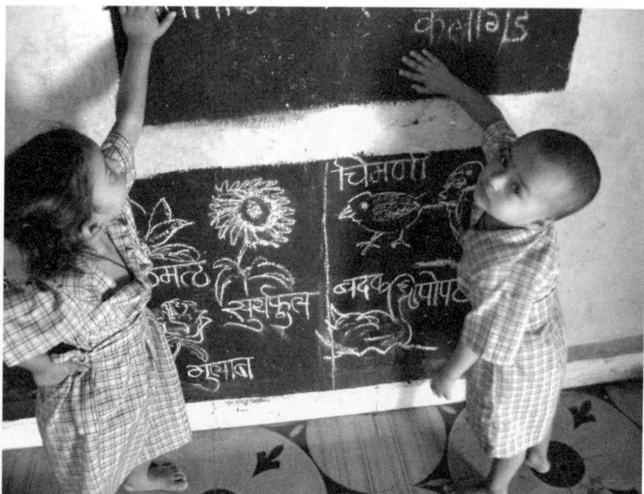
चिमणी
सूर्यफुल

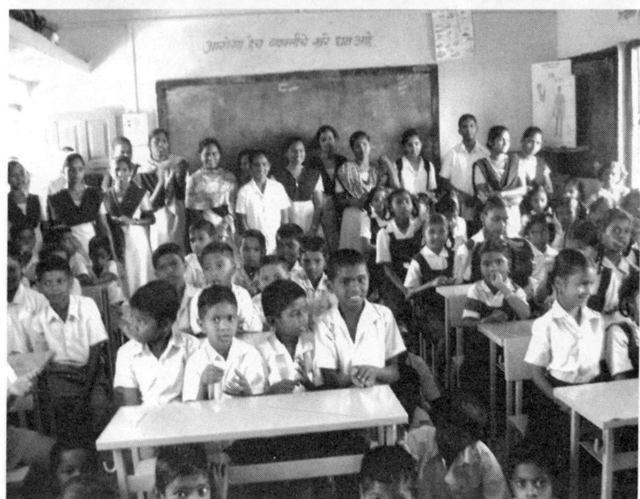

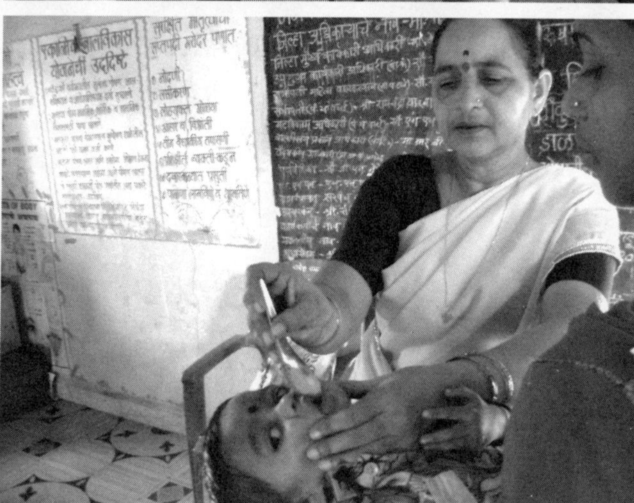

Educational Visit

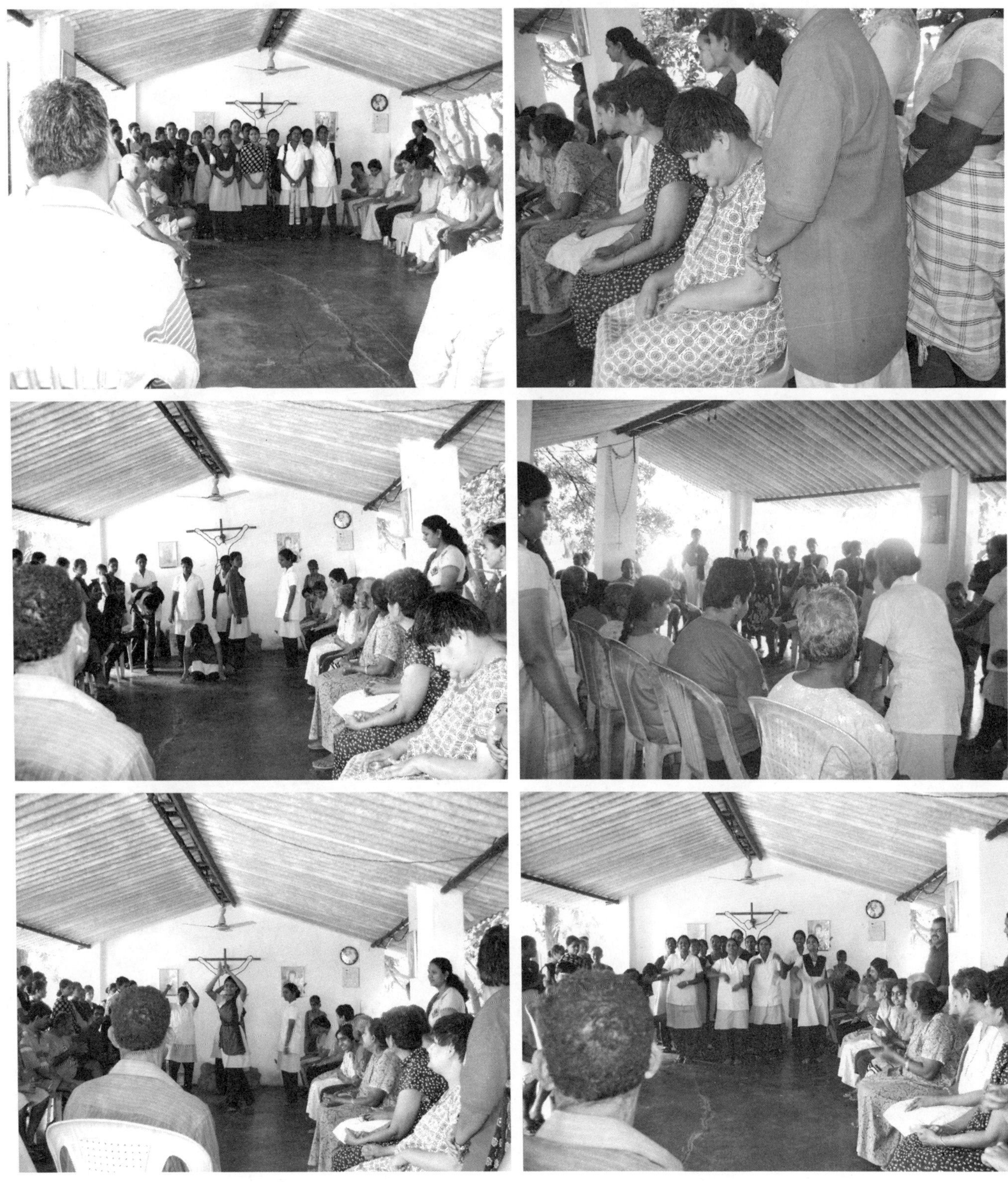

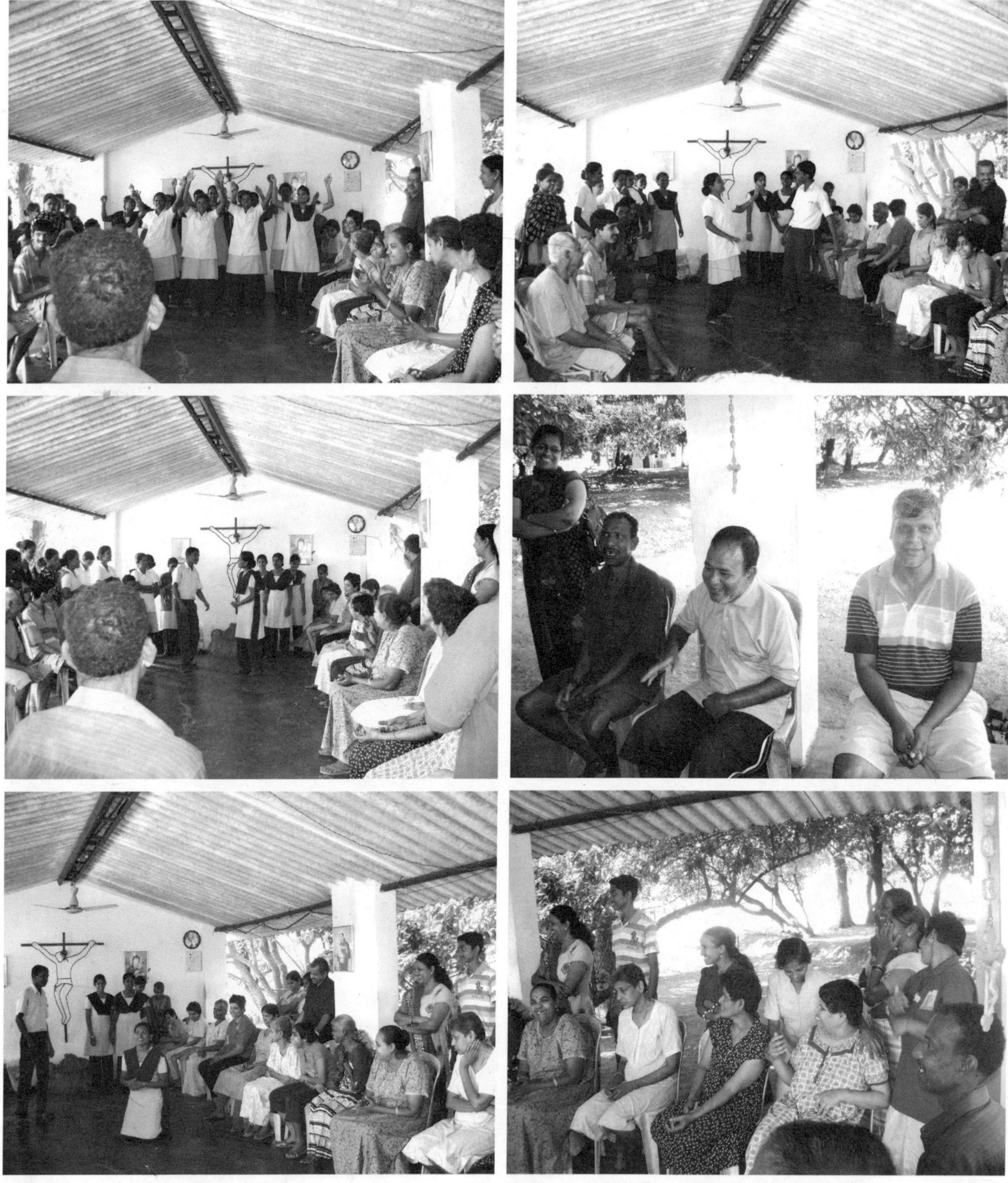

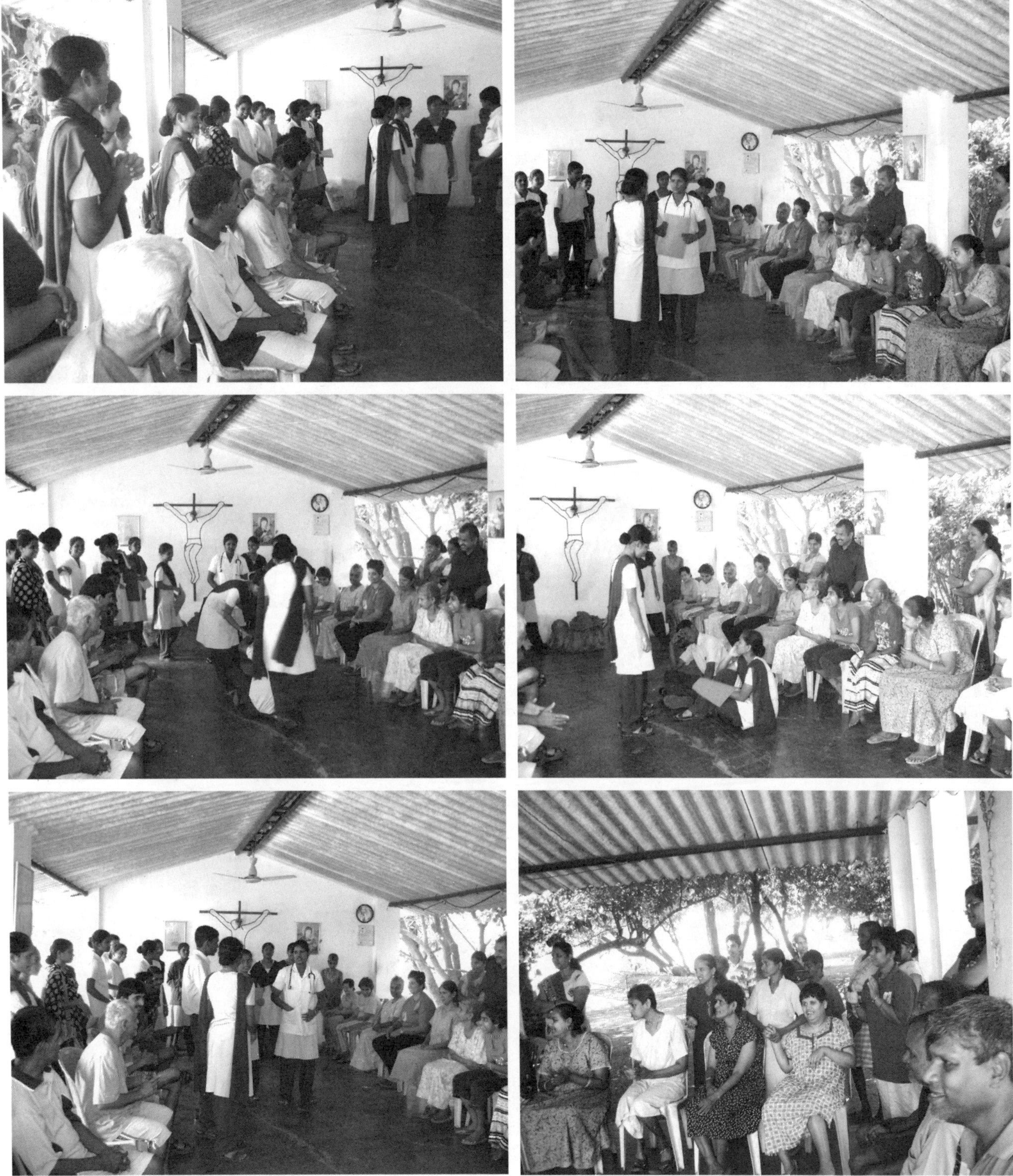

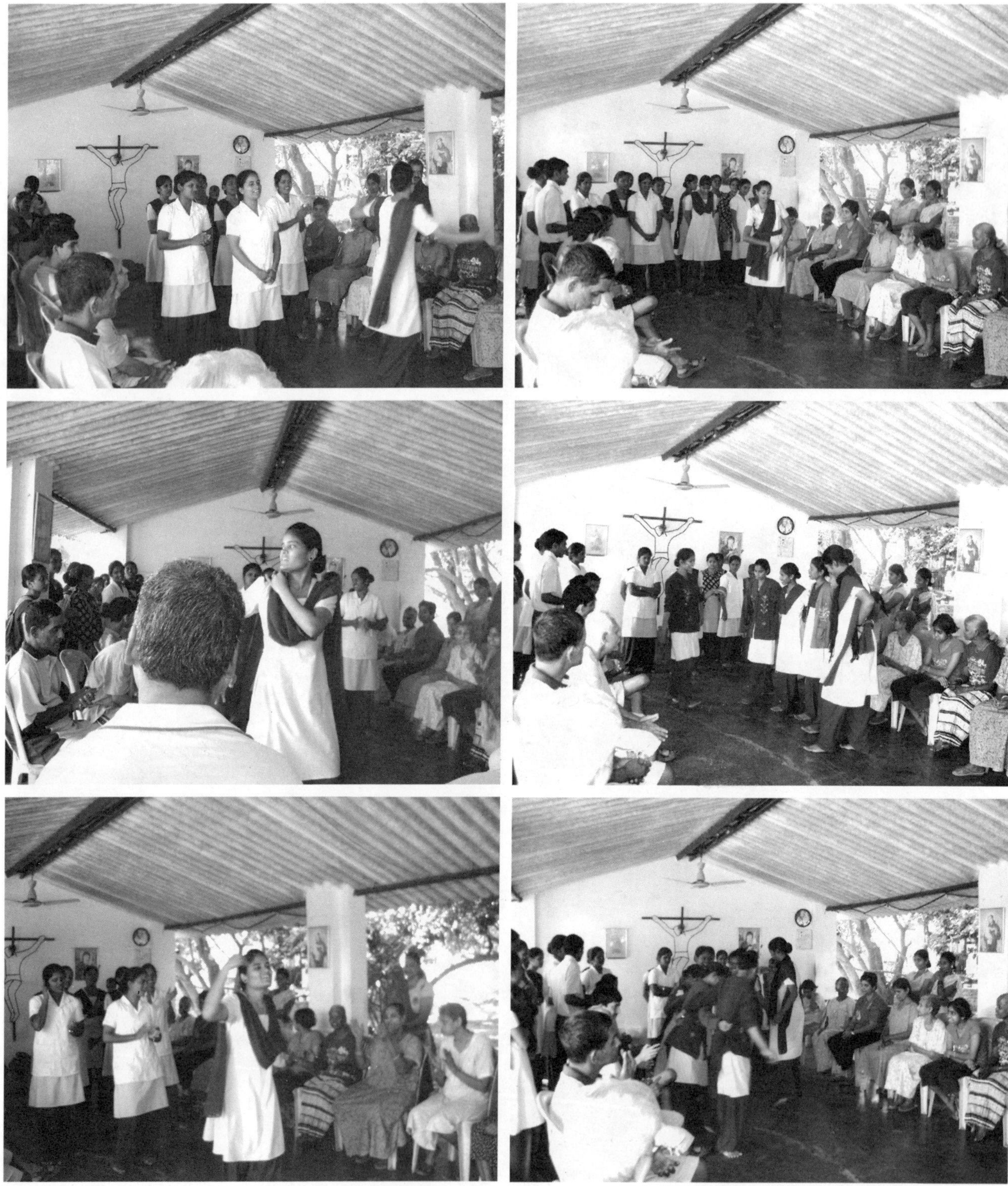

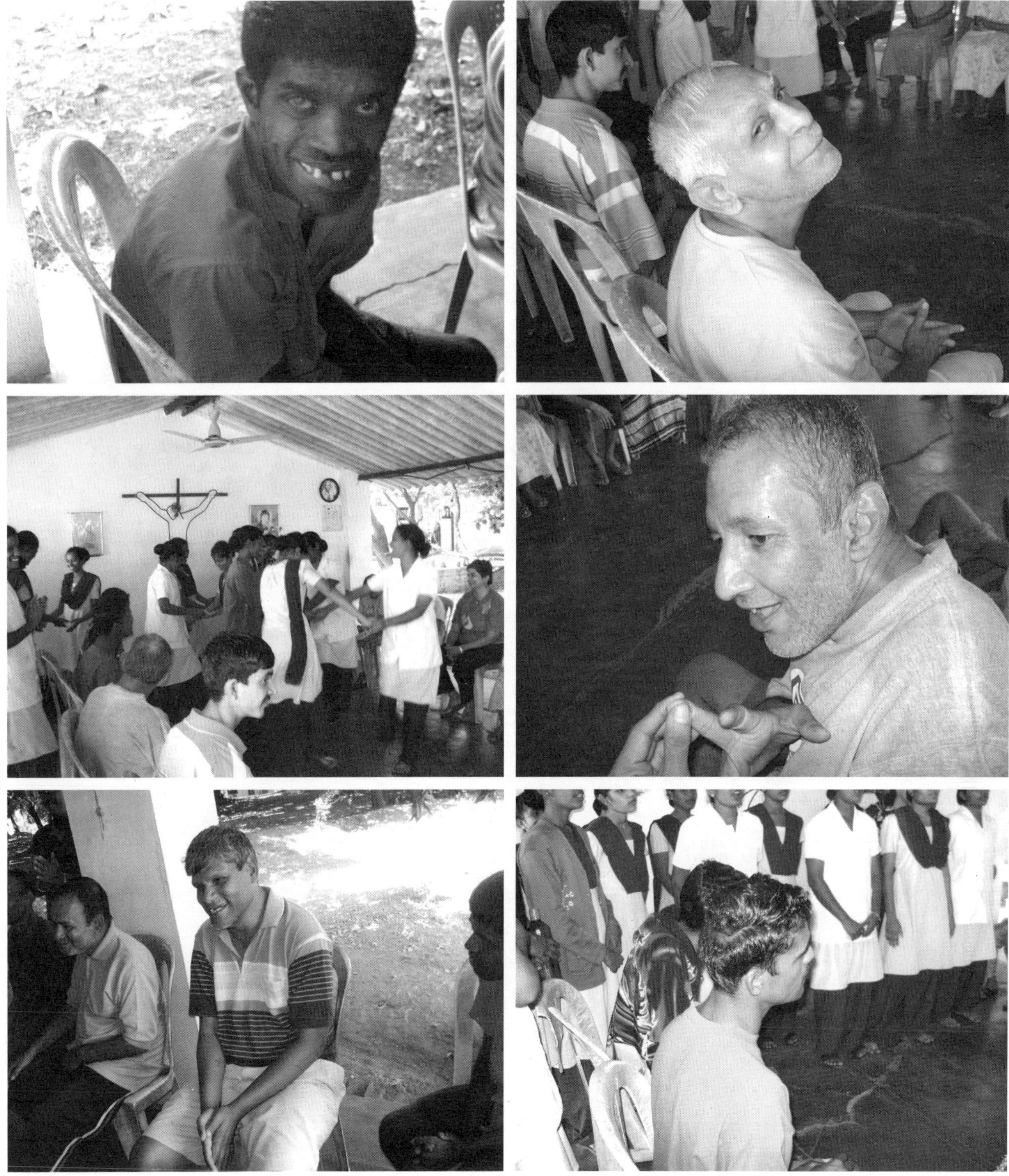

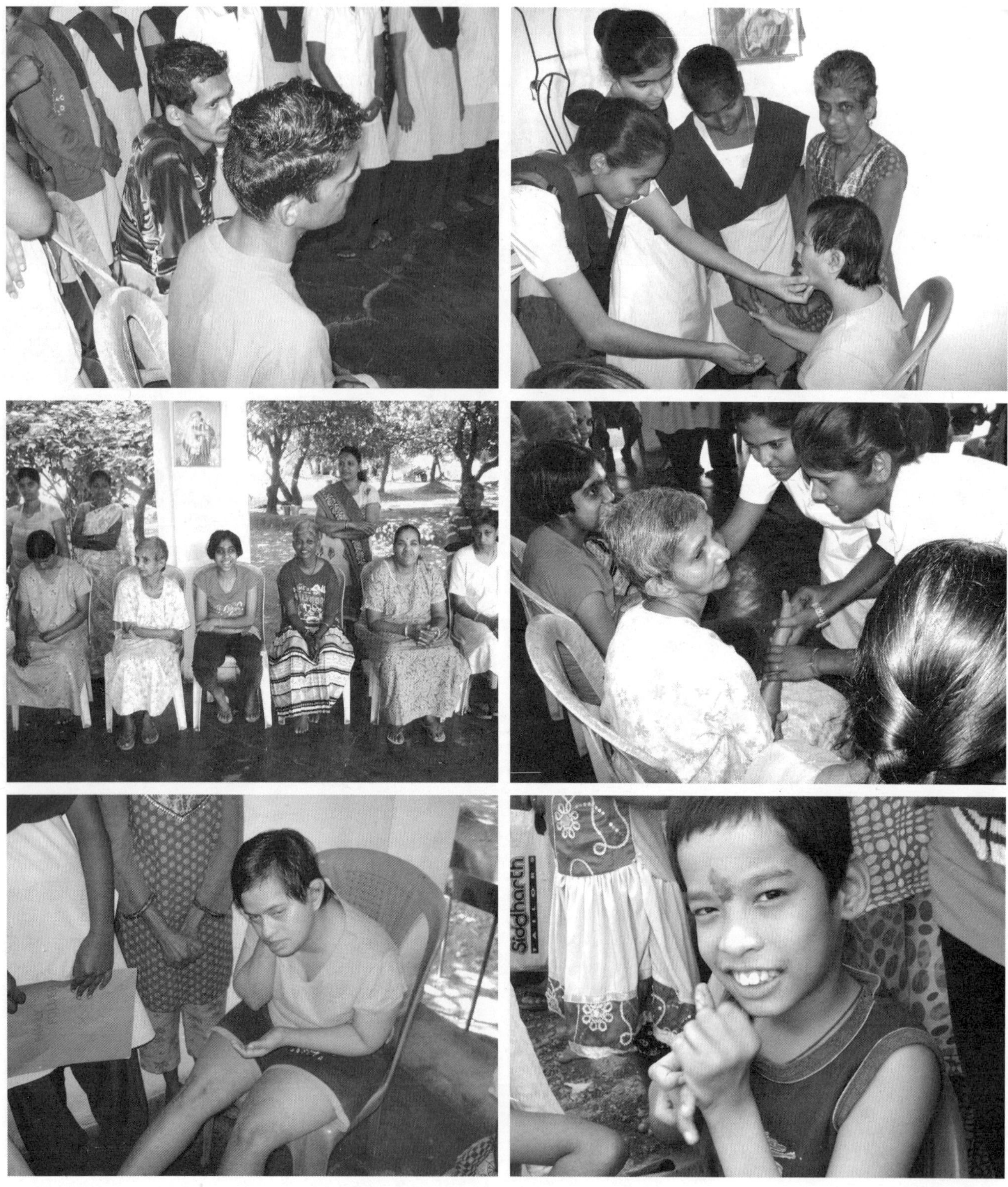
Siddharth

CHAPTER

25

Cartoons and Comics

Abstract

Health education is given through the cartoons and comics. This is also a creative method where students develop their skill and public understands better.

Comics—Are books of humorous caricature which gives a subtle message?

Popular saying on audio-visual aids as a Chinese proverb "I hear, I forger; I see, I remember; I do, I understand". One percent of what is learned is from the sense of touch, 1.5% from the sense of touch; 3.5% sense of smell; 11% sense of hearing; 83% sense of sight; 10% of what is read; 20% what is heard; 30% what is seen; 505 heard and seen; 70% what is said; **90% what you do.** Audio Visual. Aids are sensory tools which enhances clarity of communication and people get direct experience of a life situation.

Is humorous caricature which gives a subtle message? It is figurative graphic aid. It has visual-appeal and a tickling newspaper carry daily which are political or social in nature.

It is a **metaphorical presentation** of reality. It makes learning more interesting and effective as it creates a strong appeal to emotions. The carton is an interpretive illustration, which uses symbols to portray an opinion, a scene or a situation.

It makes use of personalized humor, fantasy incongruity, satire, exaggeration.

It depends on the quality of drawing. It can be useful in appraising, interesting and emphasizing the topic.

The art of comic books are not only about drawing, but telling a story through drawing. First requirement is the desire to tell a story. We can't teach, we can teach the technique to telling a story through drawing. Comics are a way of thinking that is neither writing nor drawing, but both at the service of each other. We can't remove one picture from a comic book. It is there because of the one before and after. There are 4 more options of visual arts besides comics; they are computer graphics, illustration, advertising and graphic arts.

Animation is as old as early mans drawing. In a primitive attempt at animation, prehistoric artist used cartoon like techniques to give the impression that their images were moving across cave walls.

A **cartoon** is a form of two-dimensional illustrated visual art. While the specific definition has changed over time, modern usage refers to a typically non-realistic or semi-realistic drawing or painting intended for satire, caricature, or humor, or to the artistic style of such works. An artist who creates cartoons is called a cartoonist. The term originated in the middle ages and first described a preparatory drawing for a piece of art, such as a painting, fresco, tapestry, or stained glass window. In the 19th century, it came to refer to humorous illustrations in magazines and newspapers, and in the early 20th century and onward it referred to comic strips and animated films. In modern print media, a cartoon is a piece of art, usually humorous in intent. Modern single-panel gag cartoons, found in magazines, generally consist of a single drawing with a typeset caption positioned beneath or (much less often) a speech balloon. Newspaper syndicates have also distributed single-panel gag cartoons. Noteworthy in the area of newspaper cartoon illustration is Richard Thompson, who illustrated numerous feature articles in the Washington post before creating his Cul de Sac comic strip.

Editorial cartoons are found almost exclusively in news publications and news websites. Although they also employ humor, they are more serious in tone, commonly using irony or satire. The art usually acts as a visual metaphor to illustrate a point of view on current social and/or political topics. Editorial cartoons often include speech balloons and, sometimes, multiple panels. Comic strips, also known as "cartoon strips" in the United Kingdom, are found daily in newspapers worldwide, and are usually a short series of cartoon illustrations in sequence.

In the United States they are not as commonly called "cartoons" themselves, but rather "comics" or "funnies". Nonetheless, the creators of comic strips—as well as comic books and graphic novels—are usually referred to as "cartoonists". Although humor is the most prevalent subject matter, adventure and drama are also represented in this medium. Books with cartoons are usually reprints of newspaper cartoons. On some occasions, new gag cartoons have been created for book publication: Because of the stylistic similarities between comic strips and early animated movies, "cartoon" came to refer to animation, and the word "cartoon" is currently used to refer to both animated cartoons and gag cartoons. While "animation" designates any style of illustrated images seen in rapid succession to give the impression of movement, the word "cartoon" is most often used in reference to TV programs and short films for children featuring anthropomorphized animals, superheroes, the adventures of child protagonists and related genres.

Comics are the humorous entertainers, although some comics are picture-only, pantomime strips, the term derives from the mostly humorous early work in the medium, and came to apply to that form of the medium including those far from comic. The sequential nature of the pictures, and the predominance of pictures over words, distinguishes comics from picture books, although some in comics studies disagree and claim that in fact what differentiates comics from other forms on the continuum from word-only narratives, on one hand, to picture-only narratives, on the other, is social context.

Comics as a real mass medium started to emerge in the United States in the early 20th century with the newspaper comic strip, where its form began to be standardized (image-driven, speech balloons, etc.), first in Sunday strips and later in daily strips. The combination of words and pictures proved popular and quickly spread throughout the world. Comic strips were soon gathered into cheap booklets and reprint comic books. Original comic books soon followed. Today, comics are found in newspapers, magazines, comic books, graphic novels and on the web. Historically, the form dealt with humorous subject matter, though comics are non-linear structures and can be hard to read sometimes, they are usually simply presented. However, it depends on the reader's "frame of mind" to read and understand the comic. Comics as an art form established itself in the late 19th and early 20th century, alongside the similar forms of film and animation. The three forms share certain conventions, most noticeably the mixing of words and pictures, and all three owe parts of their conventions to the technological leaps made through the industrial revolution.

Though newspapers and magazines first established and popularized comics in the late 1890s, narrative illustration has existed for many centuries. However, these works did not travel to the reader; it took the invention of modern printing techniques to bring the form to a wide audience and become a mass medium, artists were experimenting with establishing a sequence of images to create a narrative. To construct a picture-story does not mean you must set yourself up as a master craftsman, to draw out every potential from your material—often down to the dregs! It does not mean you just devise caricatures with a pencil naturally frivolous. Nor is it simply to dramatize a proverb or illustrate a pun. You must actually invent some kind of play, where the parts are arranged by plan and form a satisfactory whole.

One of the first magazines of satirical cartoons was based on the United Kingdom's Punch, A market for such comic books soon followed; the popularity of the character swiftly enshrined the superhero as the defining genre of American comics. The genre lost popularity in the 1950s but re-established its domination of the form from the 1960s until the late 20th century. Comics have been a popular source for film and television adaptations. For a list of film adaptations, see list of films based on comics. Comics have been presented within a wide number of publishing and typographical formats, from the very short panel cartoon to the lengthier graphic novel.

The comic strip is simply a sequence of cartoons that unite to tell a story. Originally, the term comic strip applied to any sequence of cartoons, no matter the venue of publication or length of the sequence, but now, mainly in the United States, the term refers to the strips published in newspapers as Sunday or daily strips. States the term "comics" is sometimes used to describe the page of a newspaper upon which comic strips are found, with the term "comic" quickly adopting through popular usage to refer to the form rather than the content.

Newspaper strips also get collected, both in Europe and in the United States. In the US, the selection of strips to be reprinted in books has often been somewhat haphazard, but there have been several recent efforts to produce complete collections of the more popular newspaper strips. The comics form can also be utilized to convey information in mixed media. For example, strips designed for educative or informative purposes, notably the instructions upon an airplane's safety card. These strips are generally referred to as instructional comics. The comics form is also utilized in the film and animation industry, through storyboarding.

Storyboards are illustrations displayed in sequence for the purpose of visualizing an animated or live-action film. A storyboard is essentially a large comic of the film or some section of the film produced beforehand to help the directors and cinematographers visualize the scenes and find potential problems before they occur. Often storyboards include arrows or instructions that indicate movement. Like many other media, comics can also be self-published. One typical format for self-publishers and aspiring professionals is the mini-comic, typically small, often photocopied and stapled or with a handmade binding. These are a common inexpensive way for those who want to make their own comics on a very small budget, with mostly informal means of distribution. Scholars disagree on the definition of comics; some claim its printed format is crucial, some emphasize the interdependence of image and text, and others its sequential nature. The term as a reference to the medium has also been disputed. While almost all comics art is in some sense abbreviated, and also while every artist who has produced comics work brings their own individual approach and art styles. Therefore the students can create her/his own style that public can understand in their lifestyle.

The purpose of comics is certainly that of narration, and so that must be an important factor in defining the art form.

Comics, as sequential art, emphasize the pictorial representation of a narrative the narration of a comic is set out through the layout of the images, and while, as in films, there may be many people who work on one work, one vision of the narrative guides the work. Artists can use the layout of images on a page to convey passage of time, build suspense or highlight action. Computers dramatically changed the industry, and today many cartoonists and illustrators create digital illustrations using computers, graphics tablets and scanners.

Digital art has replaced traditional pen-and-ink drawings on an increasing number of comic books and strips. Some illustrators do a pencil sketch, scan it and then use different software programs to execute the finished art, enlarging sections of the drawing for detailed close work. As a type of artwork, comics are prevalent and popular around the world. A growing number of universities around the world are recognizing the academic legitimacy of comic's studies, leading to a greater amount of comic's courses being offered at the college level.

Explanation of the Figures

There are figures in the chapter which in itself speaks volumes. They are very deep in their meaning as you see them. Select your topic according to the situation and apply it. You can create renovate pictures too, this only given you some basic ideas how you use cartons and comics in your educational purpose. The pictures I have given you can see that each picture has a story and a meaning in itself. It speaks volumes without words, students have to develop their imagination and express each idea of their topic in a unique way in a picture form, so that without even word each picture speaks for itself. Through the figures the student will know how the cartoons and comics prepared and used as to given public education.

Keywords

Comics, cartoons, audio, comic strips, newspaper strips, story board, digital art.

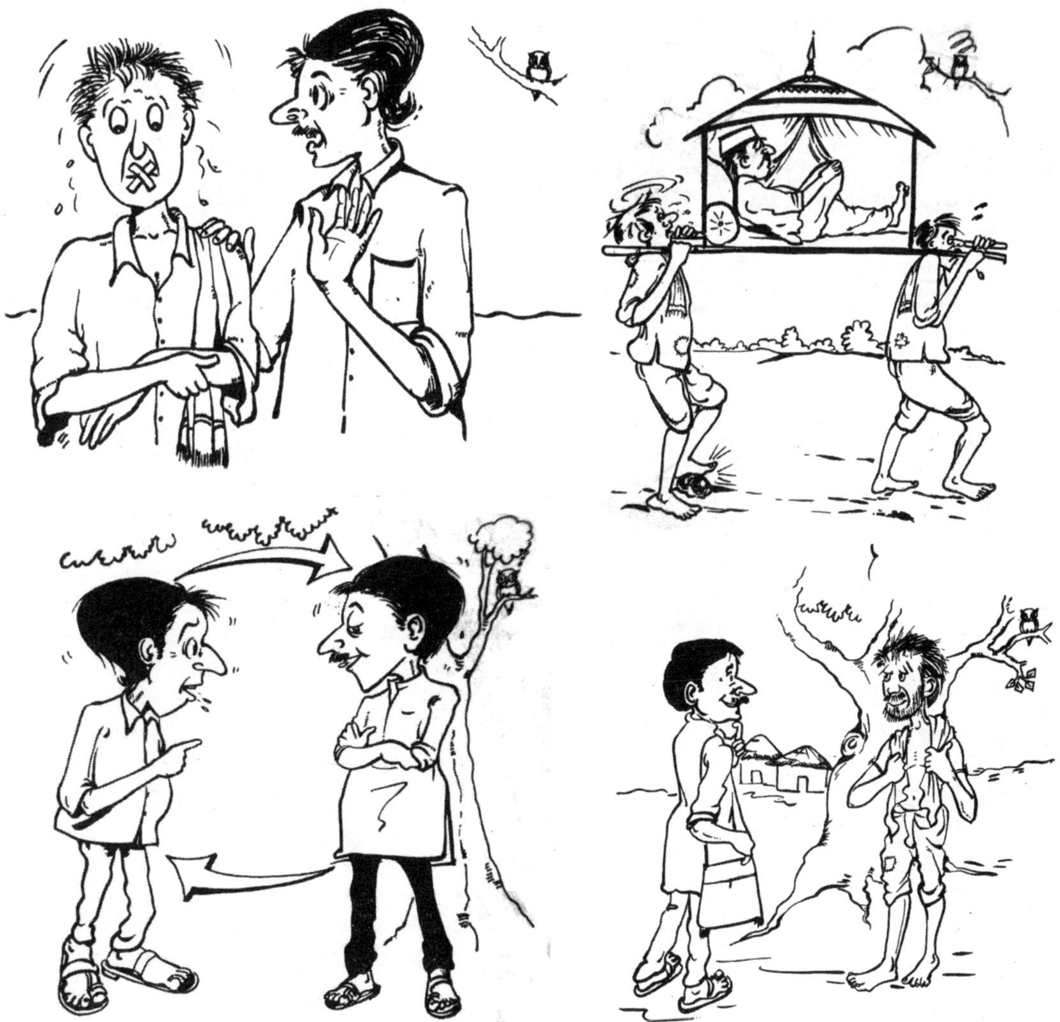

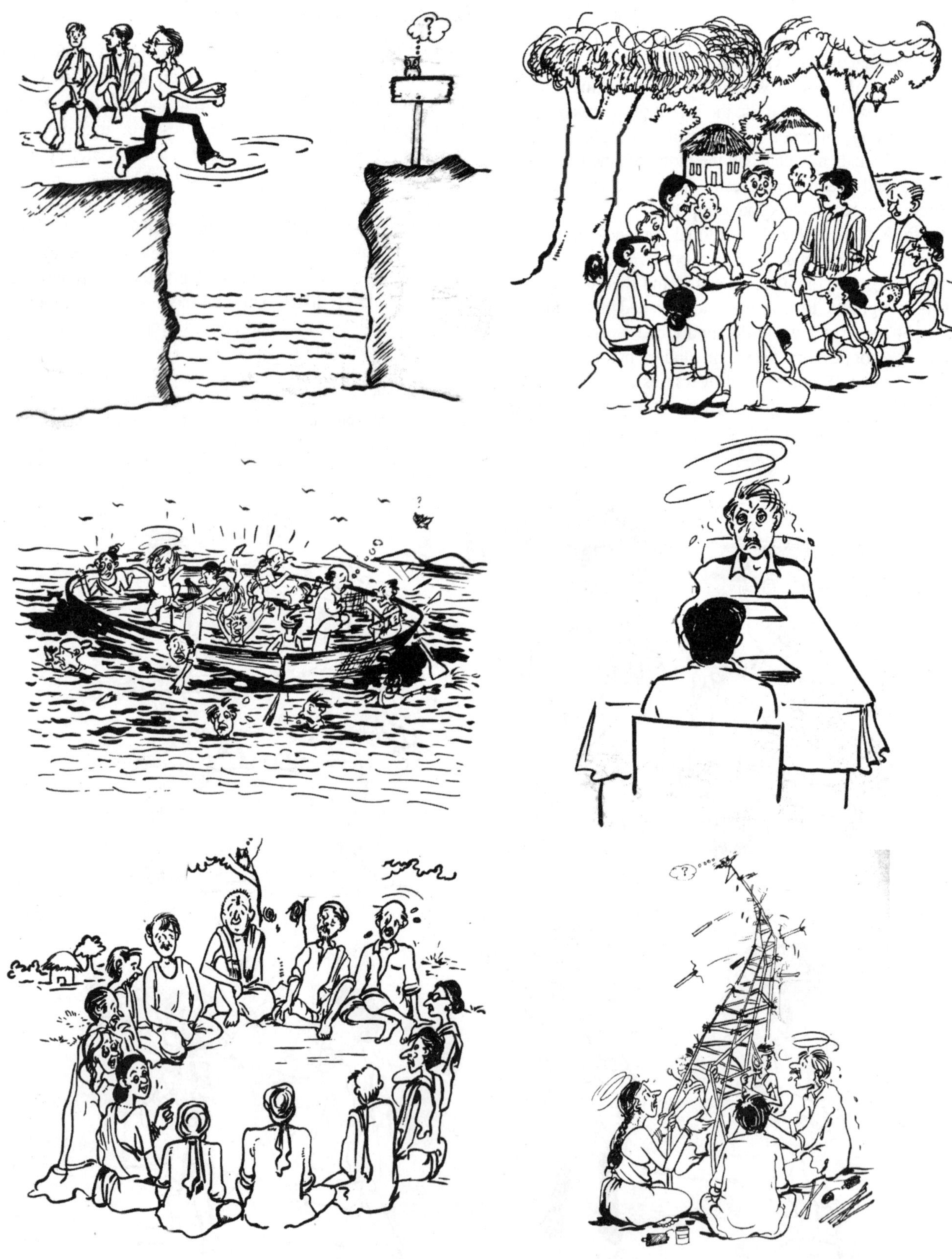

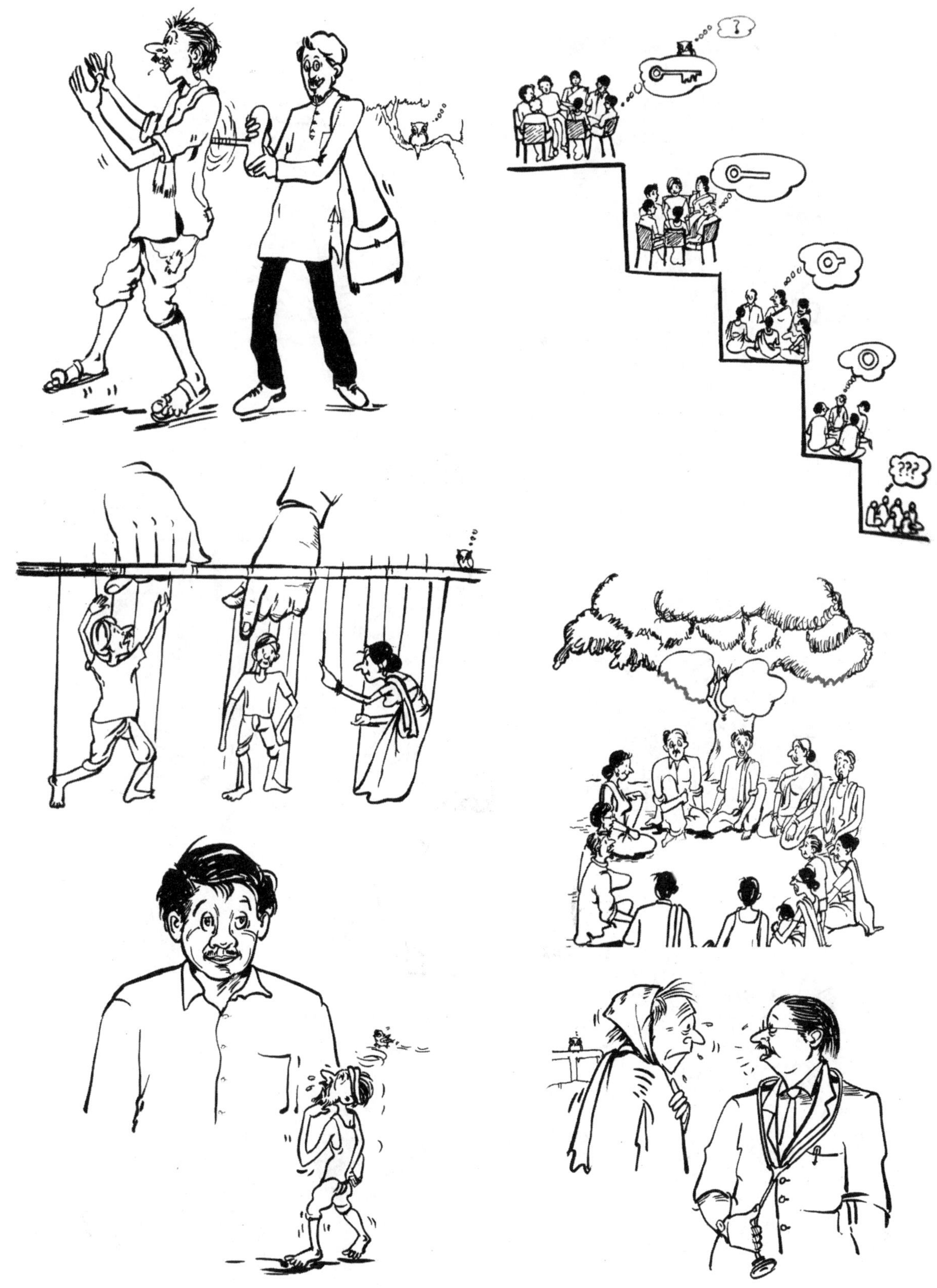

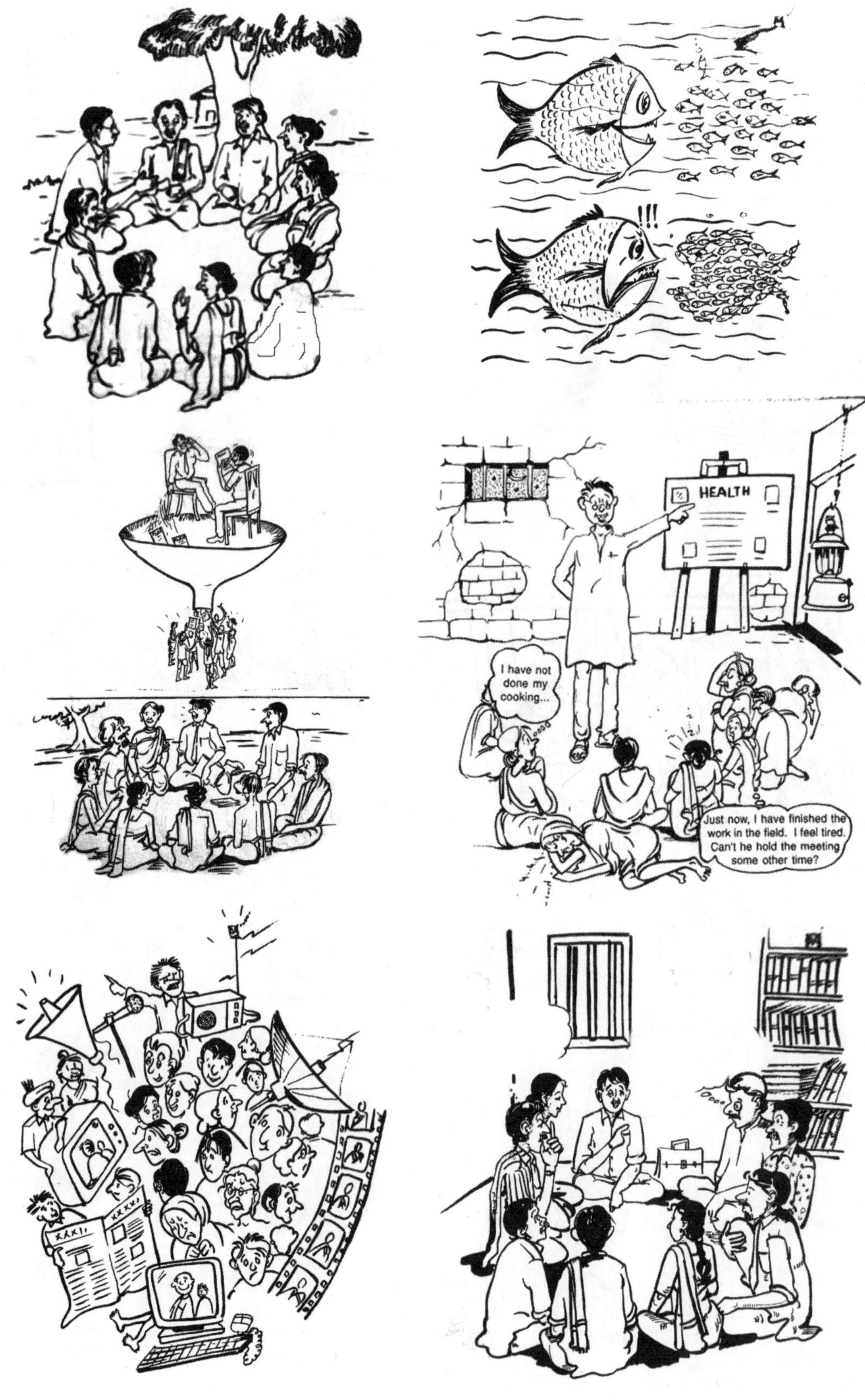
HEALTH
I have not done my cooking...
Just now, I have finished the work in the field. I feel tired. Can't he hold the meeting some other time?

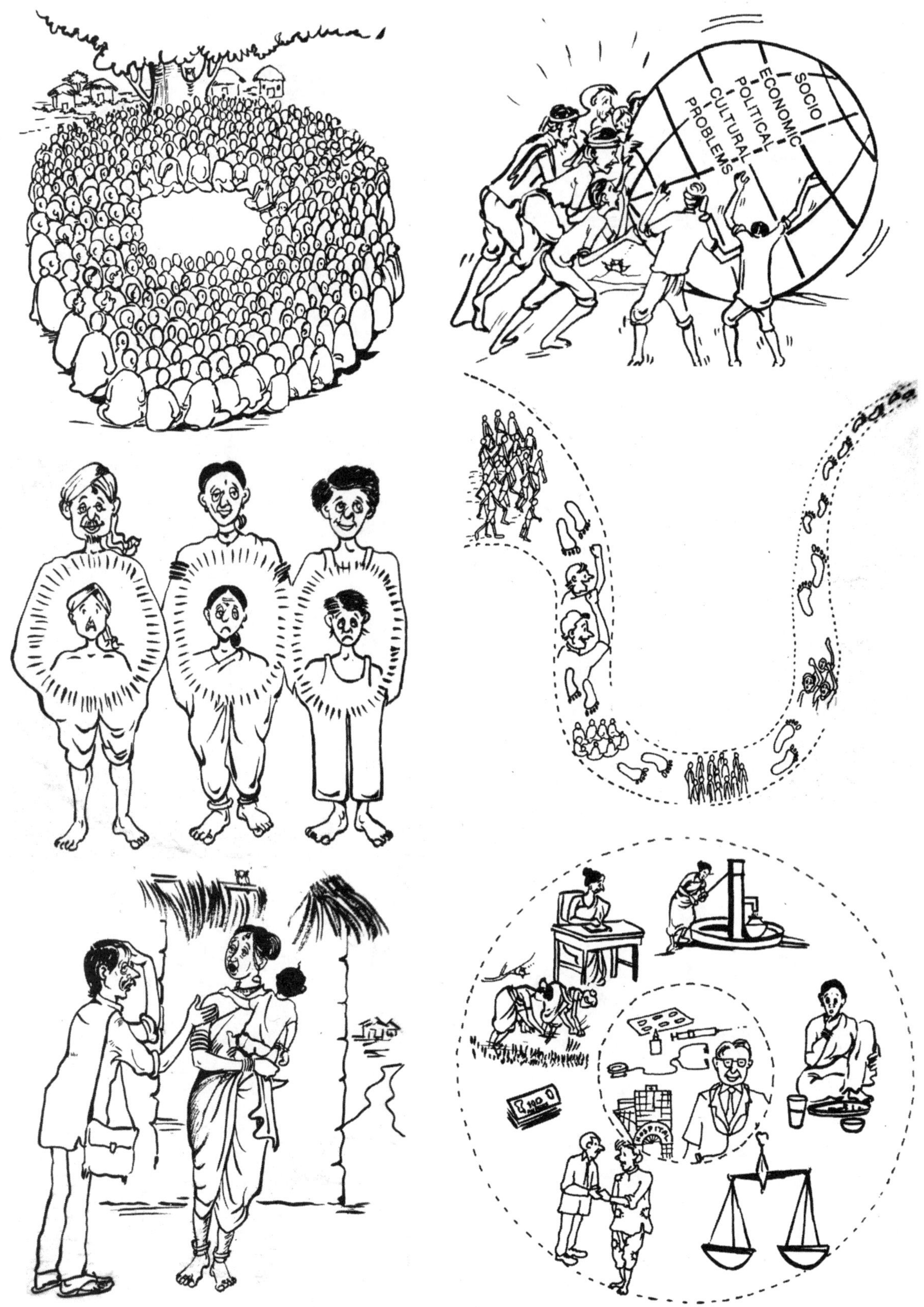
SOCIO
ECONOMIC
POLITICAL
CULTURAL
PROBLEMS

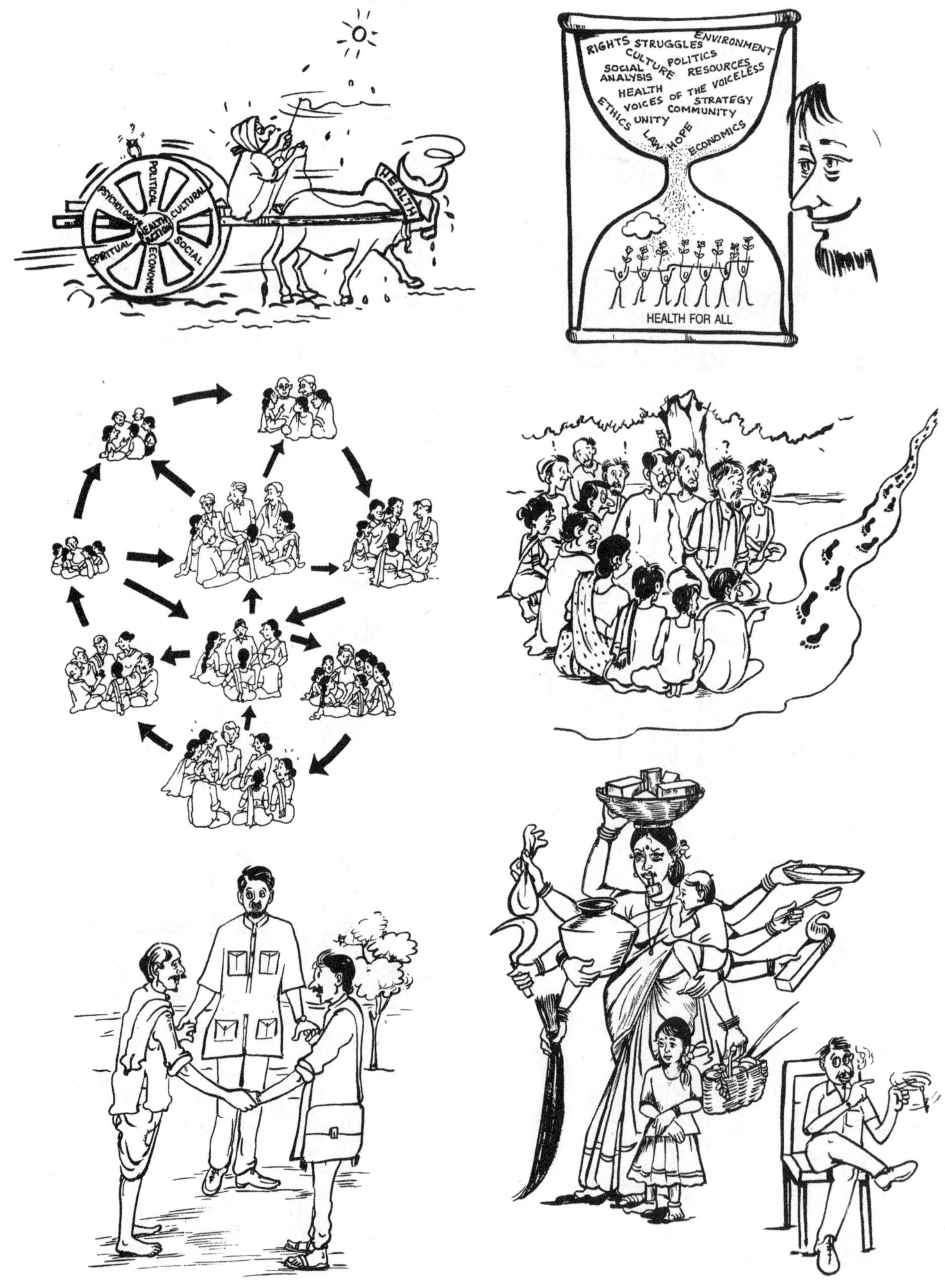
HEALTH
POLITICAL
CULTURAL
PSYCHOLOGICAL
HEALTH ACTION
SPIRITUAL
ECONOMIC
SOCIAL
RIGHTS STRUGGLES ENVIRONMENT
CULTURE POLITICS
SOCIAL ANALYSIS RESOURCES
HEALTH OF THE VOICELESS
VOICES STRATEGY
COMMUNITY
ETHICS UNITY
LAW HOPE ECONOMICS
HEALTH FOR ALL

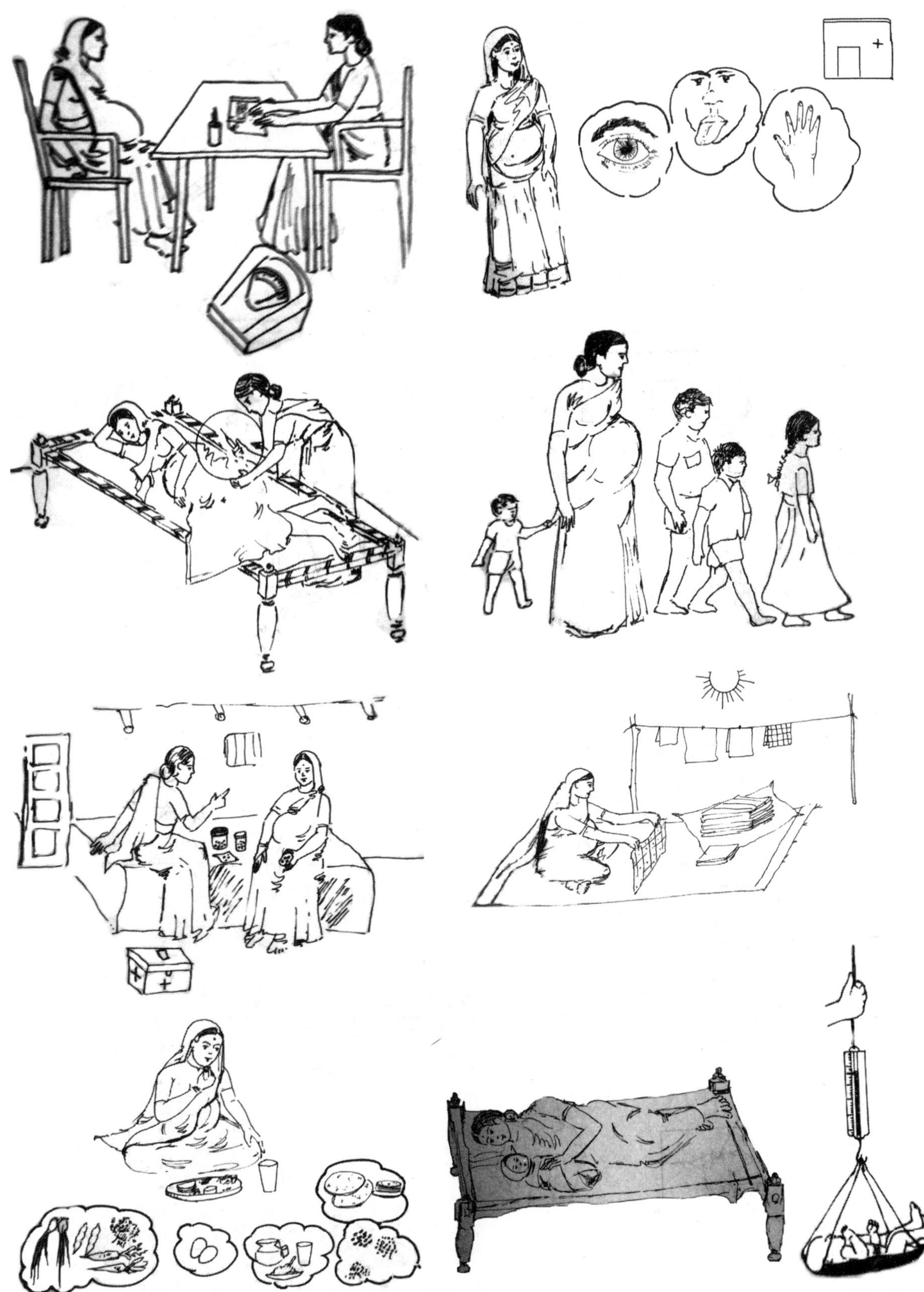

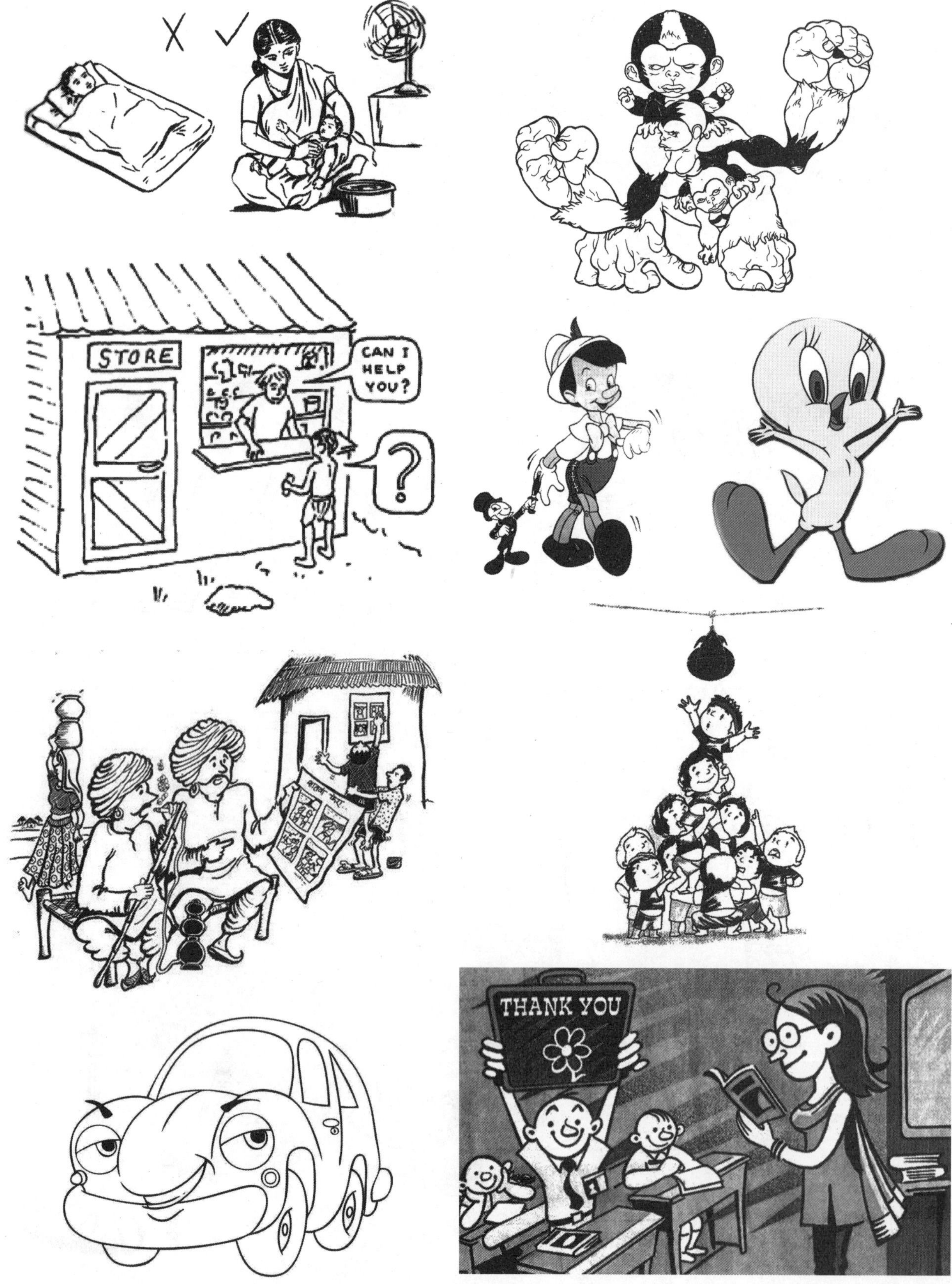
X ✓
STORE
CAN I HELP YOU?
?
THANK YOU

CHAPTER 26

Charts and Boards

Abstract

A chart, also called graph, is a graphical presentation data in which the data is represented by symbols, such as bars in a bar chart, lines in line chart, or slices in pie chart. A chart can represent tabular numeric data, functions or some kinds of qualitative structure and provides different information. A data chart is a type of diagram or graph that organizes and represents a set of numeric or qualitative data. Diagram is a symbolic representation of information according to some visualization technique. Diagrams have been used since ancient times, but become more prevalent during the enlightenment. Graphics are visual images or designs of some surface, such as a wall, canvas, screen, paper, or stone to inform, illustrate, or entertain. Boards are of different types such as lumber or other rigid materials, or plank, cutting board, cardboard, paper board, fiber board, chalkboard, white board.

DIAGRAMS, MAPS—FLIP CHART, GRAPHS, ILLUSTRATIONS

It is a combination of pictorial, which presents a clear visual summery, narrative chart, chain chart, evolution chart, cause and effect chart, tree chart? Use contrast color combination to write on chart. They can be hand drawn or machine made. Size 90×60 cm and 75×55 cm. Charts are graphic teaching materials including diagrams, posters, pictures, maps and graphs. There are tree charts, stream charts, table charts and flowcharts.

Types of Charts

1. **Tree charts**—made in the form of several branches from the trunk of a tree, such that the trunk represents the main idea while the branch represents various developments relationship or such parts of the main idea. Sometimes instead of showing various subdivision by the branches coming out of a tree trunk, it is equally peaceable to show the some by various roots starting from the bottom of the trunk. For example, complications or types of a specific diseases.
2. **Stream chart**—is the graphic cord showing the main thought idea, concept in the form of a main river and its subparts in the form of tribulctrovies among out of it.
3. **Time/table chart**—is useful for showing points of comparison distinctive and contracts between two or more things various straight columns are drawn and points are listed, while making the charts following points to be kept in kind that is chart should be 50 × 17 cm or more in size; vertical columns should be filled in short phrases, write different factors with different colors pens.
4. **Narrative charts**—arrangement of facts and ideas for expressing the events in the process of a significant issues.
5. **The chain charts**—are arrangement of facts and ideas for expressing cycles.
6. **The evolution chart**—facts and ideas for expressing changes in specific items from beginning data and its projections into the future.
7. **Strip tease chart**—enables the speaker to present the information step-by-step. It has great suspense value, which aids in holding attention and building interest. It increases imagination and interest to the very end of the presentation. The information on the chart is covered with thin paper strips to which it has been applied either by wax, tape or sticky substance or pins, tags, as points gets clear the speaker removes the appropriate strip paper.
8. **Pull chart**—consists of written messages which are hidden by strips of thick papers. The message can be shown to the viewer one after another by pulling out the concealing strip.
9. **Flowchart**—in this chart lines, rectangles, circles or other graphic representations arte connected by lines showing the directional flow.
10. **Tabulation chart**—numerical data are presented in a tabular form, used for comparisons or for listing advantages and disadvantages of an organization.
11. **Genealogy chart**—represents historical facets or growth and development of the family. Talking an analogy from the tree, the origin is shown in a single line, rectangle, circle (e.g. family tree).
12. **Job chart**—job responsibilities of specific categories will be listed.
13. **Flip chart**—a set of charts related to specific topic tagged together and hanged on supporting stand.

14. **Overlay chart**—consists of illustrated sheets which can be placed one over the other conveniently and in succession. It enables the viewer different parts and total perspective when one is placed over the other. When the final overlay is placed, the ultimate product is exposed to view.
15. **Pie chart**—a circle will be drawn and the divisions will be made into different sections and each section will be coded differently.

Chart is a mass media communication in educating small groups. The charts aim at familiarizing students with the subject in a realistic way in social contact. These delineate the process of life and of the technology that continuous.

There are 3-D leniticular charts that are printed images that show depth and motion, as you viewing angle changes to illustrate how structure changes from normal to diseases states. 3-D raised charts embark on a new dimension of learning. Transcending the world of 2-D now available in a 3-D format which heightens the reality and vividness of the image, and adds significance to the information. Each one measures 18 × 25 inches and is durable light weight, non toxic and recyclable plastic.

Map/chart display stand hangs on the stand nearest to the students. It is easy for the reach to emphasis on point highly adjustable and convenient.

Charts

1. Charts on—size 51 × 66 cm, e.g. teeth anatomy
2. Type—mounted, laminated framed charts
3. **Rigid lamination** on board and aluminum frame
4. **Flexible laminated** with rollers
5. **At a glance format** that speeds learning
6. **Clearly labeled** anatomical features that eliminate confusion
7. **Striking colorful** images that capture and hold attentions
8. **Enlarged views** of key organs and structures
9. Each chart to be **comprehensive** allowing for complete learning that is always enjoyable and accessible.

Conclusion—chart is a combination of pictorial, graphics, numerical material that presents a clear visual summary. It needs to present materials symbolically, summarize information, keep continuity, presented abstract ideas in a visual form, which can stimulate thinking. It should not have too much details written material, but give neat appreance.

Diagrams—diagrams is a simplified drawing of an object product, appliance or process to explain finger points. The following points must be kept in mind while drawing diagram-make it large enough visualization; make it outline feature sharp, include only essential and relevant parts of diagram. Is a simplified drawing, e.g. stuck figures, science forum, geometry diagram, facial expression? It should be neatly drawn in proper proportions, well labeled and explained; drawn by hand can convey ideas, concepts and situations.

Maps—a map is a graphic aid pre-presenting a diagram of surface of the earth world or such parts. A map is drawn to a scale which to movement in one corner of it. Every map showed has the following description in it. A caption or little a gird a scale, a key data which it was prepared, types of map are global flat maps and room plamktanum. Graphic representation of earth's surface or portions which convey the information by means of lines, symbols, ward and color. Types of maps are—relief, historical distribution, geographical maps, vegetation, population, economic, etc.

Graphs—depicts numerical or quantitative statistical data which are presented in the form of visual symbols.

Line graph—the data is presented through the sections or portions of a circle.

Bar graph—a graphic presentation, this extends the scale horizontally along the length of bars. Each bar must be of the same height and width which are available in two forms like vertical and horizontal. Types simple bar, compound bar histogram.

Pectoral graph—pictures are used for the expression of ideas, they are more attractive, vivid pictures with graphic messages.

Histogram or column diagram—presents accurate picture of the relative proportion.

Flip chart—set of charts tagged together and hanged on a suitable stand which carry series of messages in sequence.

Illustration—means examples, e.g. explain carbohydrate foods, show diet.

Blackboard—is more concrete and understandable. It can get standards of neatness, accuracy and speed. It can restore the alteration of the group. Many vague statements can be clarified by drawing sketches, outlines, diagrams, and summaries, initiate visual sensations. It provides many educational opportunities in all circular and co-circular activities. It can erase writing and drawing.

Explanation for the figures—Charts are also one way of educating people. Here you can see students have prepared variety of charts and displayed before the public for individual and group education media. You too can prepare such charts and use as communicate your skills and knowledge to the people. Just few examples of charts given in the figure form; which a nurse can prepare different variety of charts as give education to the public.

Keywords

Types of charts, Diagrams, Maps, Boards, Graphs, Explanation for the figures, Illustrations.

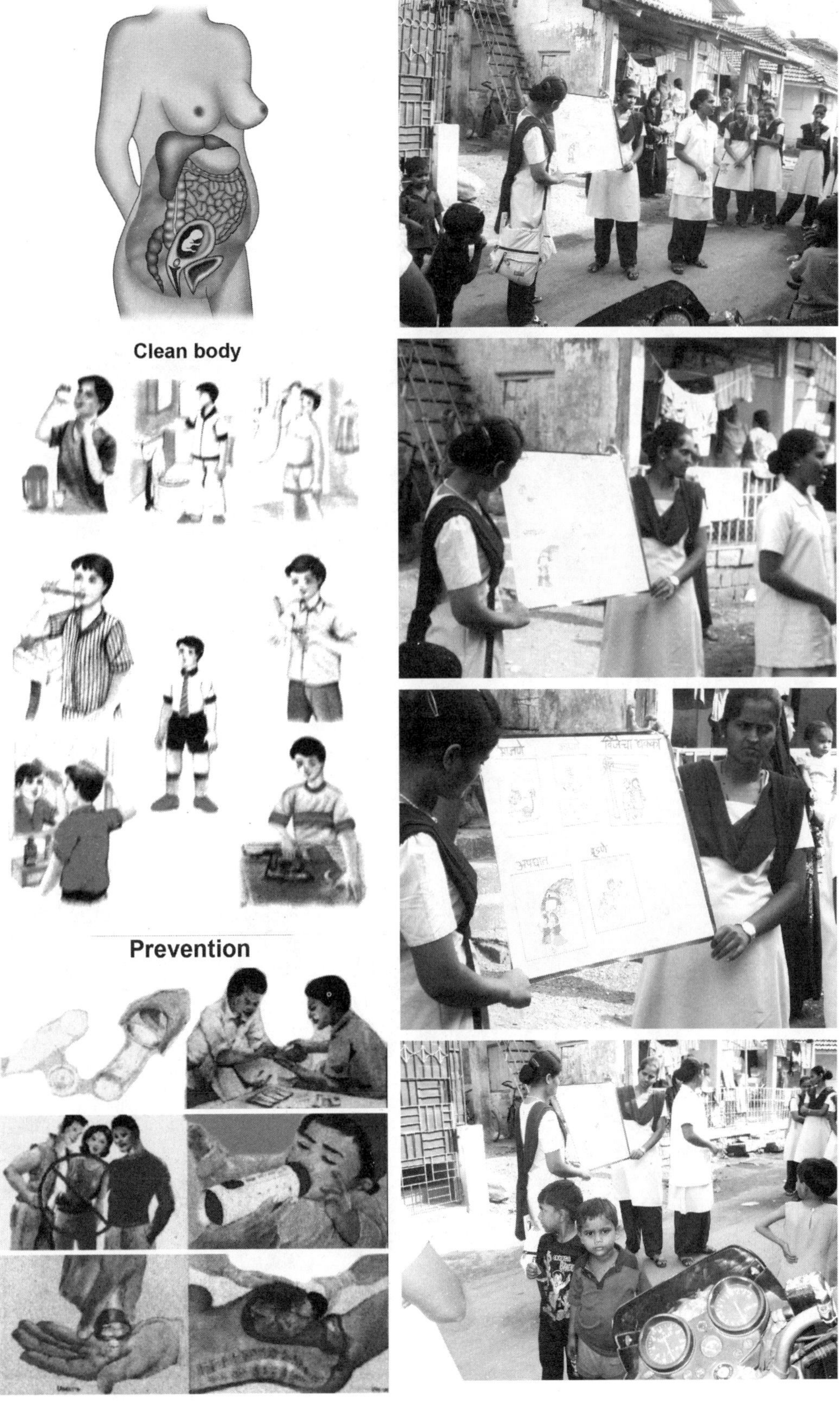
Clean body
Prevention

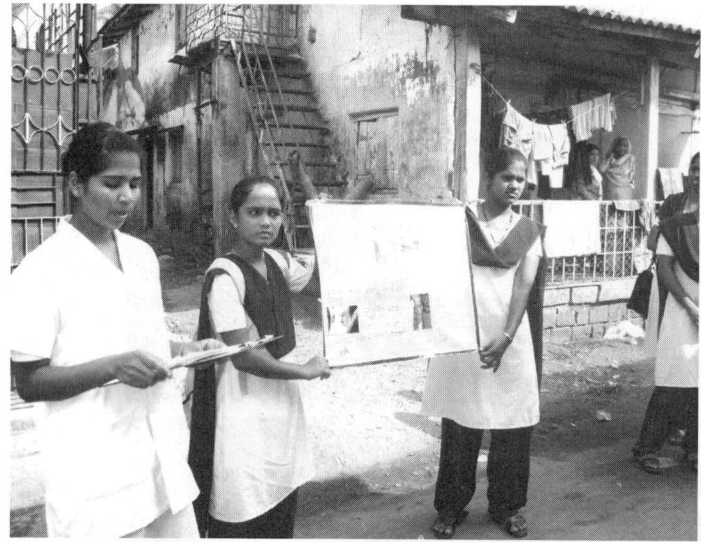

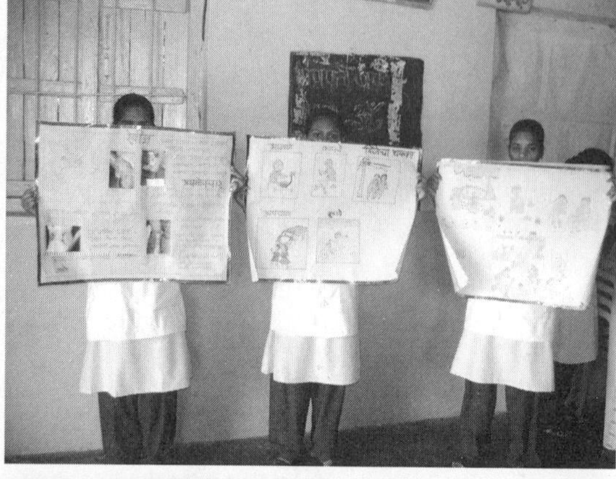

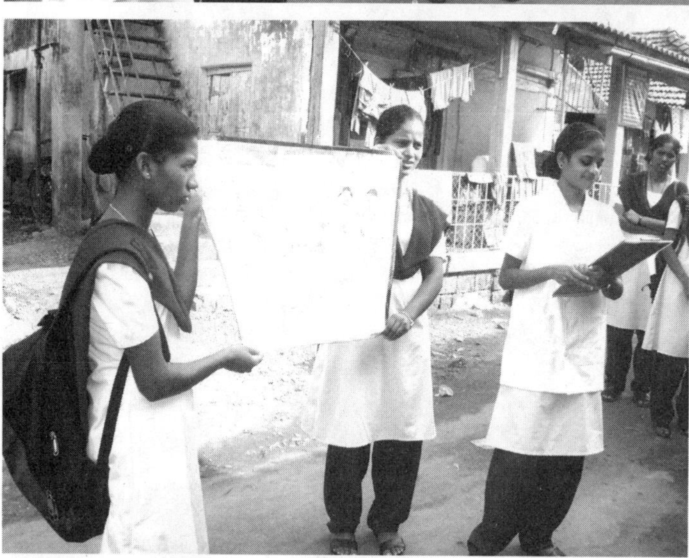

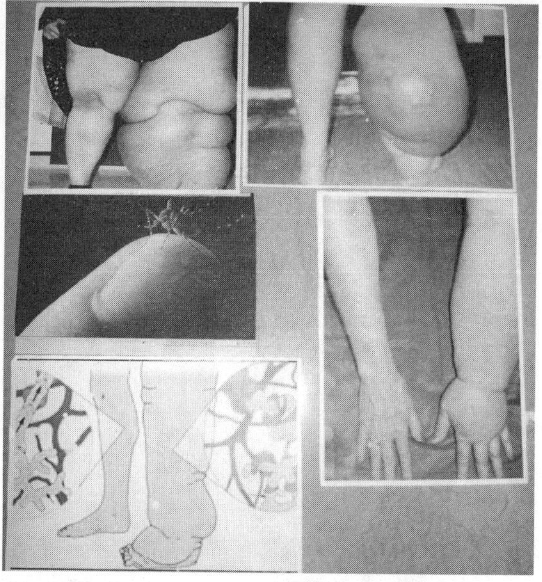

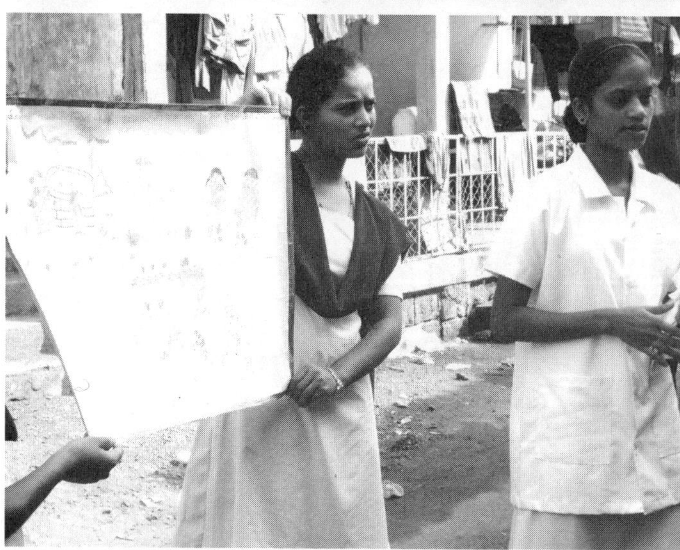

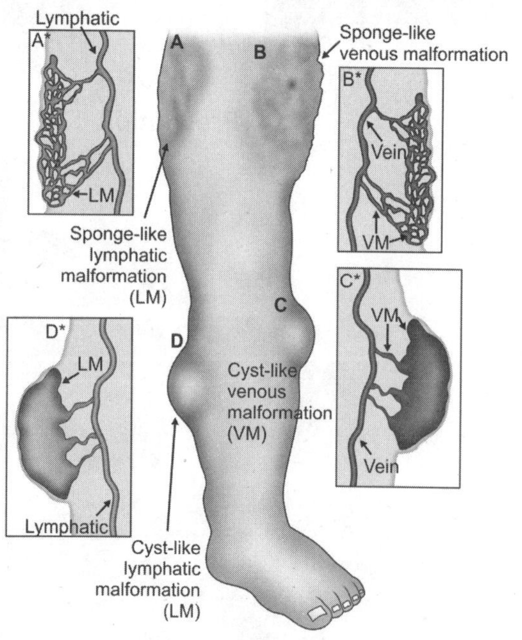
Lymphatic
A*
LM
A
B
Sponge-like
venous malformation
B*
Vein
VM
Sponge-like
lymphatic
malformation
(LM)
C
C*
VM
Vein
D
D*
LM
Cyst-like
venous
malformation
(VM)
Lymphatic
Cyst-like
lymphatic
malformation
(LM)

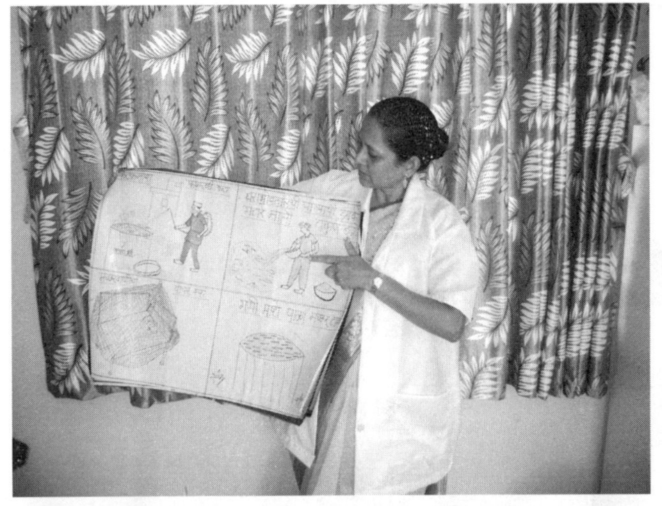

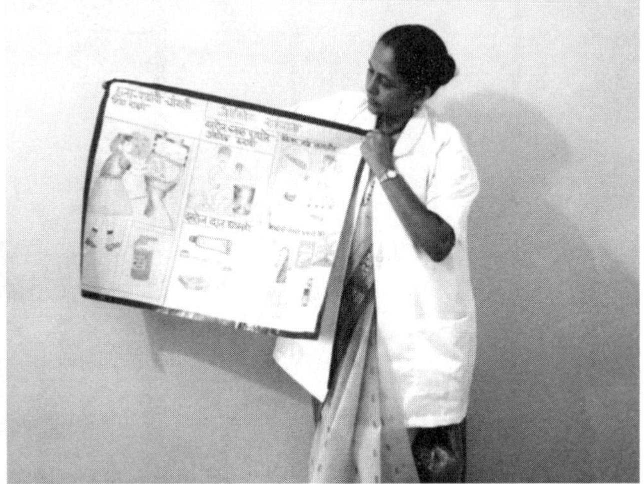

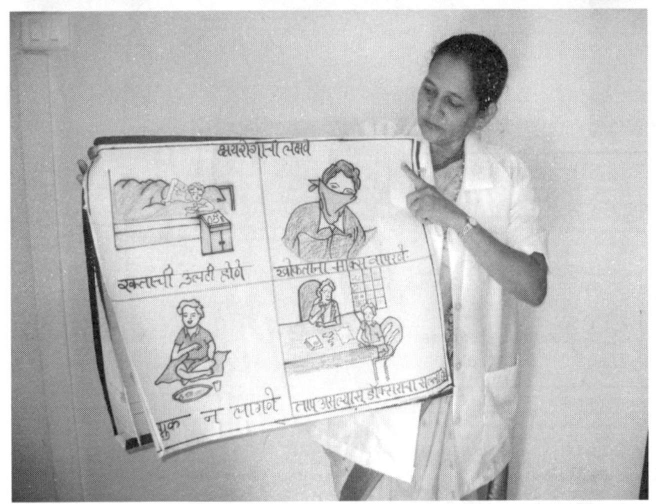
रक्ताची उलटी होणे

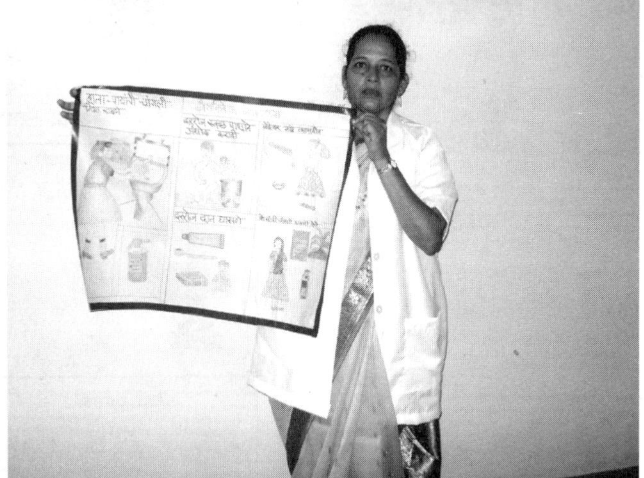

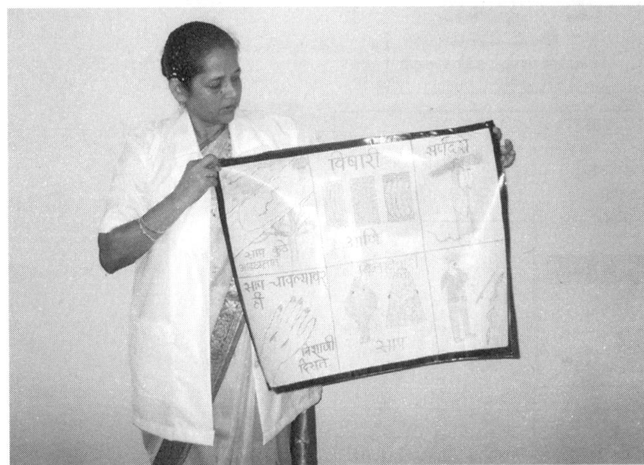
विषारी

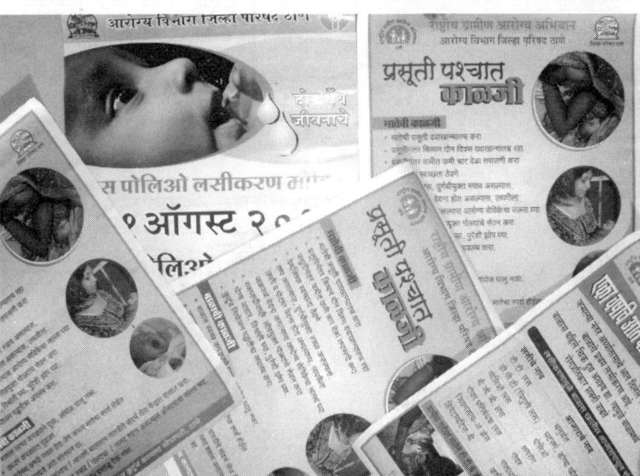
राष्ट्रीय ग्रामीण आरोग्य अभियान
आरोग्य विभाग जिल्हा परिषद ठाणे
प्रसूती पश्चात काळजी

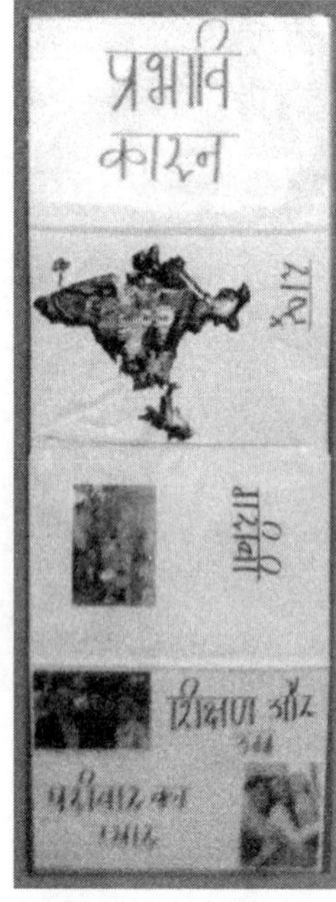
प्रभावि
कारन

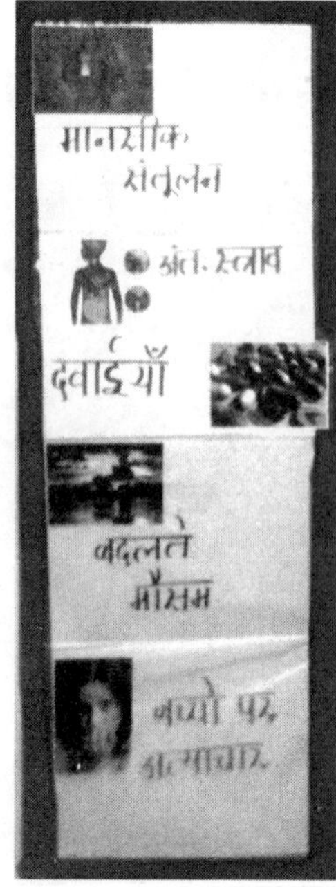
मानसिक
संतुलन
अंतः स्त्राव
दवाईयाँ
बदलते
मौसम
बच्चो पर
अत्याचार

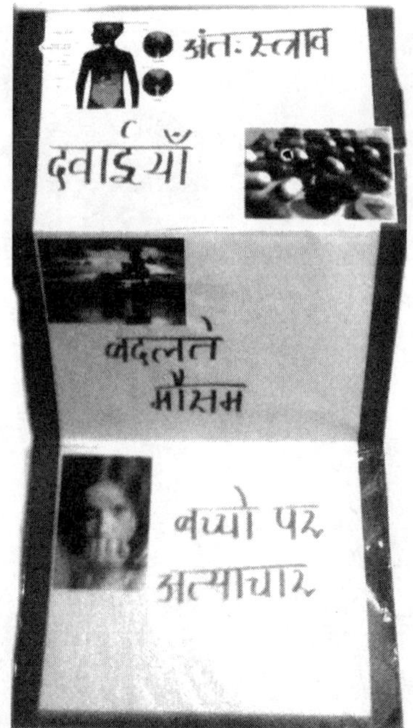
अंतः स्त्राव
दवाईयाँ
बदलते
मौसम
बच्चो पर
अत्याचार

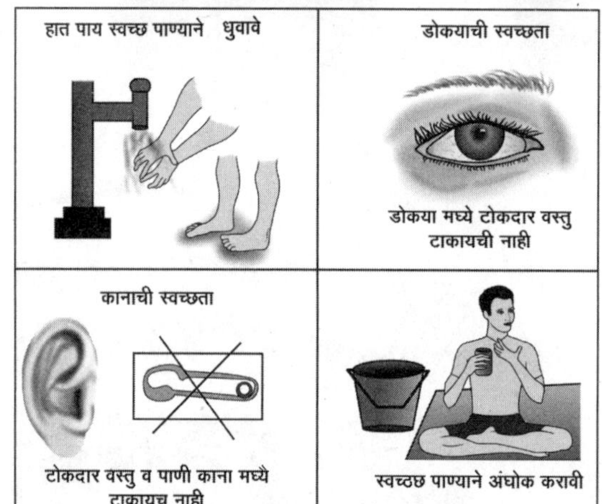
हात पाय स्वच्छ पाण्याने धुवावे
डोकयाची स्वच्छता
डोकया मध्ये टोकदार वस्तु टाकायची नाही
कानाची स्वच्छता
टोकदार वस्तु व पाणी काना मध्यै टाकायच नाही
स्वच्छ पाण्याने अंघोक करावी

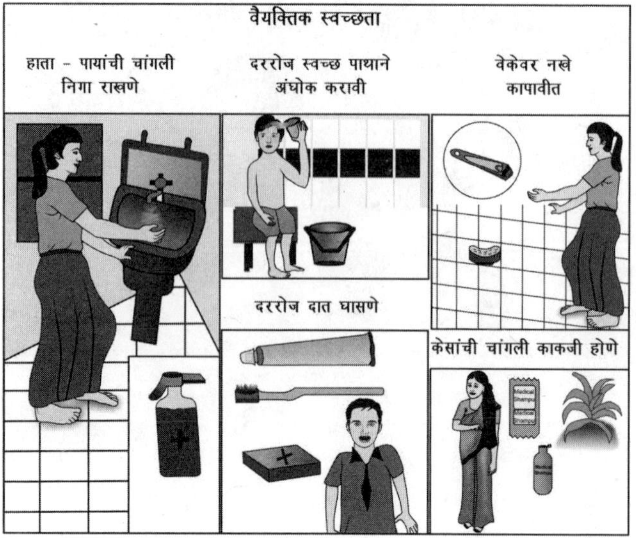
वैयक्तिक स्वच्छता
हाता - पायांची चांगली निगा राखणे
दररोज स्वच्छ पाथाने अंघोक करावी
वेकेवर नखे कापावीत
दररोज दात घासणे
केसांची चांगली काकजी होणे

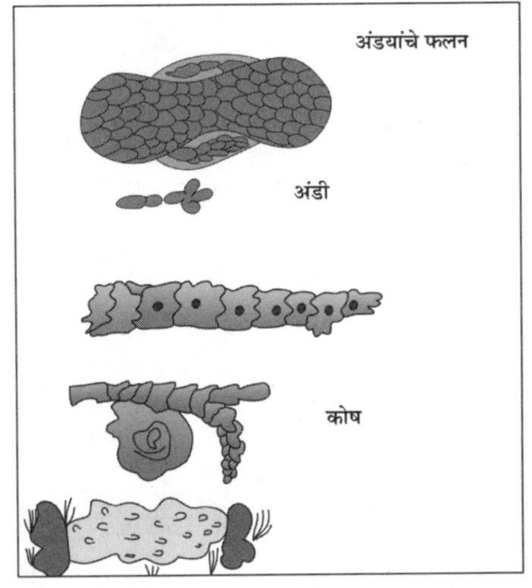
अंडयांचे फलन
अंडी
कोष

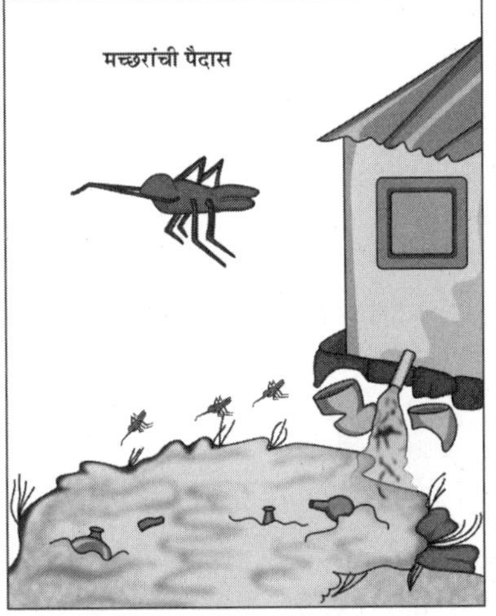
मच्छरांची पैदास

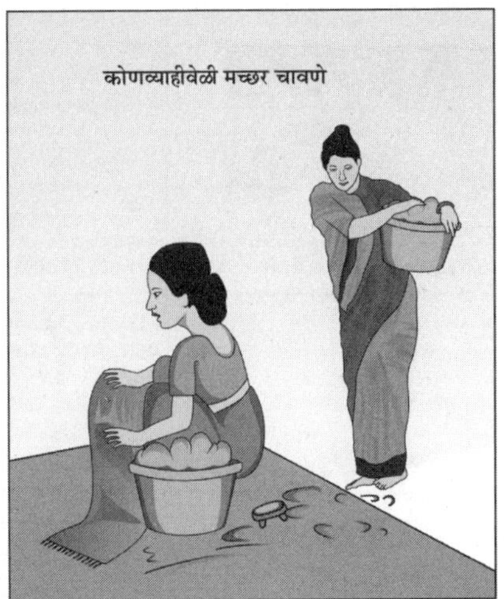
कोणव्याहीवेळी मच्छर चावणे

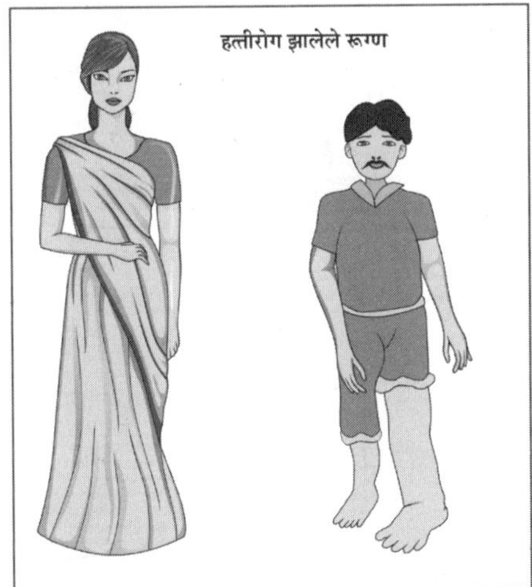
हत्तीरोग झालेले रूग्ण

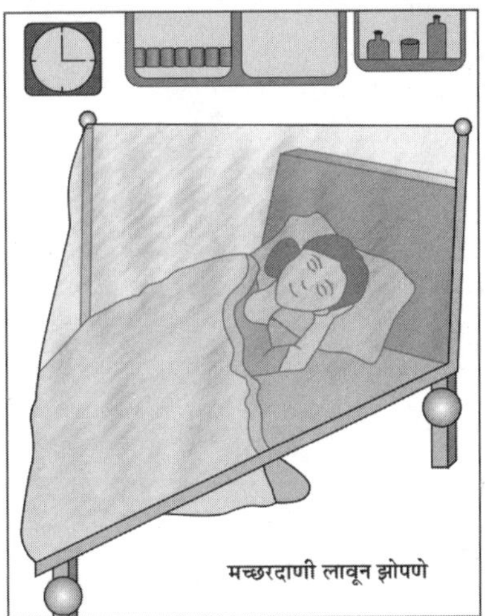
मच्छरदाणी लावून झोपणे

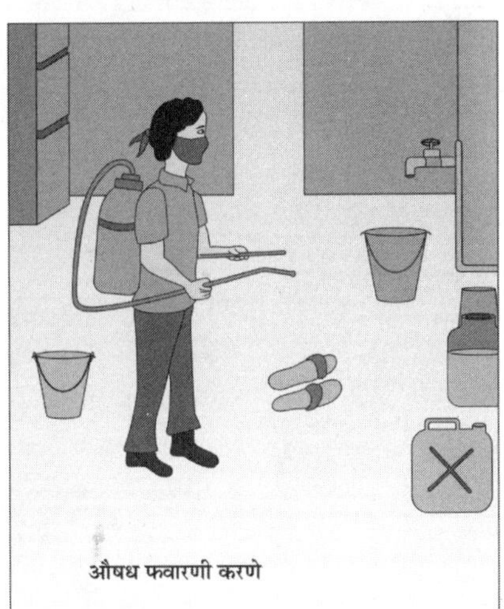
औषध फवारणी करणे

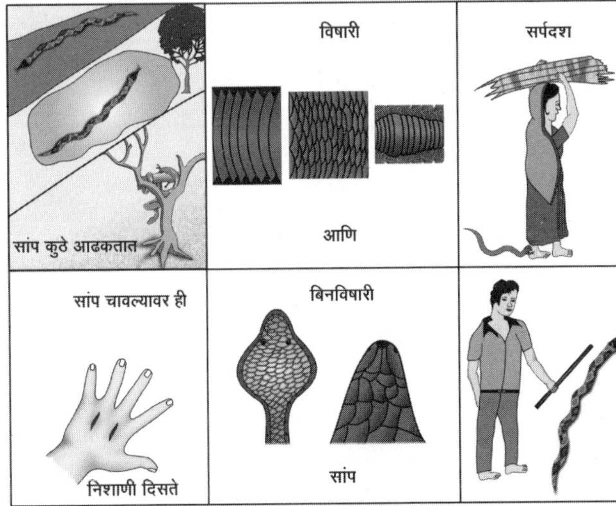
सांप कुठे आढकतात
विषारी
आणि
सर्पदश
सांप चावल्यावर ही
निशाणी दिसते
बिनविषारी
सांप

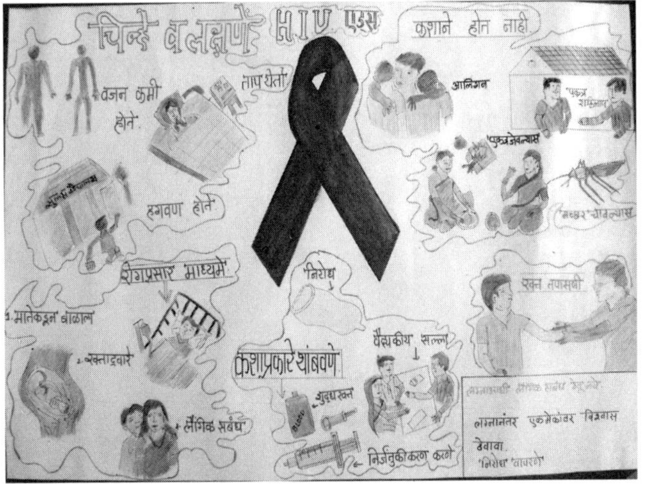
चिन्हे व लक्षणे HIV एड्स
कशाने होत नाही
वजन कमी होते
ताप येतो
आलिंगन
हगवण होते
रोगप्रसार माध्यमे
निरोध
कशाप्रकारे थांबवणे
वैद्यकीय सल्ला
निर्जंतुकीकरण करणे

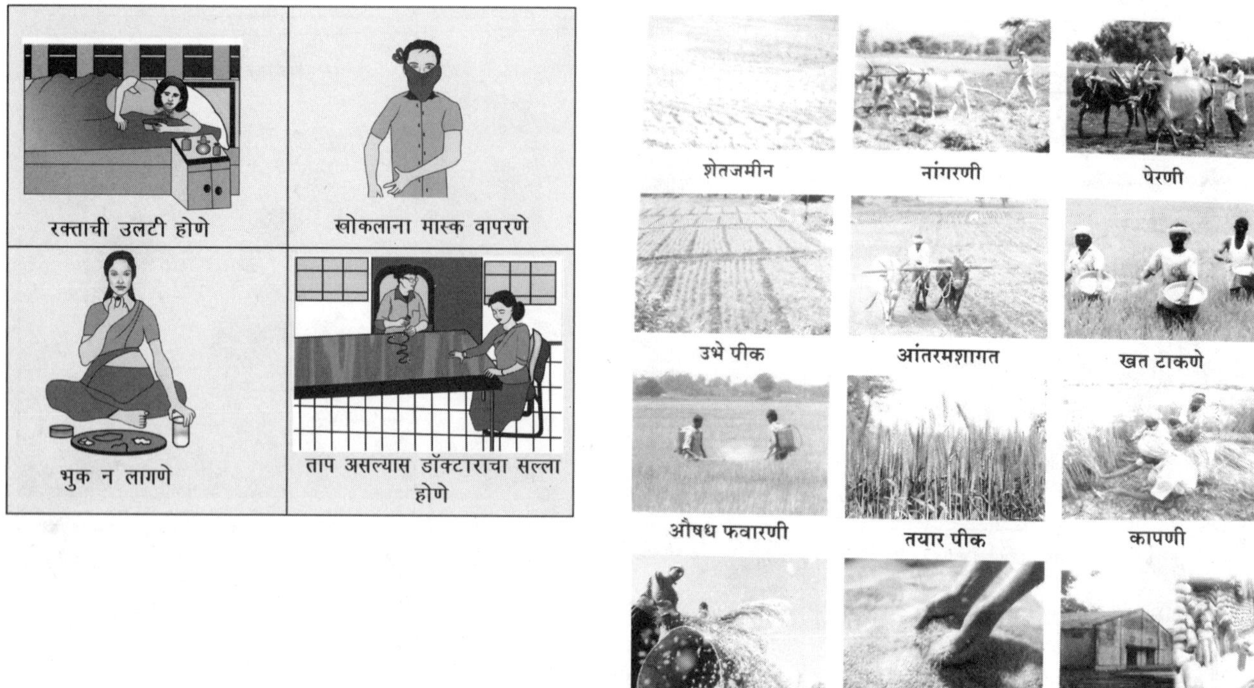
रक्ताची उलटी होणे
खोकलाना मास्क वापरणे
भुक न लागणे
ताप असल्यास डॉक्टाराचा सल्ला होणे
शेतजमीन
नांगरणी
पेरणी
उभे पीक
आंतरमशागत
खत टाकणे
औषध फवारणी
तयार पीक
कापणी
मळणी / झोडपणी
गहू
साठवण

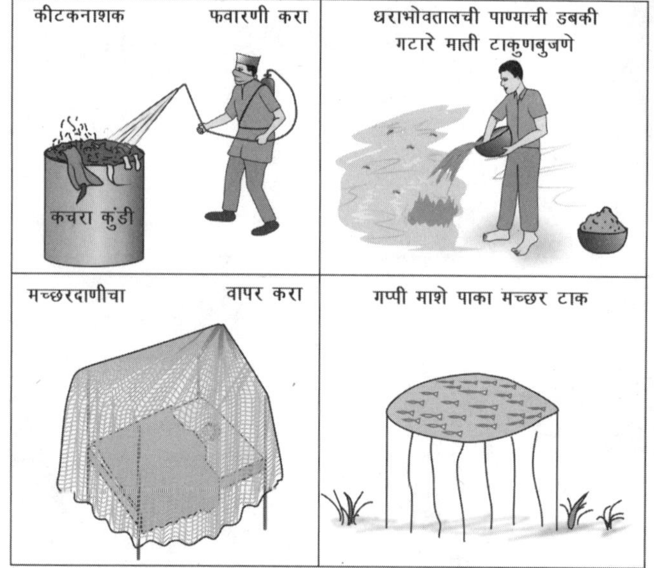
कीटकनाशक
फवारणी करा
कचरा कुंडी
धराभोवतालची पाण्याची डबकी
गटारे माती टाकुणबुजणे
मच्छरदाणीचा
वापर करा
गप्पी माशे पाका मच्छर टाक

CHAPTER

27

Demonstration

Abstract

An act of showing someone how something is used or done. It involves showing by reason or proof, explaining or making clear by use of examples or experiments.

INTRODUCTION

Demonstration is the health method of group communication-seeing is believes, a live demo often proves a very effective; it is a good way to show how to do something. It provides stimuli to all the senses of the learners, seeing, hearing, touching and may be testing and even smelling. Individual learners best when all his senses are used in the process. It enables individual/group to understand better the cause of a problem and result/consequences of an action.

It teaches by exhibition and explanation and teaches students the art of careful observation which is essential for a nurse. It is concrete illustration where students hear the explanation and see the process at the same time. It projects mental image in the mind which fortifies verbal knowledge. It activates many senses, clarifies principles and points out weather the student is able to apply her knowledge in practical way when the students does return demonstration. It is used to review and revised procedures and introduced new procedures too. Good demonstration needs advanced knowledge, all required equipments; all get good view, running comments. With apt consent demonstration is done on the live model. Here the teacher is present so students feel at ease. They get closer contact and concrete reality in front of them. It is attention catching, students can ask direct questions and clears the doubts.

Practical demonstration is an important technique of health education. We show people how a particular thing is done using a toothbrush, bathing a child, feeding an infant, disinfection of well, ORT, construction of sanitary latrine, preparing nutritional items, etc.

A demonstration leaves a visual impression or explanation of facts, concept, and procedures, in the minds of the people. Purpose of demonstration is to perform certain psychomotor skill; reproduce exactly the behavior, understand concept of principles; to provide opportunity for practice and gain skill, it can be accompany with formal lecture.

Advantage of demonstration is that it activates several senses and increases learning, it also provides the opportunity for observational, learning as it projects a mental image in the mind of the viewer which in turn help in verbal knowledge, it clarifies, creates interest by use of concrete illustration; correlate theory with practice and is a motivational force created, and students when re-demonstrate we can test the gasp of knowledge of the group.

It can be used in community to teach mother how to feed the baby, how to prepare the weaning foods, to show balance diet etc It can be shown in groups of specific people where all are able to view it, and is useful method of education.

The pictures given at the end of the chapter will give an idea to students and they can develop on there own many other situation where in different circumstances different topics can be taken in for demonstration.

Demonstration as a teaching strategy to the visual presentation of the action and activities or practical work related to the facts an principle work related to the facts and principles of a delivered lesson by the teacher in the classroom aiming to facilitate the task of teaching and learning. It is a practical form, the objects, instruments, action and events related to teaching. All get simultaneously rich practical experience with the common demonstration exhibited to them by the teacher. It helps in cultivating genuine interest and attention, it makes active participation and develops there mental faculties of observation, reasoning, deep thinking and creative imagination and principle of integration theory in practicing and readiness for practice of new knowledge evaluation of a class with demonstration of procedure—the objectives made clear, new equipment explained, steps are taken in the sequence order, procedure explained, important points noted, patients comfort and safety considered. In it the procedure done with good technique and method and it is done with skill and finished with precision, teaching aids. Skill in gaining attention.

Conclusion

Demonstrate operates to show, perform an action, activity description, illustrate an experiments or an intervention that is being tested and described. It is an practical application which is illustrated and explained, it is a technique used by teachers where students get visual representation of ideas, facts. It promotes learning by doing where they utilize the sense of sight and touch. There are different types of demonstration like individual, group, and lecture cum demonstration and return demonstration. Here students learn by doing, they can correlate theory into practice.

Explanation for Figures

Think of useful topic of useful area and demonstrate before the group, e.g. as you can see student demonstrated simple procedures, hand washing, resuscitation, attainting emergency call, doing active and passive exercise, etc. in nursing field a nurse has constantly present her topics and demonstrate and re-demonstrate every procedure either on dummy or live model. There is numberless demonstration she has to do in her career. Few examples are given just for clarity in the chapter to know what demonstration is.

Keywords
Demonstration, Explanation of figures, Conclusions.

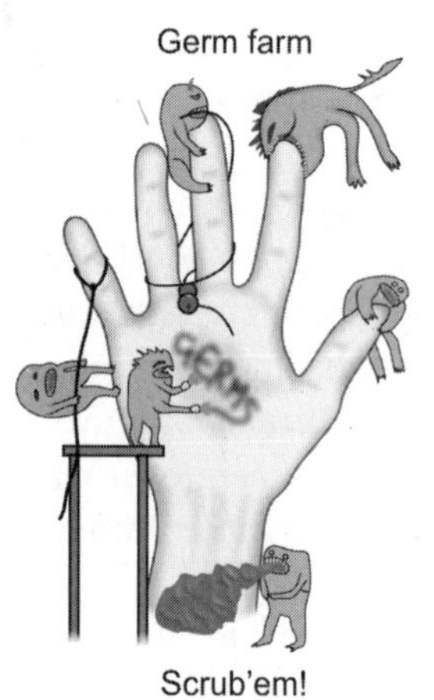

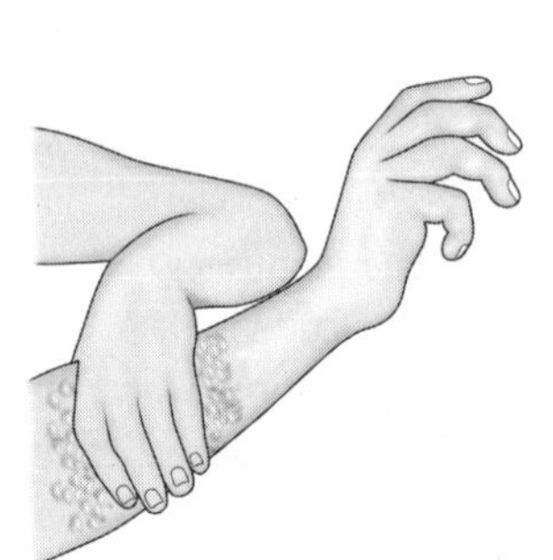

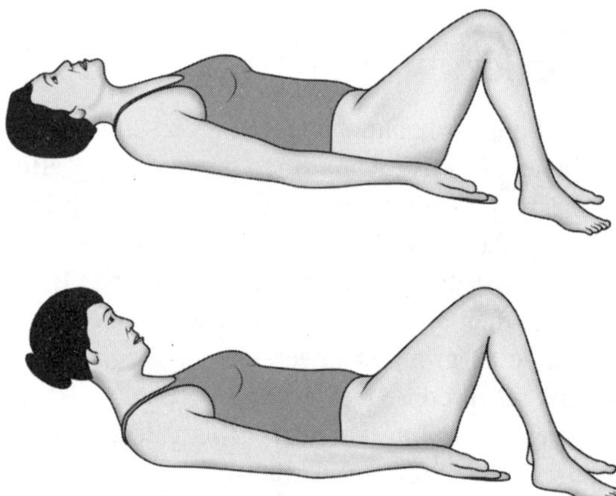

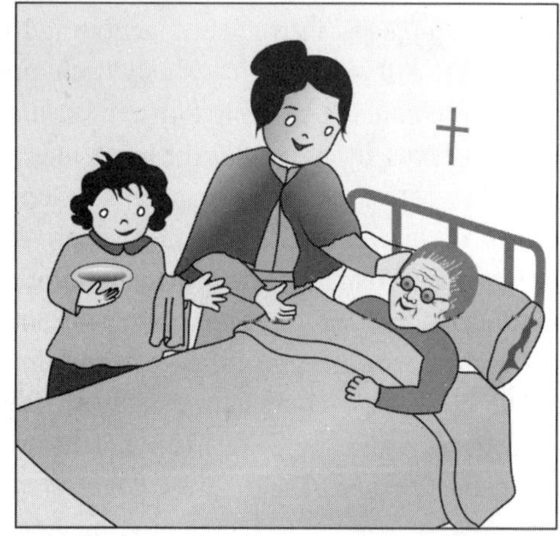

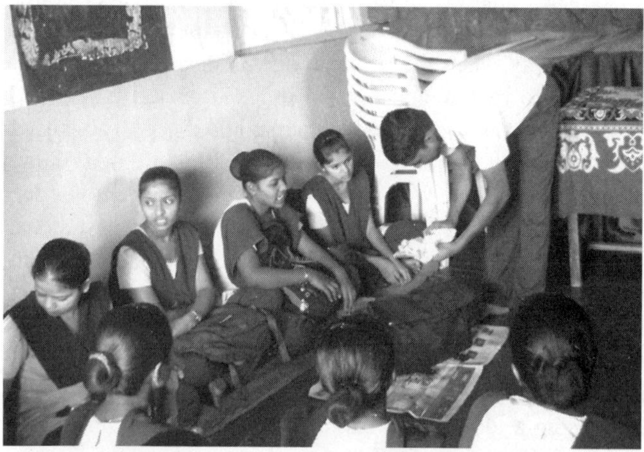

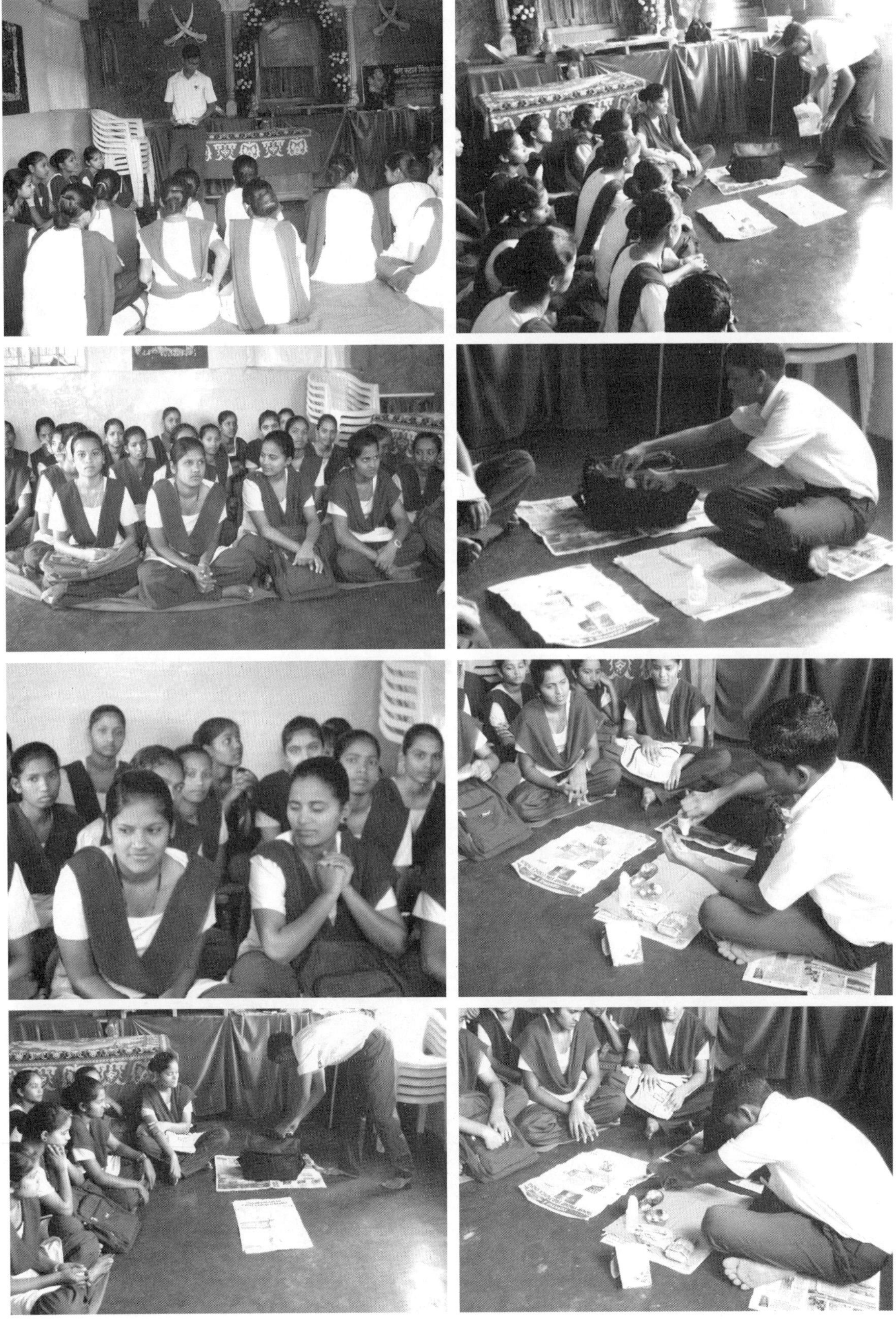

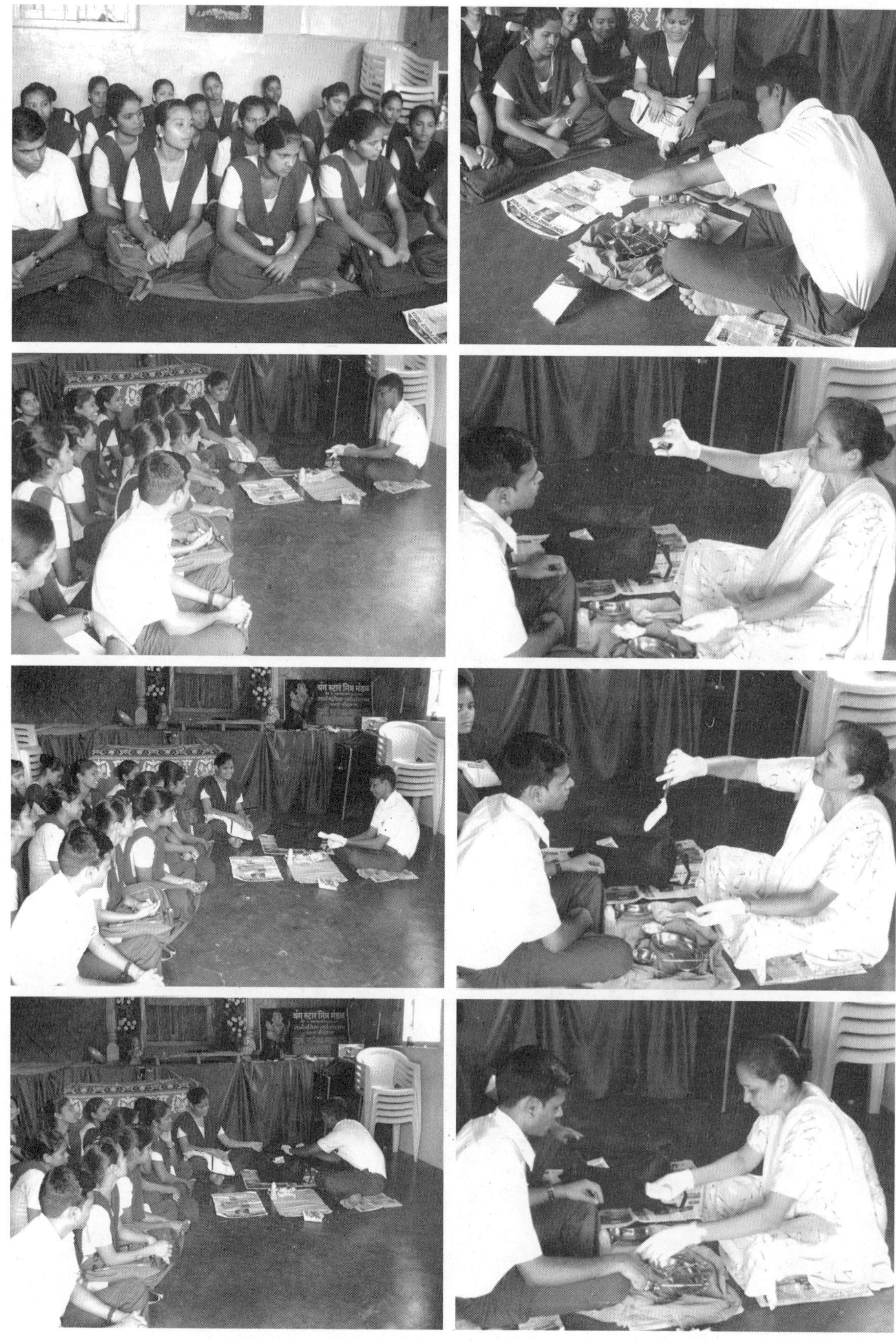

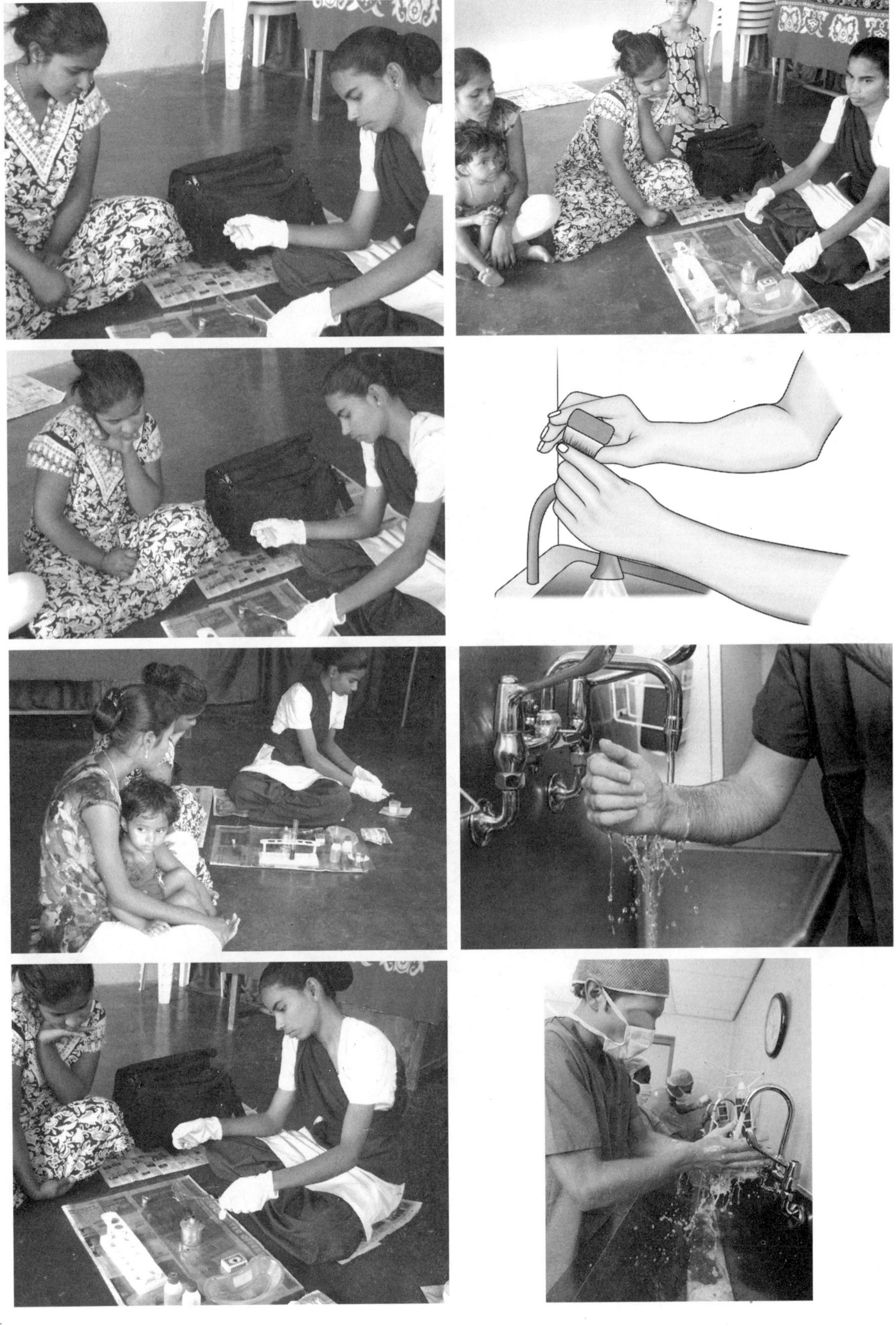

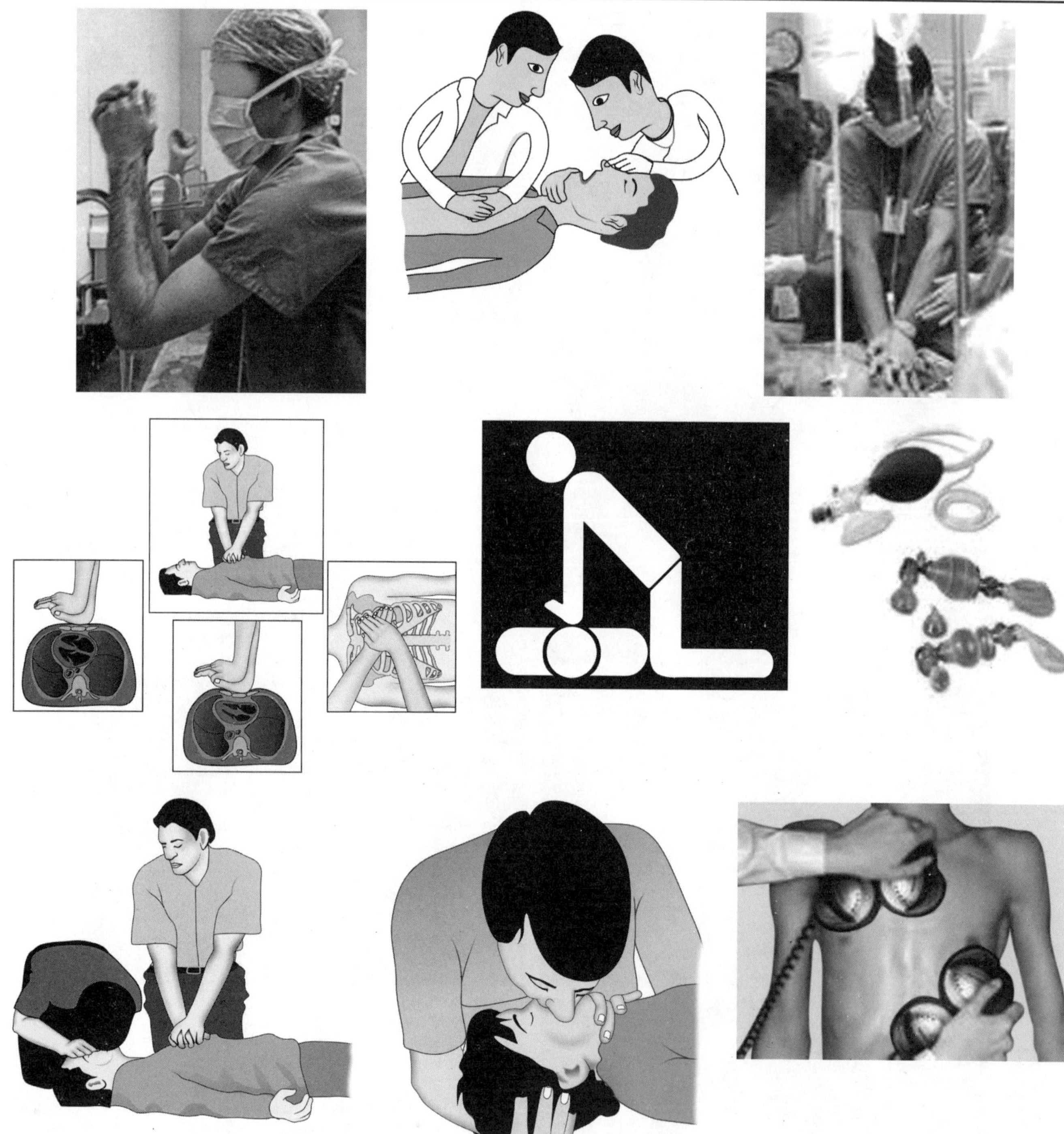

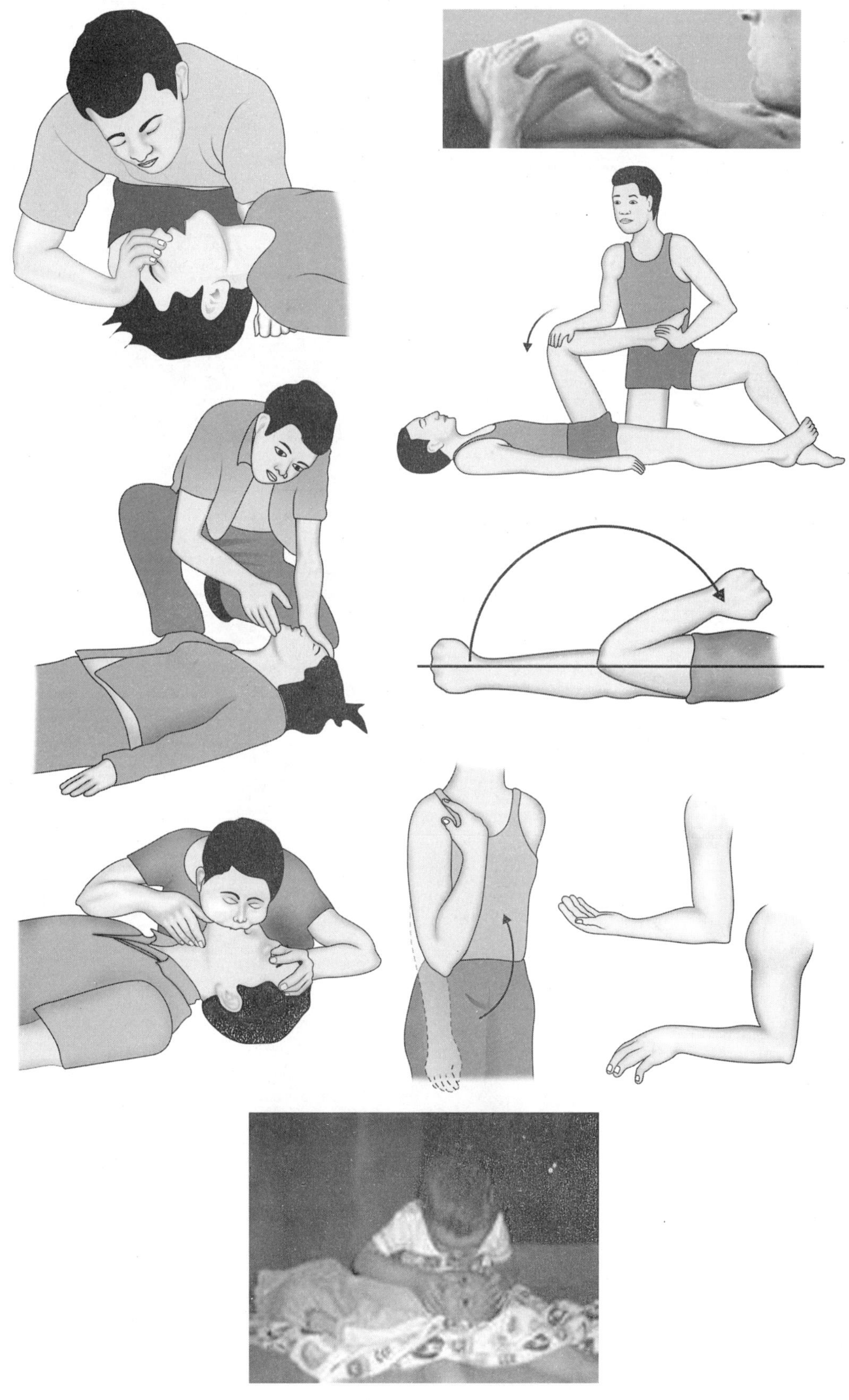

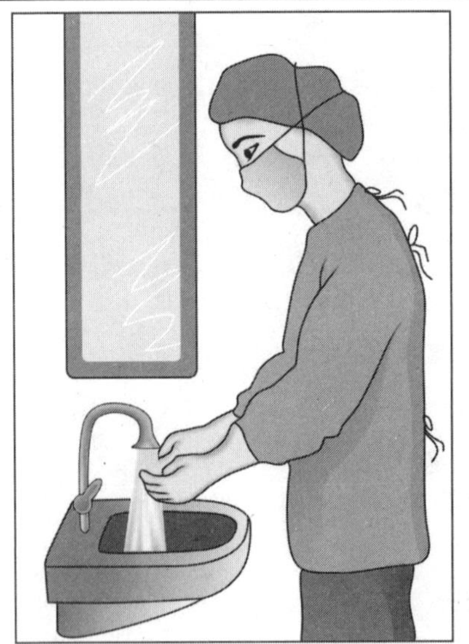

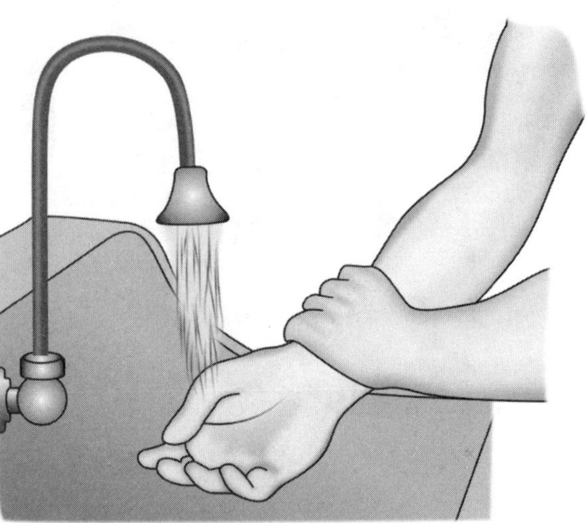

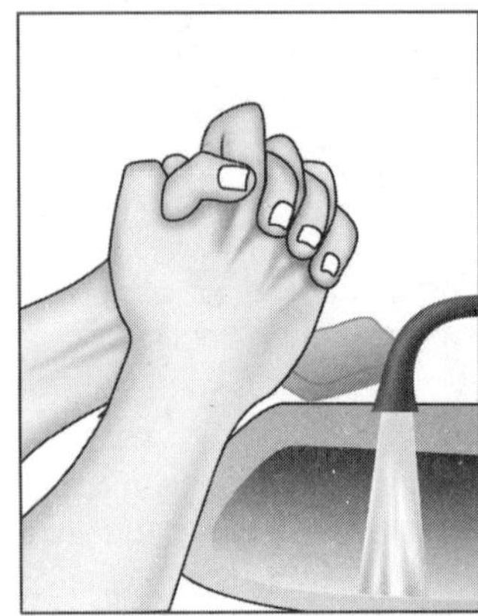

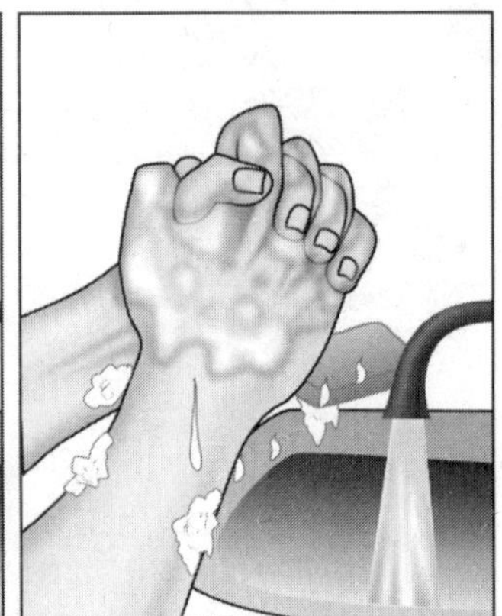

CHAPTER 28

Diabetes Control and Obesity

Abstract

Diabetes is a disease that affects your body's ability to produce or use insulin. Obesity is a condition characterized by the excessive accumulation and storage of fat in the body.

INTRODUCTION

Diabetes is here a decade early—it is bitter truth of a sweet life. Diabetes is striking Indians earlier than we think. But, there is hope yet. Lifestyle modification with the right dose of exercise can stall the onset of type 2 diabetes.

The sugar coating is off. It is a bitter pill we have to swallow. India has the unenviable title of being the diabetes capital that by 2025. India had 19 million diabetes these would increase to 57 million in 2025.

Early onset warning—diabectologists are sounding the alarm bells a decade early. What is more alarming is that the early onset of the disease has been observed 10 years early among Indians than other races. In the race to achieve our ambitions in the shortest possible time, we are driving ourselves to disaster. Besides stress leading to hypertension, we are also consuming unhealthy food high in fat and less in fiber. Our desk jobs are making us sedentary and we lack the time or initiative for exercise and outdoor recreation. Fast food on the go poses high glycemic risk and can trigger obesity even in the children.

Type 2 diabetes can occur at any age—type 2 diabetes occurs as a result of excess sugar and cholesterol in the body. This type is strongly associated with high blood pressure, high cholesterol and apple body shape, where excessive weight is carried around the waist. It is the most common form of diabetes affecting 85 to 90% of all people with diabetes. While it usually affects mature adults, younger people are also now being diagnosed in greater numbers because increase in the incidence of over weight and obesity. Type 2 diabetes used to called non insulin dependent diabetes or mature onset diabetes.

Undiagnosed diabetes is the silent killer—the statistics show that diabetes is exploding an epidemic in India, especially in the urban population. It has gone up from 5% to 18.6% from 1986 to 2009 in adult urban population age 20 and above. Today India has 61 million diabetes with almost half of them remain undiagnosed.

Exercise and diet—the best solutions—our big fat Indian weddings and festivals often celebrate the gourmand in us, with an array of tables groaning with the weight of rich food. But the potential of exercise on our health is still not embedded in our psyche. Exercise can improve insulin efficiency, lower blood pressure, and control sugar levels, bad cholesterol—all while building muscle strength and tone. Do you need another reason to exercise?

Prevention is the key—it is not the end of the road for those diagnosed with boarder line or pre-diabetes. The awareness regarding obesity and emphasis on physical activity should be start. Don't sleep over it.

Manage children with diabetes with care, commitment and compassion. While insulin is the only effective treatment for children with type 1 diabetes, they need a strong support system of the family, school and society in helping them cope with the condition.

Type 1 diabetes mellitus also called insulin dependent; juvenile or childhood onset diabetes occurs when the pancreas does not produce insulin a hormone that regulates blood sugar. The cause is unknown, but it is thought to be the result of a combination of genetic and environmental factors. Currently, there is no known way to prevent type 1 diabetes. The majority of children who develop this has no family history of diabetes.

Diabetes in children, a cause for concern—Ninety to ninety-five of children with diabetes below 16 years. If the diagnosis or treatment is delayed because of any reason, the severe lack of insulin can result in diabetic ketoacidosis and death within day. there has been alarming increase in children in the last 30 years. In below 16 years of age group, it is estimated around 70,000 new cases of type 1 diabetes are reported each year in children world wide

A strong support system is crucial to care—it is not easy to parents to accept that their child is suffering from diabetes, always believed to affect the older people. It is important for parents to remember that a child who develops diabetes will not only live with the condition for a longer period than an adult who develops the disease. Take insulin and other medicine, checking blood glucose levels, balancing activity and food choice, adds to child's challenges of physical and emotional growth.

Insulin the only effective treatment—type 1 diabetes should be treated immediately. Insulin is essential and the only treatment available. The administration of insulin will result in immediate improvement in child's health.

Symptoms of type 1 diabetes parents should recognize any symptoms below:

1. Increased thirst and appetite
2. Frequent urination or restart of bed wetting. Some times ants near the child's toilet could also be a sign of presence of sugar in urine, thus indicating type 1 diabetes
3. Unexplained weight loss and fatigue
4. Blurred vision or suffer changes in vision
5. Sweet smell on the breath, vomiting, abdominal pain and rapid breathing. All of these when present together are symptoms of diabetic ketoacidosis, is a serious condition and if not treated immediately and properly can lead to coma or death.

Children with diabetes can live a long healthy and normal life if proper and timely treatment is given. Parent's education is very important.

In India there are nearly 42.5 million diabetics as of today. CVD too is robbing our country of the young and early middle aged population. The morbidity and mortality figure too are alarming 64.2%.

In India the commonest causes of chronic kidney disease (CKD) are DM 32% and CVD 20.5%.

To prevent CKD progression is by modifying and controlling 'what you eat'. Best way to achieve is by eating 7–8 small feeds a day which are loaded with a balance of all nutrients. Burning of stored body fuel. DM is a functional disorder which cannot be restored back with use of any pathy. One can maintain correct sugar level with the help of proper diet control and medicine.

DM, CKD change body metabolism and have bad effect on the endothelial linking of blood vessels, this leads of CVD, CKD, etc.

Relevance of nutrition of health, vigor and vitality require a balanced daily diet containing adequate of all food groups. Deficiency of essential nutrients can result in serious health consequences. What is needed is will power and intelligent moderation. The new thinking allows eating delicious healthy creative food with sensible eye towards the right mix of nutrients and the right portion size spread over 7–8 small, frequent feeds, diet control means eating punctually at specific time everyday. No food should be missed. Eating balanced diet at proper times will help one remain healthy. Soyabeans is called as wonder beans.

Diet and Diabetic: CVD–CKD Patients

Instructions for Dialysis Patients

There is protein loss, amino acid loss during dialysis. They must have proteins feeds at frequent intervals. Minimum salt, just enough for taste in vegetables, restricted intake of total fluid. Hence it is advisable to swallow most of the tab with milk unless contraindicated. This would enable the patient to limit his water intake and total fluid intake.

- Develop lifestyle, habits, so that your body becomes less susceptible to having high blood sugar.
- If you are over weight, losing weight, maintain healthy weight and plenty of physical activities would help your body become less insulin resistant, the main hormone which metabolizes glucose.
- Adjust your diet, so as to ensure that you are getting the right nutrients through out the day. Eating 7–8 times, regular small meals will reduce fluctuation in your blood sugar.
- Make sure your body has enough insulin to that your cells get adequate fuel to function.

Administration of Insulin

Purpose

To temporarily restore the ability of the body to utilize carbohydrate.

General Rules

1. Keep insulin in refrigerator
2. Insulin dosage is exact and individualized, measure amount accurately a order by doctor
3. Always read the label, pay particular attention to the strength of insulin
4. Check expiration date on insulin bottle
5. Do not use insulin if it is expired date
6. Regular (un-moderated or plain) insulin and globulin insulin must always be clear as water. Protomin zinc insulin and isophane (NPH) are milky white
7. Regular insulin ordered according to specimen before meals (20–30 minutes before) protamin zinc insulin and NPH daily given 20–30 minutes before breakfast
8. Regular insulin and protamin zinc may be given together in one syringe
9. Insulin should be omitted until a fasting blood sugar is taken
10. Arms and thighs are usual sites for injecting site of injection should be rotated often
11. Insulin solutions are made in much strength. These strengths vary according to the number of units of insulin each cubic centimeter. The syringe is measured so that each line means one unit.

Equipment

1. Insulin of prescribed type
2. Sterile insulin syringe (u 40 for u 40 insulin; u 80 got u 80 insulin)
3. Sterile needles—size 25 or 26; ¾ or 1 inch in length

4. Dry sterile sponge and antiseptic sponges
5. Small tray
6. Pick up forceps
7. Medicine card with insulin order

Procedure

To prepare insulin syringe and needle

1. Using pick up forceps, remove dry 2×2 sponge and place on small tray
2. Select correct insulin syringe
3. Using pick up forceps remove barrel and plunger from container
4. Select correct size needle with forceps
5. Pick up needle at hub with forceps and attach to syringe
6. With free finger and thumb on hub fit securely to tip of syringe by giving a firm half turn
7. Test needle for burrs by drawing on dry sponge
8. Place syringe and needle on tray sponge
9. Place antiseptic sponge on tray

To withdraw solution from rubber diaphragm bottle

1. Rotate bottle gently between palms of both hands (to insure even distribution of insulin particles)
2. Clean rubber top with antiseptic sponge and discard sponge
3. Draw into syringe as much air as units of insulin to be withdrawn
4. Invert bottle, insert needle through rubber diaphragm and inject air
5. Withdraw desired units of insulin
6. Place on tray with antiseptic sponge
7. Go to the bedside and check patients name and number

To administer two types of insulin in one syringe

1. Read label on vial of protamin zinc insulin, check particularly on unit strength, and cleanse rubber top with antiseptic sponge
2. Re-read label on protamin zinc vial, check unit strength and cleanse rubber top with sponge fill syringe with same amount of air as units
3. Insert needle through center of rubber stopper, do not invert vial, and inject air into vial
4. Do not withdraw any protamin zinc insulin at this time
5. Withdraw needle from vial, fill syringe with same amount of air
6. Read label, check unit strength, clean rubber top, insert needle, invert vial and inject air into vial
7. Withdraw plunger until regular insulin in the number of units desired has entered the syringe
8. Withdraw needle from vial of regular insulin and insert needle into vial of protamin zinc insulin
9. Invert vial of protamin zinc insulin and withdraw amount of protemin zinc insulin desired.

To give insulin

1. Select site and cleanse with antiseptic sponge
2. Invert syringe and expel air
3. Pinch up fold of flesh and insert needle at 45 degree angle
4. Release pressure on skin
5. Aspirate by drawing back on plunger, if blood returns remove, change needle and insert in another site
6. Inject insulin slowly
7. Place sponge over point of injection and withdraw needle quickly

Aftercare of equipment

1. Clean syringe and needle and place with equipment to be returned to CSS
2. Return insulin to refrigerator
3. Charting—chart on diabetic record, amount, time
4. On nurses notes chart time, type, site of injection and reaction.

Obesity

Obesity is characterized by an excess accumulation of fat and reflects on the most basic level an over all positive balance between energy intake and expenditure. The causes are not fully understood but are recognized as complex and pervasive.

Overweight is expressed in terms of body mass index. It is a misconception that obesity is primarily a problem in the affluent countries. It occurs at any age. Infants with excessive weight gain in childhood results in obesity in adults, which is extremely difficult to treat with conventional methods. Men gain weight age 29 to 35 years, while women at the age of 45 to 49 years of age. Genetic factors, physical inactivity, socioeconomic status, eating habits, eating in between meals, preferences to sweet, refined food and saturated fats, food eaten and calories produced equivalent energy needs to be spent or else it deposits in to fat. When people have psychosocial problem, emotional disturbances depression, anxiety, frustration and loneliness they tend to eat more. Excessively obese individuals are withdrawn, self-consciousness secret eaters.

Obesity has a family tendency, which runs in certain family. Due to endocrine factor where growth hormone reduces and dries thus, its deficiency causes obesity in certain people. Women do gain a lot of weight after menopause as that has a lot to do with hormones and lifestyle exercise and talking calcium can help. In obese, person fatty mass increased and content of water not increased. Obesity can easily be identified at first sight. The longer your waistline, the shorter your lifeline. Extra weight could be due to extra eating. Extra fat puts a strain on your heart, kidneys, and liver and also on the large weight-bearing joints, such as the hips, knees and the ankles. Either we must increase the output of work, or we must reduce the food intake. Putting those large leg muscles to work burn up unwanted calories. Small quantities of food, balance food and regular eating are important. Do not go hungry for long. It takes real will power to lose weight, but it is certainly worthwhile, find value of losing weight.

Watch for those high calories. Such as cashew nut, coconut, cake, chocolate, butter, ghee, ice cream. Your children watch more television, eat more junk food and get more pocket money to spend. Hazards of obesity are coronary heart disease, diabetes, gallbladder disease, and low fertility, lowers life expectancy. Prevention begin in childhood with diet control/changes fiber increase, increase physical activities, one should not expect quick, tangible result. Health education, motivation, helps the patience. Ten years ago, people took the stairs up to their offices. Today they prefer elevator even if they work on first floor. Earlier lunch brought from home today power lunch. Ask yourself; is your job hazardous to your health? You do not have to be sumo wrestler to risk your life. Health is least priority today. Everyone has feeling that they are healthy, but feeling healthy and being healthy two different things. Health is only capital that is difficult to regain, better to invest in fitness programme today. Fit person has optimal immunity, alertness, a good attention span, flexibility and high energy level. So fit vs fat.

Obesity places an extra burden on the heart, requiring the muscle to work harder to pump enough blood to support added tissue mass. In addition, obesity is often associated with a sedentary lifestyle elevated serum cholesterol and high blood pressure.

Problems with body image affect both men and women. Most people face it at some stage of their life. Men face pressure to tone up, muscle up and look strong. While women face pressure to slim down, tone down and look good. If one wants to achieve a weight loss of few kilograms, it should be done under tight discipline and authoritative governance.

A composite and holistic plan to be adopted with the help of a professional. Therefore, they may exercise vigorously and not eat properly to achieve the result and hence their body suffers, they become weak and there may arise health problem, so one must consult a proper fitness professional. Fresh fruits to be consumed and workout at any point of time should not exceed. Consume natural foods, no medicines or drugs should be taken to lose weight, over exercise should be avoided, there should not be starvation, slow breathing exercise should be done and fluids like coconut water, fresh fruit juices taken, electrolyte loss also should be monitored.

Obesity—has been well documented that obese parents often have obese children, parental attitude towards food and eating habits are readily passed on to their children, the nurse must help parents to understand the unique food requirements. In Obesity, specific weight is gained. in women changes of lifestyle could be the reason. Females do gain weight during the age of 26–50 years due to physiological and pathological changes.

Discovering Healthier and Wealthier Tomorrow

Balanced life yields good health—it has been estimated that **diabetes** which is one of the most prevalent non communicable diseases in India and witnessed a steady increase over the last decade due to the economic transition and increased changes in lifestyle. Healthy lifestyle with regular exercise can help you stay hale and hearty. All have been learning prevention is better than cure—thin and apply this global phenomenon to our lives. Diabetes is the most common metabolic disorder fiercely affecting population in all geographical region of the world and is posing an enormous health problem due to lack of physical activity, desk bound work, sluggish lifestyle, obesity, stress and consumption of diets rich in sugar, fat and calories. It was formally prevalent in adults, is now found in younger generation and children due to changes in lifestyle and imbalanced eating habits. if proper care not taken it can tune hazardous. Control diabetes before it controls you; people must take ownership of their health by making right choice of food. Diabetes is a complex disease, but we can live with it with proper treatment, diet and exercise. Indians have lower muscle growth and higher fat growth; it is right from birth of baby. Even the people in India have diabetic because of low metabolism rate. This is due to sitting job and no physical movement which lads to fast accumulation in liver, lading to diabetes, do not outsource your heath to take care of it yourself. Prevention of diabetes is not just about treatment or medication, it is also about education. The use of maniple phone technology can be of great benefit in spreading awareness about the prevention and cure and this diseases. Schools to bay soft drinks and junk food in school canteens, it is in to sensitive policy makers about spreading health awareness right from school level, screening, early intervention and new medical treatment there by reducing the burden of chronic diseases.

Human body is work of art observing the artistic manner in which all the muscles are attached to the bone by tendon, joints balanced with the help of ligaments, fat deposited in manner that imparts good shape to the limbs, trunk and abdomen, the skin, pigment that makes the body look attractive, bone is nothing but earth or clay, blood is water, the radiance of skin and eyes is fire and the prana or breath that moves through the nostrils and lungs is nothing but air which drives its support from ether. They go back to their source, body gets dissolved with its five material components of earth, water, fire, air and ether from where it originally emanated. God dwelling in innermost chambers of the heart—men cling to perishable body, decaying so self-realization is important.

Most people are skipping exercise; even teens are turning to be victims of junk food addiction. We are nursing the growing diseases of an unhealthy lifestyle. The nation now to deal with a new breed of developed world obesity, coupled with sedentary lifestyle and urban youth getting affected with it.

Explanation

The figure shows how today lifestyle can also gives you diabetes and which food we have to avoid.

Keywords

Introduction, Early onset warning, Type 2 diabetes, silent killer, Exercise and diet, prevention, type 1 diabetes, children and diabetes, symptoms, CVD–CKD patients, insulin administration, purpose and general rules.

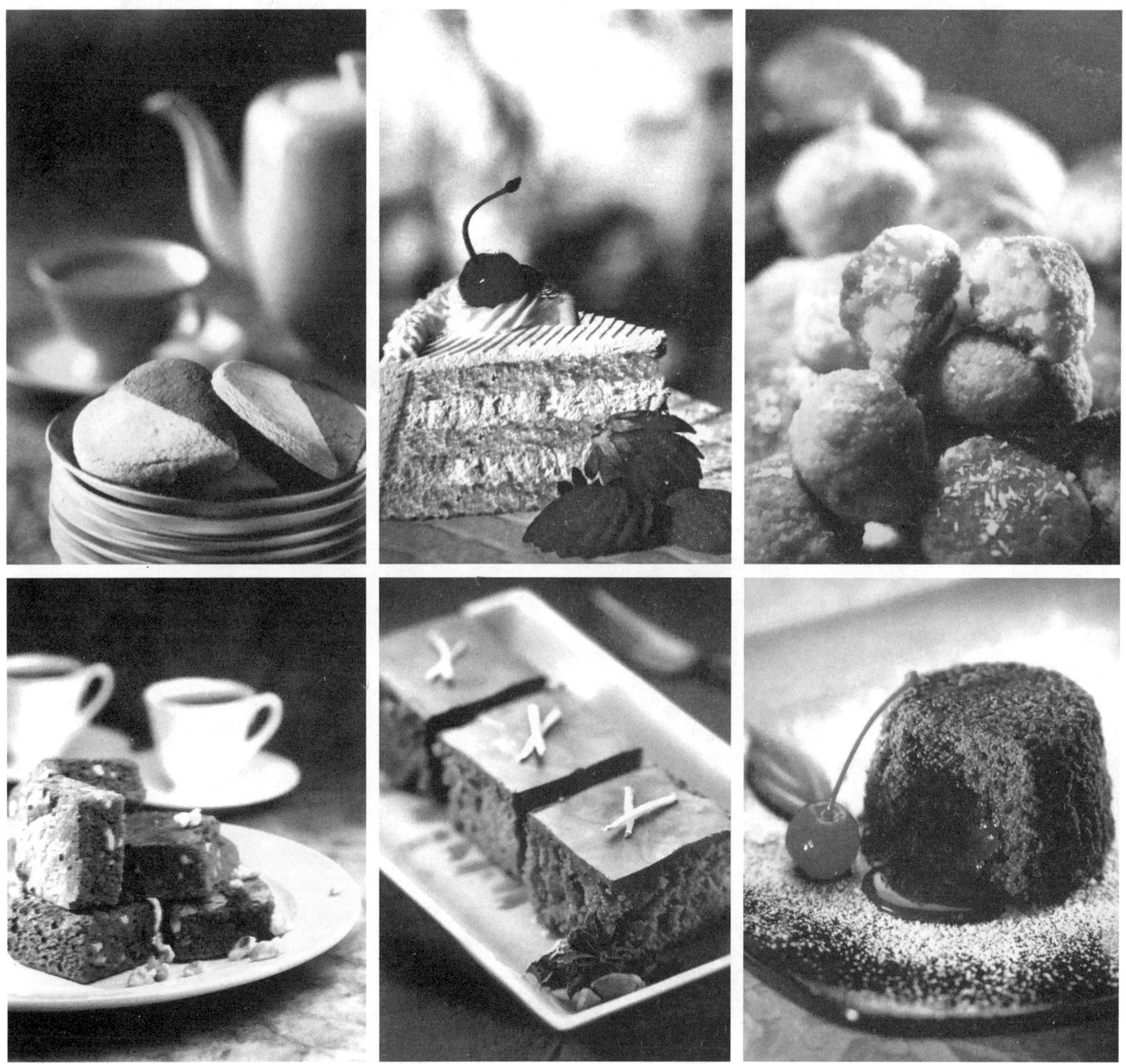

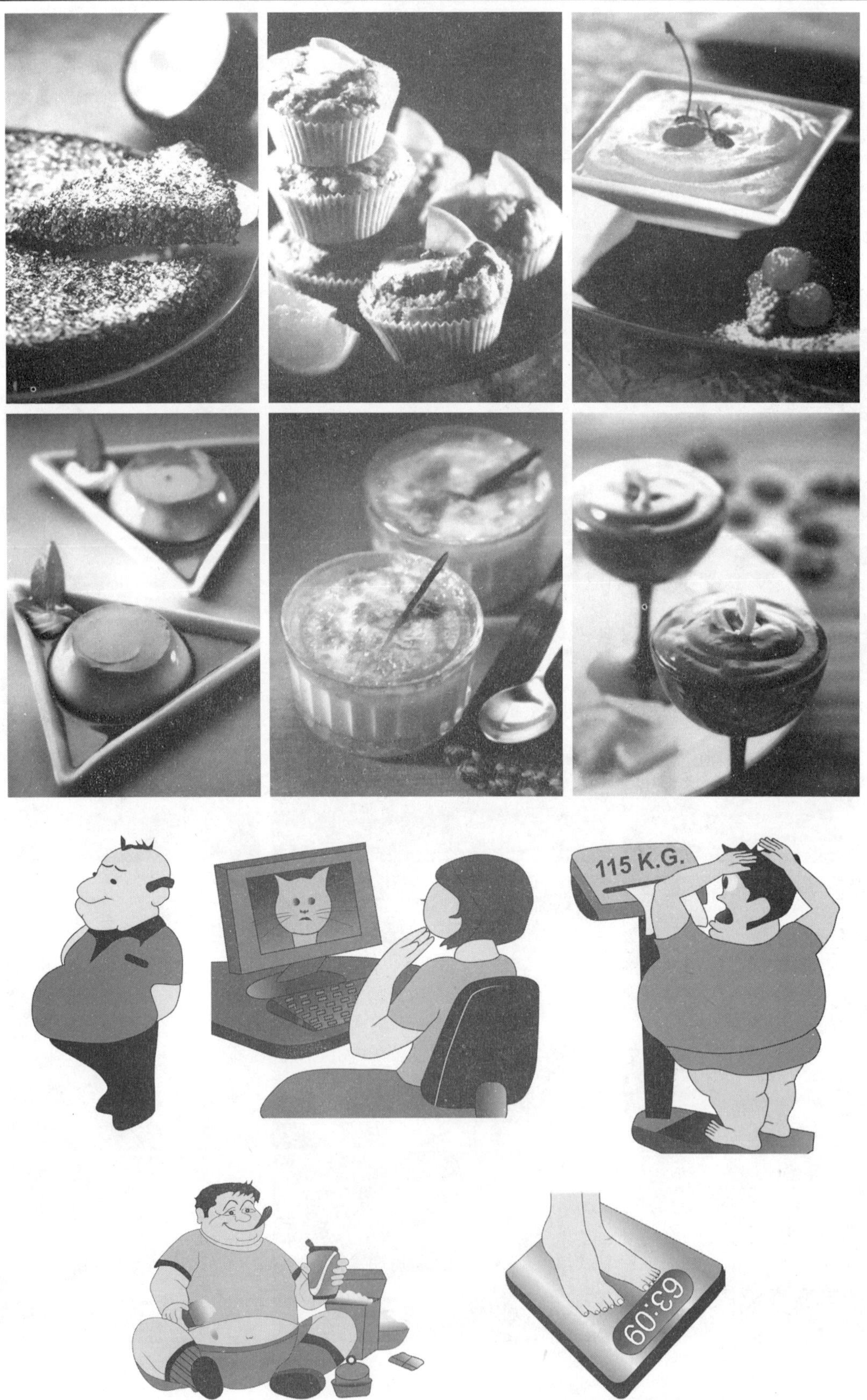
115 K.G.
63:09

CHAPTER

29

Flannel Graph

Abstract

Flannel graph is a story-telling system that uses a board covered with flannel fabric, usually resting on an easel.

INTRODUCTION

A flannel graph consists of a wooden board over which is pasted or fixed a piece of rough flannel cloth. It provides excellent background for displaying cut out pictures and other illustrations. These illustrations, and cut-out pictures are provided with a rough surface at the back by pasting pieces of sandpaper, felt or rough cloth, and they adhere at once, when put on the flannel. Flannel graph is a very cheap medium, easy to transport. The pictures must be arranged in proper sequence based on the talk to be given.

It holds interest of students, helps in lesson development. It enables teacher to talk along with changing illustrations.

The flannel board of 1.5 × 1.5 meter is most widely used. Collect the pictures, light objects or cutouts and back them with sandpaper pieces. Display material on the flannel board in a sequence to develop the lesson plan, change the picture or cutout as you talk to the patient. It can be used for telling a story. It display holds the interest and arrest their attention, it provides continuity in the lesson development, it provides quickness and easy to tell a story.

Graphs are visual teaching aids for presenting statistical information and contributing the trends or changes of certain attributes. There are four main types of grapes such as bar graph, line graph, picture graph and pie graph. A graphic material is a combination of graphic and pictorial material designed for the orderly and logical visualizing of relationships between key facts and ideas. It includes graphs, charts, maps, and diagrams.

Flannel Graph Definition

Flannel graph (sometimes called a flannel board) is a storytelling system that uses a board covered with flannel fabric, usually resting on an easel. It is very similar to Fuzzy Felt, although its primary use is as a storytelling medium, rather than as a toy.

Description of use—The flannel board is usually painted to depict a background scene appropriate to the story being told. Paper cutouts of characters and objects in the story are then placed on the board, and moved around, as the story unfolds. These cutouts are backed, either with flannel, or with some other substance that adheres lightly to the flannel background, such as coarse sandpaper.

Plain, undecorated flannel boards can also be used as a visual aid during presentations, allowing the speaker to display and remove charts and graphs as needed.

Flannel graph has been (and continues to be) a popular medium for telling Bible stories to young Sunday school students in Christian (and particularly Evangelical) churches. Indeed, it is used as a storytelling method almost exclusively in elementary-level Christian education. This may be attributed, in part, to the fact that flannel graph is relatively inexpensive, yet provides a more vivid alternative to storytelling without visual illustration.

Explanation

You can see how in the field students used the flannel graph and educated people on different topics allotted to them.

Keywords

Introduction, flannel graph, description, explanation.

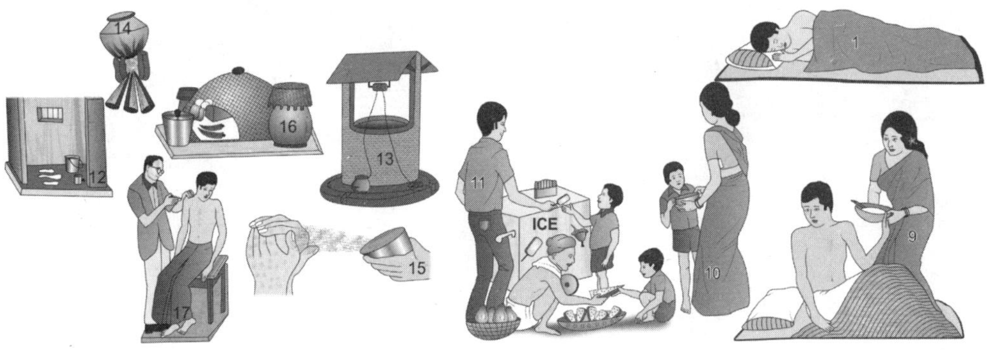

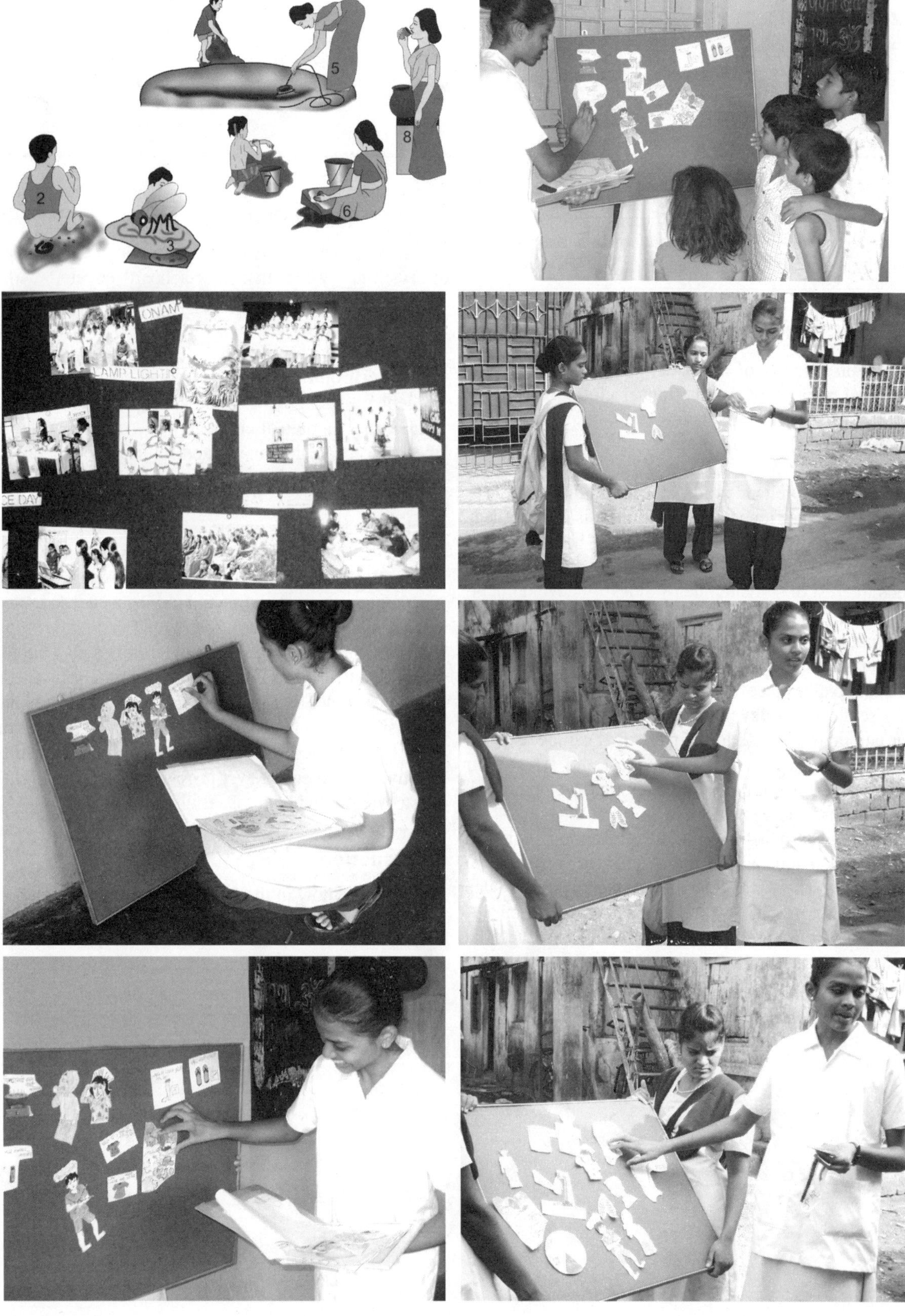
5
8
2
7
6
3
ONAM

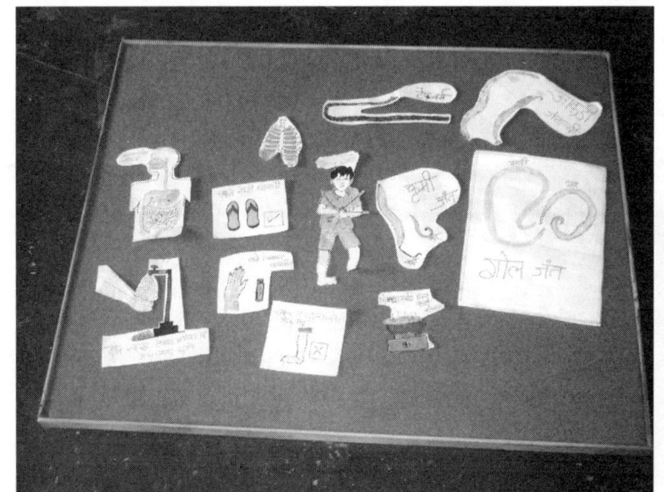
गोल जंत

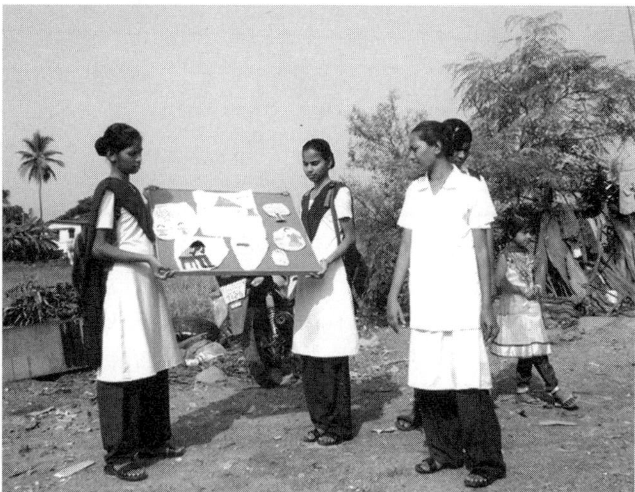

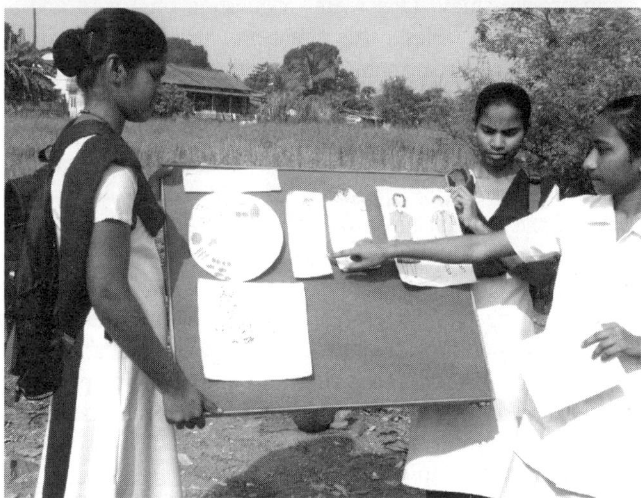

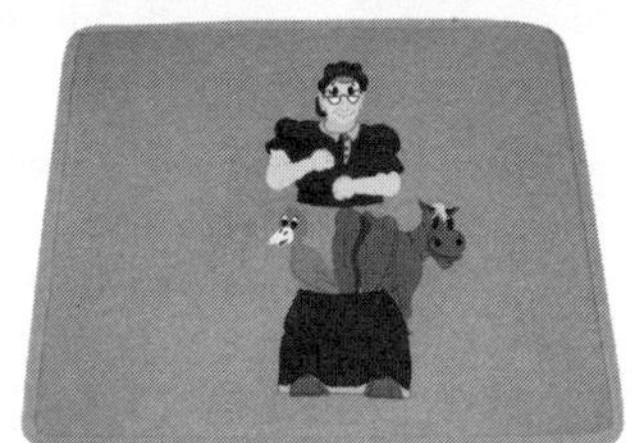

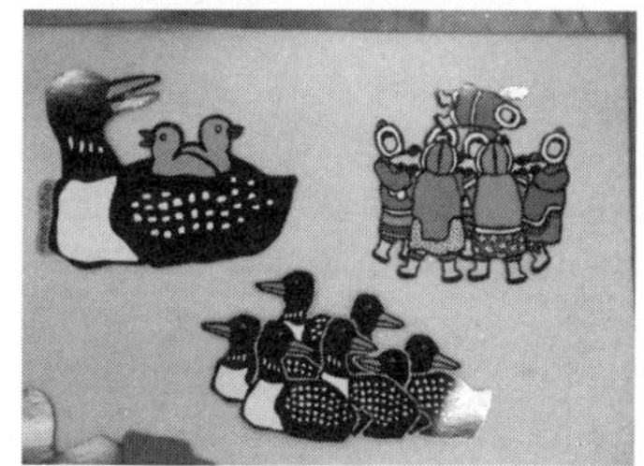

CHAPTER 30

Flashcards

Abstract

A flashcard is a set of cards bearing information, as words or numbers, on either or both sides, used in classroom drills or in private study for gaining rapid response from students.

INTRODUCTION

A set of picture compact paper cards of varying size flashed one by one in logical sequences. They can be self-made or commercially prepared. It conveys messages quickly, is dynamic and flexible. Maintains continuity, easy to prepare, portable, exosmic, can be used for illiterate people. They are small cards of generally 25–30 cm in size which are shown for a few moments before the class to send across a message or impart an idea. Idea in the flashcard must be brief preparation of flash. A chart paper cut into four equal parts, write the content in it either with free hand using stencils or sketch pens. Also the height of writing in the flashcard should be approximately 5 cm. closing flash cards give brief introduction about the lesson. Flash the cards in right time hold it in away so that all can see it.

They consist of a series of cards, approximately 10 × 12 inches—each with an illustration pertaining to a story or talk to be given. Each card is "flashed' or displayed before a group as the talk is in progress. The message on the cards must be brief and to the point. The size of the group should not be more than 25. Small compact cards which flashes before the class to bring any idea, 10" × 12" or 22" × 28" in size. For one health talk, students can make at least 10 to 12 cards. Prepare a picture for each idea, which will give visual impact to the idea. The message can be brief, content will be written in few lines at the back of each flash card also. Adapted to local condition, use plenty of colors.

A set of cards can be prepared on a single topic, put in sequence manner, before starting the explanation. The story on each card must be familiar, in simple words and local terminology. Hold the cards at the chest level where people can see clearly, hold against body and not in the air, and face different parts of the group to show cards to all.

Glance down at cards, as you are ready to explain and make sure to give correct information. Use pointer, do not cover the matter with hands, and enjoy explaining the matter. Important points to be written backside, if you forget can see easily.

It can be used for drill and practice in elementary classes, It can be used to introduce a topics, to develop recalling ability, it can be used to review topic, it is useful supplementary aid and can be effectively used with other materials, graphic aids are helpful in arresting students attention. Conveying information into a condensed matter. Stimulating interest presenting information efficiently.

A flashcard is a set of cards bearing information, as words or numbers, on either or both sides, used in classroom drills or in private study. One writes a question on a card and an answer overleaf. Flashcards can bear vocabulary, historical dates, formulas or any subject matter that can be learned via a question and answer format. Flashcards are widely used as a learning drill to aid memorization by way of spaced repetition.

Flashcards exercise the mental process of active recall: given a prompt (the question), one produces the answer. Beyond the content of cards, which are collected in decks, there is the question of use—how does one use the cards, in particular, how frequently does one review (more finely, how does one schedule review) and how does one react to errors, either complete failures to recall or mistakes? Various systems have been developed, with the main principle being spaced repetition–increasing the review interval whenever a card is recalled correctly.

It is used for small group not more than 30 people. It provides variety and activity in the class. The messages can be brief, drawing or photographs or cartoons, and adapted to local condition. Each idea can be prepared in picture form and can be used individually or with other charts. Prepare 10–12 series of cards on one topic and give appropriate numbering before starting your explanation and hold it at chest level for the people to view using pointer to avoid blocking with hand.

Two-sided—Physical flashcards are two-sided; in some contexts one wishes to correctly produce the opposite side on being presented with either side, such as in foreign language vocabulary; in other contexts one is content to go in only one direction, such as in producing a poem given its title or incipit (opening). For physical flashcards, one may either use a single card, flipping it according to the direction, or two parallel decks, such as one English-Japanese and one Japanese-English. For electronic flashcards, cards going in the opposite direction can easily be produced, and may be treated either as two unrelated cards, or being related in some way, as in the program Anki, which enforces a minimal time spacing between opposite sides of a card. They have a number of uses that can be very simple or very elaborate for the person to memorize.

There are various systems for using flashcards, many based around the principle of spaced repetition—reviewing information at increasing intervals. Manually managing interval length can add greatly to the overhead of using flashcards: the Leitner system is a simple spaced repetition system designed for paper flashcards, based on a small number of boxes and a simple algorithm, while the Super Memo algorithms are more complicated, tracking each card individually, and designed for implementation by computer.

Three-sided cards—Physical flashcards are necessarily two-sided. A variant, found in electronic flashcards, is what is known as a three-sided card. This is a particular kind of asymmetric two-sided card; abstractly, such a card has three fields, Q, A, A*, where Q & A are reversed on flipping, but A* is always in the answer—the two "sides" are thus Q/A, A* and A/Q, A*. Concretely, these are most used for learning foreign vocabulary where the foreign pronunciation is not transparent from the foreign writing—in this case the Question is the native word, the Answer is the foreign word (written), and the pronunciation is always part of the answer (Answer*). This is particularly the case for Chinese characters, as in Chinese hanzi and Japanese kanji, but can also be used for other non-phonetic spellings, including English as a second language.

Purpose—The purpose of three-sided cards is to provide the benefits of two-sided cards—ease of authoring (enter data once to create two cards), synchronized updates (changes to one are reflected in the other), and spacing between opposite sides (so opposite sides of the same card are not tested too close together)—without the card needing to be symmetric.

One can generalize this principle to an arbitrary number of data fields associated with a single record, with each field representing a different aspect of a fact or bundle of facts.

History—Paper flashcards have been used since at least the 19th century, with Reading Disentangled in 1834 a set of phonics flashcards by English educator Favell Lee Mortimer being credited by some as the first flashcards. Previously, a single-sided hornbook had been used for early literacy education.

Explanation

You can see you can prepare flash cards on important topics and use as a communication media. We have tried, it was very useful, and you too try and experience the result of powerful media.

Keywords

Two-sided cards, various systems, purpose, three-sided cards, history, explanation.

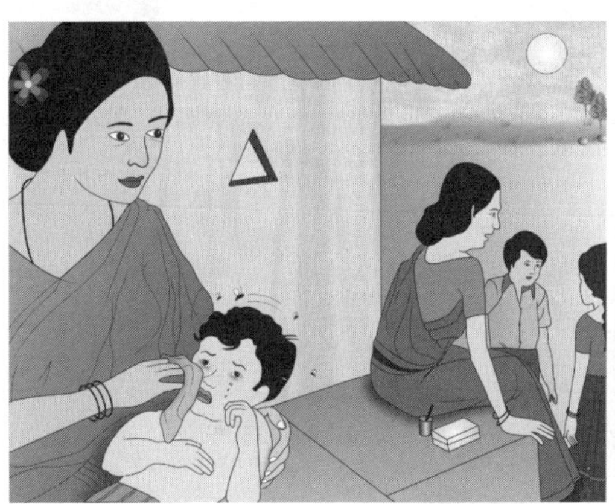

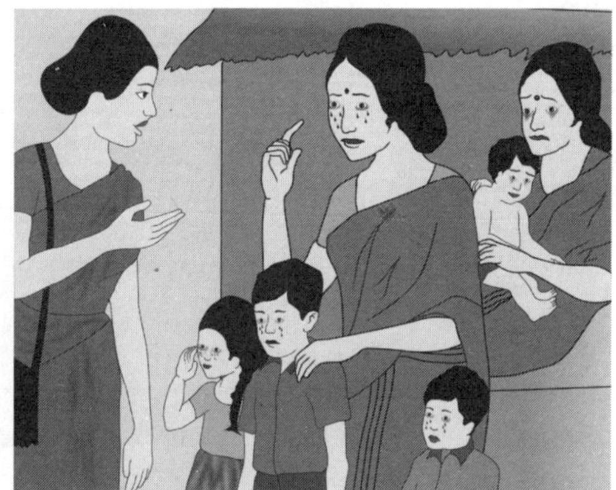

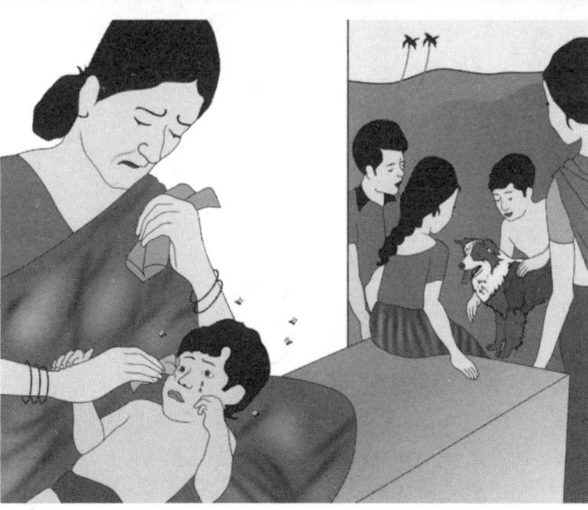

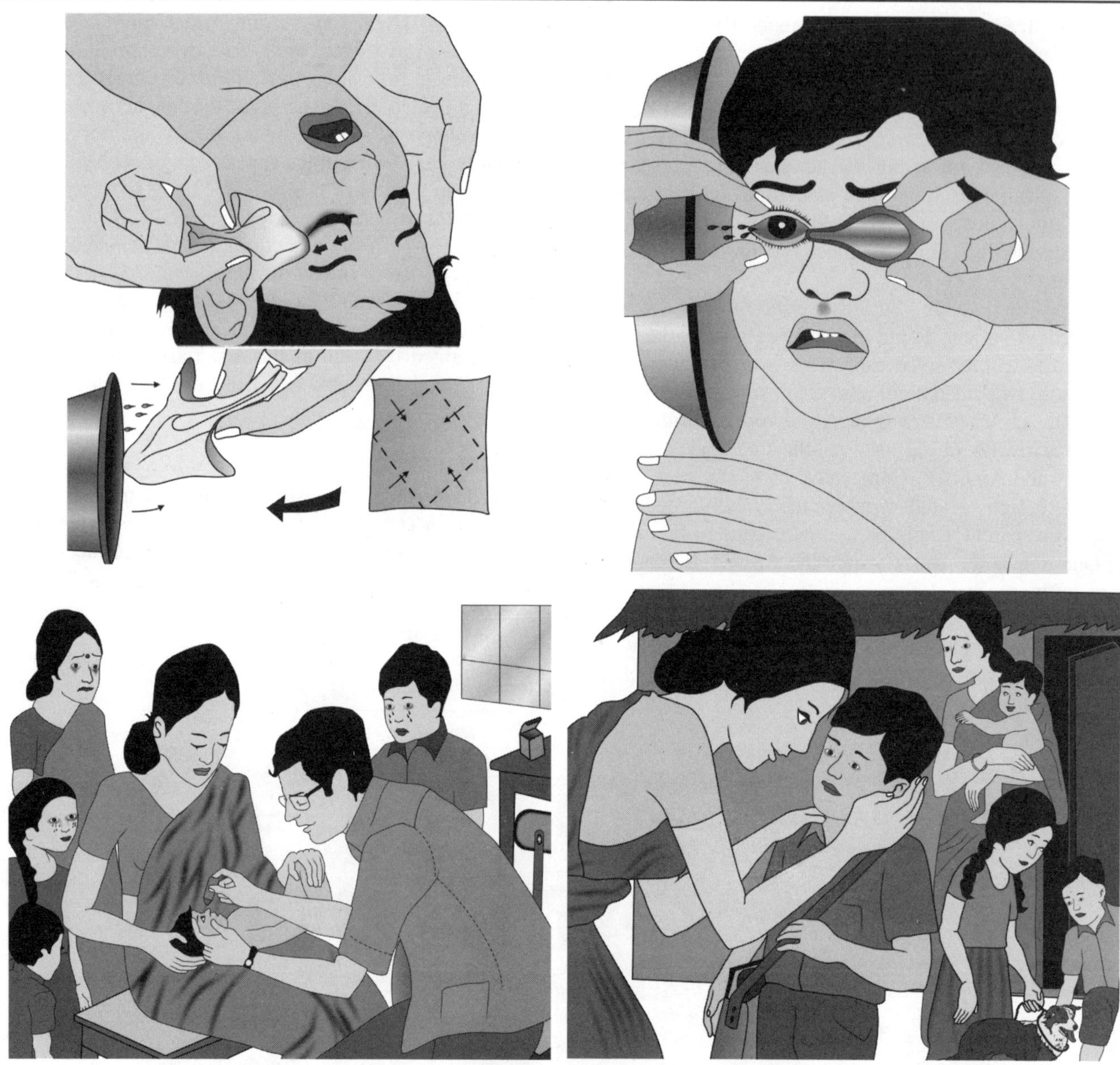

AIDS AND HIV AWARENESS

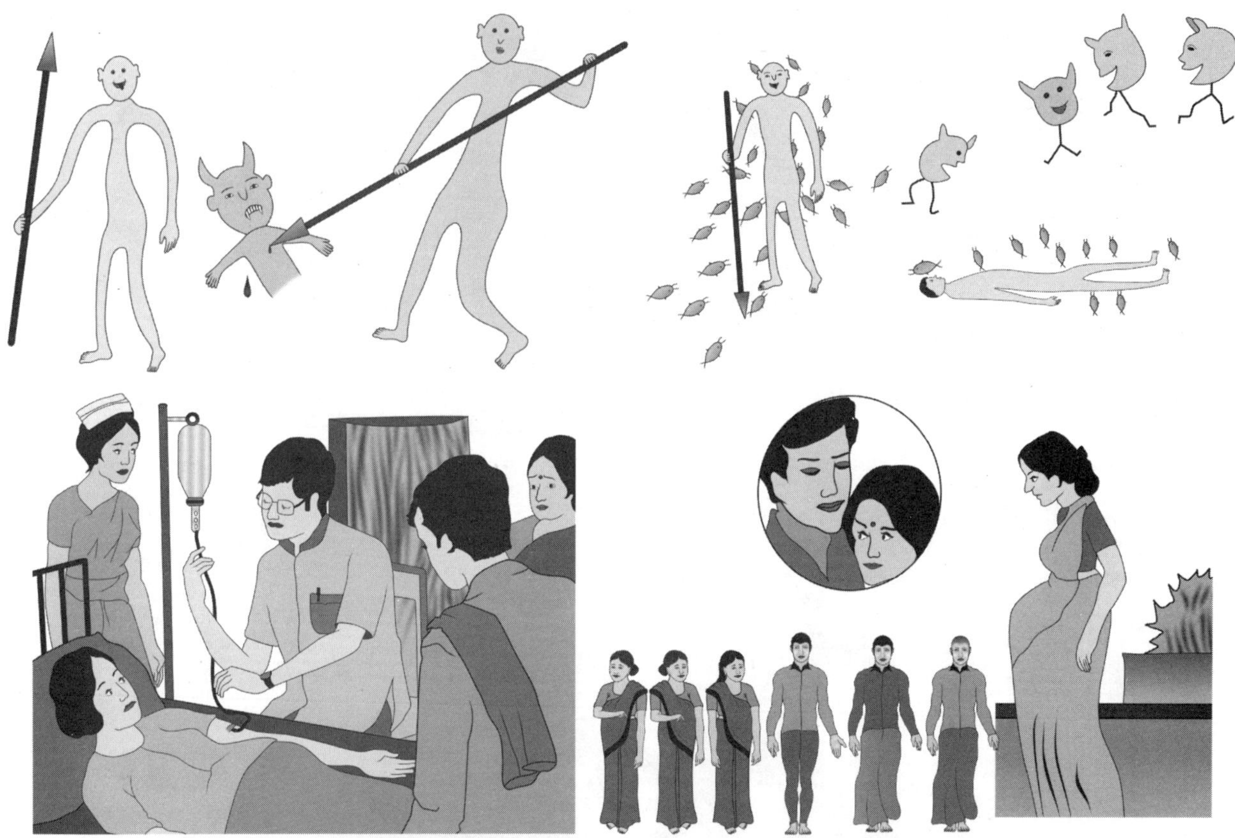

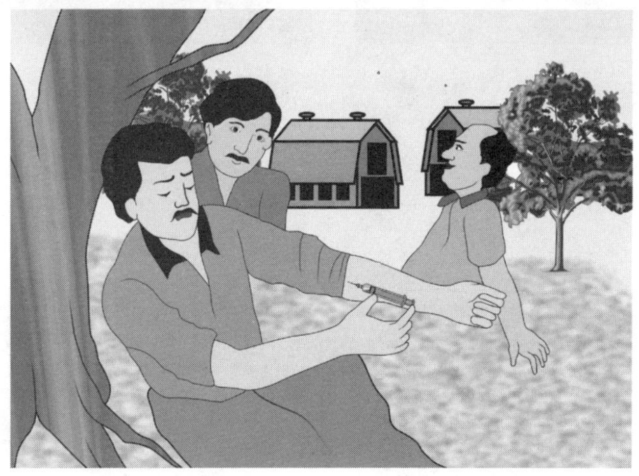

PLANNING FOR SAFE DELIVERY

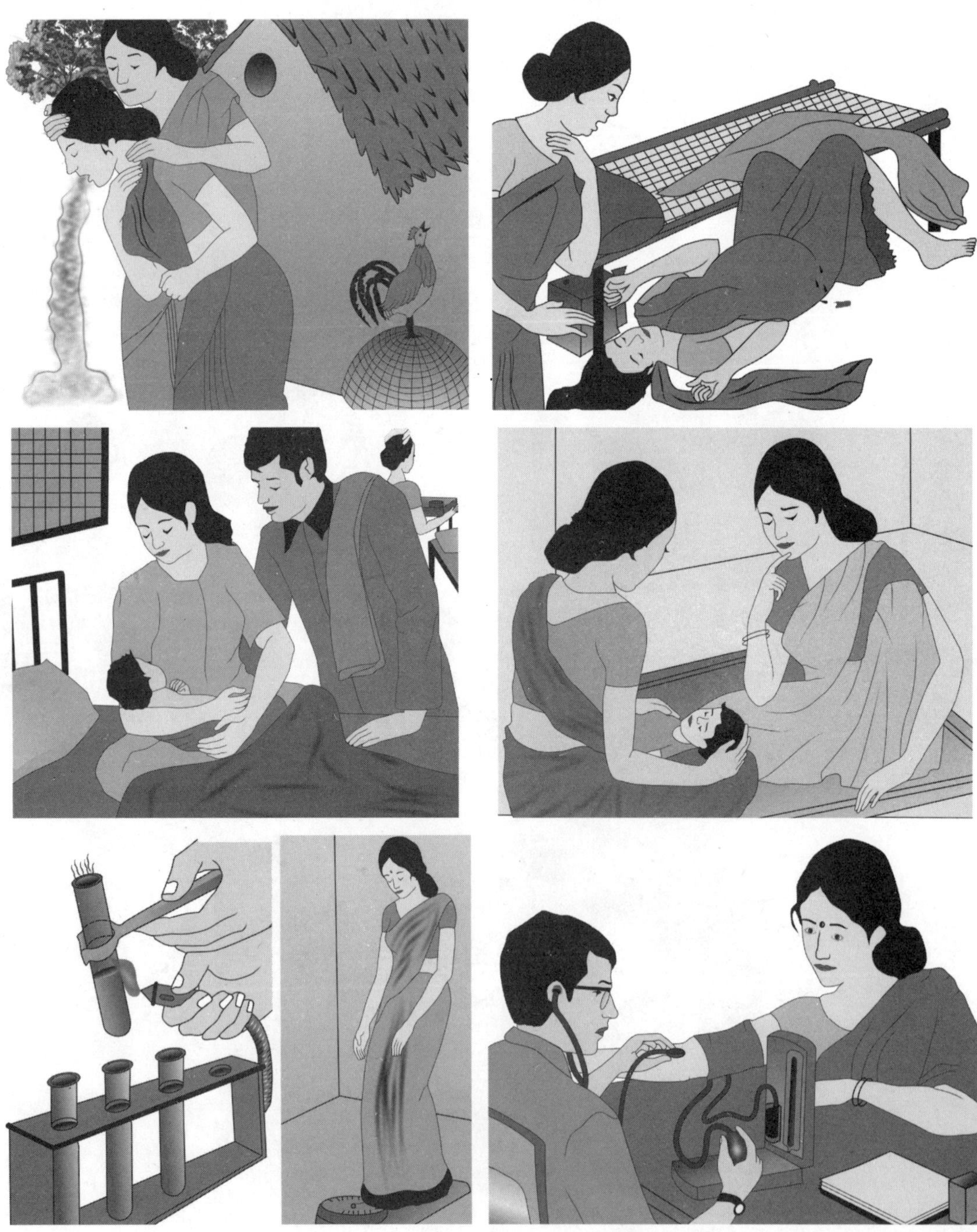

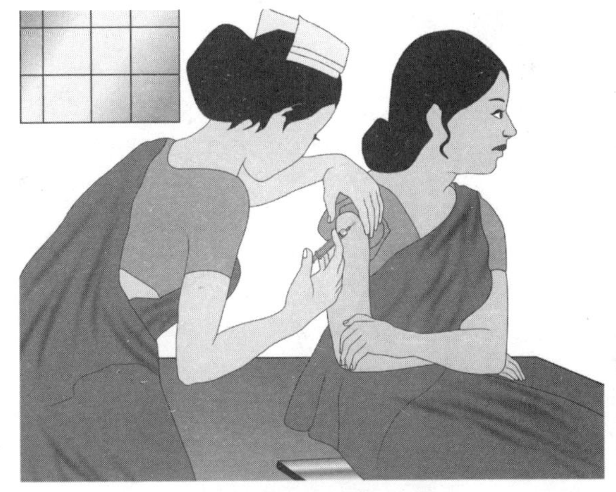

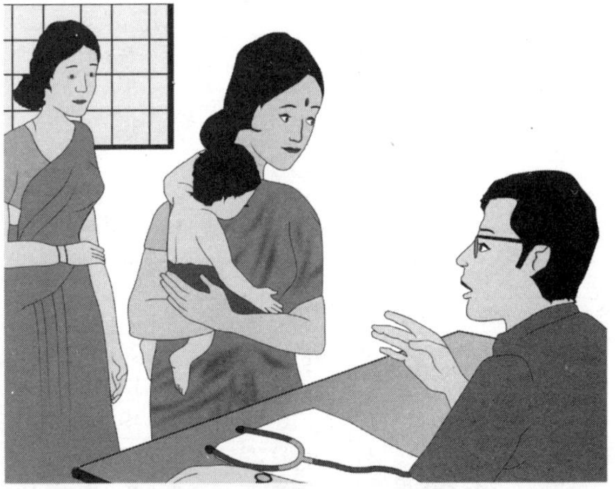

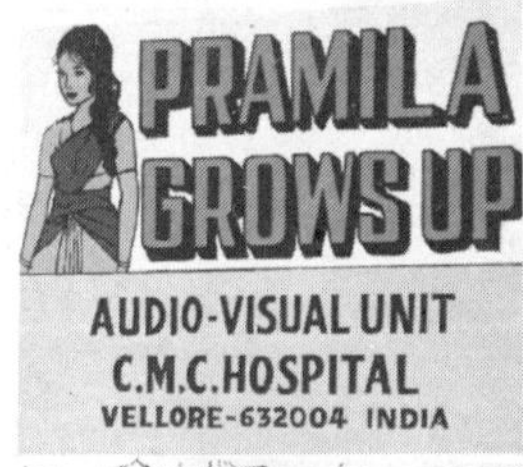
PRAMILA
GROWS UP
AUDIO-VISUAL UNIT
C.M.C.HOSPITAL
VELLORE-632004 INDIA

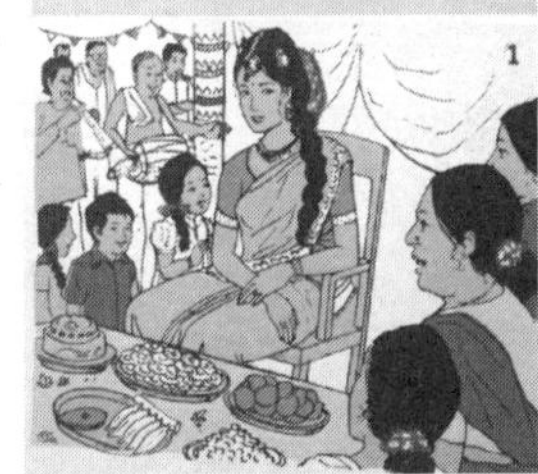
1

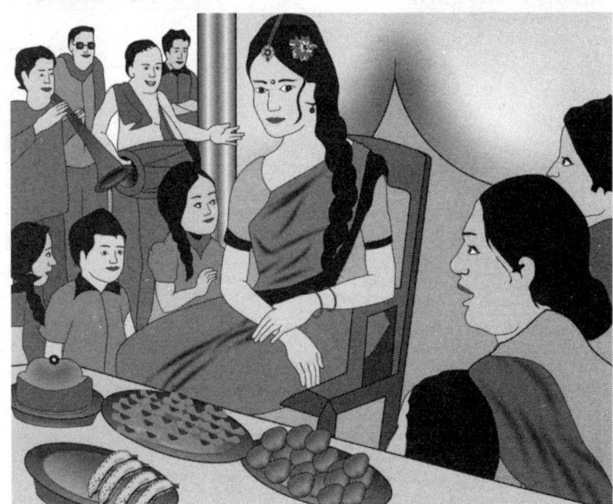

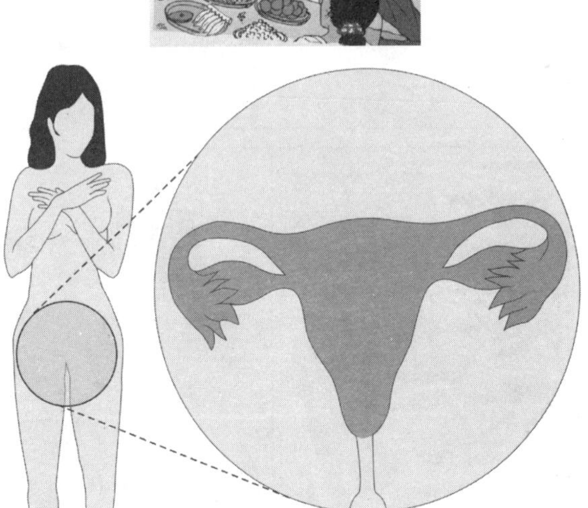

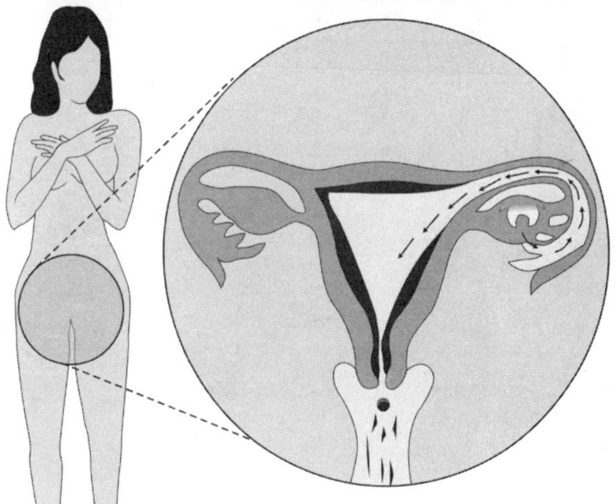

MAY						
S	M	T	W	T	F	S
30	31	●	●	●	●	1
2	3	4	5	6	7	8
9	10	11	12	13	14	15
16	17	18	19	20	21	22
23	24	25	26	27	28	29

JUNE						
S	M	T	W	T	F	S
●	●	1	2	3	4	5
6	7	8	9	10	11	12
13	14	15	16	17	18	19
20	21	22	23	24	25	26
	28	29	30	●	●	●

JULY						
S	M	T	W	T	F	S
●	●	●	●	1	2	3
4	5	6	7	8	9	10
11	12	13	14	15	16	17
18	19	20	21	22	23	24
25	26	27	28	29	30	31

AUGUST						
S	M	T	W	T	F	S
1	2	3	4	5	6	7
8	9	10	11	12	13	14
15	16	17	18	19	20	21
22	23	24	25	26	27	28
29	30	31	●	●	●	●

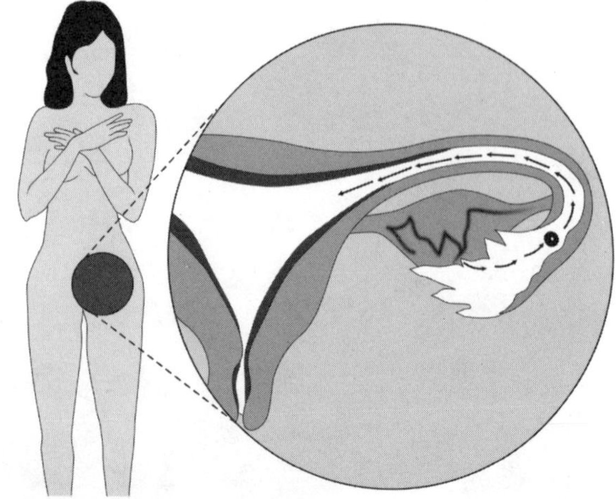

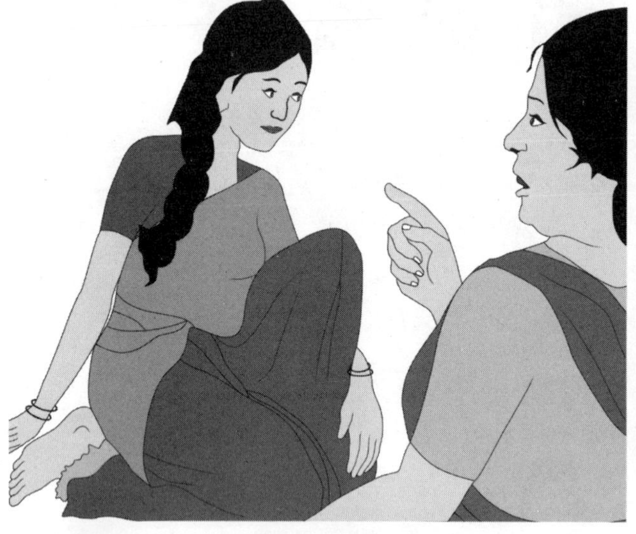

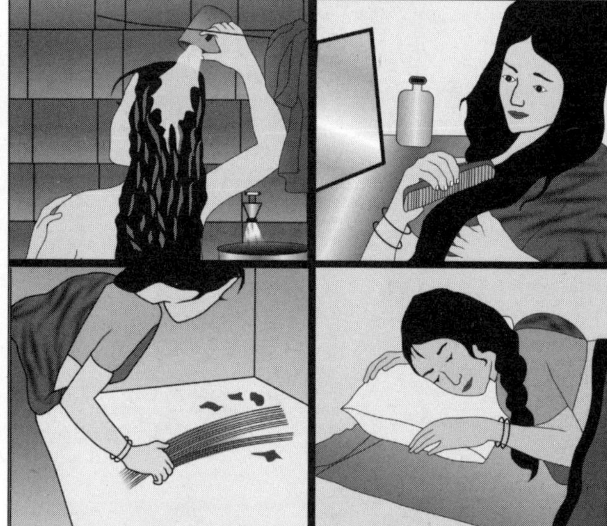

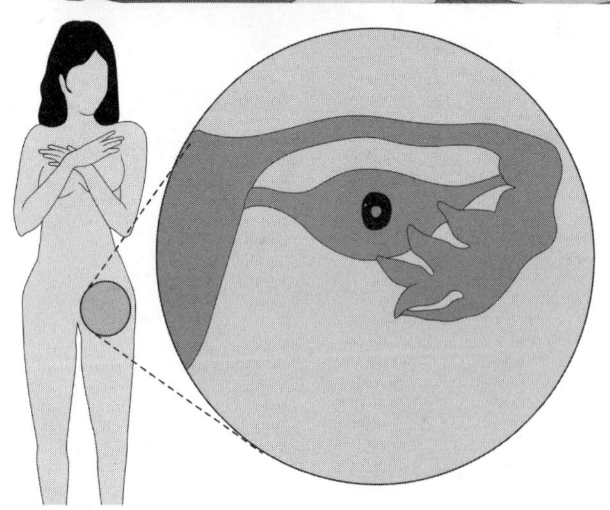

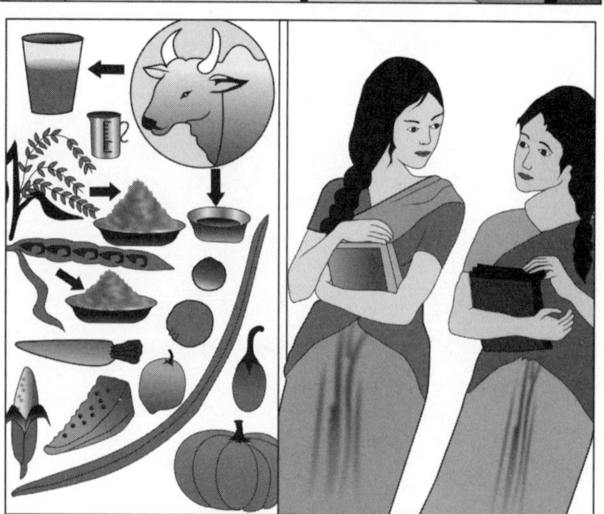

HOW? LIFE BEGINS

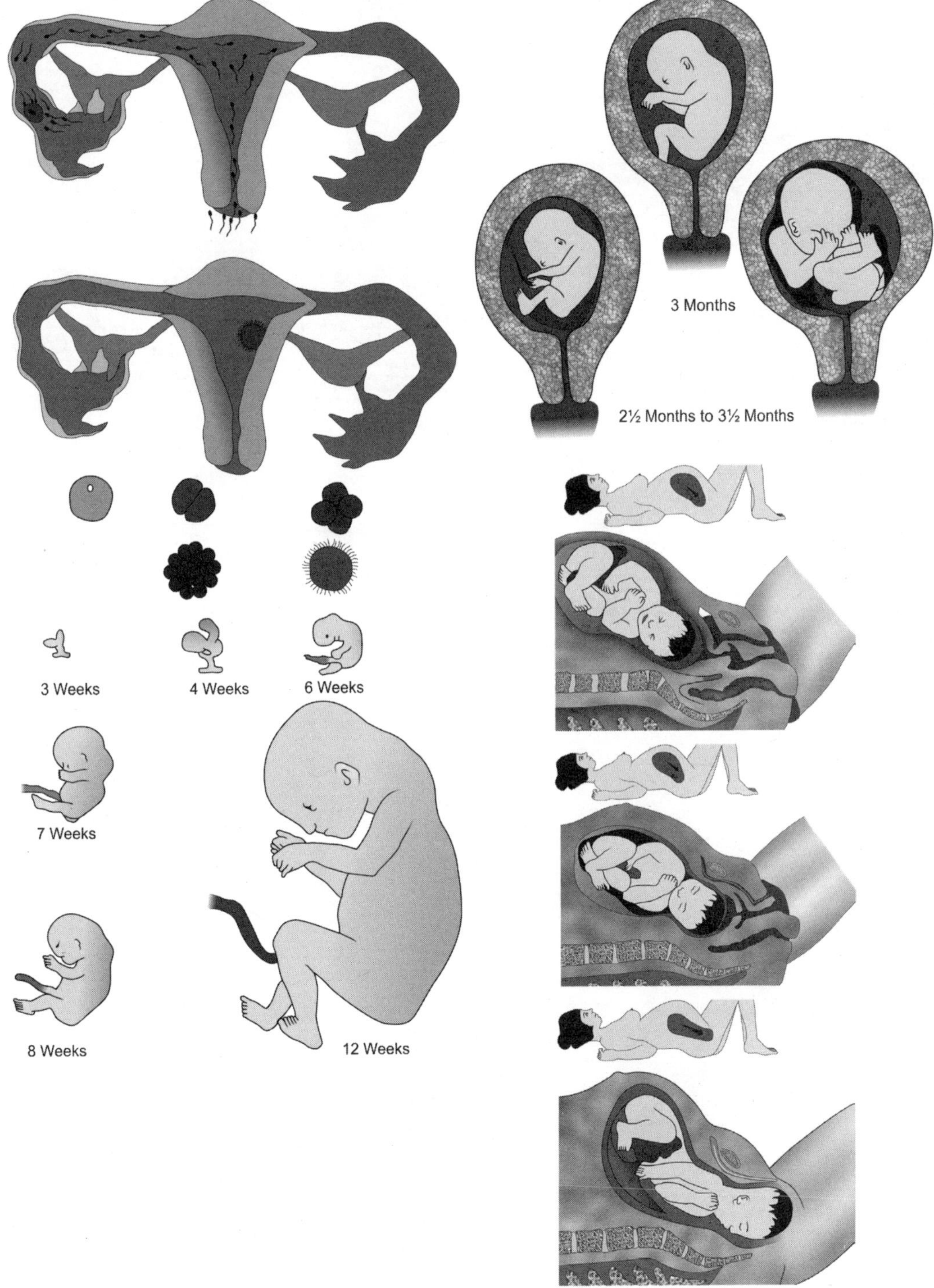

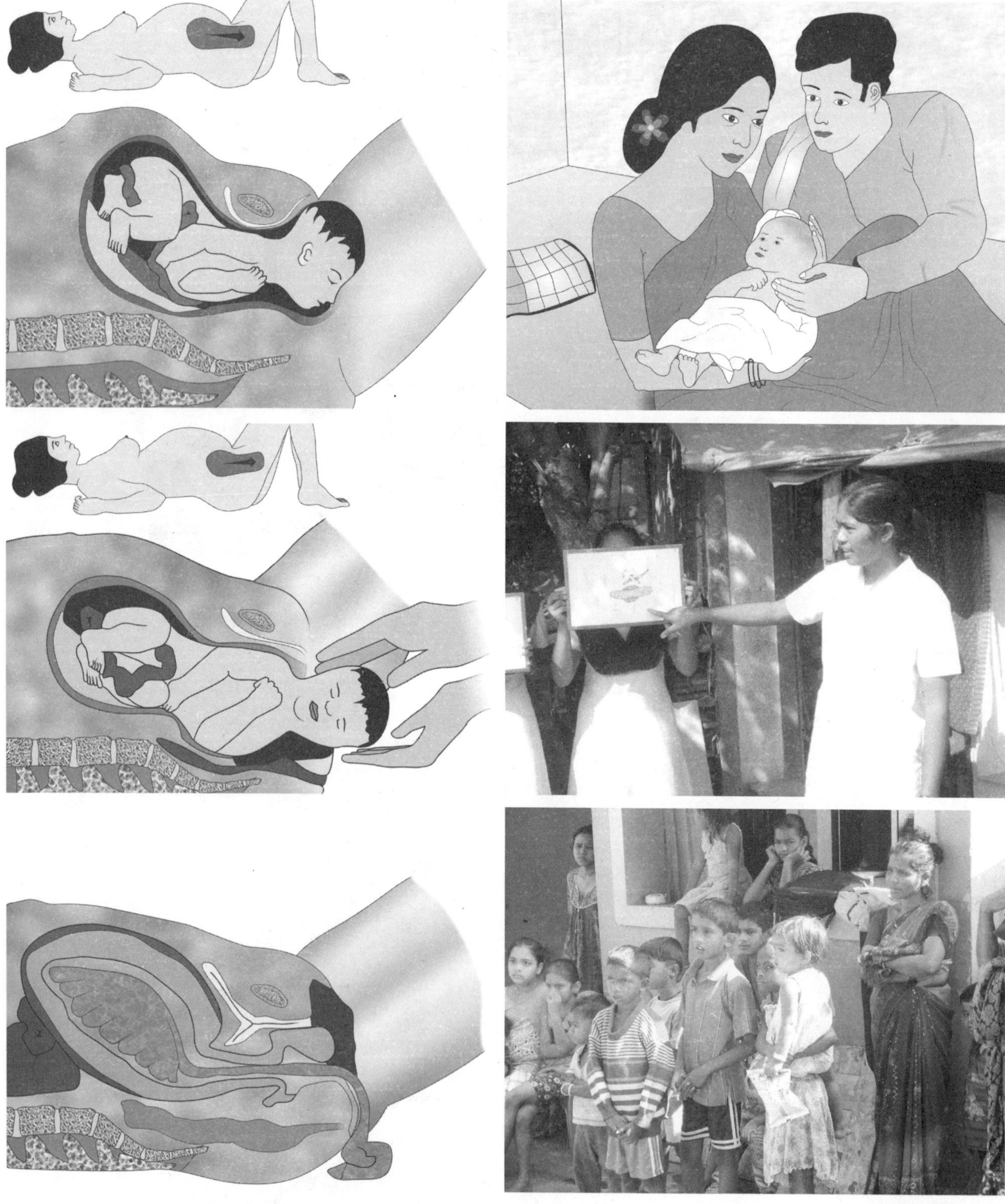

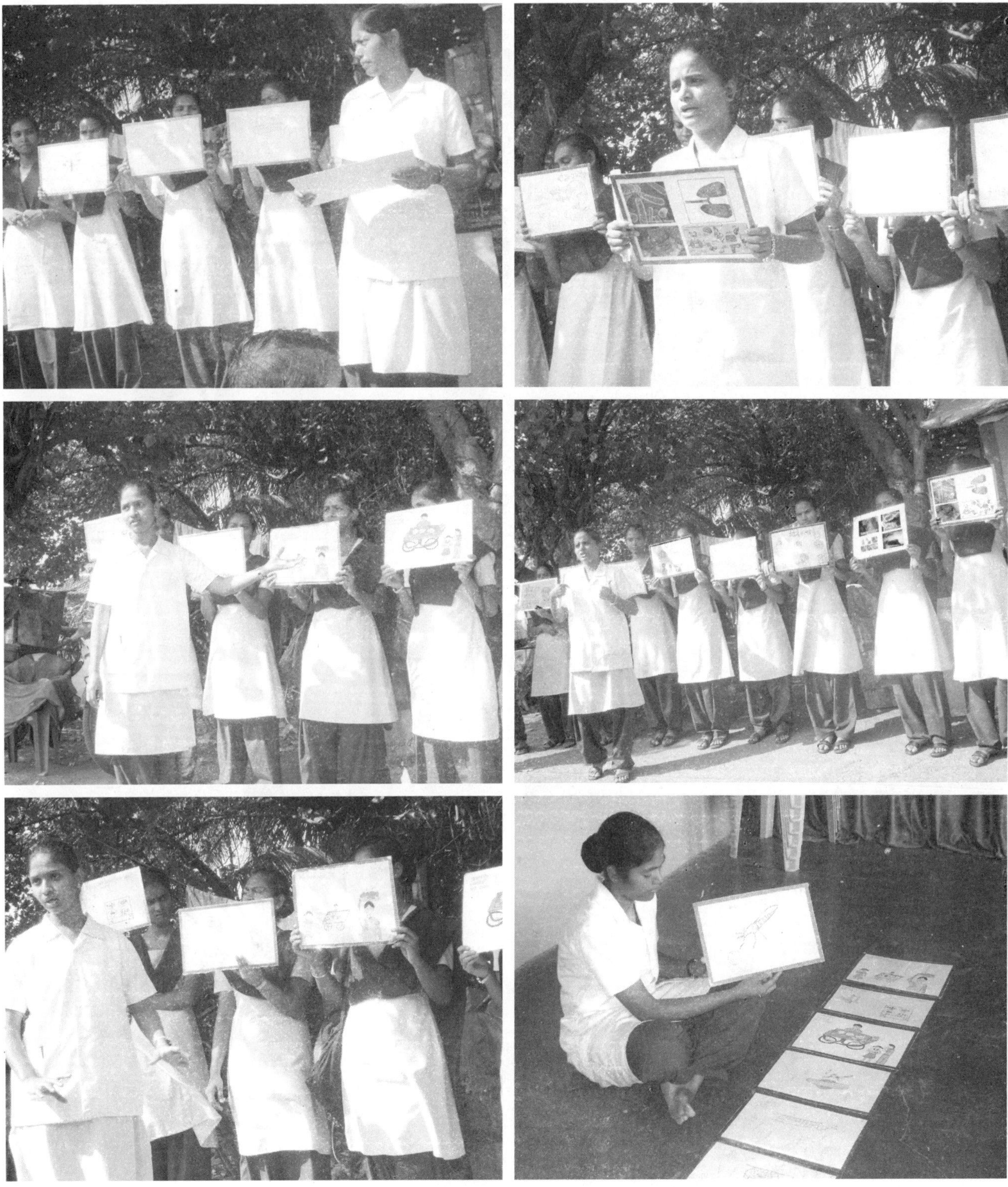

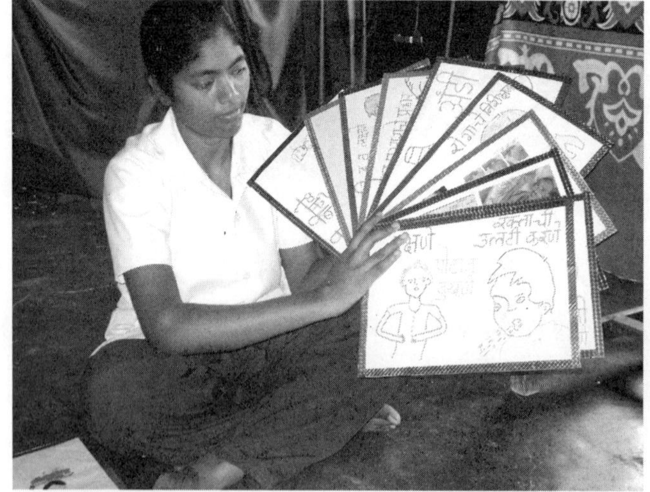

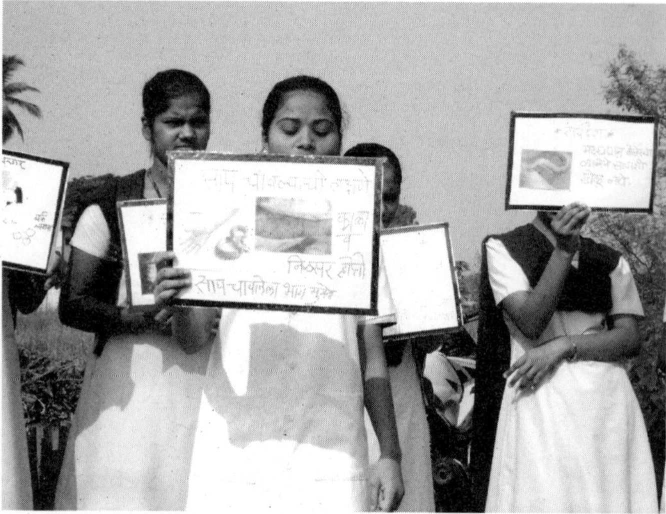

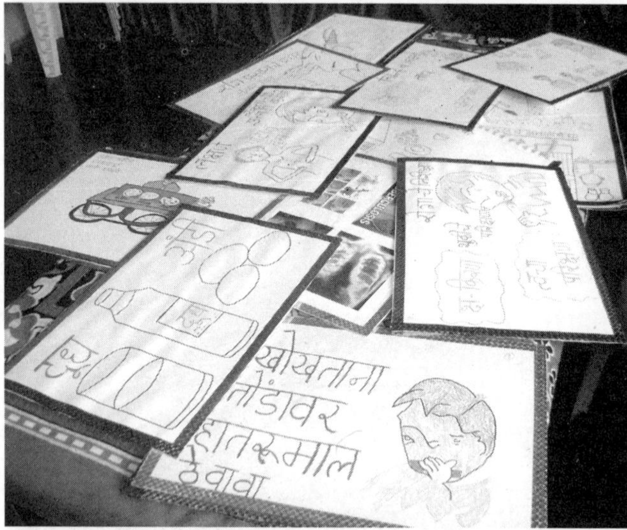

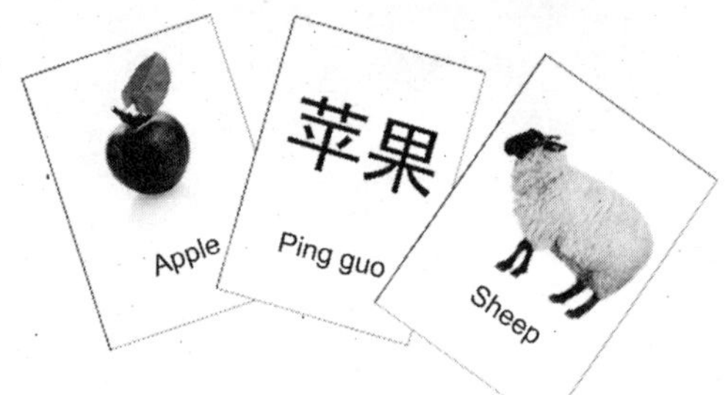
Apple
苹果
Ping guo
Sheep

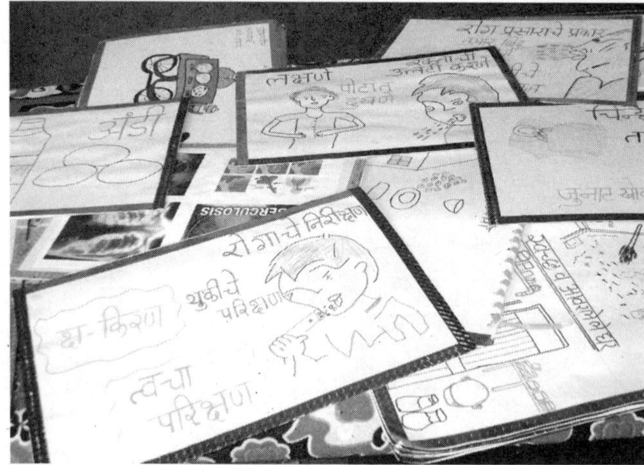

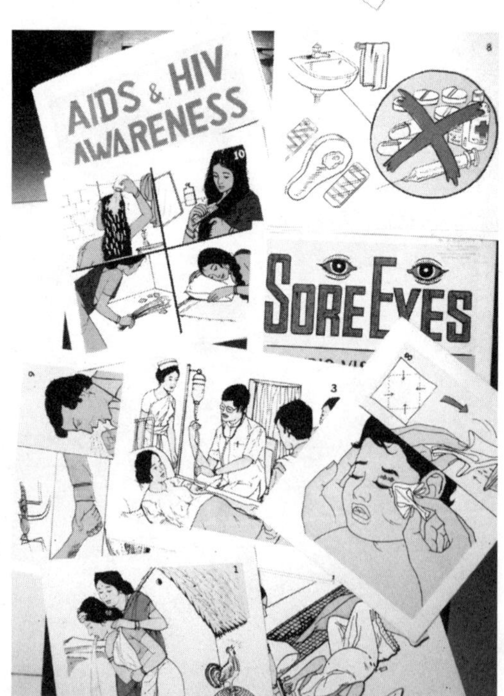
AIDS & HIV
AWARENESS
SORE EYES

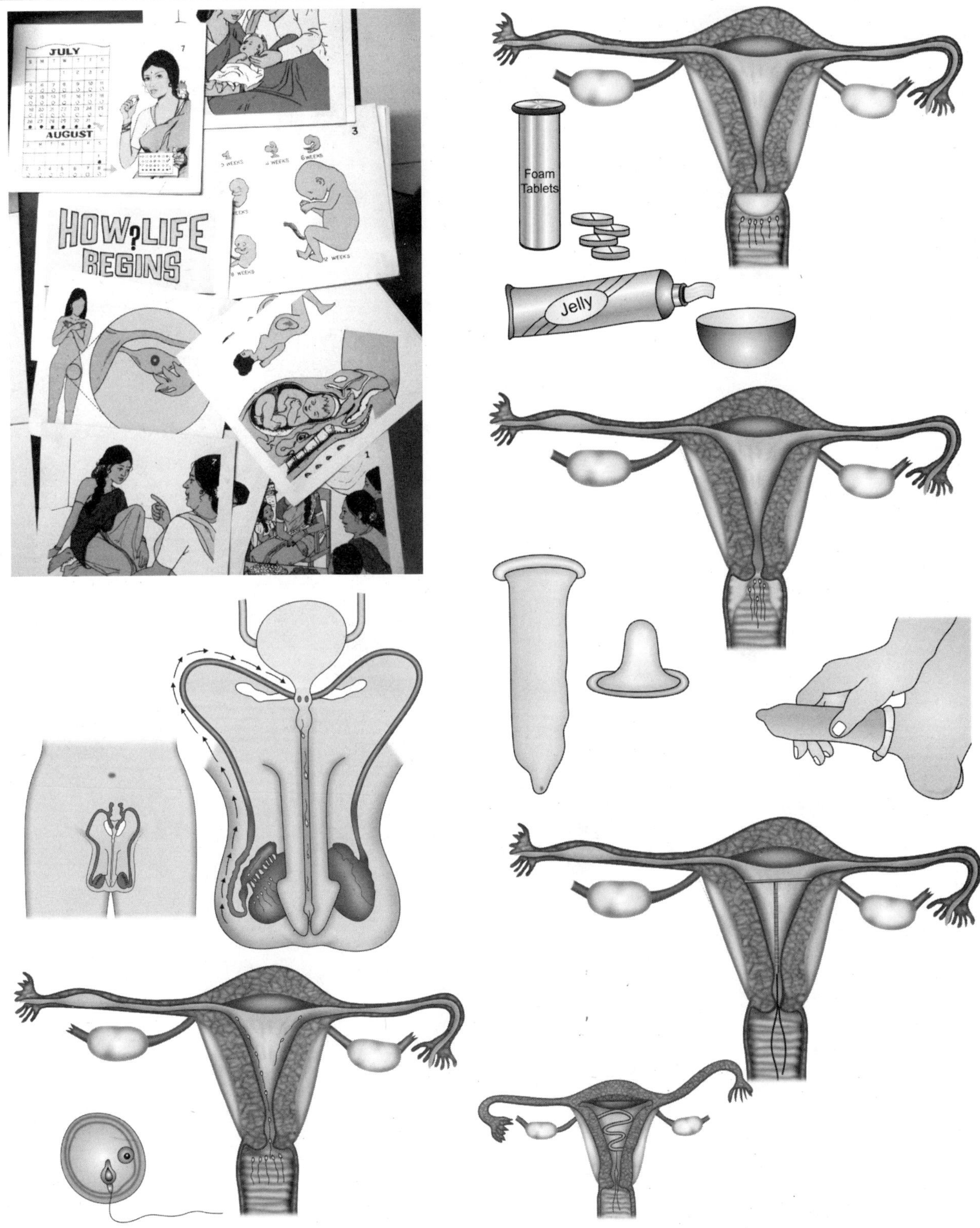
JULY
AUGUST
HOW LIFE BEGINS
Foam Tablets
Jelly

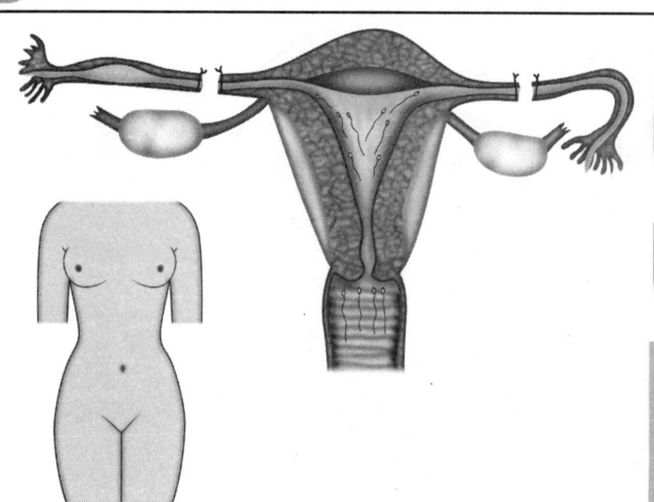

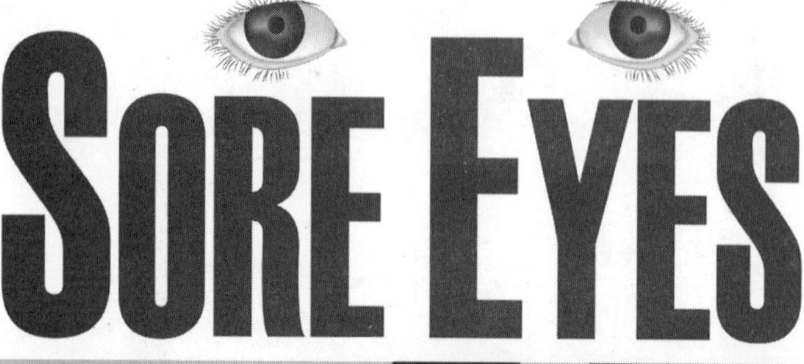
SORE EYES

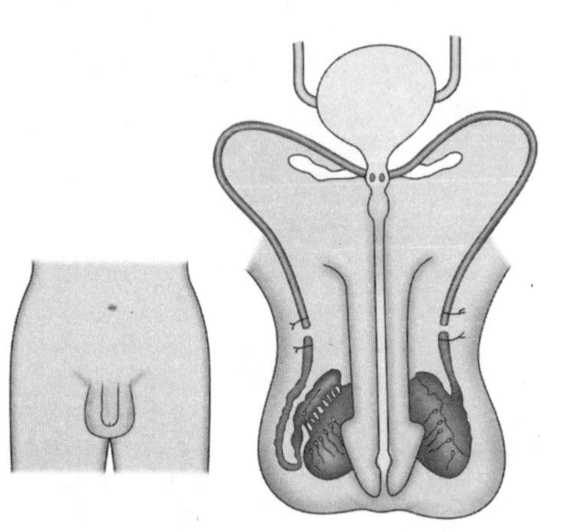

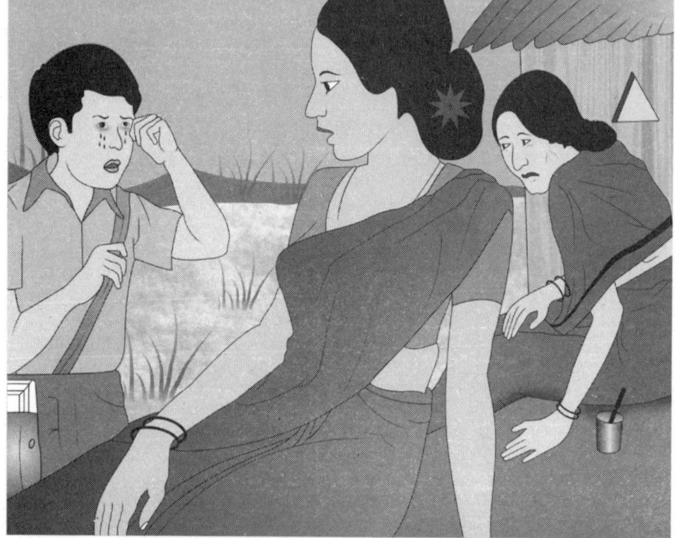

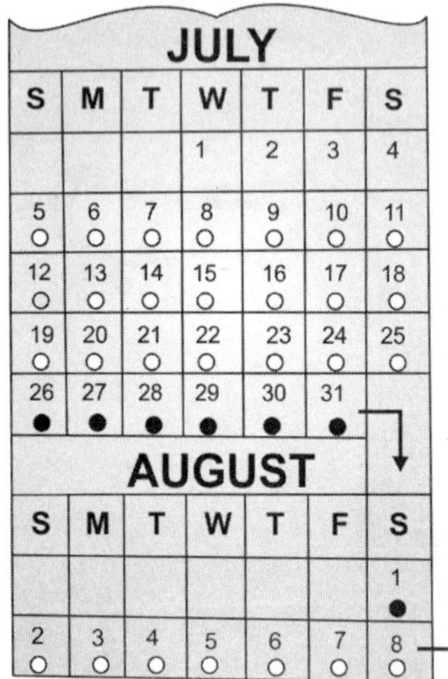
JULY
S M T W T F S
1 2 3 4
5 6 7 8 9 10 11
12 13 14 15 16 17 18
19 20 21 22 23 24 25
26 27 28 29 30 31
AUGUST
S M T W T F S
1
2 3 4 5 6 7 8

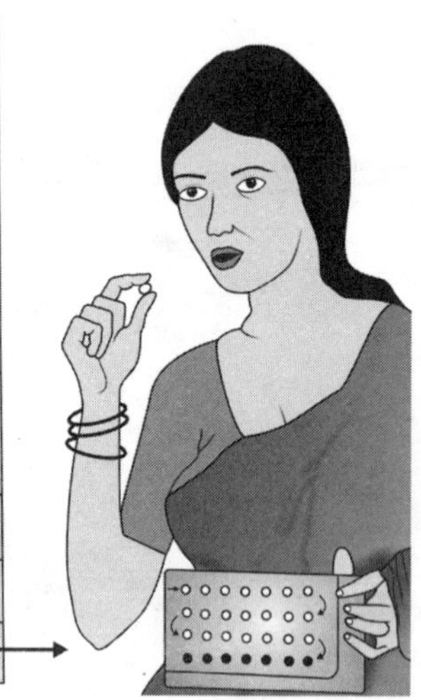

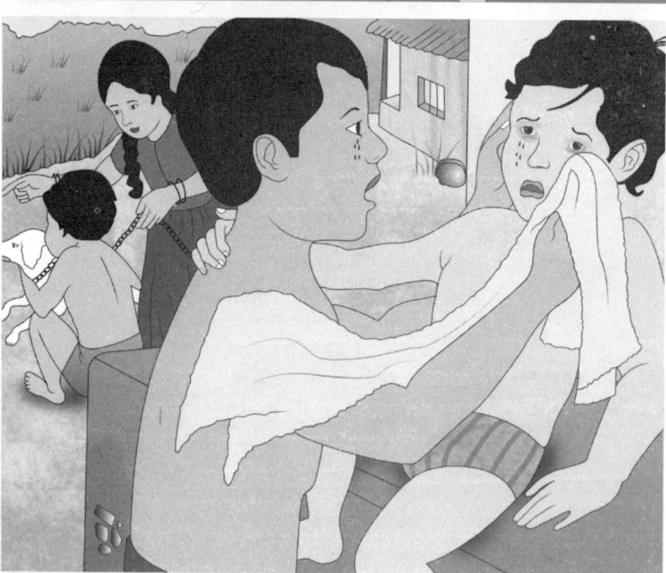

CHAPTER

31

Flip Books

Abstract

Flip book is an online interactive format for presenting traditional print documents, books, magazines, catalogs. Flip books have been around since the late 1800s and are now recognized as one of the earliest forms. Flip books make animation easier to learn because they are so easy to use.

Flip book is a small booklet, spiral binding type. You can prepare the figures and tie them artistically in a booklet types and use as a aid of education. It is useful for smaller group. As you explain, you keep turning pages in sequence of your topic as you can see in the figures how our students used them as communication aid.

A flip book is a book with a series of pictures that vary gradually from one page to the next, so that when the pages are turned rapidly, the pictures appear to animate by simulating motion or some other change. Flip books are often illustrated books for children, but may also be geared towards adults and employ a series of photographs rather than drawings. Flip books are not always separate books, but may appear as an added feature in ordinary books or magazines, often in the page corners. Software packages and websites are also available that convert digital video files into custom-made flip books. Flip books are essentially a primitive form of animation. Like motion pictures, they rely on persistence of vision to create the illusion that continuous motion is being seen rather than a series of discontinuous images being exchanged in succession. Rather than "reading" left to right, a viewer simply stares at the same location of the pictures in the flip book as the pages turn. The book must also be flipped with enough speed for the illusion to work, so the standard way to "read" a flip book is to hold the book with one hand and flip through its pages with the thumb of the other hand. Flip books are now largely considered a toy or novelty for children; they continue to be used in marketing today, as well as in art and published photographic collections. Vintage flip books are popular among collectors, and especially rare ones from the late 19th to early 20th century have been known to fetch thousands of dollars in sales and auctions.

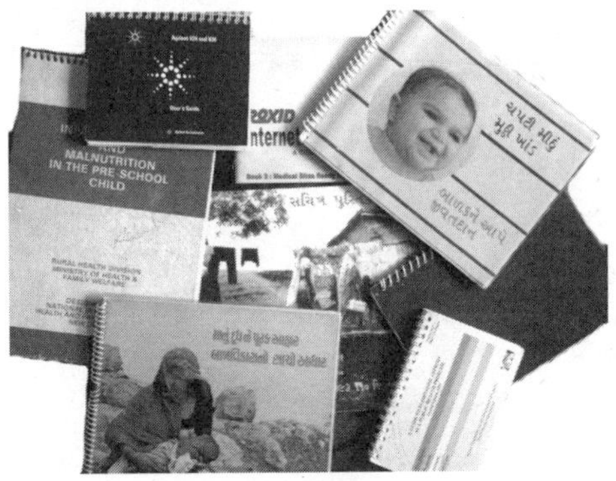

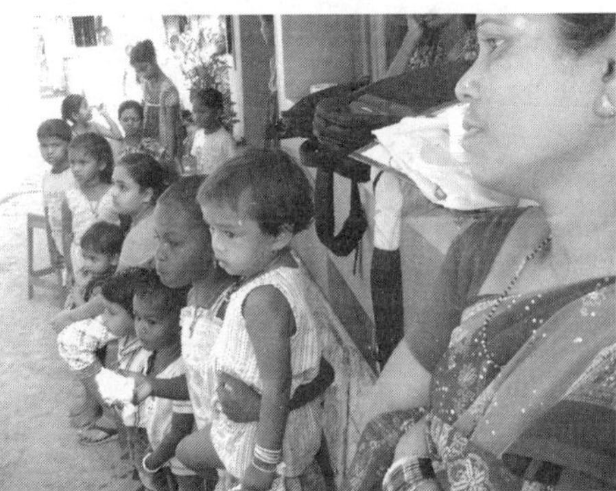

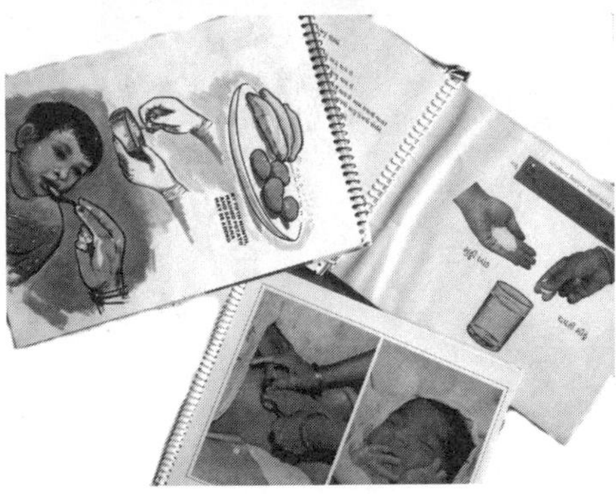

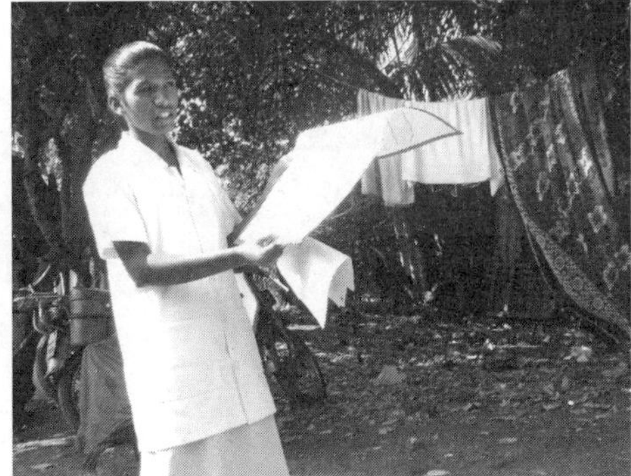

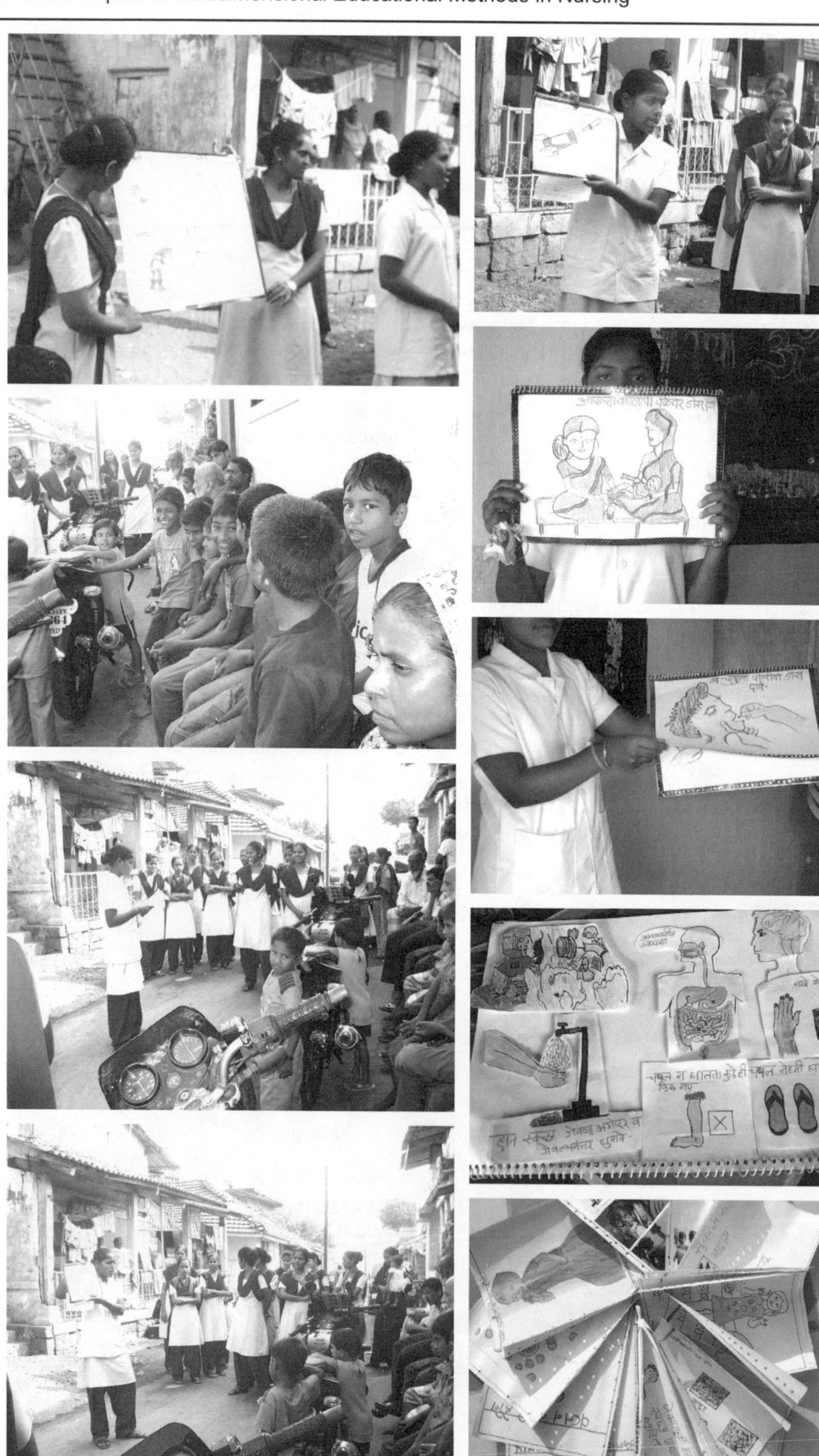

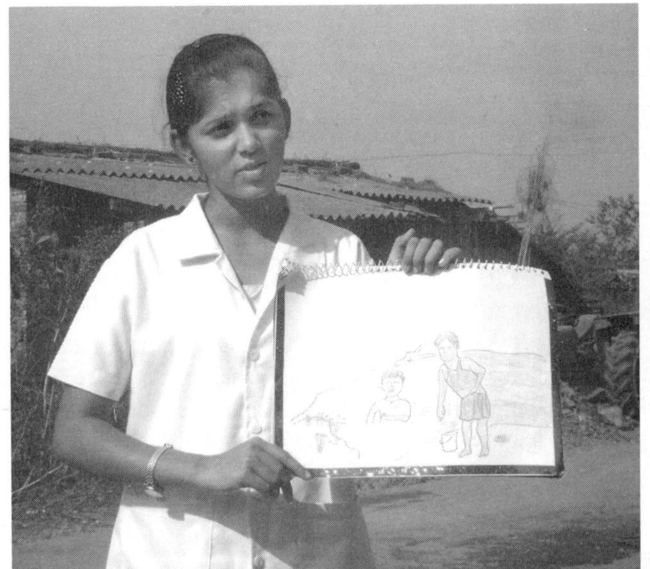

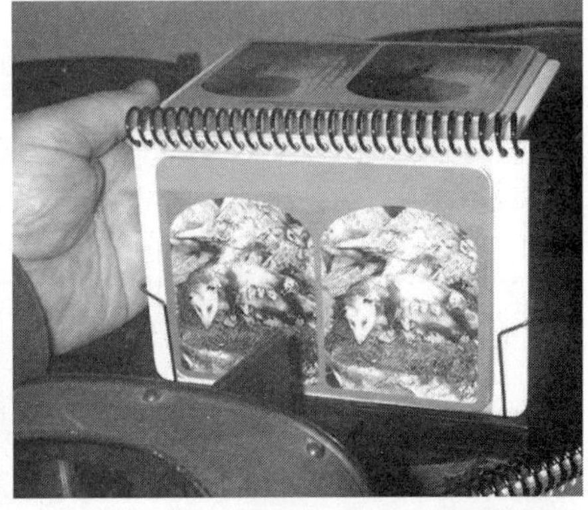

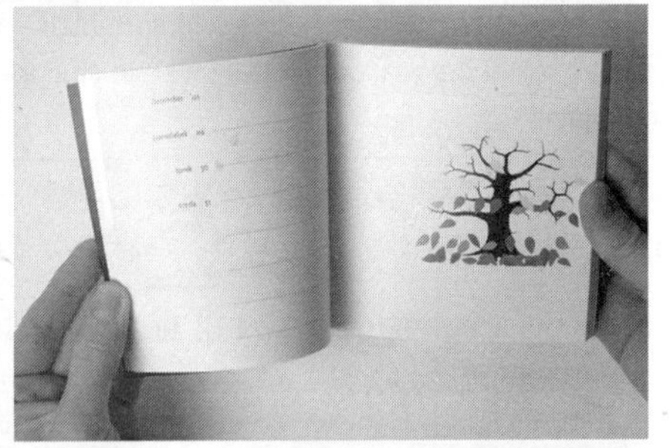

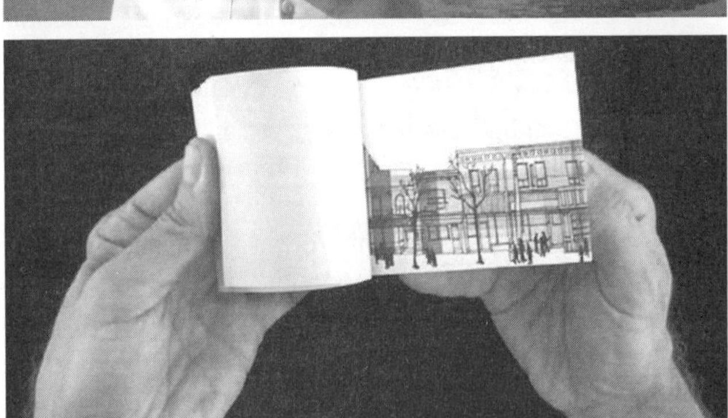

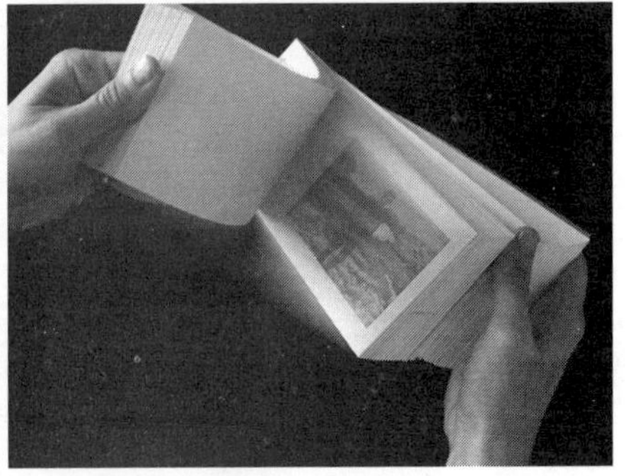

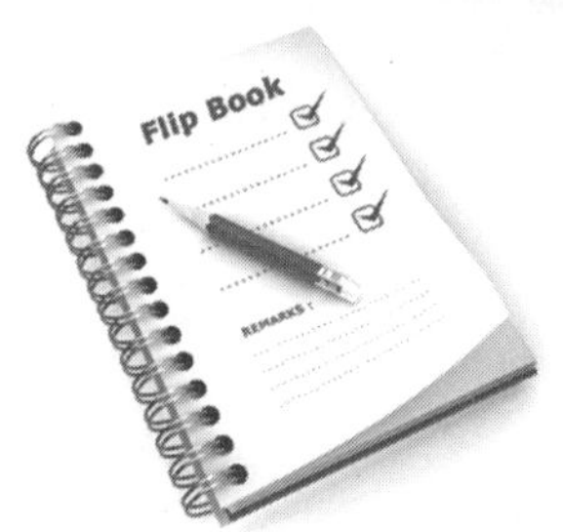

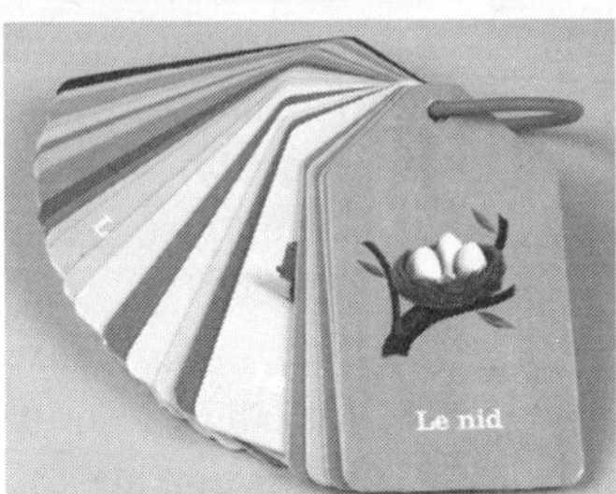

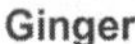

Ginger

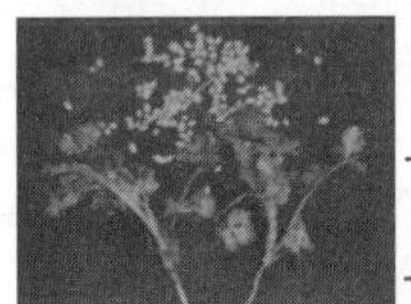

- Urine always very yellow
- Skin allergy due to bilava seed oil
- Burning micturition

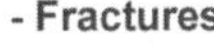

- Fractures

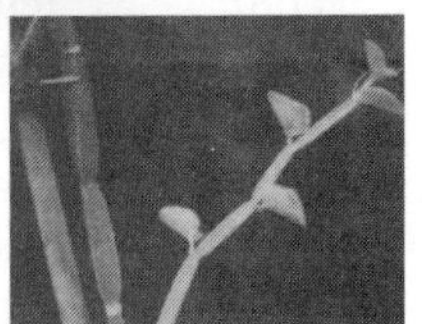

Custard Apple

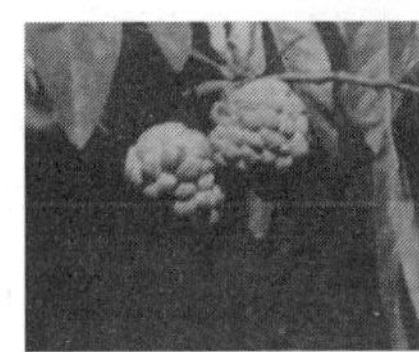

- Abscess not ripening
- Head lice
- Cattle not eating

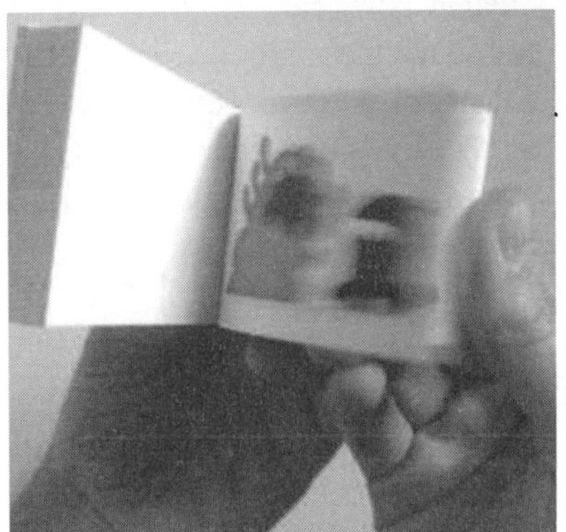

CHAPTER 32

Lectures

Abstract

Lecture is an educational talk with an audience, especially with students in a university or college. It is an oral presentation intended to present information or teach people about a particular subject. Lectures are used to convey critical information, history, background, theories and equations. A talk given to student about a particular subject.

MEANING

Lectures are the most popular method of health teaching. In this the communication is mostly one way, the people are only passive listeners, and there is no active participation on their part in learning. The effectiveness and impression depends on the personality and the reputation of the speaker. Lecture provides basic information on the subject. Lectures have important place in health education of small group.

Lecture is the oldest method of teaching. Almost all subjects can be taught by lecture. Lectures are the most popular method of health teaching. In lecture system the communication is mostly one way. The group can be controlled and can be kept before her eyes. This helps oneself to mange the activities. Limited resources are needed. Can teach many people at a time with wide range of topics within a limited time, it provides basic information of subject.

In lecture a teacher transmits information to the students. In lecture clarification or explanation of points, facts, principles for the students to understand, doubts can be clarified. Lecture can be supported by teaching aids, if illustrative material is used it should be prepared and tested before lecture. The lecture is written in outline form, and teacher builds rapport with the students. Her voice must be clear and tone of voice natural, gestures natural with total expression, address students with apt eye contact, have good questioning skill and wind up and summery at the end.

Lecture is an efficient method of teaching where a large number of students she can communicate. Teacher can plan the lecture in advance so she can well present and increase the motivation level in students for learning. She can present new knowledge and students get inspired with new ideas and new concepts, new content.

In this communication people are passive listeners. A lecture does provide basic information on the subject. Lectures have an important place in the health education of a small group.

It does not pay attention to the interest ability of the group. It is a one sided affairs. The teacher talks and the group listen. No practical activities, experimentations or demonstration is possible. There is no active participation on the part of the learning. The impression and effectiveness of lecture depends on personality and reputation of the speaker, as well as the technique of lecture strategy and planning stage:

1. Decide what you want to communicate
2. Identify the nature of the learners potential provides knowledge or problem of the group.
3. Choose appropriate language; prepare notes for highlighting new concepts and points. Try and find out appropriate examples, prepare av aids to support teaching.

It is a teaching activity where by the teacher presents the contents in a comprehensive manner by explaining the facts, principles and relationships during which the teacher is expected to elicit student participation by employing appropriate technique.

Purpose

1. To provide structural knowledge.
2. To motivate guide in hunting knowledge by means of electrifying lecture, collect more information, guide them, give main or list of books which are common followed.
3. To arouse interest in subject orient them to subject.
4. Introduce term to new areas of learning innovation that are occurring on a regular basis, this innovations have created new learning areas and lecture method helps to introduce these areas.
5. Clarify difficult concepts lecture method helps in creating a contusive atmosphere for discussions.
6. To promote critical thinking a thoughtful designed it can be challenge and critically and analytically by modifying the thinking process.

Techniques

1. Spontaneity is the essence instead reading continuously from a prepared notes, converse freely, look in-between at the prepared notes, practice before class as sudden outflow of information which is enriched with life experience.

2. Voice gradation and voice quality, periodical alteration of both pitch and volume, more high lighting as monotonous makes them passive.
3. Adequate pacing—slow, fast, crease boredom and later leads to confusion dealing with difficult areas go slow pace.
4. Proper body language, action speaks louder than words, maintaining eye contact, occasionally more towards them.
5. Use aids which helps to facilitate learning in this method.
6. Due to the hurry in finishing the content do not neglect feedback which helps to know the effectiveness of lecture
7. Helps in further classification of difficult concepts, any doubts to be rectified.
8. Manage time and manage content within the stipulated time.

Explanation

They get more information by lecturing than reading books. It enhances the listening capacity. Emphasis high level intellectual skills, link between sections like what is coming next and what has been just and when has been just completed. Summarize, review, highlights key ideas, interact with each other and explore issue and report back. Interactive lectures class time can be logically and effectively divided into section for lecture, discussion, questioning, etc.

Keywords

Meaning of lecture, purpose, techniques.

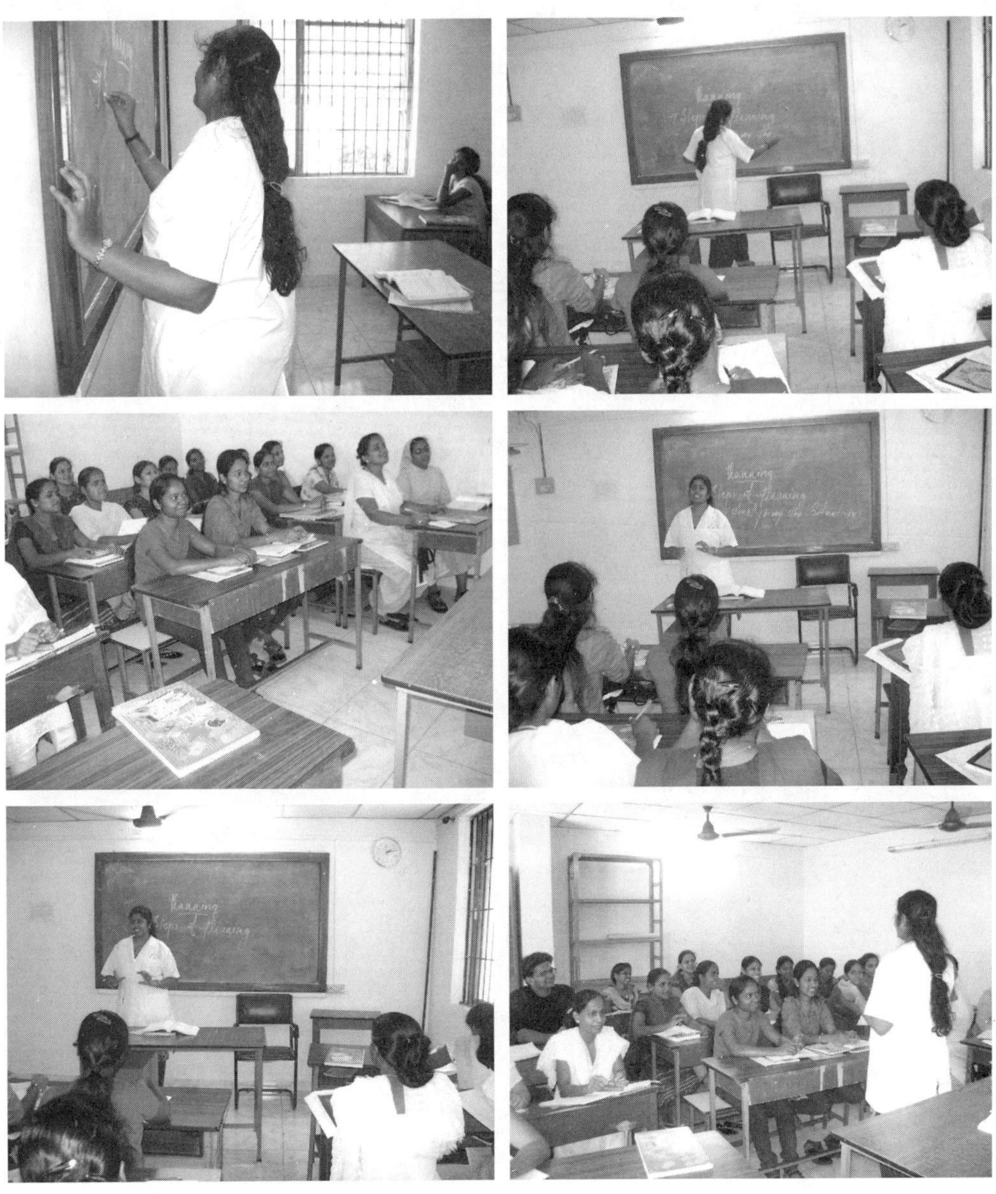

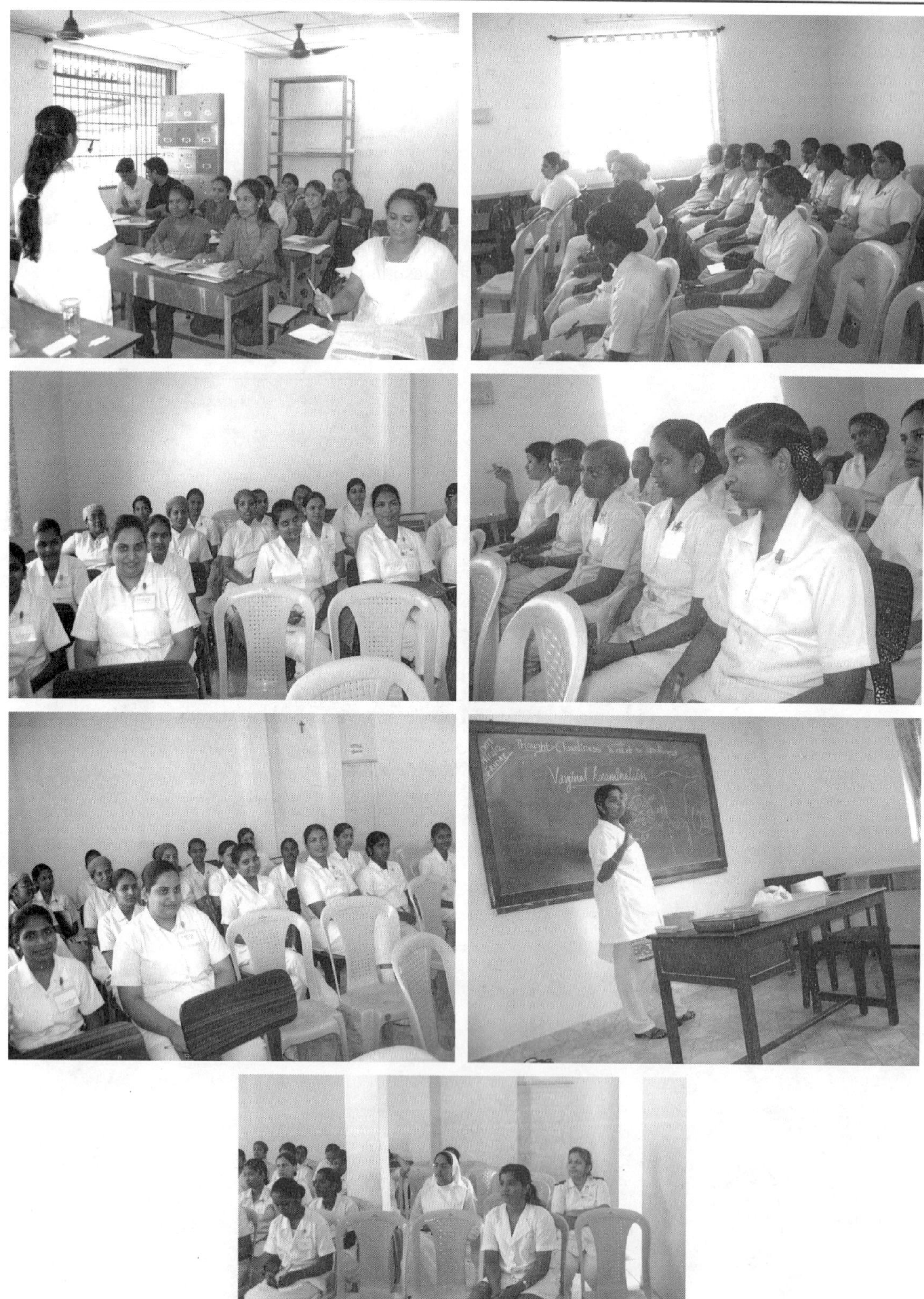
FRIDAY
Vaginal Examination

CHAPTER

33

Health Magazines/Books/ Press/Technological Education

Abstract

Health magazine: provides motivation and inspiration on health, gives latest information and expert advice about a healthy and active lifestyle. The **printing press** was invented in the Holy Empire by the German Johannes around 1440.

Technological education: Is the study of technology in which students learn about the processes and knowledge related to technology. As a field of study, it covers the human ability to shape and change the physical world to meet needs, by manipulating materials and tools with techniques. It is the study of technology, in which students learn about the processes and knowledge related to technology. As a field of study, it covers the human ability to shape and change the physical world to meet needs by manipulating material and tools with techniques.

Book: Book is a set of written, printed, illustrated, or blank sheets, made of ink, paper, or other material.

HEALTH MAGAZINE

Good health magazines can be an important channel of communication. The material needs expert presentation. The health magazines stimulate awareness among people.

Health magazines such as health action, health for million, Anubhav, nursing journal, world health, to name the few, are good important health magazines. Good writers and authors who are experienced and intellectual give good articles. It is food for the thought; it can satisfy intellectual craving and thirst for knowledge. It will develop your mental capacity and thinking power, your reflective power, your wisdom and will make you self confident.

Life can change with just one novel idea. You can develop hobby of reading, you will spend your time constructively, and they will become your friends. Choose good literature, they are expensive but worth investing and spending as it will give you knowledge and knowledge is power.

Aid of any kind can help to achieve objective and make teaching more effective. Be thorough and familiar with material. The aids helps in introducing a subject, create an exciting curiosity and stimulating interest in the people. It is a vehicle for transmitting the new information. In this the students should get full benefit from aid so prepare them in advanced. Present well, evaluate and do follow-up, it will help to establish the new impression in child learning.

Effective health education lays a solid foundation for individual. The goal of health education is to teach people to live life to its healthiest. Teaching helps other person to learn. Good method used health education can promote, protect, prevent and enhance well-being and improve quality of life. You are known by your education. To get education is expensive in today's world. Education has a higher values, it is a power and weapon in your hand in life.

Publications—to communicate information like an article can be published.

Press

Newspapers are the most widely distributed of all forms of reading material. They are an important channel of communication to the people. For example, newspapers give us daily news of the fresh happenings in and around the planet. There are daily news, midday news, and evening news. We get each news paper in any language. There are as many languages spoken that many languages news paper printed and communicated. News paper is a paid channel of the communication. If you want to give any add of your business you will have to pay and get it printed to reach the vast public. News papers have large public we can reach to all yet it can get out dated the next day, therefore it has short life. There are columns and space and pages reserved for specific news. It gives us variety of information that is educative. We get latest researches done, discoveries, etc. There is so much served for everyone's test to be satisfied. All kinds of knowledge is served. It is good habit to read news paper daily. You get self taught information. It is cheap, fresh, valuable, recycled and sold. There are certain press conferences with good prepared questionnaire which is kept open to the public to see and hear and vast larger amount of people can get benefited with it.

Postal direct mailing—sending health educational material by post to the village leader, to the remotest area and reach to the un-reached to become the voice of the voiceless.

Printed material like weekly, monthly, periodic news letters bulletin.

Printed Aid

Photo books are main source of knowledge.

Publication of books on health, pamphlets, handouts, powerful and popular media of communication.

Newspapers—health messages can be published which can reach to the people easily. It can be published in local language with low cost and easy to read and understand.

Pamphlets

Can be folded into 3, 3, 5 printed either single or both sides, conveys a lot of information at a time. Holds interest of the group, makes lecture interesting.

Pictures—are most commonly used graphic aids. Pictures include photograph, paintings, illustration form, magazines, news paper, news letter, etc. If the pictures collected are small they can be enlarged and drawn in a chart paper-sketches, crayons are used for it. For preserving pictures for repeated use for teaching they should be mounted. A thick cardboard frame used for this purpose. First cut out a portion slightly smaller than the size and paste the pictures using adhesive behind the cardboard frame. The picture should be captioned and labeled.

Technological Education

Internet transfer of knowledge by e-mail, SMS, pager, website.

Technology results in new design and also devices anew ideas in process. Education technology is the application of scientific knowledge in a systemic way to improve the efficacy of process of learning and instruction. All AV aids have advantages and disadvantages, so one should select appropriate one.

IEC (information, education and communication)—we all communicate all the time, there is not a single moment when we are not communicating. Communication plays a vital role in our day today life. It is a central to all the progress that human being have made. No progress is possible in absence of communication. There is close association between communication and development. It creates awareness about new thing it equipping people with new information and skills.

Messages proper and appropriate may be designed to convey facts, alter attitudes, change behaviour or encourage participation in decision making. It should be in audience interest, it has to draw and retain attention, should be creatively designed, have clarity, simple, short, easily comprehended, clearly convey required information, maintain consistent, avoiding confusion, facilitating understanding, reinforcing learning and relating the them of your message. It should be truthful, honest, complete, worth effort, help to improve efficacy. Change is not easy to bring about as people resist it.

Due to low literacy, low purchasing power, poor means of transportation that hampers timely delivery of newspapers or repair or maintenance of TV/radio sets in rural areas. Irregular supply of electricity makes its operation problematic. Of late BCC behaviour communication change is emphasized to bring about development change.

It is a dynamic process and exchange of information and ideas. Communication and human interaction go together. It imparts, conveys and exchanges ideas, knowledge, and transfers, through, exchanges information. it is two way process, the communication process is essentially a function of brain. Interpersonal communication is face to face with person, instantly you get feed back. Today mass communication has become global in nature.

Effective teaching aids need not be elaborate or expensive. Many of them can easily be made from local materials at little or no cost, with the participation of local people. Making teaching aids is often part of the learning process, and should be included in the dialogue between the health worker and the community: It is important to remember, however, that all teaching aids should be carefully tested to make sure that the message they are intended to convey is well understood and accepted. If people are not used to learning from pictures, another way should be found to help them understand basic health messages. Images or activities that are not culturally acceptable may do more harm than good. The best way to ensure that they are appropriate is to involve members of the community in making them.

Indirect learning takes place

1. Reading accounts or description or discussions in books, magazines, journals, newspapers
2. Observing pictures, photos, maps, charts, models
3. Listening oral description, lectures, talks.

Book Writing

How the inspiration of writing a book thought was born?

Writing medical book is not like writing a spiritual book. In spiritual books we have meditation, reflections, life experiences, and God experiences, etc. whereas in medical books we have lot of extensive reading, research, clinical practice, continuous medical updates and education, attending workshops, training, experiences, internet references, newspapers and other educational method integrated. For me personally. People have inspired me with their pain and struggles of life. The spark that is born to do something and reach to the people through your experience and knowledge was deeply felt. And I feel it is inspired by God and spirit lead. It is also inspired by number of people whose hard work I have enjoyed and got enriched with whom I owe my knowledge and all that I am today. I feel each person has something unique to offer and her point of view is unique which can suit to certain categories of people who are like minded and similar wavelengths. To write a book needs lot of seriousness, responsibility. Lot of time, energy, hard work, sacrifice needed to spend valuable time that could have been used for other purpose. In last 27 years working in nursing field has given me a lot and I want to return in hundred fold in my own way back to the society. Thus this book is written in full faith with humble attempt; I hope it will be appreciated and benefited in nursing faculties in number of ways.

Explanation

One life is not enough to dive into the depth of the wisdom and knowledge. Read books, magazines, daily newspaper, etc. and enrich your educational field and give them back to the society which is thirsty for it.

Reading a newspaper—you select a newspaper that you read, new items you read interpret matter.

Keywords

Health magazine, press, Postal direct mailing, Printed aid, Pamphlets, Pictures, Internet, IEC, Message popper, Book writing, Reading a newspaper.

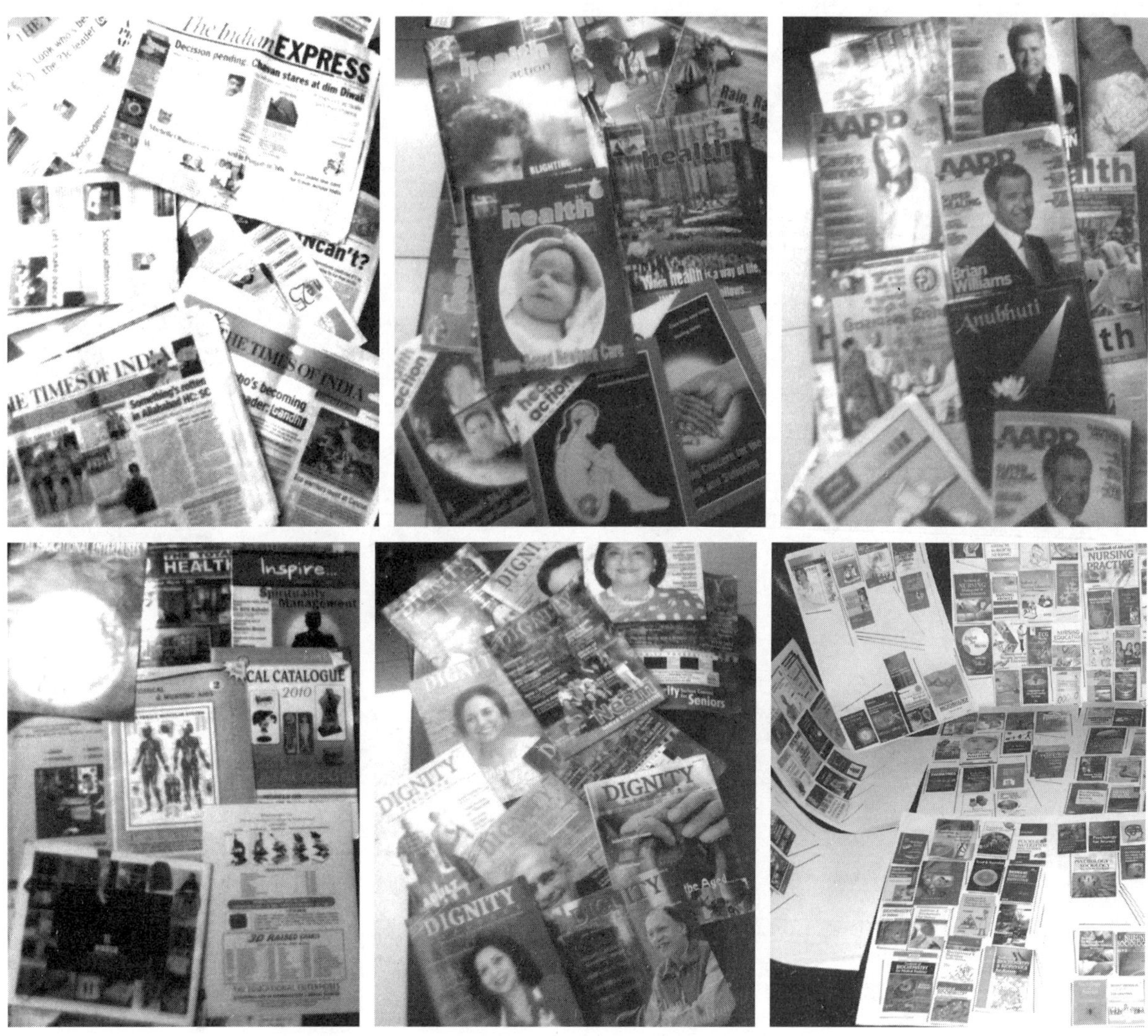

Psychiatric Mental Health Nursing
Psychiatry for Nurses
Textbook of Psychiatric Mental Health Nursing
Textbook of Postgraduate Psychiatry
Psychiatry & Mental Health Nursing
A Short Textbook of PSYCHIATRY
A Guide to Mental Health & Psychiatric Nursing
Textbook of Mental Health Nursing
Practical Guide to Mental Health Nursing
COMMUNITY MENTAL HEALTH IN INDIA
Psychiatric Mental Health Nursing
Practical Record Book for Psychiatric/Mental Health Nursing
MENTAL HEALTH NURSING

Fundamentals of Nursing for General Nursing and Midwifery
Fundamentals of Nursing
NURSING
Practical Nursing Procedures
Principles & Practice of NURSING
Basic Concepts on Nursing Procedures
Practical Standard Prescriber
Application of Nursing Process & Nursing Diagnosis
Essentials of NURSING
Nursing Care Plans
Textbook of NURSING FOUNDATIONS
NURSING PROCESS
Common Diagnostic Procedures for Nurses
Clinical Nursing Procedures: The Art of Nursing Practice
Foundations of NURSING
History of Nursing

Textbook of Midwifery
Obstetrics for Nurses and Midwives
Manual of MIDWIFERY
OBSTETRICS & GYNECOLOGY
TEXTBOOK OF GYNECOLOGY
Textbook of OBSTETRICS
Maternity Record Book
Textbook of Midwifery & Reproductive Health Nursing
A Guide to Midwifery Students
MIDWIFERY
Obstetrics Drug Handbook
OBSTETRICS & GYNECOLOGY
MIDWIFERY & GYNECOLOGICAL NURSING
Essentials of Midwifery & Obstetrical Nursing
Domiciliary Care in Midwifery

Samta Soni
Short Textbook of Advance NURSING PRACTICE
JAYPEE
OPHTHALMIC NURSING
Midwifery Record Book for BSc Nursing Students
Medicine for Nurses
ECG in Medical Practice
Textbook of Communication and Education Technology for Nurses
Orthopaedics for Nurses
Smart Life @ 40+
Nursing Theories & Nursing Practice
Textbook of Nursing Education
The Short Textbook of NURSING EDUCATION
Manual of Operating Room

मिडवाइफरी
MEDICAL SURGICAL NURSING
शिशु परिचर्या
Textbook of NURSING ADMINISTRATION for BSc Nursing
Textbook of NURSING Management in Service Education
NURSING PROFILE
Textbook of Nursing Education
KP Neeraja
JAYPEE
English for Nurses
Management of Nursing Services & Education
ECG Made Easy
NURSING EDUCATION Principles and Concepts

Essentials of MEDICAL PHARMACOLOGY
PHARMACOLOGY for Nurses
PHARMACOLOGY
Pharmacology for Nurses
Calculating Drug Dosages
Introduction to NURSING PHARMACOLOGY
Human Genetics in Nursing
Textbook of PATHOLOGY
PATHOLOGY & GENETICS FOR NURSES
Textbook of PATHOLOGY & GENETICS

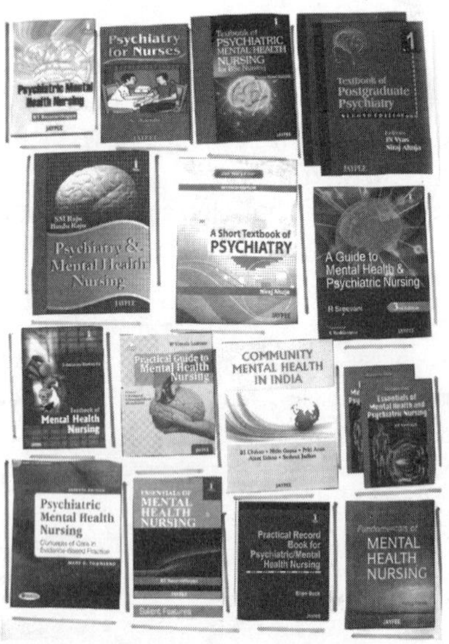

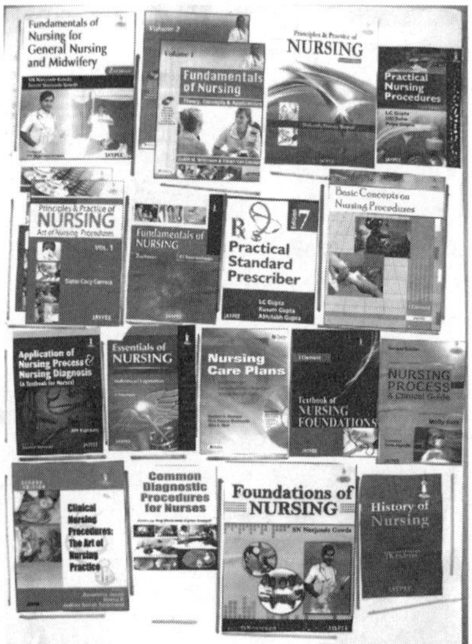

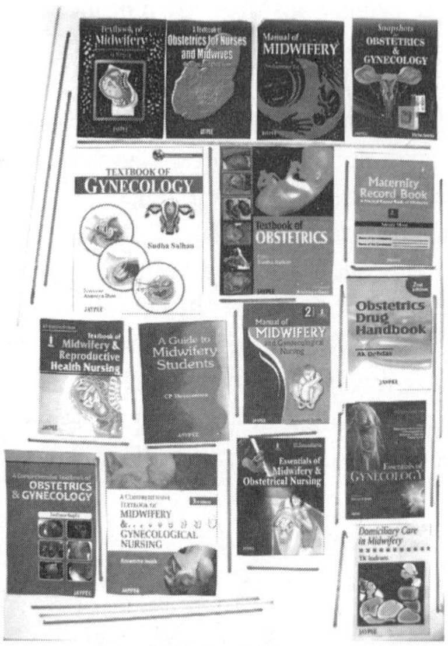

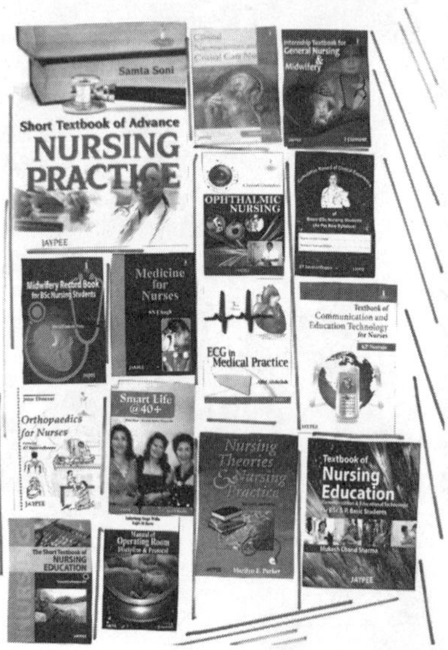

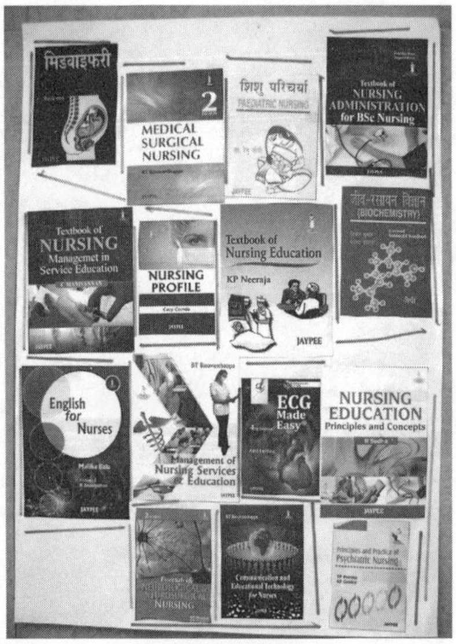

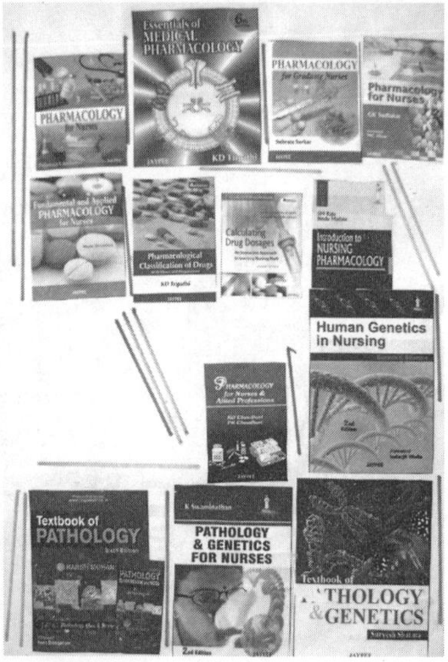

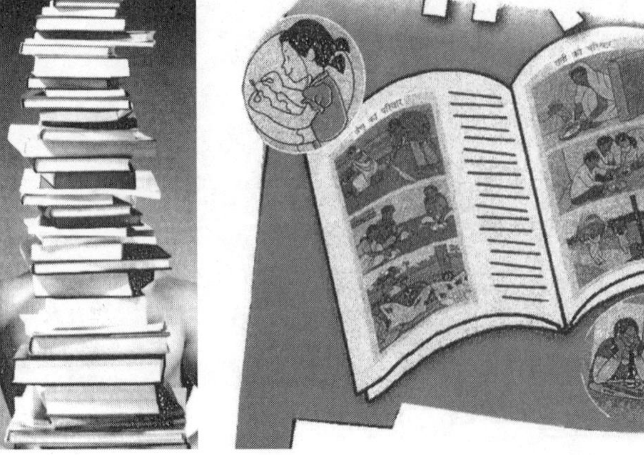

CHAPTER

34

Model

Abstract

Models are human muscle torsos, full size and half-sized human torsos, anatomical models are a great educational tool to study and explain the internal and external structure of the human body. Explore the organs of the human body and their functions in this 3-D model. Easy to assemble richly detailed miniature.

Model is a visual aid for teaching structures in schools and colleges. The model is made of PVC plastic with natural size dimension.

It helps concrete objects to explain structure and function of real things, made up of clay, pulp, cotton, cardboards, cloth and wood, etc. It is an enlarge objects to an observable size, promotes creativity interest in people.

Model enhances clarity in communication and enriches learning. Model provides direct, concrete, and purposeful experience, it gives opportunity to touch, to feel, to see a model. It brings remote events of either space or time in classroom. Model is a life-size miniature substitute for real things which is concrete object. Model is a representation of real thing low cost models are made up of clay, pulp, plaster of Paris, cotton, cardboard, thermacole, cloth, wood etc. models enables students to have a correct concept of the object. It should be accurate, simple, and useful. It thus creates creative interest among pupil, explains various processes of objects and machines, etc. scale models can display a dam for instance; simplified model gives an idea of an external form of an object like fish, working model can demonstrate in a simple way an process such as fetal circulation and a cross-section model inside of an object is visible.

Models are:

1. Still models
2. Working models
3. Sound models
4. Cross-sectional models
5. Solid models
6. Cut away X-ray models
7. Sand models.

It is a life-size miniature or cover size or original size. They are substitutes for real things. Models enable patient to have a correct concept of the object. It simplifies the reality and direct, meaningful learning. Concretizes abstract concepts; enables us to reduce or enlarge objects to an observable size; it provides the correct concept to a real object like dam, bridge. A working model explains the various processes of objects and machines. It promotes creative interest among pupil; it heightens reality of thing. It explains complex concept. It is expansive and need to be made properly.

Models used in nursing training—e.g. human skeleton with stand, size 170 cm life size. Different size mini made of PVC plastic. It is removable arms and legs and other parts mounted on a sturdy base washable, unbreakable, and ideal for teaching the basics of human anatomy. It has detachable joints and durable parts. It is a visual aid for instruction and encourages students to learn bones. Some human skeleton shows the nerves and blood vessels. Depicts the position and better equipments give better results. Shoulder joint can illustrate abduction, adduction, ante version, retroversion and internal and external rotation. It has flexible artificial ligaments. A knee joint demonstrates flexion, extension and internal and external rotation. Hip joint demonstrates ante version, retroversion, and abduction, internal and external rotation. It is vivid display will go deep down the memory. Better education is a great national gain. So you have eye model, liver, DNA. Larynx, lungs, ear, stomach pumping heart, etc.

Visual aids attract the students. PVC models have long-lasting life.

Demonstration room nursing Manikin can teach basic nursing procedures. You can explore, show the important parts of the human body. You learn how your body works, how different organs work and how the different organs work together to keep us alive and healthy. Everything in the body is there for a reason. From skin to heart to finger prints. Each organ does a specific thing to keep human alive.

Medical model is the "set of procedures in which all doctors are trained." This set includes complaint, history, physical examination, ancillary tests if needed, diagnosis, treatment, and prognosis with and without treatment.

After use of AV aids they should be placed safely, away from dampness, dust, insects. Regular servicing done for projected aids.

Keywords

Model, Models in.

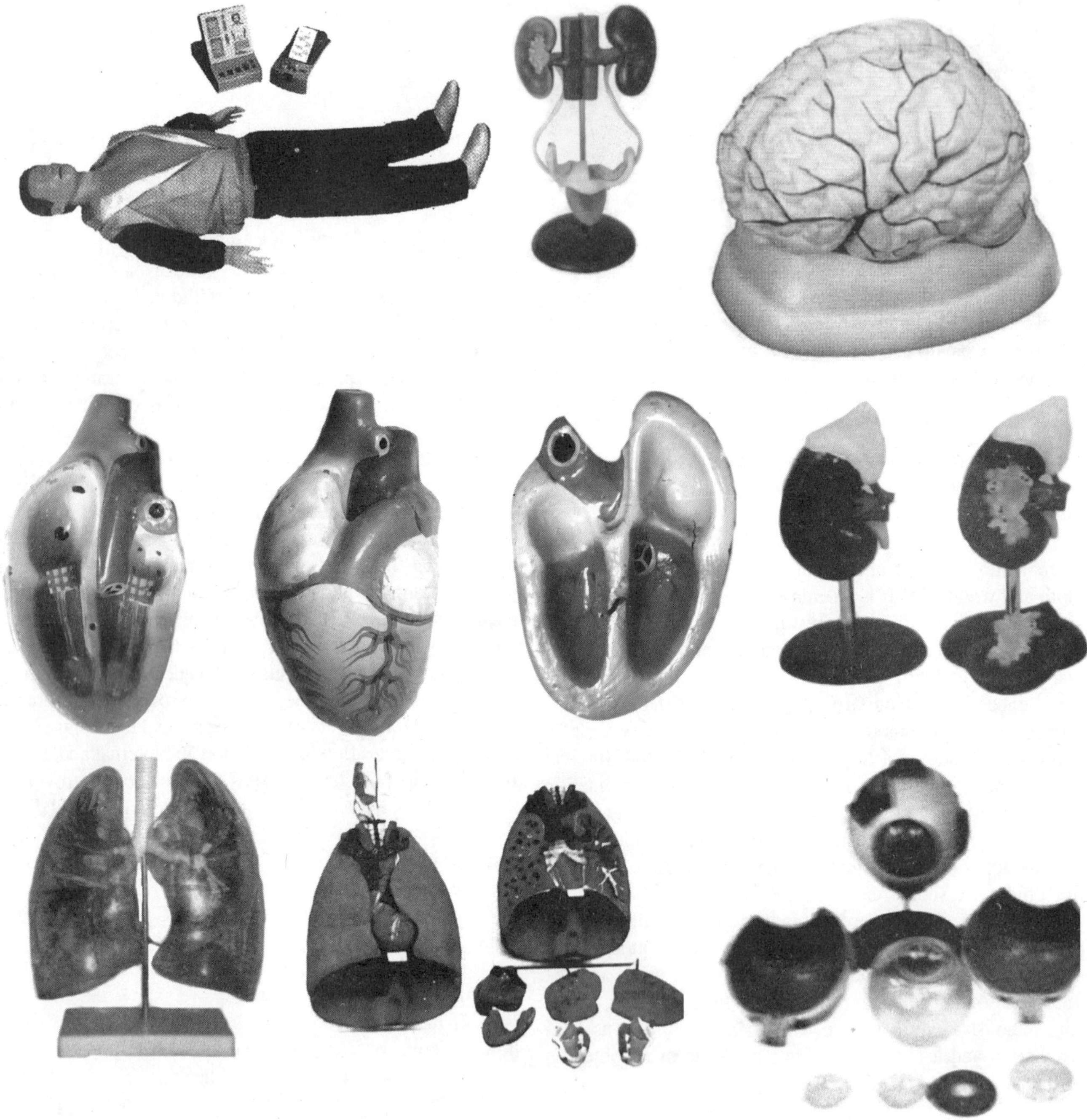

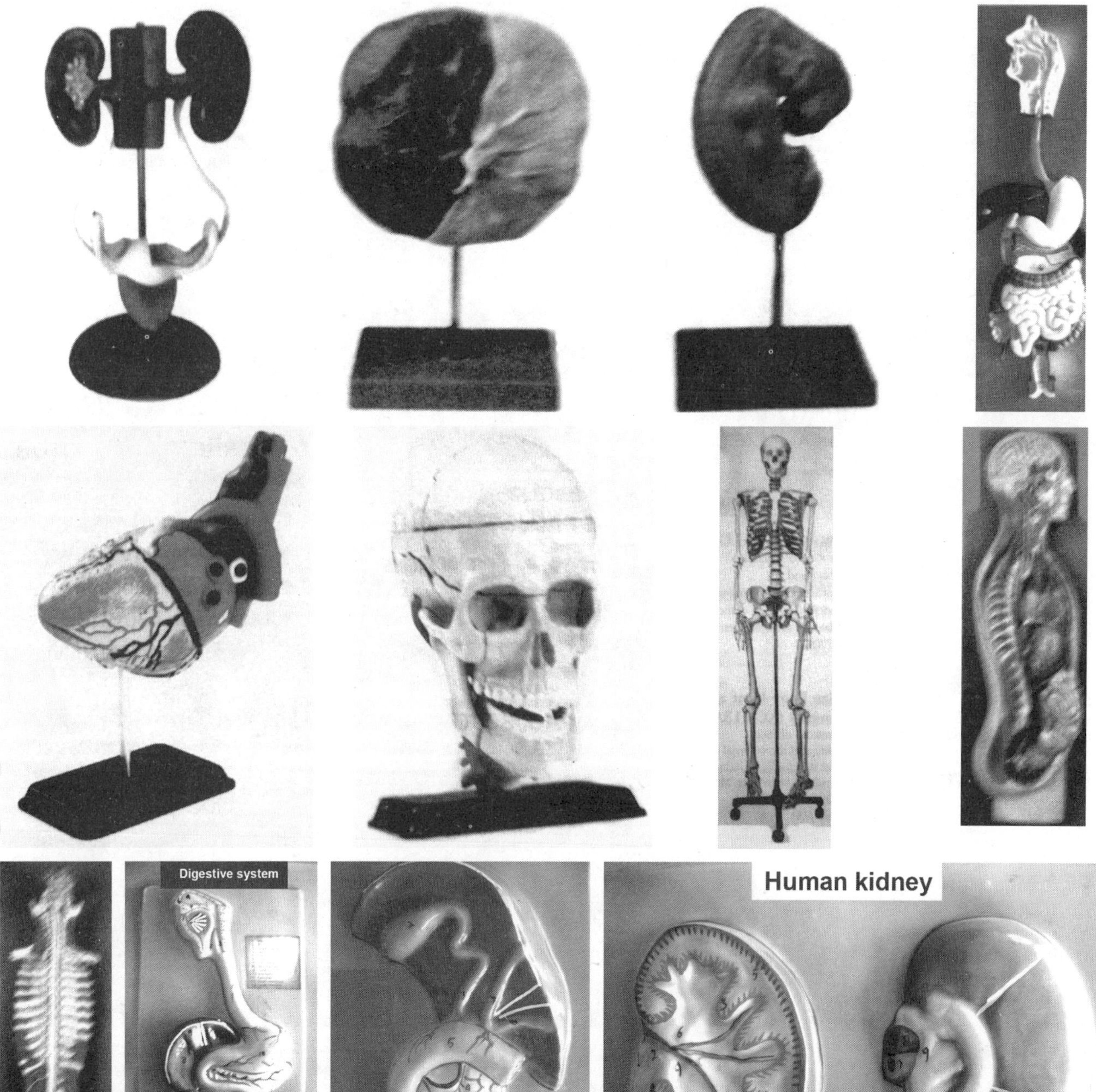
Digestive system
Human kidney

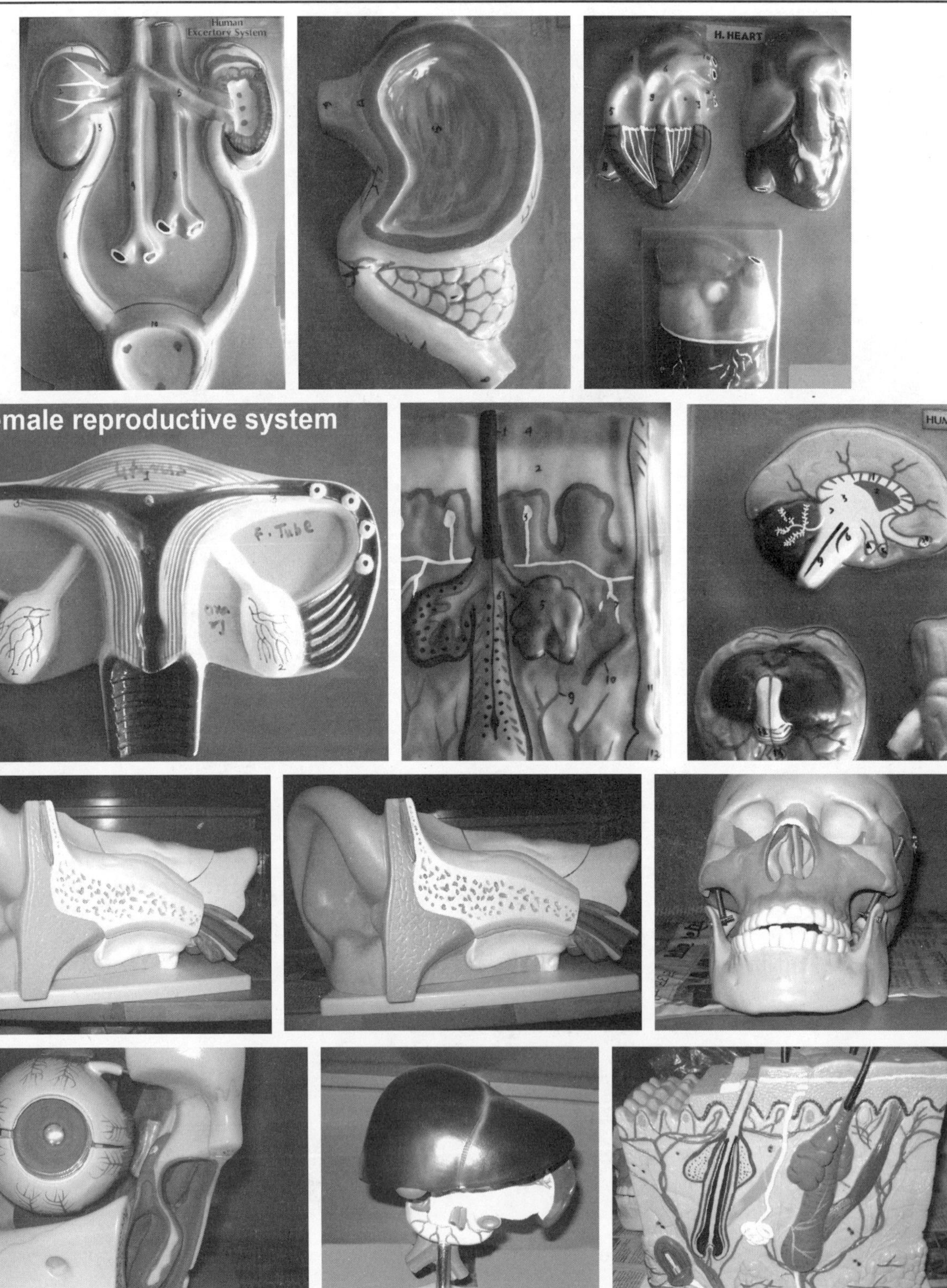
Human Excertory System
H. HEART
Female reproductive system
Uterus
F. Tube
Ovary

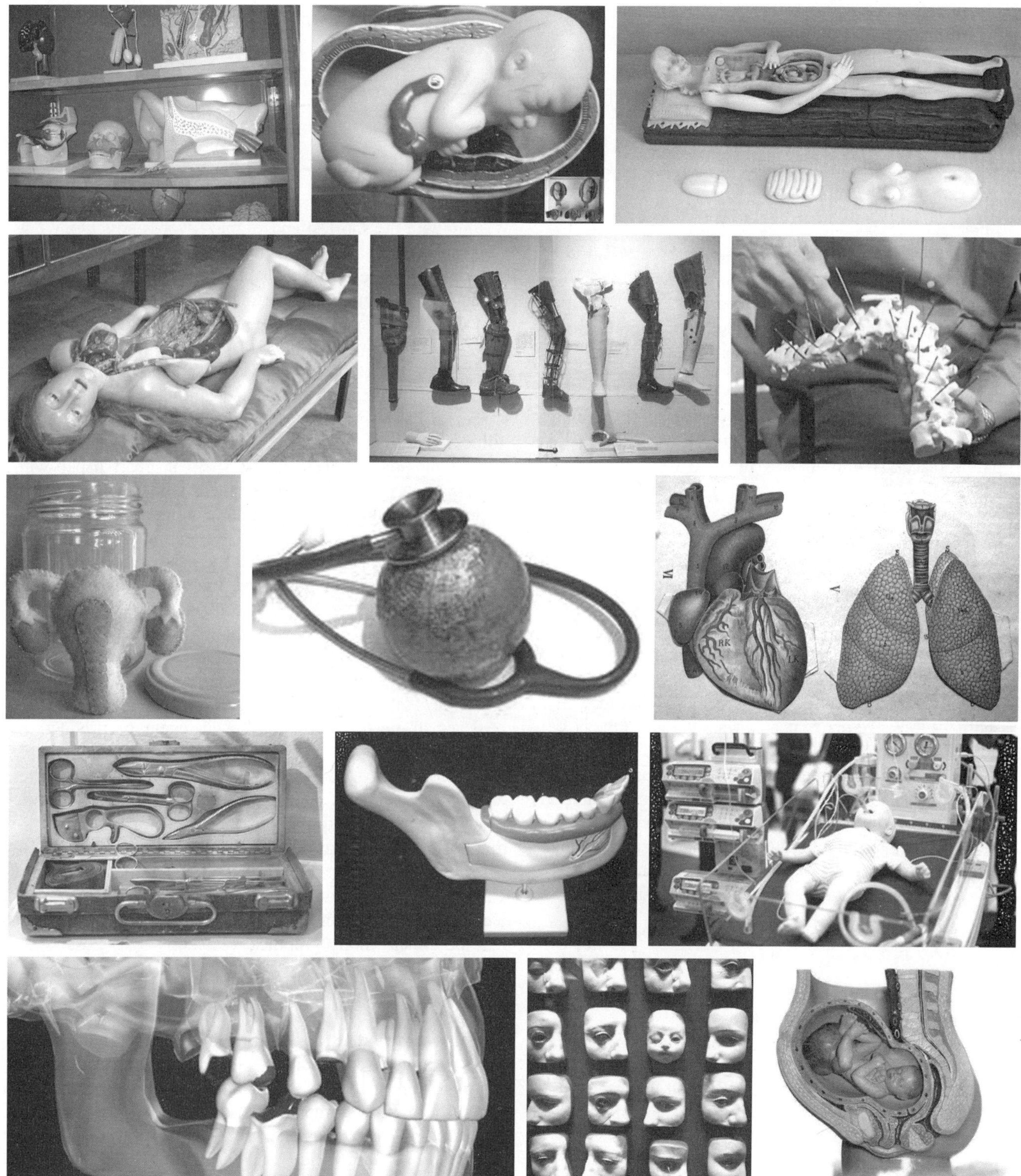
RK
LK

CHAPTER 35

Making Posters

Abstract

Poster is a piece of printed paper design to be attached to a wall. Education posters are eye-catching and visually appealing. Posters are great visual cues for students. It gives short and forceful message. Posters can be visually striking and are usually designed to make an immediate impression from a distance.

Posters can convey a single, simple message very strongly. They can be displayed in health centers, clinics, schools, or in public places. Points to bear in mind when designing a poster are:

- Choose large, clear images
- Avoid too much unnecessary detail or background
- Include only the relevant details which are essential to the message
- Avoid complex ideas which are hard to represent visually
- Avoid the use of objects shown larger than they really are within a picture—this may be misleading
- Do not use technical drawings
- Select colors, where used, with care, so that they fit in with the message, make people want to look at the poster, and are culturally acceptable.

Different cultural groups will respond to different types of visual image. In some countries photographs are familiar, in others it may be better to use outline drawings. Careful use of color is important because, although it can help make a poster more attractive and effective, certain colors have significance in themselves which may undermine the message of the poster.

Using Words

It is important that any writing used is clear and easy to read:

- Make the letters big enough to be easily seen
- Keep the style of the letters simple-printed capitals are usually best
- Leave enough space between words and lines
- Be sure that the contrast between the color of the background and of the letters is clear so that they are easy to see.

Where it is appropriate to use written materials for health education, try to choose or make those which are as clear as possible. Written materials should be:

- Attractive, easy to read, with plenty of space and pictures
- Broken into short sections
- As short as possible, with the most important points at the beginning.

Written with the shortest and simplest words possible.

Display one aid at a time and remove all unrelated materials to make an instant appeal and convey few ideas. It should be Comprehensible and clear to understand at a glance. Plan for specified people, it should stop people and make them look, use bold letters.

Posters are graphic aids which sent quick and typical message with attention capturing paintings. A good poster is said to have simplicity depiction, dramatic action, color fullness, eye catching design. Posters simple, inexpensive way of making pictures can be stick on chart paper with accompanying idea can be written with a marker pen Posters are intended to attract public attention. The material needs artistic preparation to catch attention of public. The message can be taken at a glance and easily understood. We find different types of posters at bus stop, railway station, hospitals, health centers, and streets, etc.

The message on the poster should be short, simple, and direct and one can see at a glance and easy to understand. It is Colorful and eye catching, Short message, Simplicity in depiction, Placed where people gather.

Uses of posters—Advertising an event or product; to make an instant appeal.

To conveys single idea or few ideas. Giving a directive, warming. Suitable for patient education, presenting scientific facts, showing a safety measures, symbols or signs, the life of a poster is short and needs frequent replacement.

A **poster** is any piece of printed papers designed to be attached to a wall or vertical surface. Typically posters include both textual and graphic elements, although a poster may be either wholly graphical or wholly text. Posters are designed to be both eye-catching and informative. Posters may be used for many purposes. They are a frequent tool of advertisers (particularly of events, musicians and films), propagandists, protestors, and other groups trying to communicate a message. Posters are also used for reproductions of artwork, particularly famous works, and are generally low-cost compared to original artwork. "For over two hundred years, posters have been displayed in public places all over the world. Visually striking, they have been designed to attract the attention of passers-by, making us aware of a political viewpoint, enticing us to attend specific events, or encouraging us to purchase a particular product or service." The modern poster, as we know it, however, dates back to 1870 when the printing industry perfected color lithography and made mass production possible.

Posters, in the form of placards and posted bills, have been used since earliest times, primarily for advertising and announcements. Purely textual posters have a long history: they advertised the plays of Shakespeare and made citizens aware of government proclamations for centuries.

Posters soon transformed the thoroughfares of Paris into the "art galleries of the street." Their commercial success was such that some of the artists were in great demand and theatre stars personally selected their own favorite artist to do the poster for an upcoming performance. The popularity of poster art was such that in 1884 a major exhibition was held in Paris. Many posters have had great artistic merit and have become extremely collectible. Many printing techniques are used to produce posters. While most posters are mass-produced, posters may also be printed by hand or in limited editions. Most posters are printed on one side and left blank on the back, the better for affixing to a wall or other surface. Pin-up sized posters are usually printed on A3 Standard Silk paper in full color. Upon purchase, most commercially available posters are often rolled up into a cylindrical tube to allow for damage-free transportation. Rolled-up posters can then be flattened under pressure for several hours to regain their original form. It is possible to use poster creation software to print large posters on standard home or office printers.

Many posters, particularly early posters, were used for advertising products. The film industry quickly discovered that vibrantly colored posters were an easy way to sell their pictures. Today, posters are produced for most major films, and the collecting of movie posters has become a major hobby.

Poster advertising or proposing a travel destination; or simply artistically articulating a place have been made tremendous impact on people like in Railway **posters; event posters, etc.**

Posters advertising events have become common. Any sort of public event, from a rally to a play, may be advertised with posters; a few types of events have become notable for their poster advertisements. Boxing posters were used in and around the actual venue to advertise the forthcoming fight, date, ticket prices, and usually consisted of pictures of each boxer. Boxing posters vary in size and vibrancy, but are not usually smaller than 18 × 22 inches. Pinup posters, "pinups," or cheesecake posters are pictures of attractive women designed to be displayed, first coming to popularity in the 1920s. Book text on poster is a type of poster design where the entire text of a book (usually a novel) is printed in legible form. This unique and modern design style is commonly characterized by a wall of text with a depiction of an important element of the book by use of negative space, which in this case is also known as white space.

Comic book posters; educational posters: Posters are used in academia to promote and explain research work. They are typically shown during conferences, either as a complement to a talk or scientific paper, or as a publication. They are of lesser importance than actual articles, but they can be a good introduction to a new piece of research before the paper is published. Poster presentations are often not peer-reviewed, but can instead be submitted, meaning that as many as can fit will be accepted. Posters are a standard feature of classrooms worldwide. A typical school in North America will display a variety, including: advertising tie-ins (e.g. an historical movie relevant to a current topic of study); alphabet and grammar; numeracy and scientific tables; safety and other instructions; artwork and displays by the students.

Explanation—posters should stop the people and make them to look that attractive; so as to get message at a single glance and place in a place where people pass or gather together. So that it can make instant appeal, make it sufficiently clear. It is suitable for patient education, presenting scientific facts, showing safety measures and many other facts relating to health it varies from a simple printed card to a complicated and artistic design.

Slogans for posters may be as follows:

1. A healthy child a sure future
2. Smoking or health—the choice is yours
3. Add life to years
4. Children health tomorrows wealth
5. Healthy youth our best resource
6. Healthy living everyone is winner
7. Immunization a chance forever child
8. Health for all—all for health
9. Our planet—our health
10. Think globally act locally
11. Should disaster strike be prepared
12. Heartbeat—the rhythm of life
13. Handle life with care prevent violence and negligence
14. Oral health for a healthy life
15. Target 2000 and a world without polio
16. Laugh everyday its like inner jagging
17. Healthy village for better life
18. Safe motherhood and breastfeed the best for child
19. Global alert global response
20. Active aging makes the difference
21. Healthy environment for children
22. Better understanding appropriate care
23. Prevention is better than cure
24. Smoking is injurious to health eat healthy live healthy
25. Towards tomorrow together.

Reflection—What is good education? What is meaningful education? Mould students into good human beings, critical thinking and the leaders of tomorrow. What are the new directions needed to make education broader, bolder and better? What changes are necessary to make envy child feel special and to bring out best. What roles can a teacher, parents play in shaping a new more meaningful educational home and school and society?

Keywords

Posters, using words, use of posters, comic book posters.

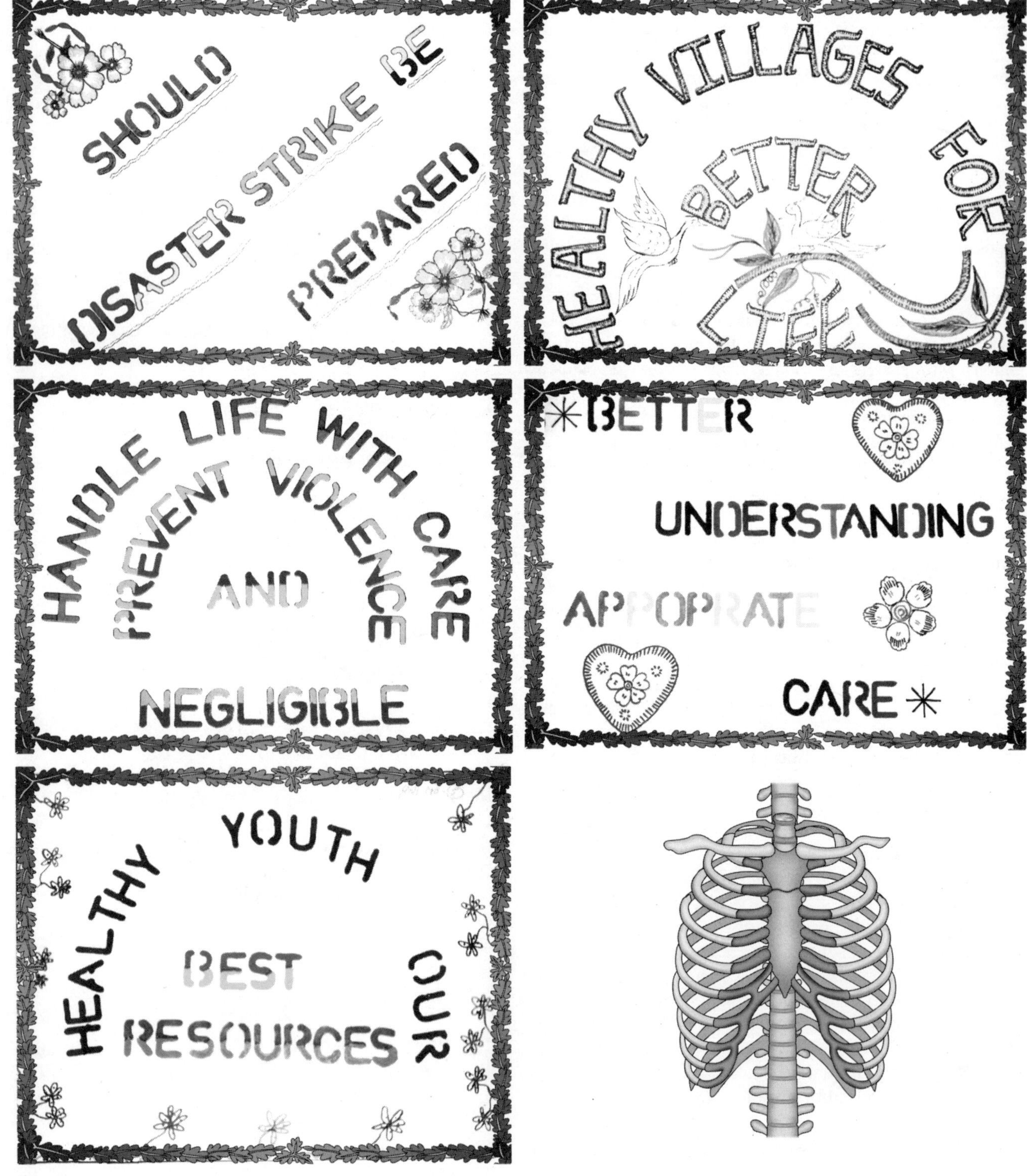
SHOULD
DISASTER STRIKE BE
PREPARED
HEALTHY VILLAGES FOR
BETTER
HANDLE LIFE WITH CARE
PREVENT VIOLENCE
AND
NEGLIGIBLE
BETTER
UNDERSTANDING
APPOPRATE
CARE
HEALTHY YOUTH
OUR
BEST
RESOURCES

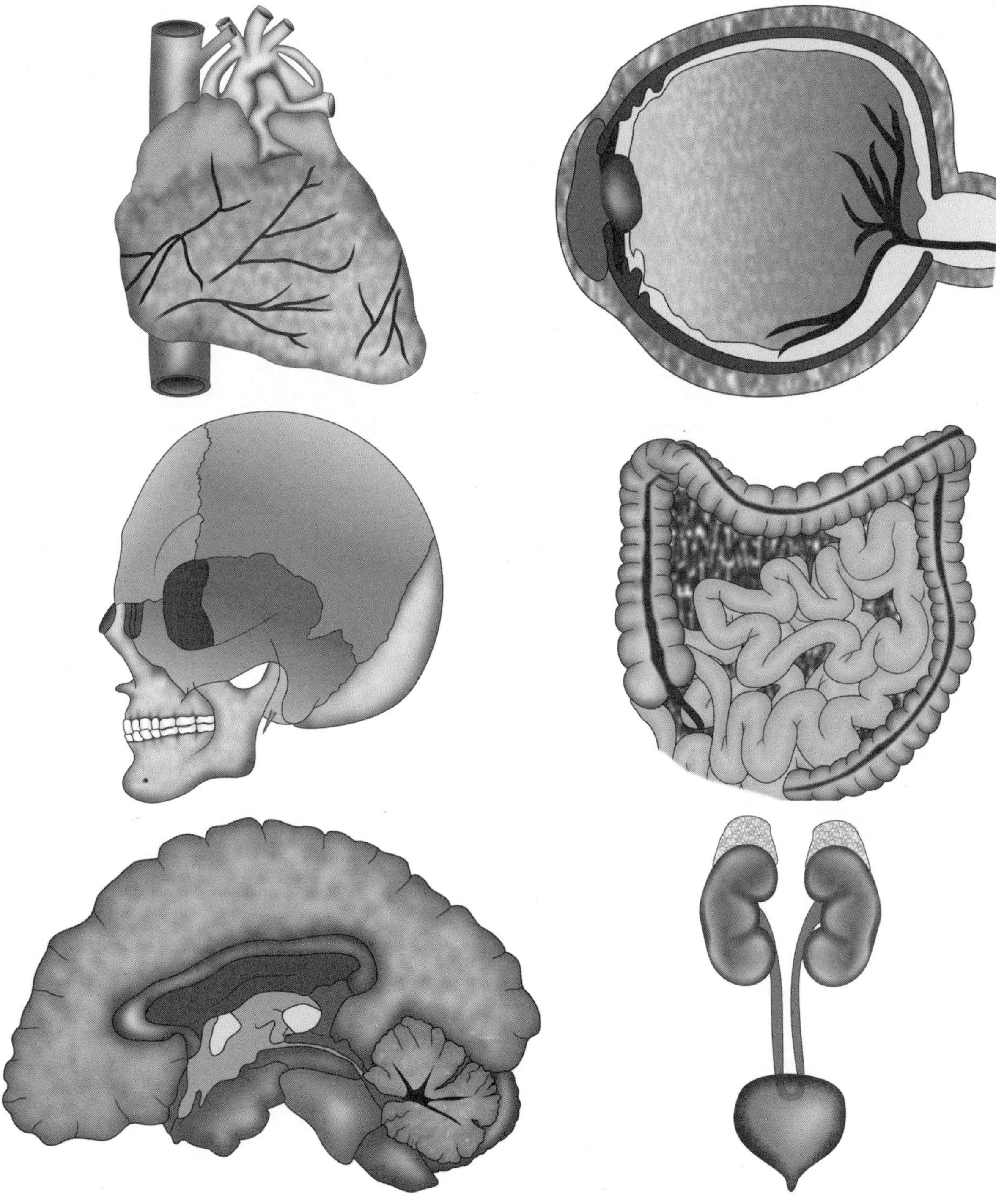

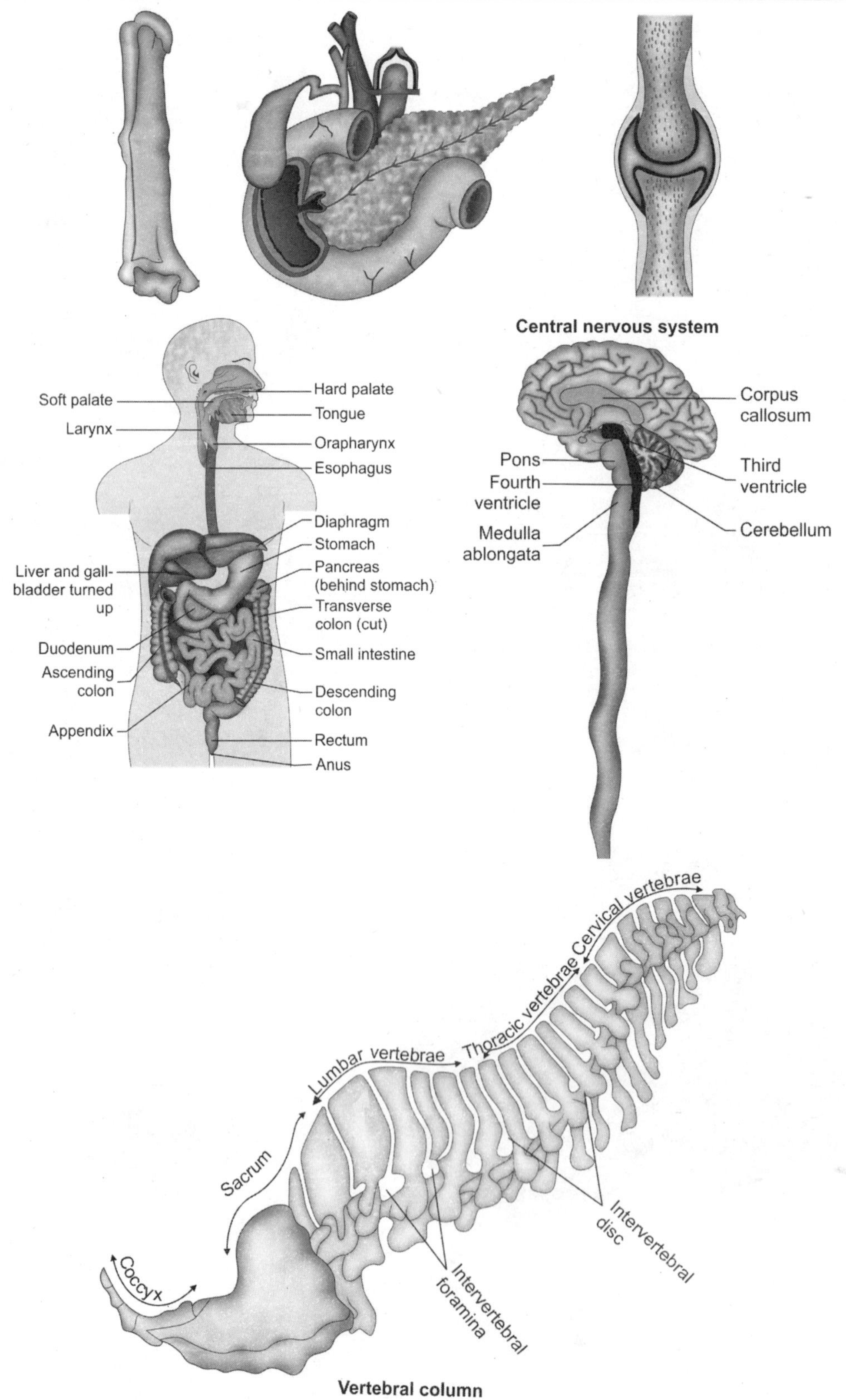

Central nervous system

Vertebral column

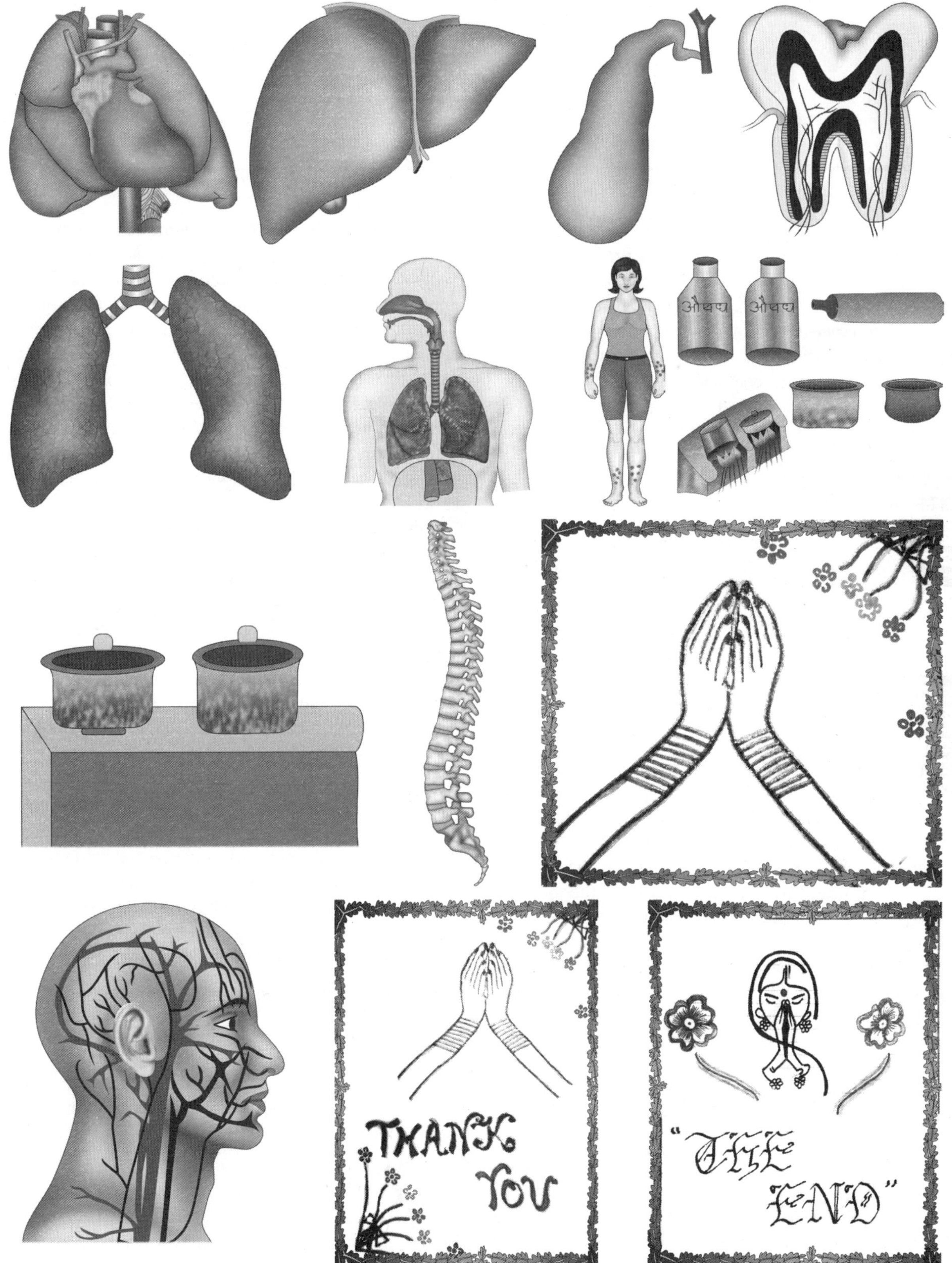
औषध
औषध
THANK
YOU
"THE
END"

CHAPTER 36

Project Exhibits

Abstract

Project: Plan set of inter-related task to be executed over a fixed period and within certain cause. It is a temporary endeavor undertaken to create the unique product, service or result, something that is contemplated, deviced, or planned.

Exhibitions: Public display of works of art or other items of interest held in an art gallery or museum or at a trade fair. It is in most general sense to an organized presentation and display of a selection of items.

INTRODUCTION

Audio-visual aids are those devices by the use of which communication of ideas between persons and group in various teaching and training situation is healed.

They are learning devices that help the teacher to clarify, establish, co-relate and coordinate accurate concepts; interventions and appreciation enable them to make learning more concrete, effective, interesting, inspirational, meaningful advice.

Purpose of communication—is to transmit information from one person or group of persons to other persons or groups with a view to bring about behavioral changes.

It is an direct or indirect exchange of information, ideas as a means of understanding and education.

Share ideas, facts, feelings or impression is the core.

One who communicates should know the need of information, its importance detailed knowledge, methods of communication.

It should be clear, relevant, correct, attractive, acceptable and specific.

It is the medium by which message is transmitted.

Daily we receive lot of information; our ability to influence others depends upon our ability to communicate. Good communication is the essence of good leadership, politicians excel in these skills. It will help you to score higher marks in the examination.

Audience should be apt to the topic you have selected. Not like women's topics discussion with kids. The group will accept or reject the message, or forget it is all depends on how you have presented the information. the process of learning is active.

Communication is essential to all human association. All of us are engaged most of the time in receiving information. Our ability to influence others depends upon our ability to communicate. Good communication is a complex process. It should be specific, accurate, and timely and appealing, objectives clearly defined and channel properly selected.

Educational exhibit offers in an interesting and unique manner of combining multiple media into small area which gives creative thinking and face even the big gathering.

A project is a problematic act carried to completion in its natural setting. Learning by living. Intellectual activity in natural setting in social environment the whole hearted purposeful activity is essential of project method. It should be problematic in nature.

Directed and planned by students, practical in nature with emphasis on a single complete unit of purposeful activity, resulting in a concrete achievement. The undertaking must be complete in itself, and the goal must be definite and objectives measurable. To get best out of life and gives opportunity for self expression by relating self to the community. It is like play activity. In which a solution to a problem is to be found out. Training and learning through practical problem solving, think of a problem, write reasons for selecting, creative expression, educational value.

Exhibits

It can be commercial/educational in nature. It introduces new unit of work and develops imagination and help visualization.

Types—there are simple exhibition which can illustrate various foods, e.g. carbohydrates, fat, proteins. Specimen exhibits, e.g. circulatory system of the heart. Complex exhibits-2–3 dimensional, motion pictures.

How is the exhibition useful in nursing education?

Exhibits consist of objects, models, specimens, etc. they convey a specific message to the observer. They are essentially mass media of communication. Many times a department of the school or class put up their works for showing it to people out side the school such as a show is called exhibition.

Requirements for Exhibition—it should have a central theme. It should be clean and labeled properly. Proper placement so that it is visible to everyone. It attracts larger number, key point of interest displayed in fairs, festivals, mass campaign etc. It inspires students to learn by doing things themselves as they get a sense of involvement. It develops social skills of communication; cooperation and coordination. It fosters creativity. A health exhibition attracts large numbers of people. They are used in connections with key points of interest. For example, fairs, festivals, mass campaigns, etc.

It should have—

1. Actual plan of action.
2. Have educational objectives, goals, visualization.
3. Utilization of appropriate method.
4. Student's needs guidance, instructions, and student's activities.
5. Method to evaluate weather the goal is achieved.
6. Understand sociocultural background.
7. Ensure active learning and avoids boredom, variety and a novelty in this type of presentation.
8. Topic properly illustrated.
9. Stimulate interest in pupil.
10. The principle, continuity, sequence and integration of ideas during presentation, problem solving approach during exhibition.
11. The place of arrangement for presentation or display of exhibition or a room should be well ventilated, lighted, pleasant and free from noises.

Teaching aids are projected and non-projected.

Objects

Makes direct appeal to senses, e.g. splints, forceps.

In group project students needs steps in developing, presentation and evaluation of group project. They have to know the essentials, objectives, limitations, usage, resources, classification, advantages, selection criteria, and place of conduct.

The concept of health is mostly focused on health awareness regarding promotion of health, prevention of diseases at the end, treatment of diseases, information, education, communication for which the mass media is utilized and the community setting is an ideal area for the students of group projects. It is a task that requires cooperation. It is whole hearted purposeful act competed in natural setting. It has purposeful goal and practical in nature. For example, individual projects say: to prepared poster on malnutrition. Group project integrate with role play, safe motherhood model. Learning project is like learn to operate monitor in ICCU. The objective is at the end of any project the student is able to develop leaderships qualities and achieve expected goal. It should arouse interest, practical action and provide opportunity to develop skill, bring out hidden talents. It can be used for different variety of groups like industrial workers, schools, urban and rural area, clinics, old age homes etc. It provides opportunity for creative expression and self activity, it has educational value.

Questions

1. What is the purpose of the project or the exhibition?
2. What are you suppose to learn?
3. What skills are you suppose to capture?
4. How will you decide project exhibition work in the field?
5. What are you suppose to produce?
6. Will you know the group of beneficiary?
7. Will you work cooperatively with other groups?
8. Will you need any help or resources?

An **exhibition,** in the most general sense, is an organized presentation and display of a selection of items. In practice, exhibitions usually occur within museums, galleries and exhibition halls, and world's fairs. Exhibitions include whatever as in major art museums and small art galleries; interpretive exhibitions, as at natural history, for example; and commercial exhibitions, or trade fairs. The word "exhibition" is usually, but not always, the word used for a collection of items. Sometimes "exhibit" is synonymous with "exhibition", but "exhibit" generally refers to a single item being exhibited within an exhibition. Exhibitions may be permanent displays or temporary, but in common usage, "exhibitions" are considered temporary and usually scheduled to open and close on specific dates. While many exhibitions are shown in just one venue, some exhibitions are shown in multiple locations and are called traveling exhibitions, and some are online exhibitions.

Though exhibitions are common events, the concept of an exhibition is quite wide and encompasses many. Art exhibitions include an array of artifacts from countless forms of human making: paintings, drawings, crafts, sculpture, video installations, sound installation, performances, interactive art, etc. Art exhibitions may focus on one artist, one group, one genre, one theme or one collection; or may be organized by curators, selected by juries, or show any artwork submitted. Fine arts exhibitions typically highlight works of art with generous space and lighting, supplying information through labels or audio guides designed to be unobtrusive to the art itself. Interpretive exhibitions are exhibitions that require more contexts to explain the items being displayed. This is generally true of exhibitions devoted to scientific and historical themes, where text, dioramas, charts, maps and interactive displays may provide necessary explanation of background and concepts. Interpretive exhibitions generally require more text and more graphics than fine art exhibitions do. Commercial exhibitions, generally called trade fairs, trade shows or expos, are usually organized so that organizations in a specific interest or industry can showcase and demonstrate their latest products, service, study activities of rivals and examine recent trends and opportunities. Some trade fairs are open to the public, while others can only be attended by company representatives (members of the trade) and members of the press.

Medical Fair India is India's No. 1 Trade Fair for hospitals, healthcare centers and clinics. Held annually alternating between New Delhi and Mumbai, it provides best opportunities to cover the enormous Indian healthcare market as well as considering the special potential of the two big metropolitan areas with its growing demand and rising investments in the public and private healthcare sector. The highlight of the industry is the most successful event in the fair's history, with 322 exhibitors and 6,721 visitors; held in 2012, the International Exhibition and Conference on Diagnostics, Medical Technology, Rehabilitation, Medical Equipment and Components, ended on 4 March 2012 as a resounding success, having seen 322 exhibitors from 17 different countries welcome 6,721 visitors. The event, which focused on the topics of medical technology, rehabilitation, accessories and services in the health sector, lasted for three days in total—and it is going from strength to strength! Medical Fair India offers a new platform for technology and service solutions for use in the medical engineering industry—from new materials, components, intermediate products, packaging and services all the way over to more complex micro system technology and nanotechnology.

Conclusion—good teaching aids should be meaningful, purposeful, accurate, simple, cheap, up to date, and easily portable and motivate the learner. It should be clear image, helpful, vivid.

Explanation—pictures of students who had to exhibit their project in rural and urban area for health education purpose. As part of syllabus they have to prepare individual and as a group project books.

Keywords

Introduction, Exhibits, Requirements for exhibition, objects, questions, exhibition, medical fair, conclusion.

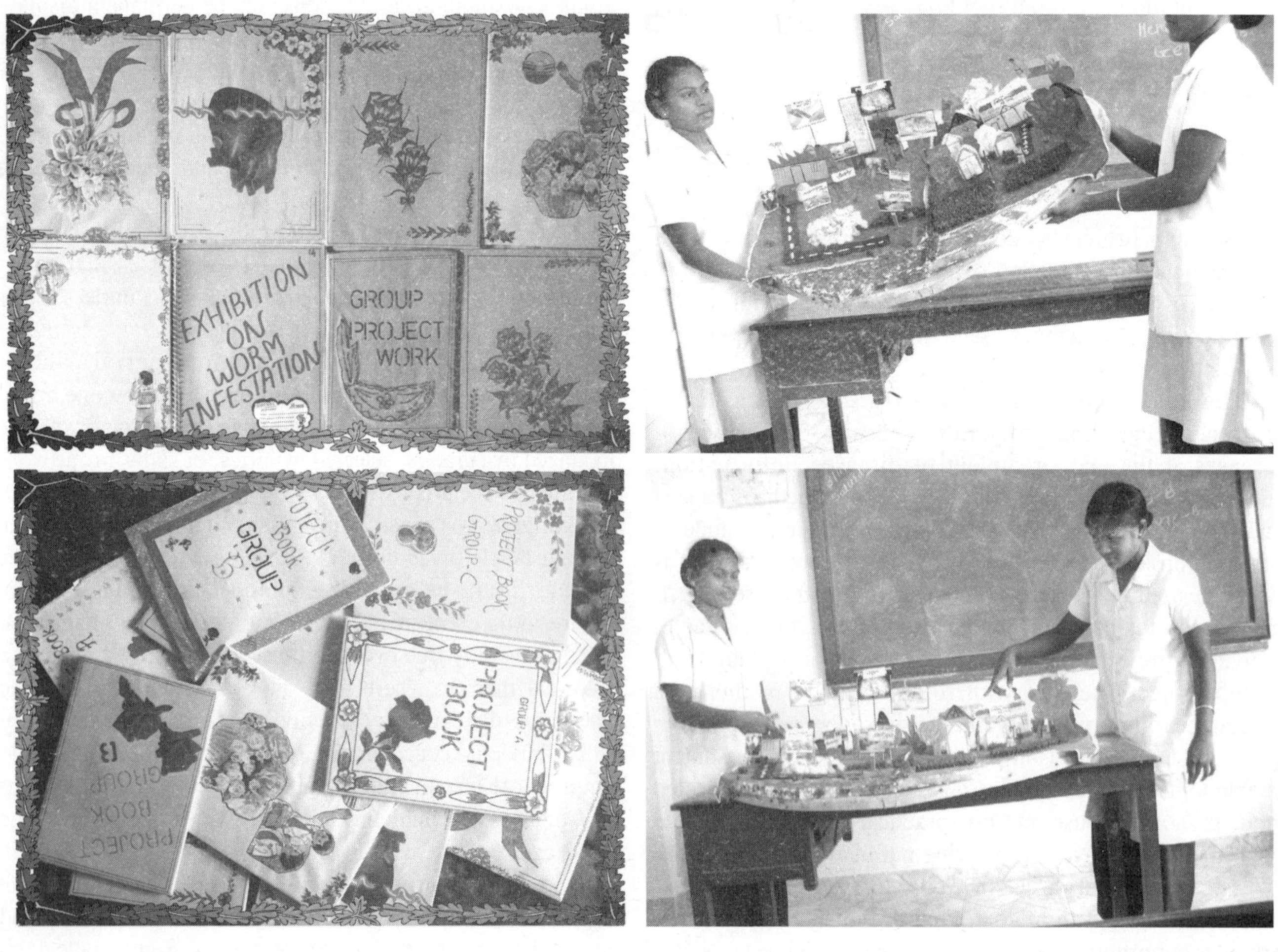

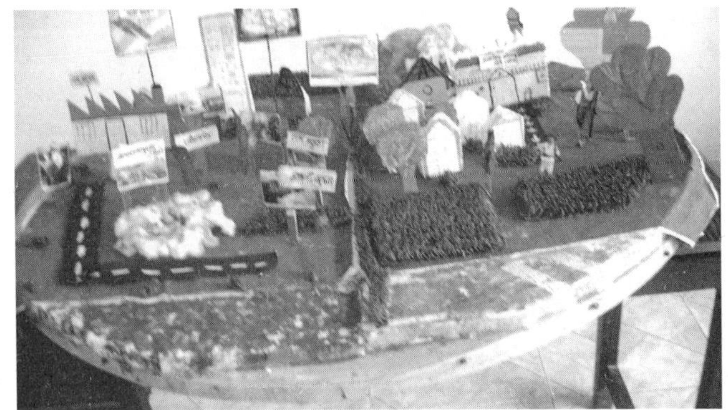

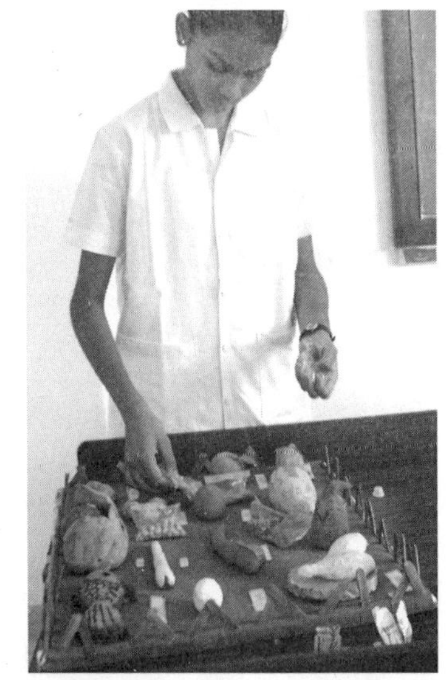

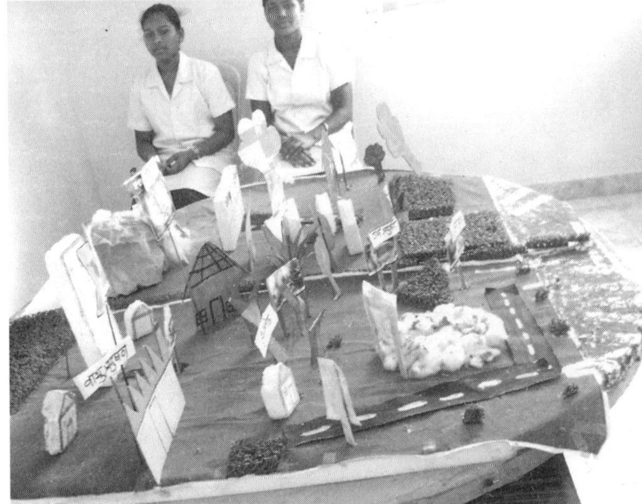

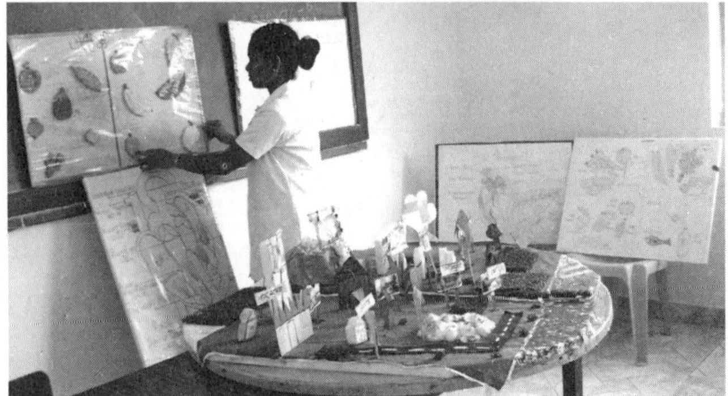

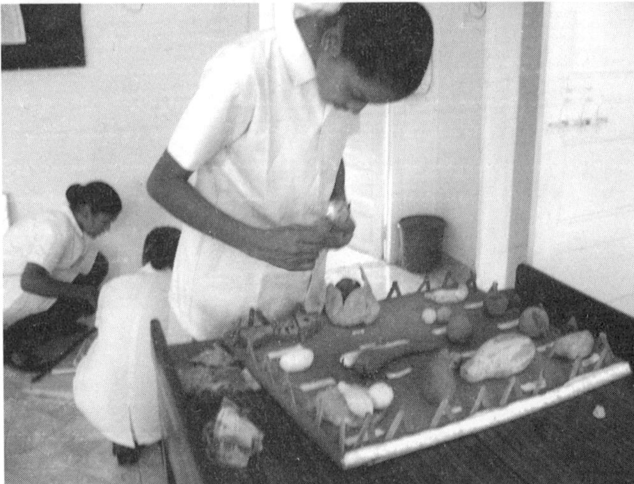

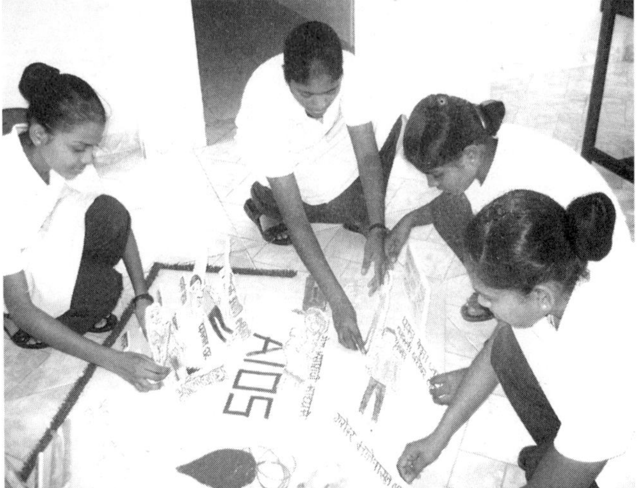
AIDS

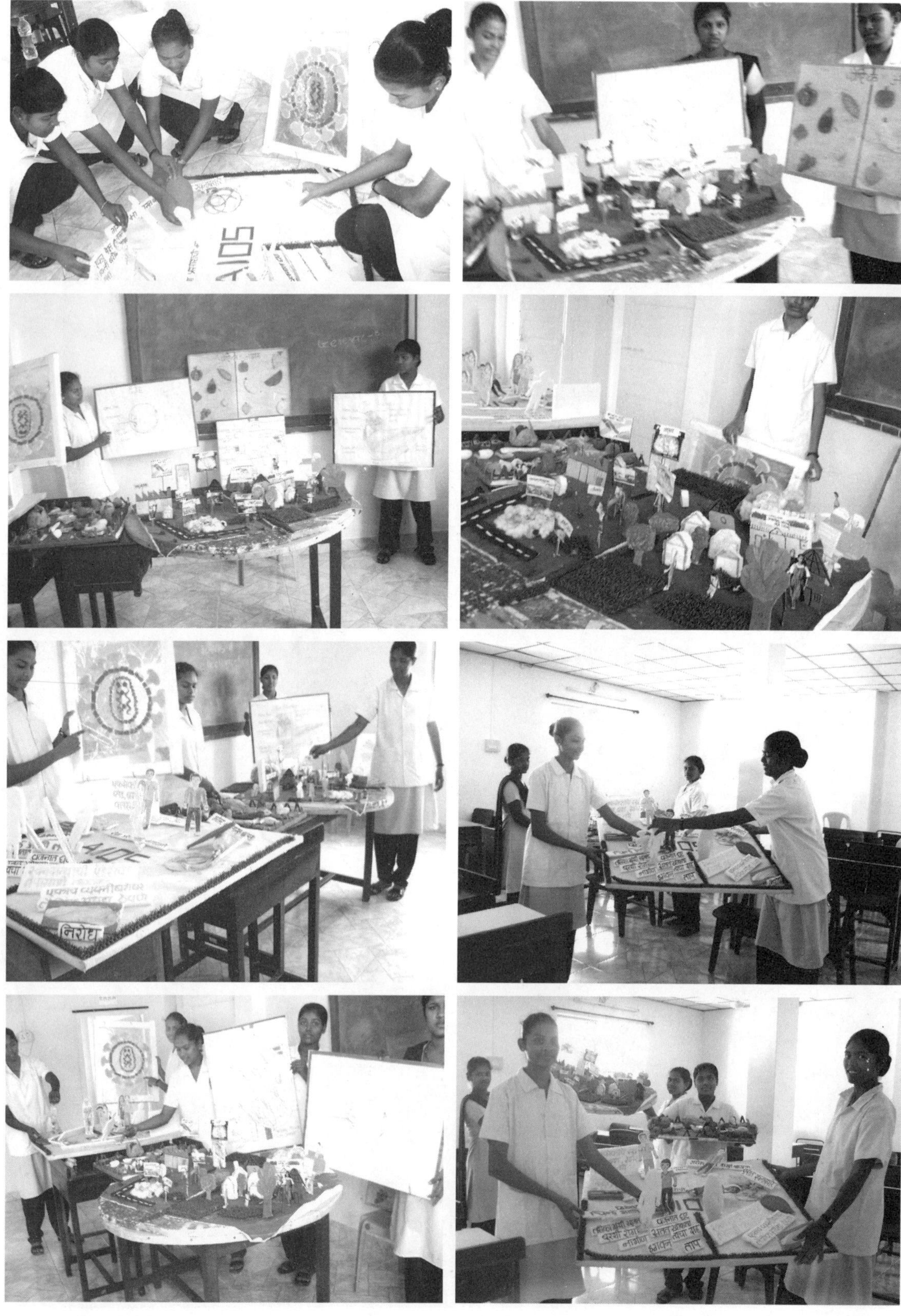

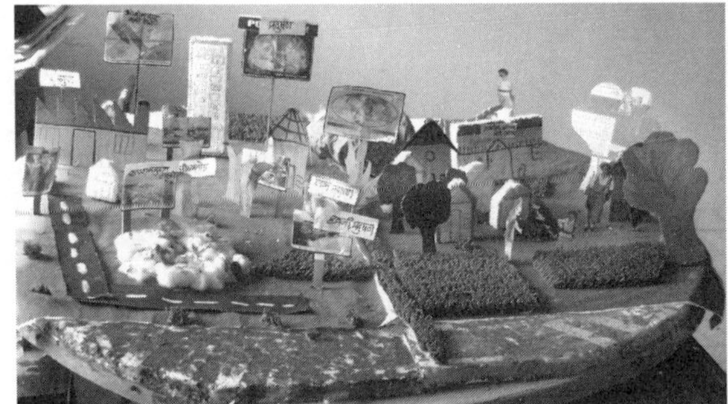

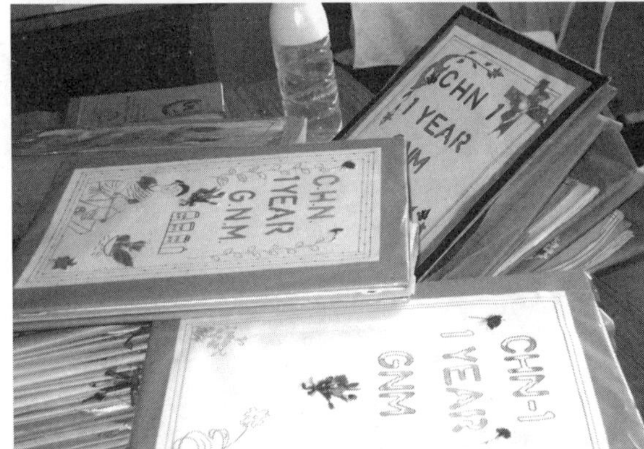
CHN I
1 YEAR
CHN
1YEAR
G.N.M.
CHN-1
1 YEAR
GNM

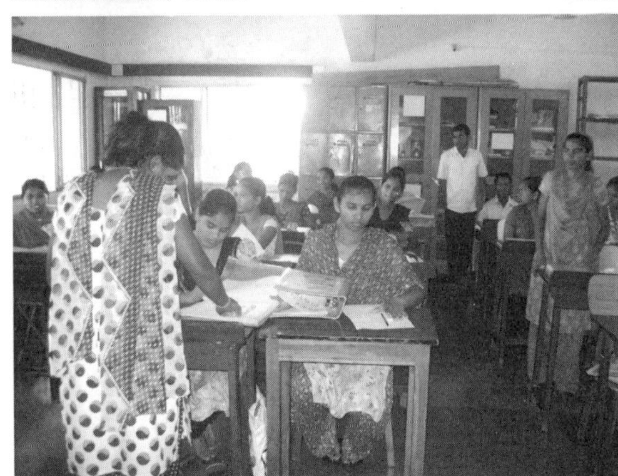

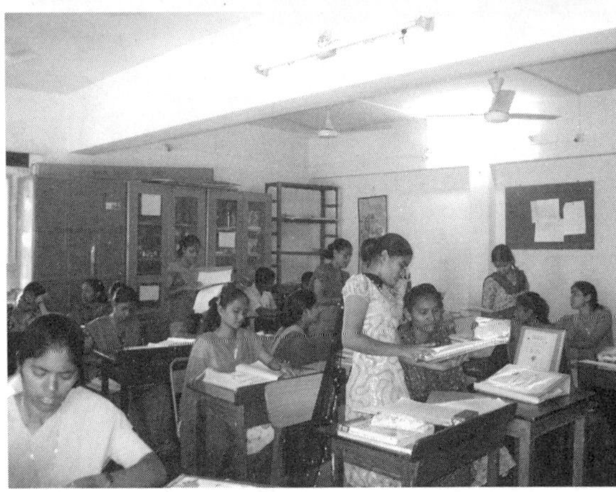

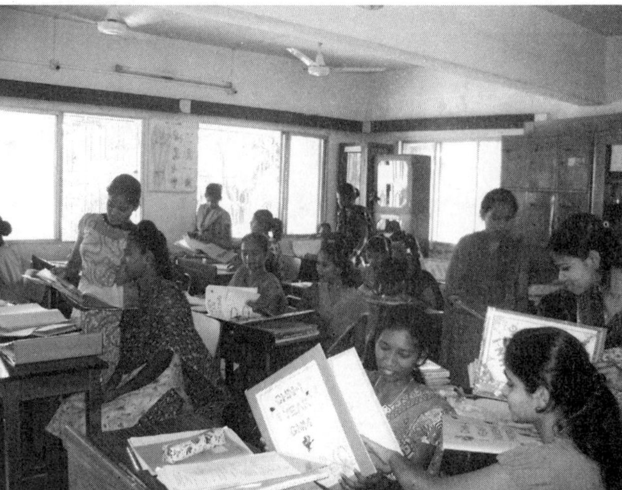

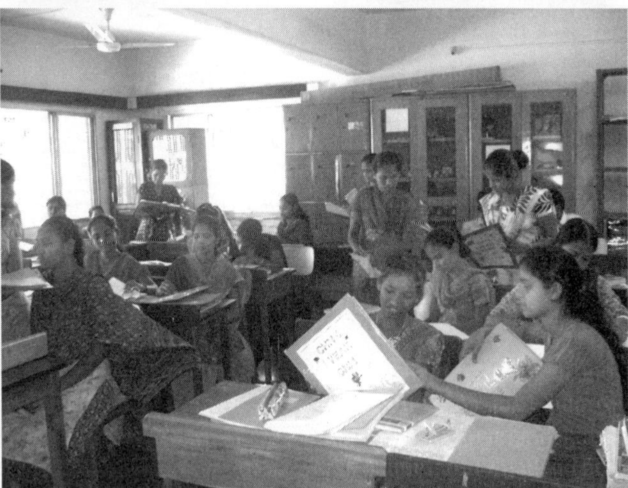

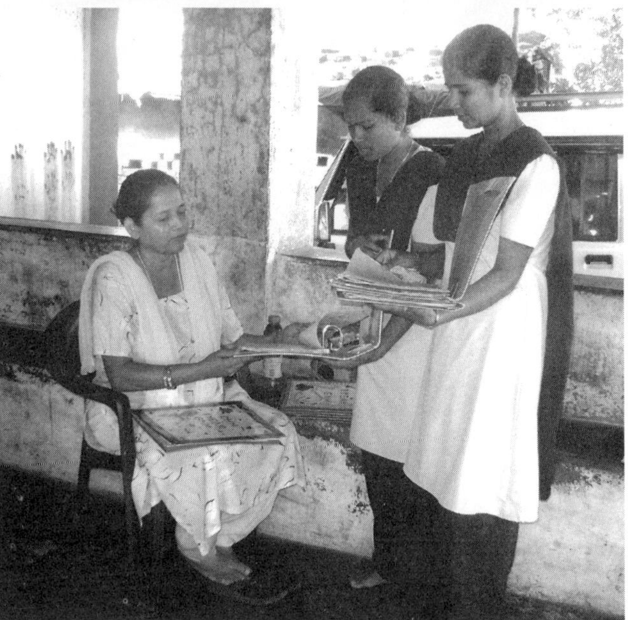

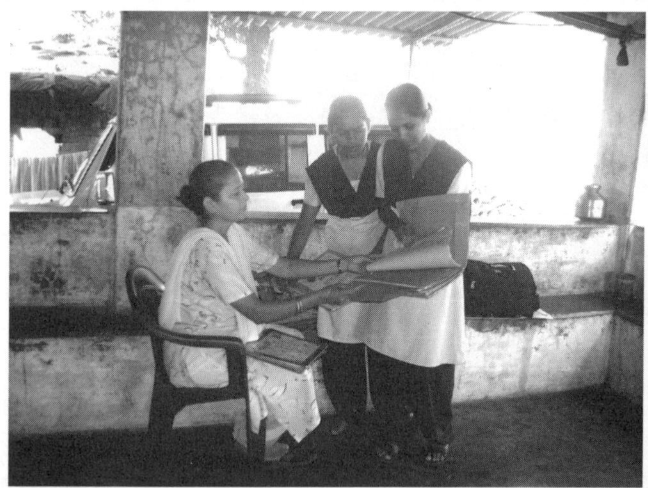

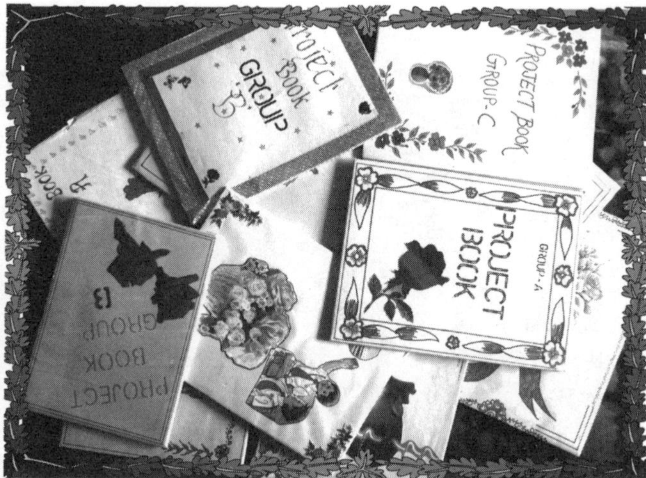
Project Book GROUP
PROJECT BOOK GROUP-C
GROUP-A PROJECT BOOK
PROJECT BOOK GROUP

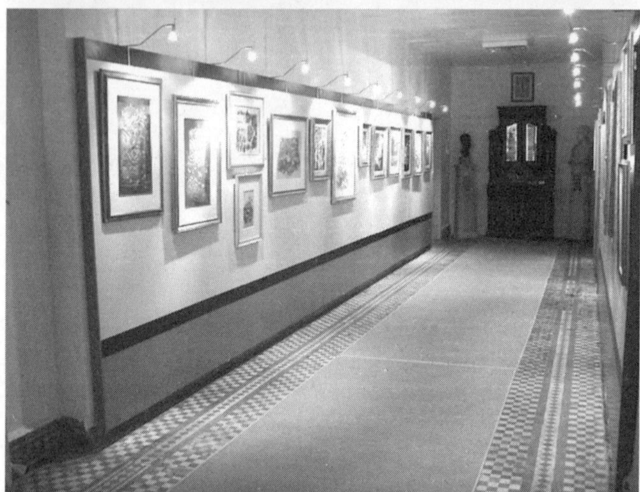

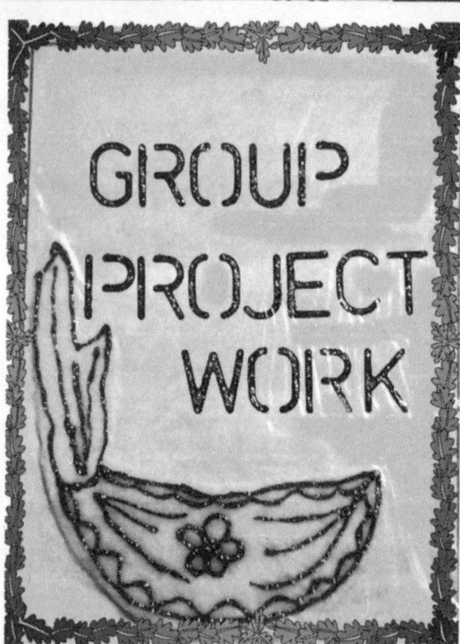
GROUP PROJECT WORK

CHAPTER

37

Preparing and Using Puppets

Abstract

Puppet is a movable model of a person or animal that is typically moved either by strings controlled from above or by the hand inside it. It is a small figure of a person or animal having a clothed body and a hollow head designed to be fitted over and manipulated by the hand.

INTRODUCTION

Puppetry is one of the old and poplar method in Indian villages. It is an effective method of learning. There are hand puppets which fit in the hand like a glove and are used in form below by finger. Road puppets operated from below the stage by a combination of rods and strings. It provides amusements and entertainment and learning as well. Puppets show can heighten the human emotions and capture attention.

It is one of the old and popular art in Indian village has been puppetry. It serves an effective aid to learning can help to illustrate lessons. There are hand puppets and string puppets (figures with moveable limbs operated through strings).

A puppetry has all advantages of dramatization along with providing amusements and entertainment. Also, a puppet show can heighten the human emotions and capture attention. In nursing peppery used in health education.

If you are planning to use puppets for health education, ask yourself:

- What story will be used, and who will make it up?
- What information will be used in building up the story?
- What is the aim or result hoped for?
- How will you find out whether this has been achieved?
- What support and follow-up will there be?

Appropriate stories can be developed using local experience, beliefs and culture. Be careful to appeal to what people understand, or—better still—ask community members to develop stories, Identify the major health problems in your area and explore ways to help people to overcome them through the puppet show. It is very important to be responsible about the message contained in the show: unrealistic drama will either raise false hopes or be ignored by people. Plan what follow-up there will be after the puppet show or series of shows.

Making Puppets

There are various types of puppet, some of which are extremely simple to make, and others which, although more work is needed, can still be made at very little cost. Children usually enjoy making puppets. Different types of puppet are:

- Glove puppets with papier mache or clay heads
- Rod puppets
- Paper bag puppets
- Vegetable puppets
- Jointed puppets
- Shadow puppets.

Puppet Stage or Theater

A puppet stage can be just a wall or curtain for the puppeteers to stand behind while they operate the puppets. You can hang a blanket or large piece of cloth between two trees, or across a doorway, or use the window of a house. Or, you could make a simple box theatre using wood or mats which could be taken apart and easily transported.

For shadow puppet shows, all that is needed is a large sheet of thin fabric that light will shine through. This can be hung between trees or poles. Remember to position the light source so that the puppets will cast shadows in the way you want. It is important to position the light safely, particularly if you are using paraffin or kerosene lamps, or candles.

Puppet show put up:

For an effective show, remember to:

- Use music and dance
- Have plenty of action: people are not interested in puppets which just talk
- Keep your speeches short and clear
- have a mixture of emotions (happiness and sadness)—this gives variety and holds the attention of the audience.
- Aim for clarity of plot; have a single idea at the centre of the drama, with all action contributing to this
- Be appropriate to the local culture and use local languages
- Use sound effects and props if you can make them
- Involve the audience: have the puppets ask them questions and demand a response.

What Do People Think of the Show?

Questions which should be asked after the puppet show include:

- Can the performance itself be improved? Was it well received?

- Did people get involved—in planning and at the time of the performance?

Has the show changed knowledge or behavior?

Using puppetry programme uses face-to-face encounters to provide existing and potential puppeteers with the necessary skills to empower community and peer-group educators to reach out to their communities with specific performances and workshops.

Communication Strategies

This programme works by enabling communities to perform their own educational theatre programme for their peers. These productions provide information that is designed to change patterns of both thought and behavior. The program is based on the following tenets:

Puppetry can bridge gaps of misunderstanding and bring people together to examine community social issues. Productions combine both music and humor in an effort to cross cultural and language barriers and reach people.

The puppet is a visual metaphor, representing 'real life'—at the same time, it is one step removed from the real world. Puppets can become alive and interactive, and, when combined with humor and music, generate both an entertaining and educative experience.

Puppetry holds up a mirror to society and gives people a chance to look objectively at themselves and especially enables people to laugh at themselves. It is less threatening than the human performer.

Puppetry breaks down barriers—It can be used to challenge social and political barriers as well as stereotypes because it represents the 'neutral' aspect of the human, exaggerating 'larger than life' issues. The puppet does not necessarily have to belong to any particular culture or language group or social class, as these can be researched and adapted.

Puppets can say more than the 'live' actor—They can get away with being highly controversial and thus often 'say more' about taboo issues like sex, dying, and racism. The puppet can form a 'buffer' between the performer and his audience, delivering a strong message in a light-hearted manner without offending or frightening the audience.

This programme relies on partnership. It is implemented in conjunction with both government and local community-based organizations.

Explanation

You can choose the one that suits your topic and situation the best. Even in the advanced technological ultra modern world this communication media is still highly estimated in villages as well as in the cities and class rooms was my experience. When I conducted the puppet show in the different areas even so called highly educated people too joined the show and enjoyed and got the message in simple yet forceful manner. Puppets create interest in public and make them grooved to the place until the show is over. Try it you yourself will experience the difference even in the class room if you cover the lesson plan on the particular topic by puppet show, all the happy smiling faces and work done in optimal satisfaction. So I advice you to do puppet show and give your topic full justice.

Keywords

Introduction, Puppet stage or theater, Making puppet, Communication strategies, Explanation.

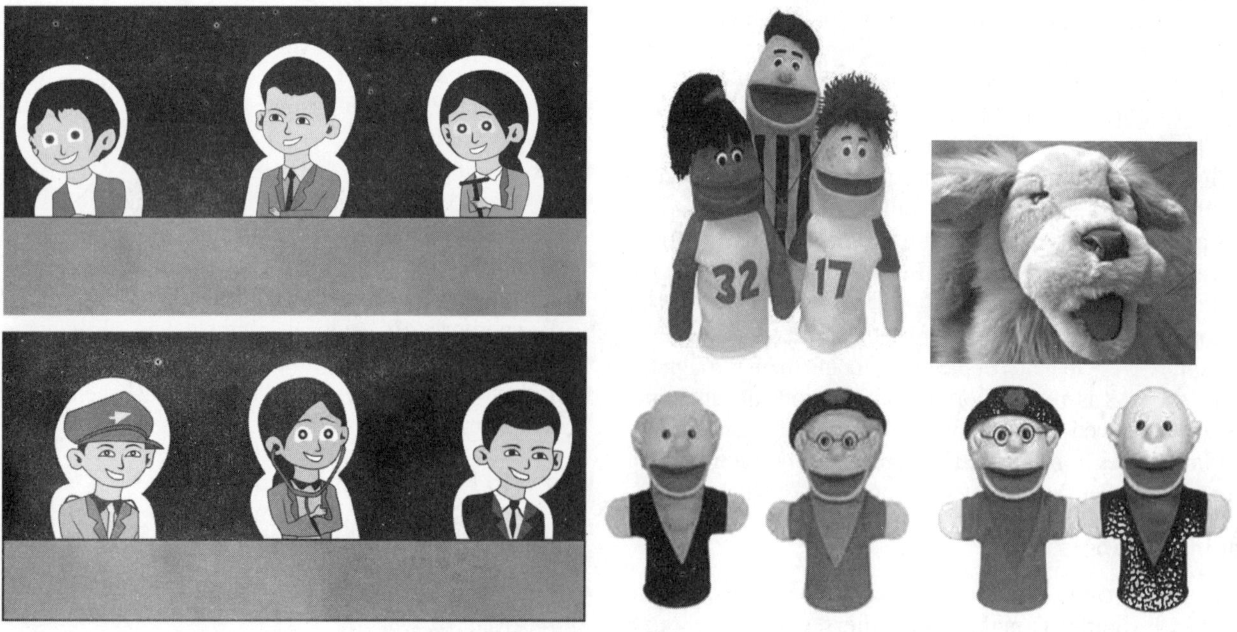

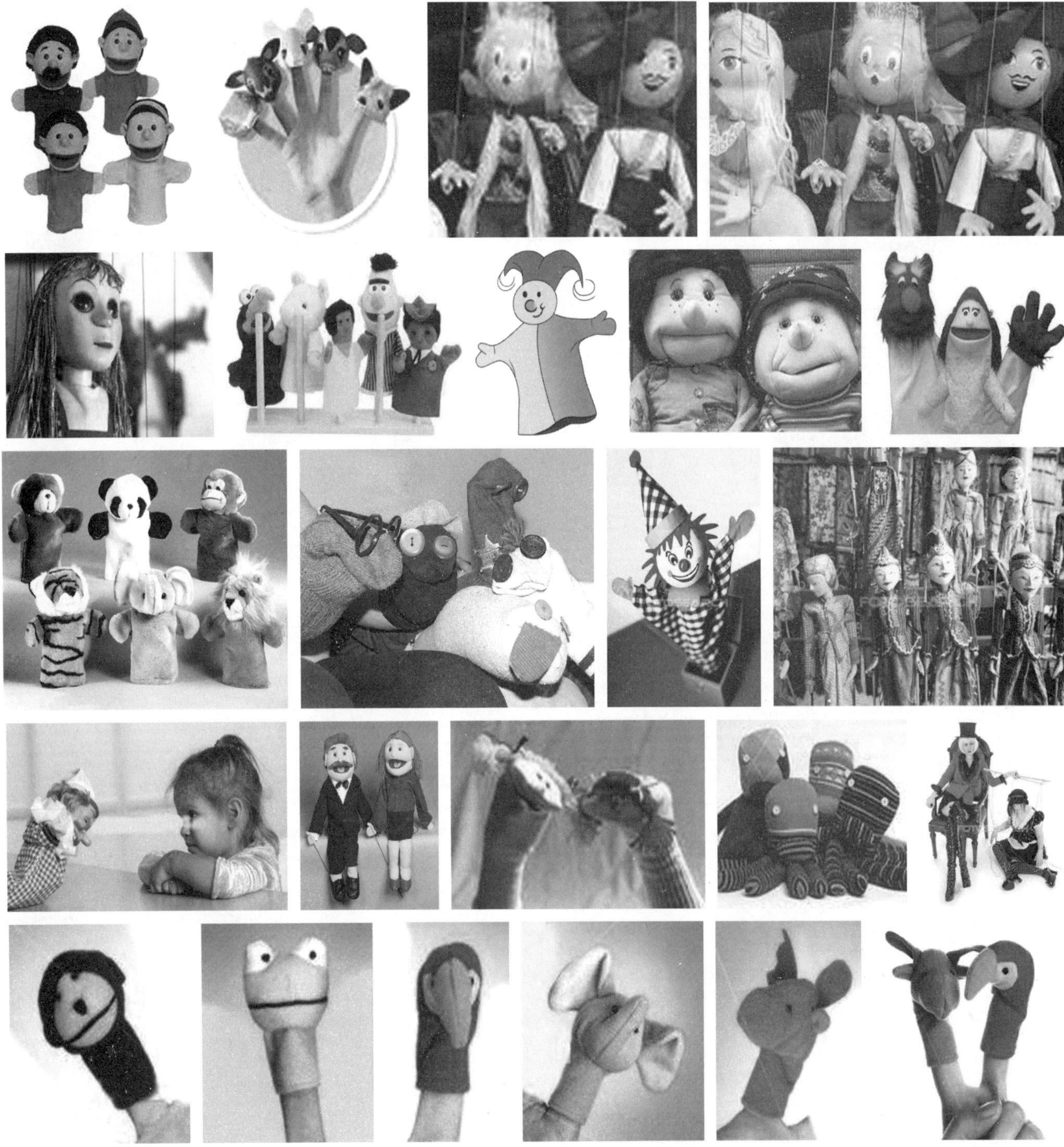

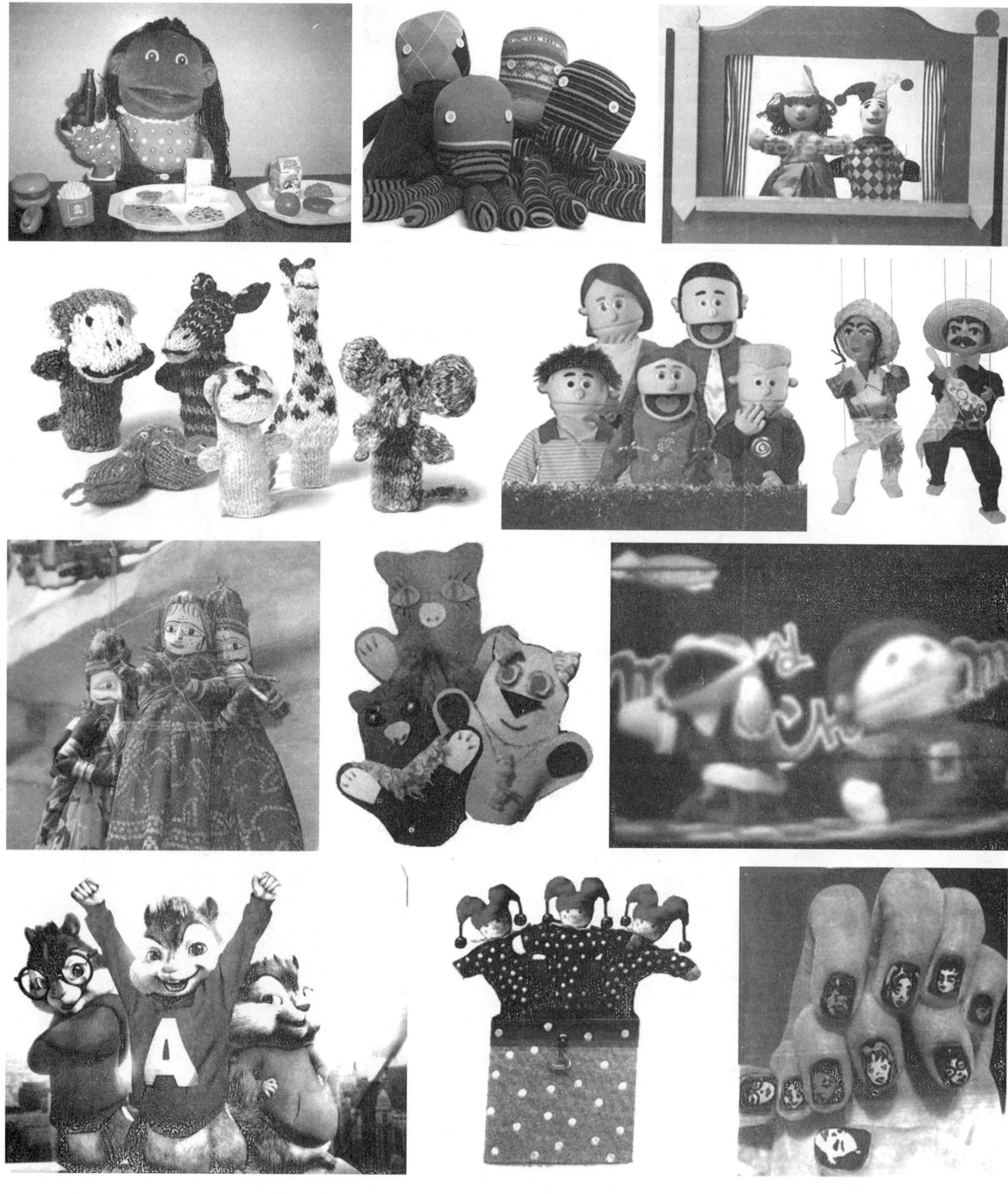

CHAPTER

38

Songs and Dances

Abstract

Song and dance are a musical comprising two acts, one entirely song and one entirely dance.

Students prepared lot of folk songs and awareness songs that would give message to the people in simple manner. They danced and sang songs to make the education interesting and people enjoyed the motivational awareness songs and dances. The songs had very melodious catchy tune that by the end of the education they started to sing themselves, e.g. we had prepared a song on hygiene how to wash hands after and before defecation, how to wash legs when come from out, how to wear clean clothes, drink clean water, not to spit anywhere, not to smock and drink, etc. In simple dances and songs, the message was reached and practiced.

Creative people show their creativity in everything and do not wait for a particular cause of action or event. The best way to start is to start working in the area that you are so passionate about and stop evaluating others' work. However, the success or failure of an individual largely depends on his performance. Conviction will inspire confidence in our abilities; let our creative personality surface... We do not know how much power we have deep within us until we try to discover it.

We need good nurses/leaders to take the nation forward towards 21st century. The success of every organization depends upon the leadership qualities. Good leadership is a motivating factor, higher the motivations better the performance. It builds morale of the group, which leads to stability.

So I hope what we do will help us to cope up in profound changes occurring in nursing and in health care. Time never waits—progress is impossible without change. The quality and competency should be motto.

Music has life-saving effect—the power of music restores maintains and improves emotional, physical, psychological well-being. It alleviates and helps cure various ailments. It has a supernatural and amazing power. It brings peace to heart; it gives physical as well mental solace. Magical effect on human body and mind. Hearing you forget the world around.

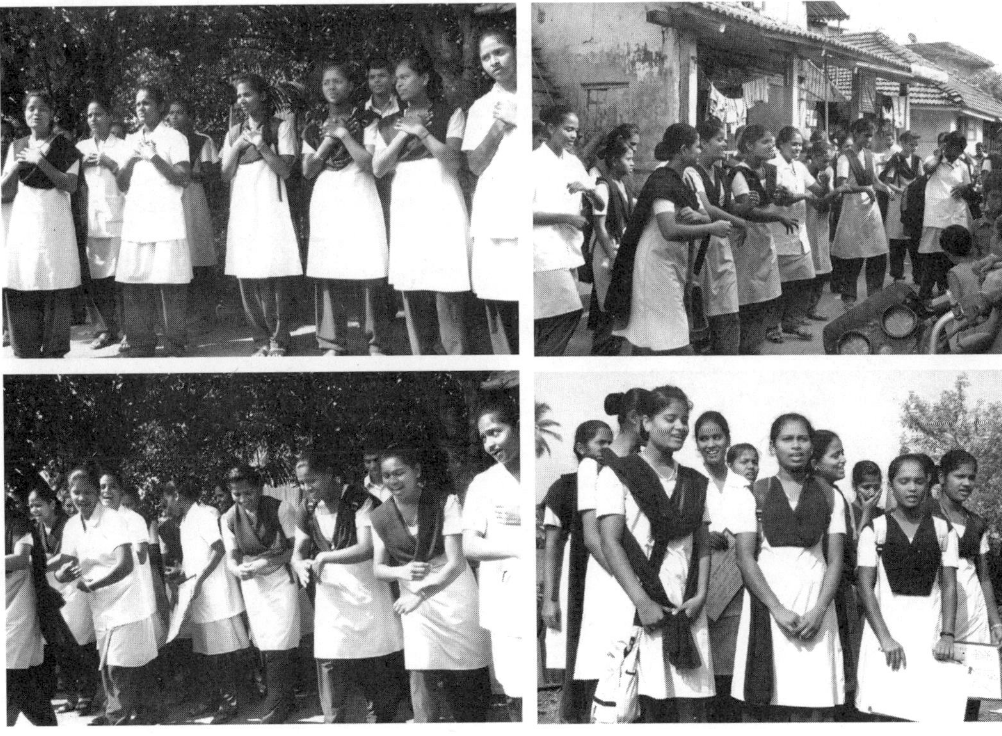

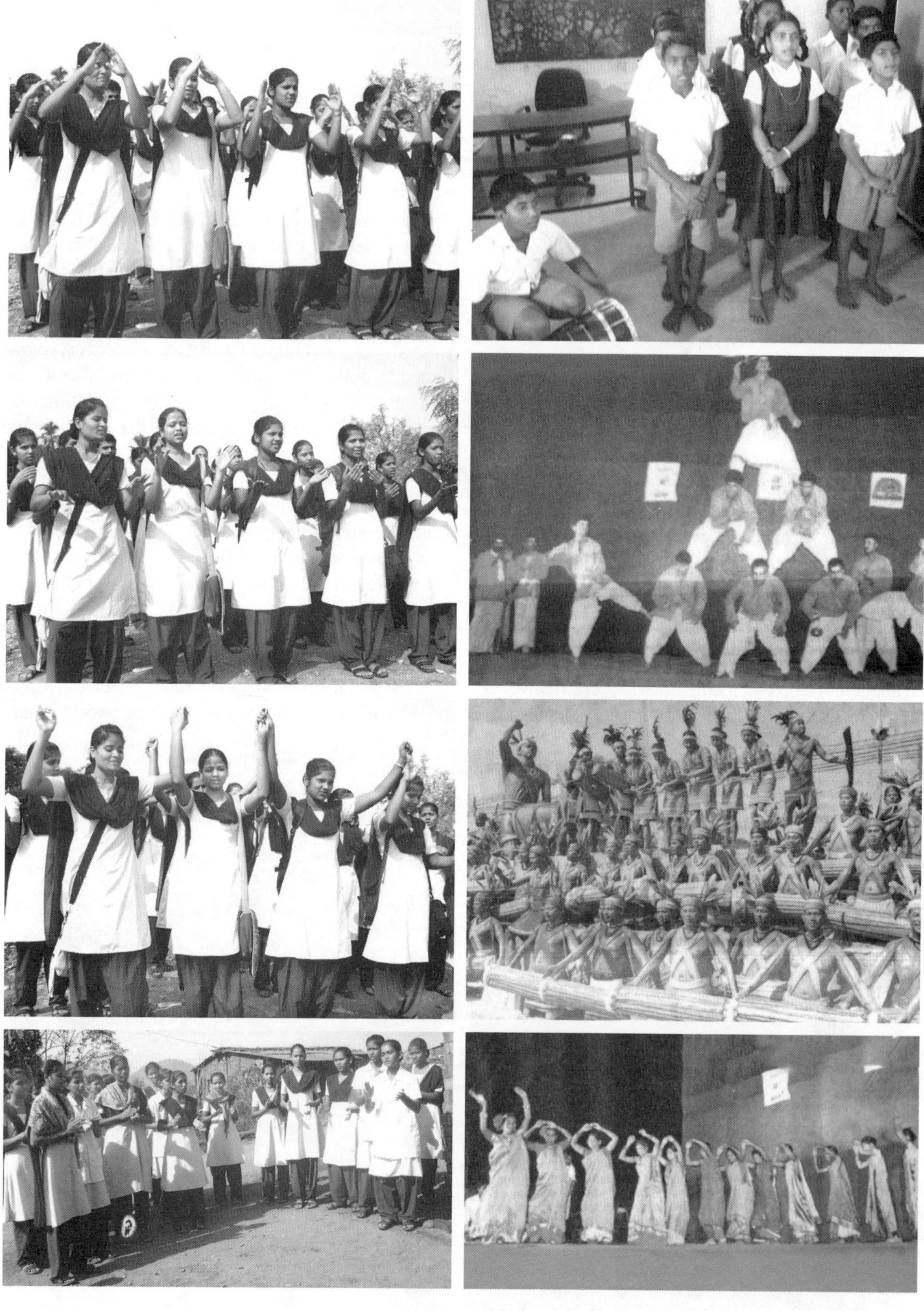

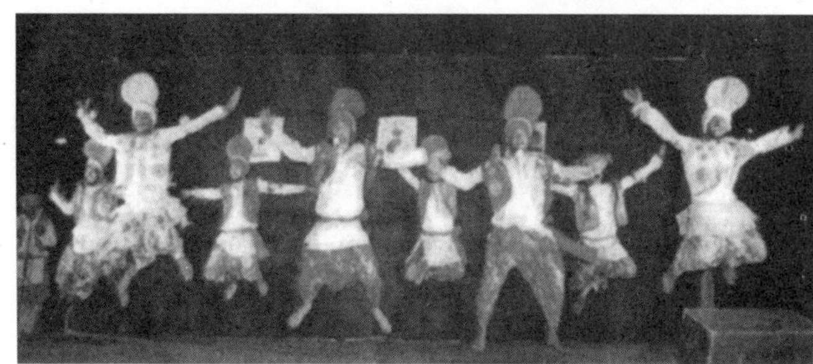

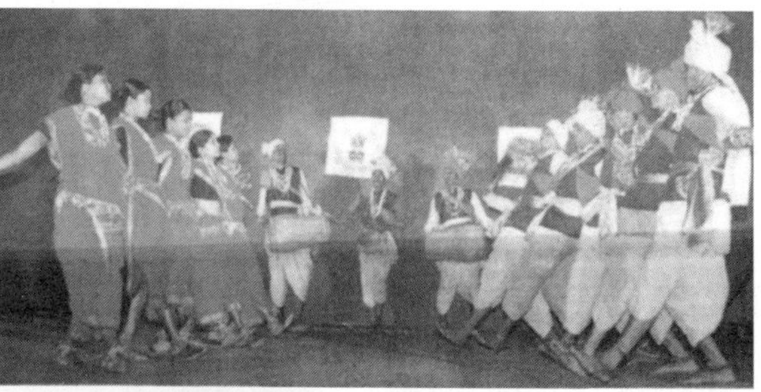

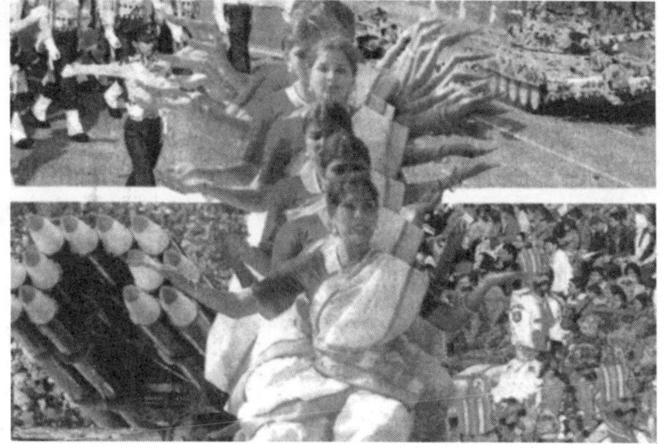

CHAPTER

39

Specimens

Abstract

An individual animal, plant, piece of minerals, etc. used as an example of its species or type for scientific study or display. A specimen is a sample of something like a specimen of blood or body tissue that is taken for medical testing.

Objects and specimens are collection of real thing. It develops social skills. Collection of object as specimen by students requires interaction. For example, you know urine, blood specimen.

For example, hytro-pathological specimens which are taken out from body like appendix, uterus, pre-mature still born infant, etc.

Specimens are of real objects taken from the natural setting. It is simple that shows quality or structure, e.g. section of a lung.

They arouse interest in learning.

They involve all five senses in the process of learning.

They make teaching lively.

Mounting and displaying specimen and object—small objects and specimen can be mounted by pasting them with adhesive wire nails, cello tape, etc. on cardboard. The collection of grain and sand seeds can be kept in small bottles or polithine bags. Discard cardboard can be divided into small rectangular or squire compartment to hold a specimen.

Specimen is an individual, object, or part regarded as typical of the group or class to which it belongs; a sample of tissue, blood, urine, etc., taken for diagnostic examination or evaluation (Life Sciences and Biology); the whole or a part of an organism, plant, etc., collected and preserved as an example of its class, species, etc. An individual, item, or part representative of a class, genus, or whole.

A sample, as of tissue, blood, or urine, used for analysis and diagnosis.

Explanation to understand what is specimen some figures are given for clarity and concept to be clear.

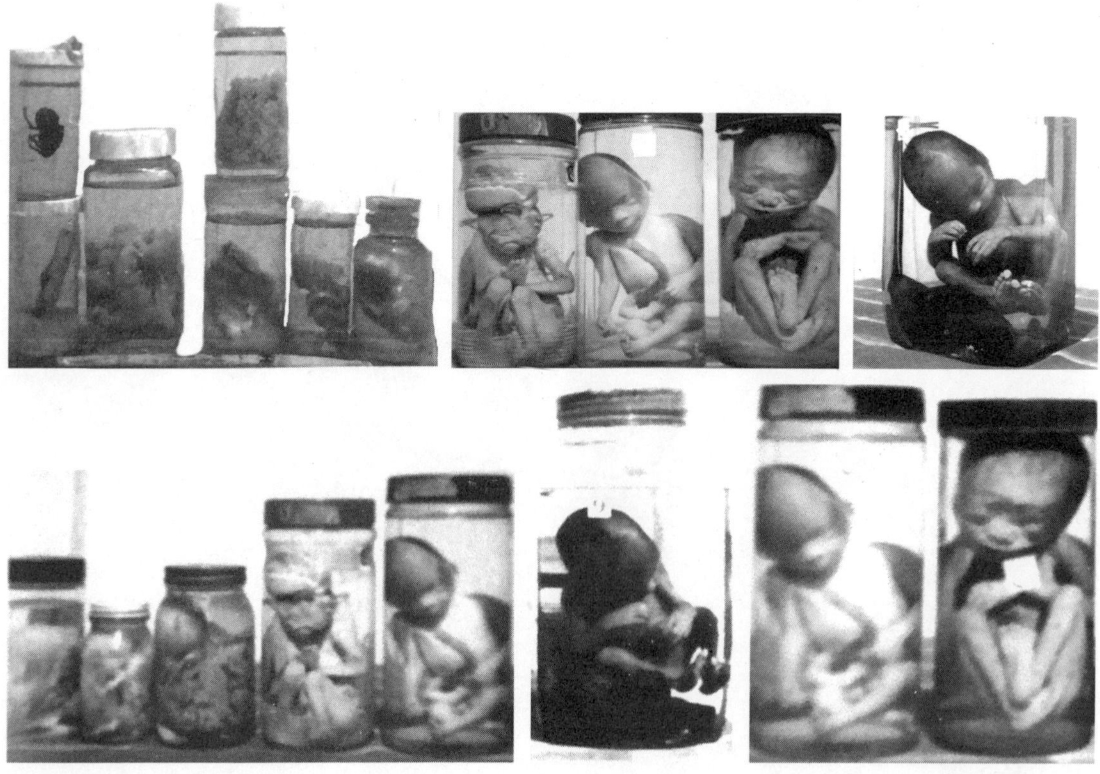

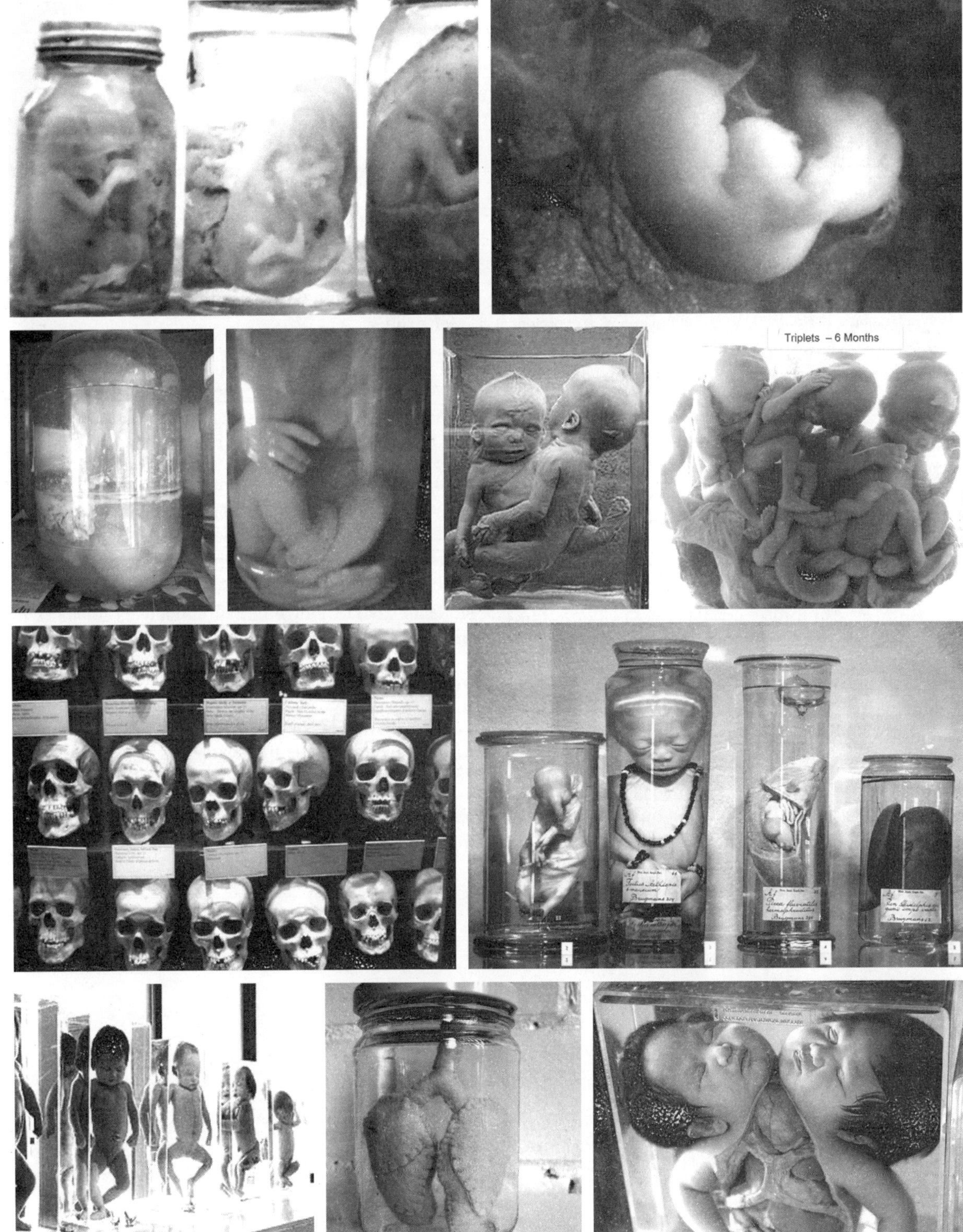
Triplets – 6 Months

CHAPTER

40

OHP Transparency

Abstract

Overhead projectors used to be fixtures in classroom, conference rooms and boardrooms. They consisted of three major parts—light, a place to rest a transparent or other translucent media to be projected, and a lenses' assembly to focus the image and project it at a screen. OHP panels allow you to use an overhead projector to share your computer display. An OHP is a variant of slid projector that is used to display images to audience.

INTRODUCTION TO OHP

It is popular instruction medium? Simple, light and easy to use permits face to face interaction can be used in day light condition, can present information in a systematic developed sequence. Projected transparencies on screen images in lighted room; overhead projector (OHP) use can write/draw diagrams on transparencies.

Dry-Lam Transparency Film for Plain Paper Copiers—Produces a crisp black image on a clear background. Presentation visuals are easily made with your plain paper copier. Just insert the transparency film into your copier instead of paper. The copier will place a sharp black image on the clear transparency film for your overhead projector presentation. With removable stripe.

Dry-Lam Ink Jet Transparency Film—The ideal material for creating colorful presentations. A special coating on the print side ensures quick drying time and less "bleeding". Works with virtually any color or monochrome inkjet printer.

Dry-Lam Transparency Film for Laser Printers—Make presentations for your overhead using your laser printer. Our transparency film produces sharp black images on a clear background. Works with virtually any monochrome laser printer.

Dry-Lam Write-on Film (also referred to as Acetate Film)—Reusable writes on sheets for overhead presentations. It can be wiped clean to use again. Comes in medium weight and heavy weight sheets and rolls in two sizes.

In projected aids, a bright light is shown though a transparent picture, an enlarged picture is projected on a screen by means of lenses; in opaque projection it is not transparent. It can capture attention towards bright picture in a dark room. There are OHP mark pens which are easily erasable with damp cloth, students have to follow certain guidelines for marking OHP transparencies.

Types of Transparencies

1. Teacher-made transparencies
2. Commercial-made transparencies
3. Xeroxed transparencies

Explanation—some of the examples of transparency are given in figures for students just to understand.

Keywords

Dry-Lam Transparency, Ink Jet Transparency Film, Film for Laser Printers, Acetate Film, Types, Explanation.

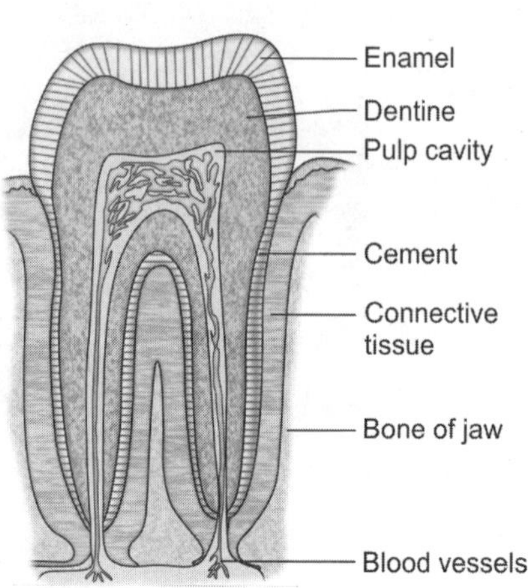

Human immunodeficiency virus

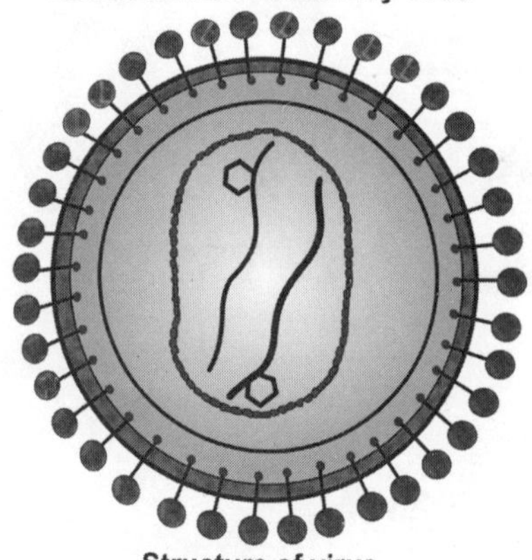

Structure of virus

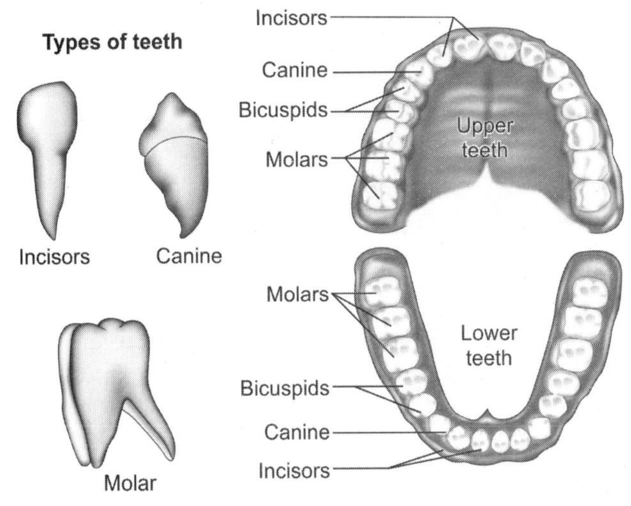

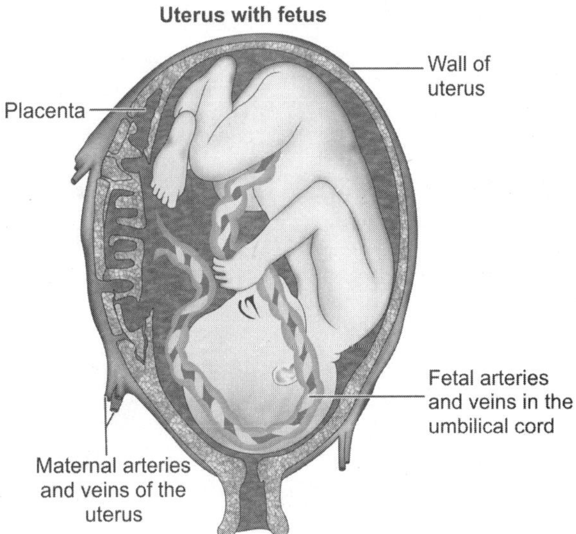

Sector of the human uterus with a fetus connected by the umbilical cord to the placenta

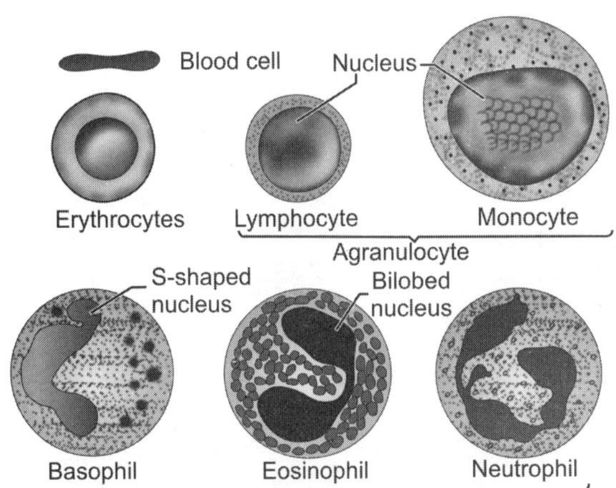

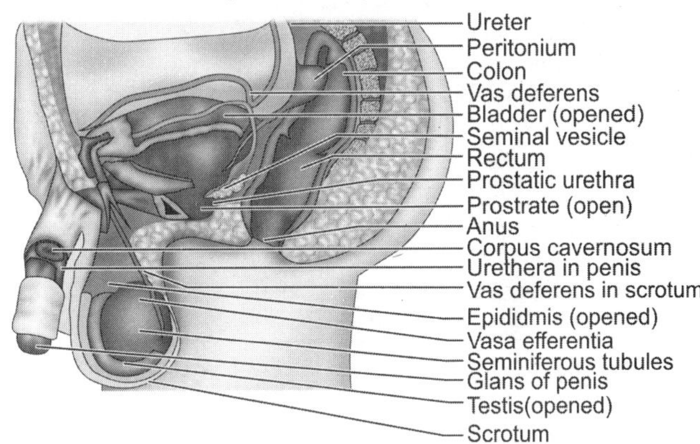

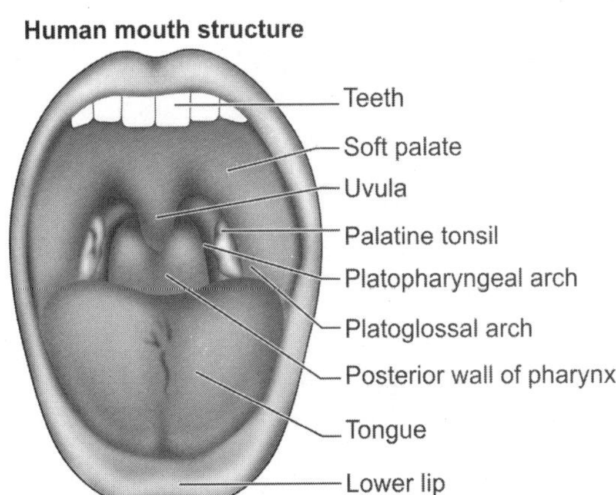

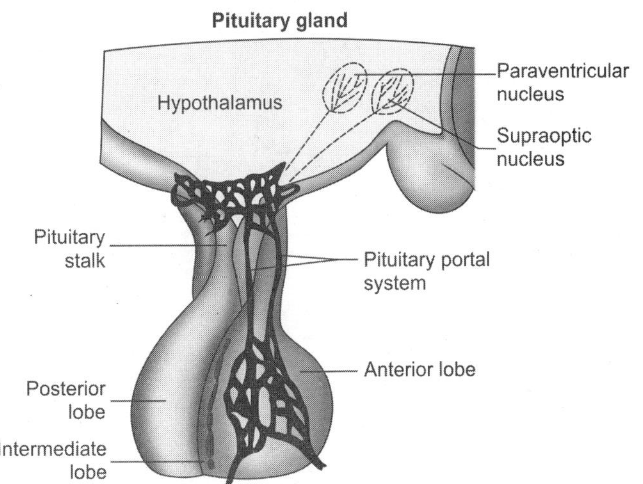

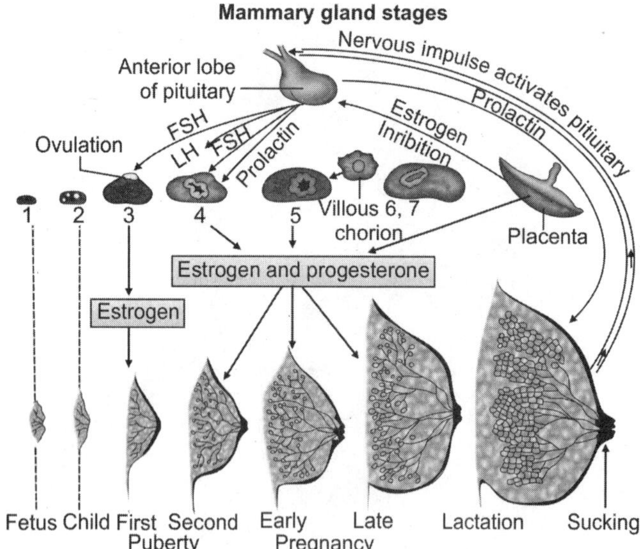

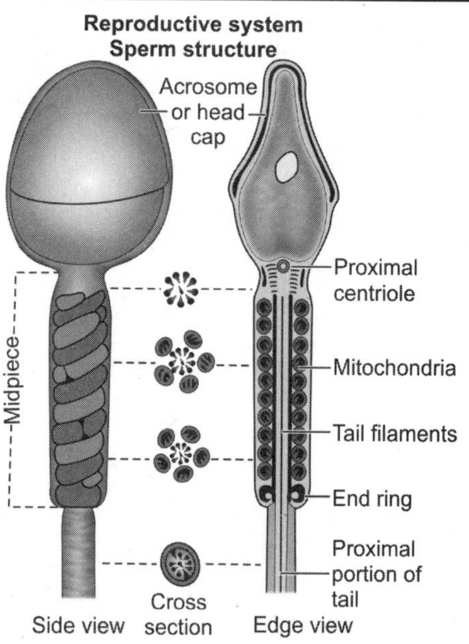

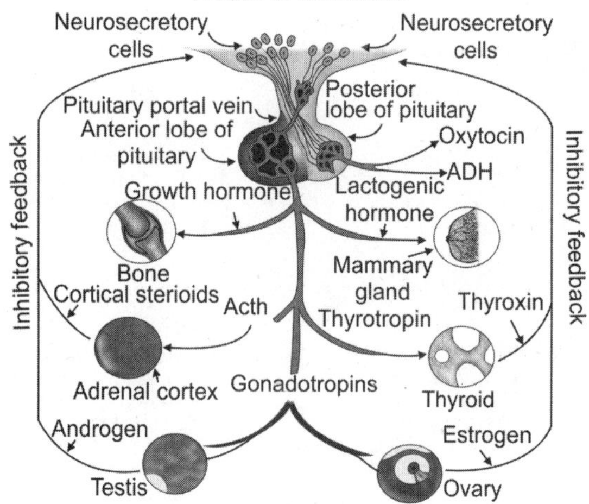

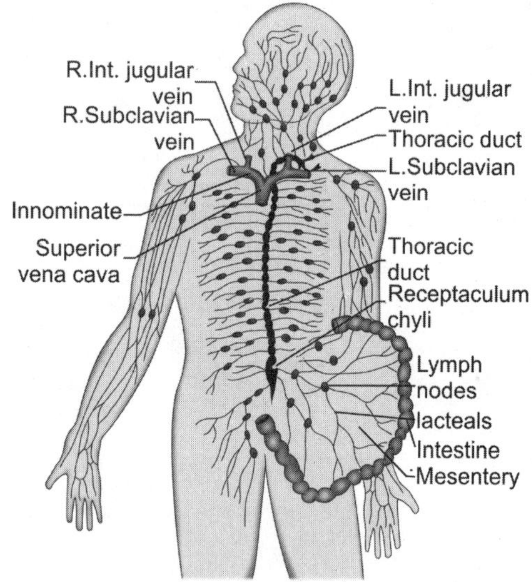

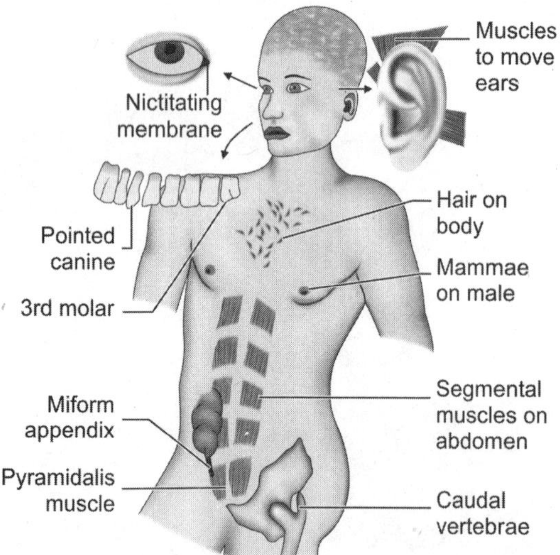

Some vestigial structures in the human body

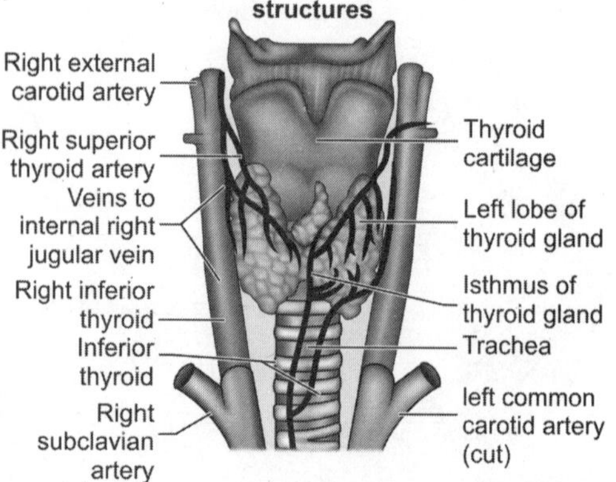

Position of thyroid gland and its associated structures

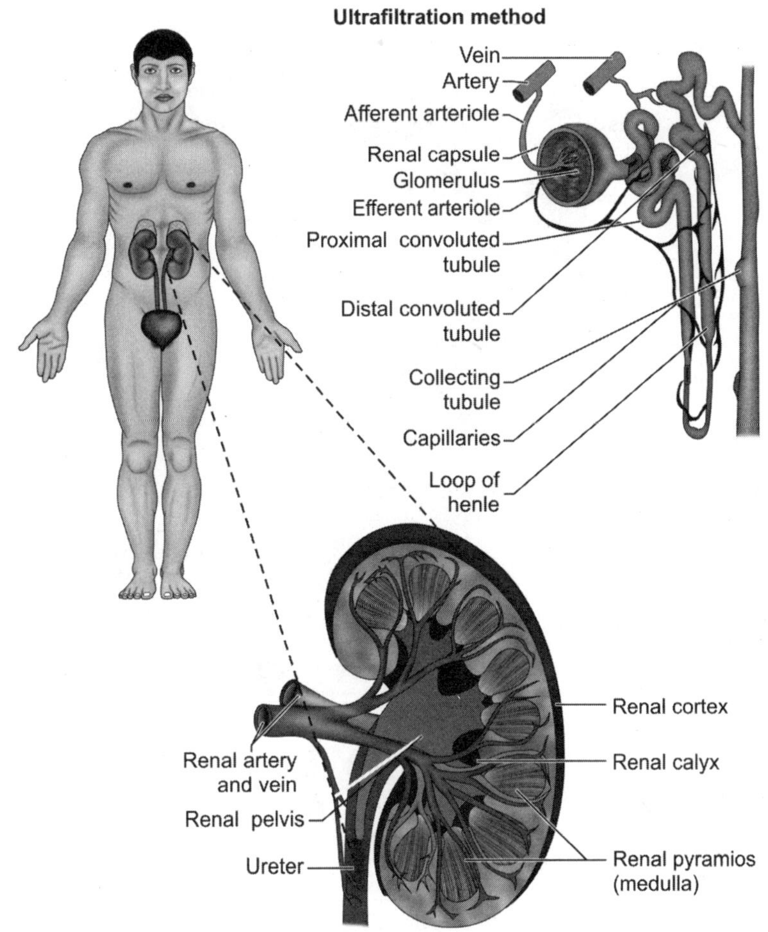
Ultrafiltration method
Vein
Artery
Afferent arteriole
Renal capsule
Glomerulus
Efferent arteriole
Proximal convoluted tubule
Distal convoluted tubule
Collecting tubule
Capillaries
Loop of henle
Renal cortex
Renal calyx
Renal artery and vein
Renal pelvis
Ureter
Renal pyramios (medulla)

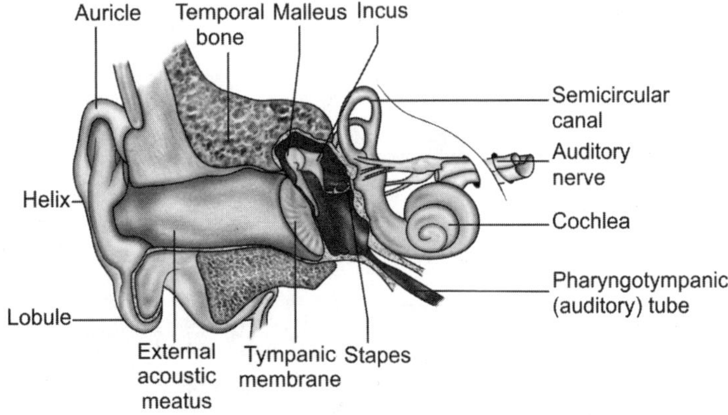
Structure of human ear
Auricle
Temporal bone
Malleus
Incus
Semicircular canal
Auditory nerve
Helix
Cochlea
Pharyngotympanic (auditory) tube
Lobule
External acoustic meatus
Tympanic membrane
Stapes

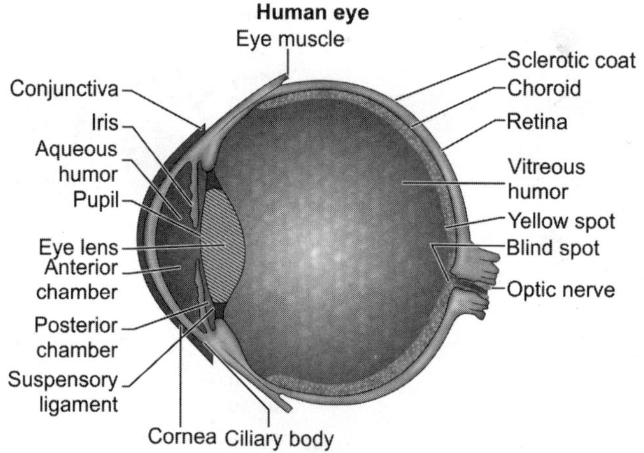
Human eye
Eye muscle
Conjunctiva
Iris
Aqueous humor
Pupil
Eye lens
Anterior chamber
Posterior chamber
Suspensory ligament
Cornea
Ciliary body
Sclerotic coat
Choroid
Retina
Vitreous humor
Yellow spot
Blind spot
Optic nerve

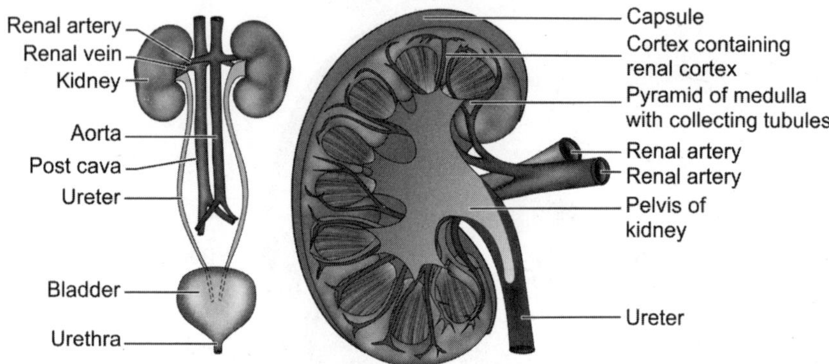
Human urinary system
Renal artery
Renal vein
Kidney
Aorta
Post cava
Ureter
Bladder
Urethra
Capsule
Cortex containing renal cortex
Pyramid of medulla with collecting tubules
Renal artery
Renal artery
Pelvis of kidney
Ureter

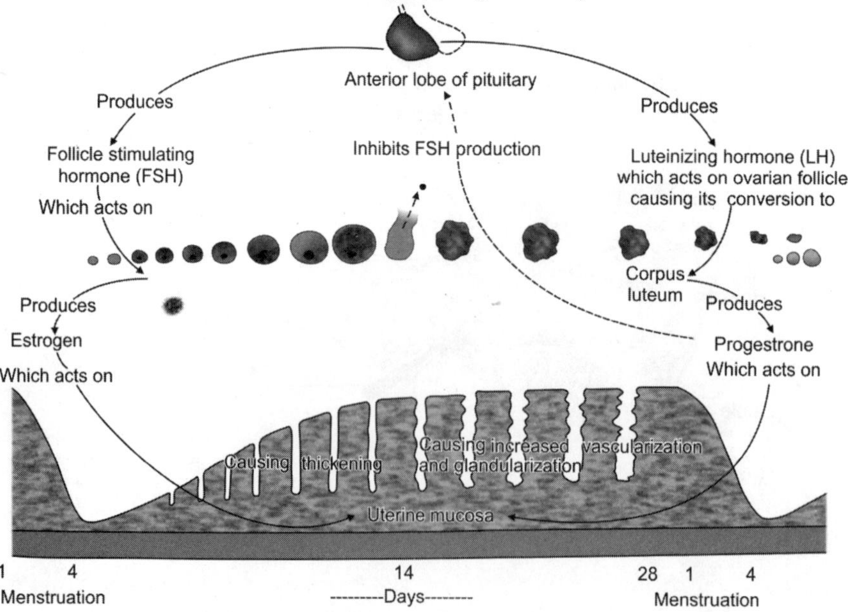
Menstrual cycle (Diagrammatic)
Anterior lobe of pituitary
Produces
Follicle stimulating hormone (FSH)
Which acts on
Inhibits FSH production
Produces
Luteinizing hormone (LH) which acts on ovarian follicle causing its conversion to
Corpus luteum
Produces
Progestrone
Which acts on
Produces
Estrogen
Which acts on
Causing thickening
Causing increased vascularization and glandularization
Uterine mucosa
1
4
Menstruation
14
---------Days--------
28
1
4
Menstruation

Developing ovum

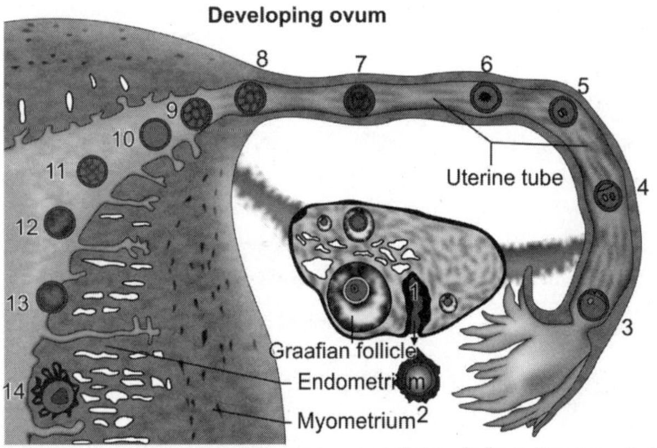

Stages of the developing human ovum as it travels from the ovary to the uterus developing ovam

1. Follicle bursts, 2. Ovum with adhering granulosa cell, 3. Sperm enters egg, 4. Male and female pronuclei present, 5. Pronuclei fuse, 6. First cleavage division 7,8,9. Early cleavage, 10. Morula, 11. Early gastrula, 12. Later gastrula, 13. Start of implantation, 14. Growing embryo fully implanted

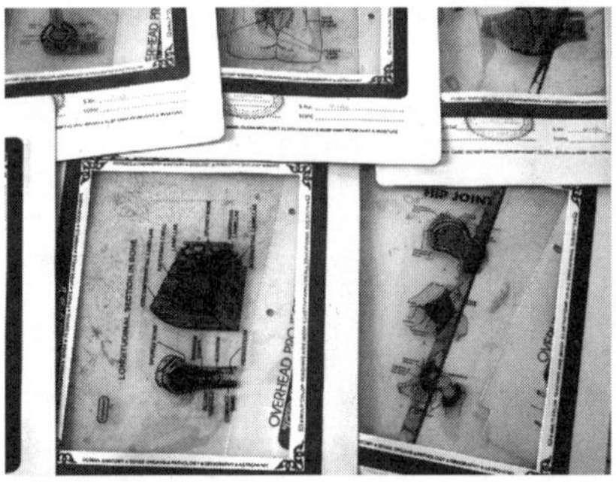

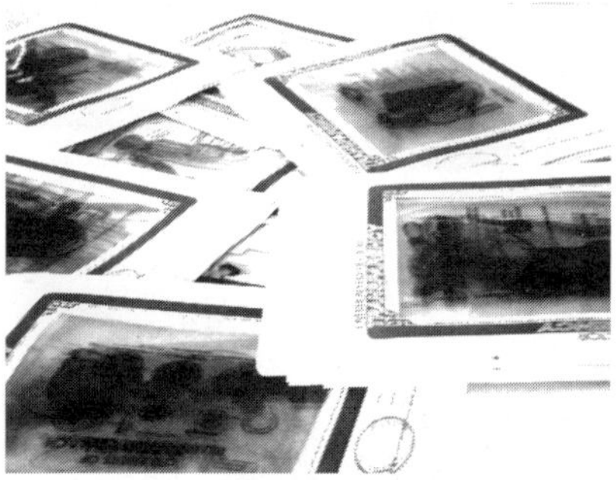

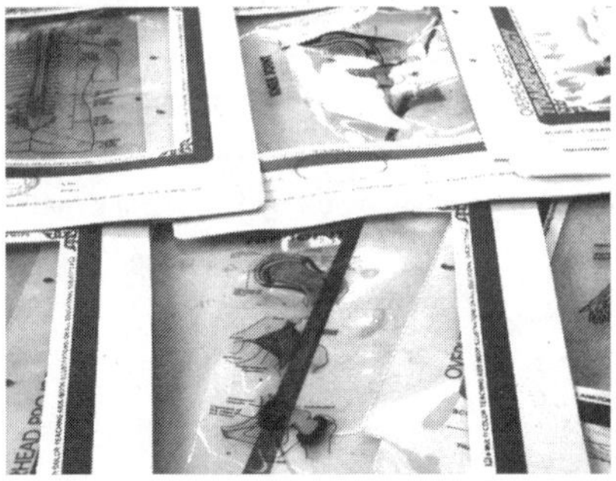

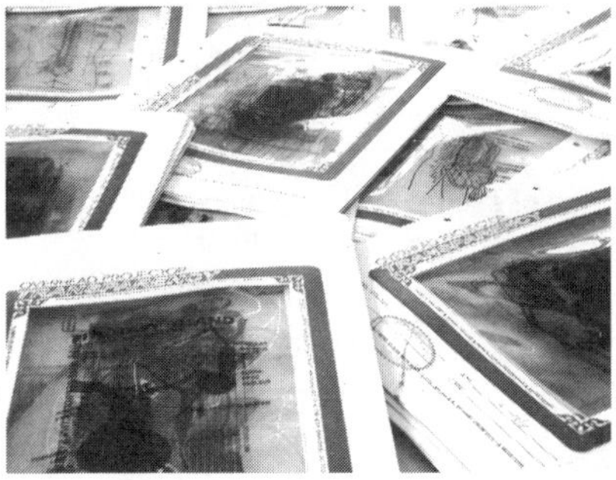

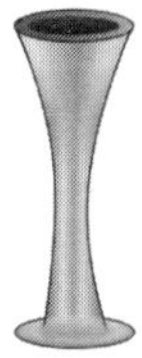

Fetoscope

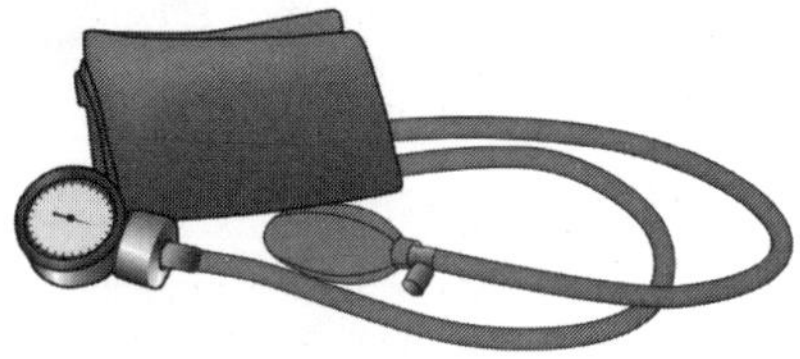

Aniroid blood pressure apparatus

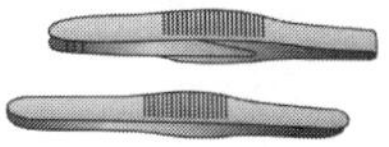

Thumb forceps

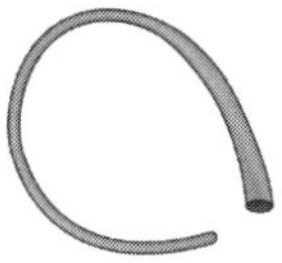

IR catheter

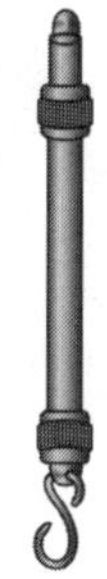

Spring balance

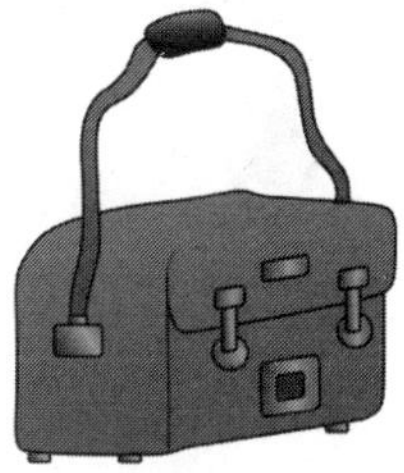

Bag

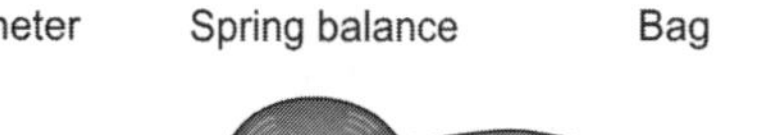

Mucous sucker

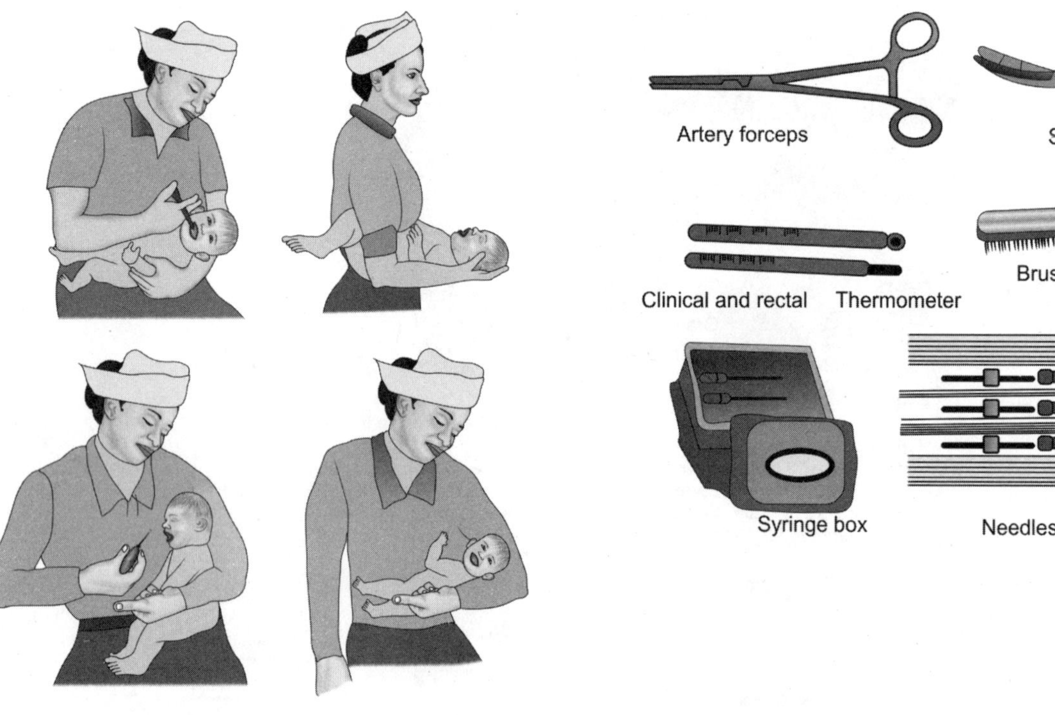

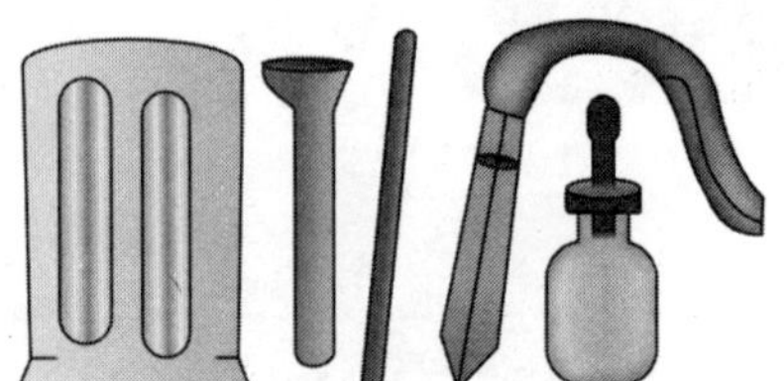

Materials of hemoglobin estimation by Sahli method

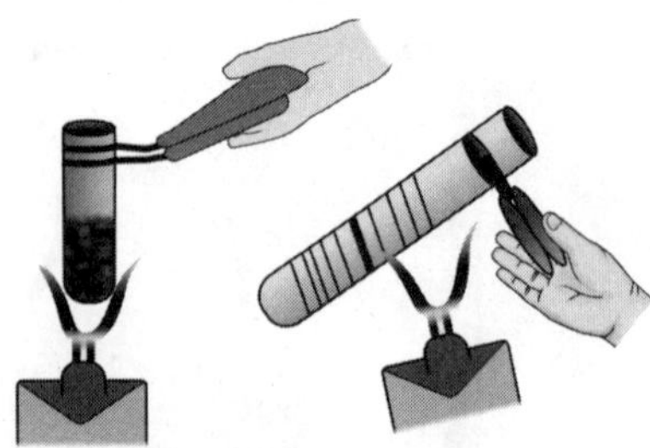

Urine for sugar Albumin test

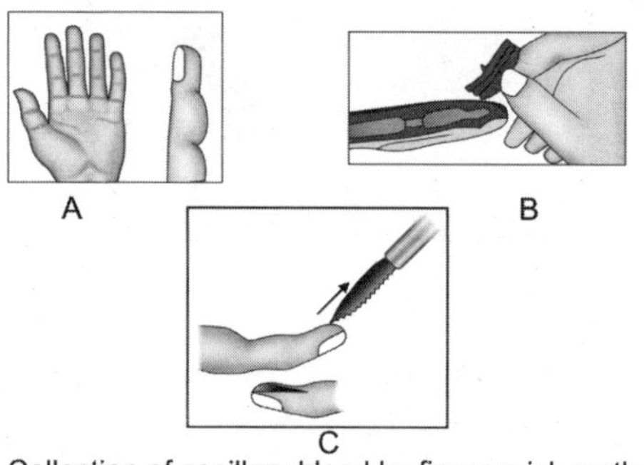

Collection of capillary blood by finger prick method

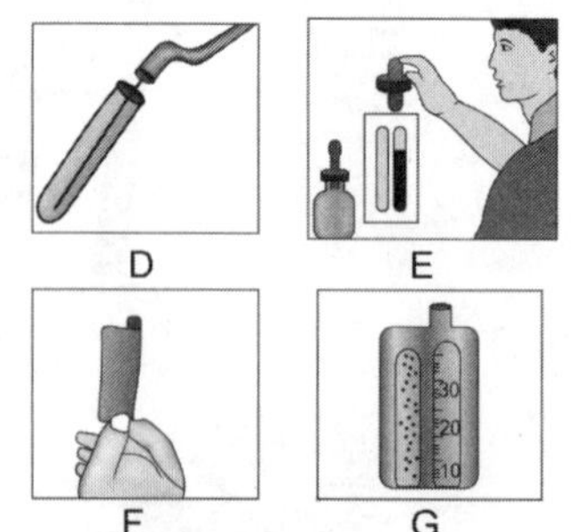

Method of estimating HB in blood collected by finger prick method

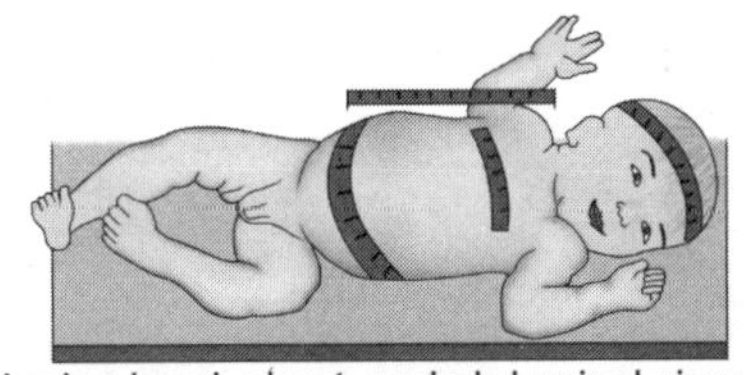

Meaburing head, chest, and abdominal circumference

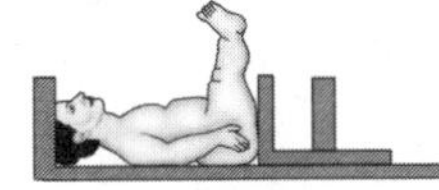

Position infant measuring body length

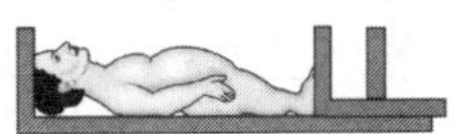

Position body length

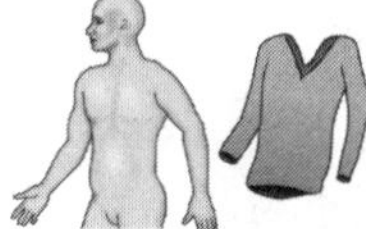
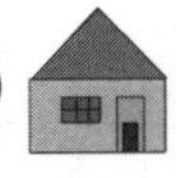
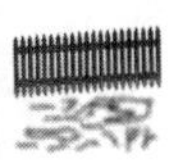

Four things which we must keep clean

Procedure of anthropometry

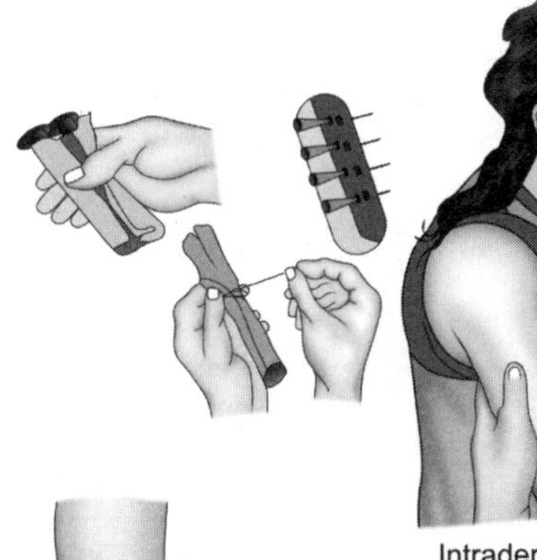

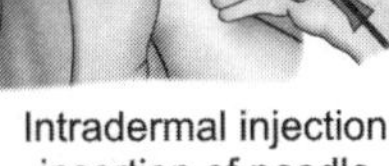

Intradermal injection insertion of needle

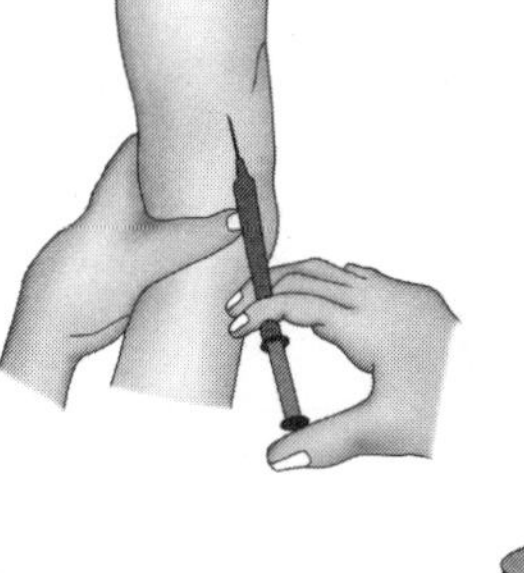

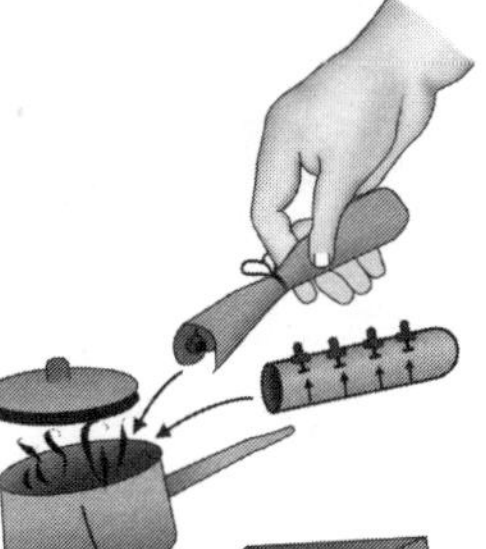

Procedure of injecting subcutaneous injection and its sterilization technique

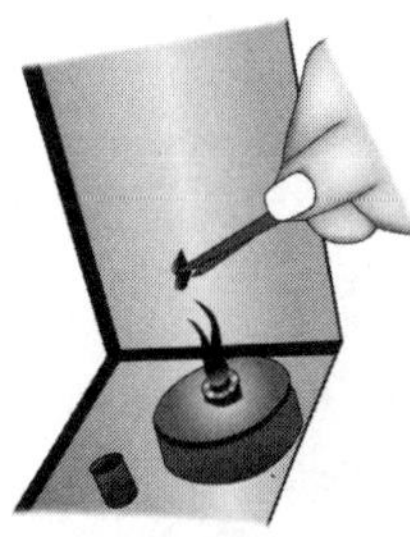

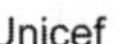

Unicef

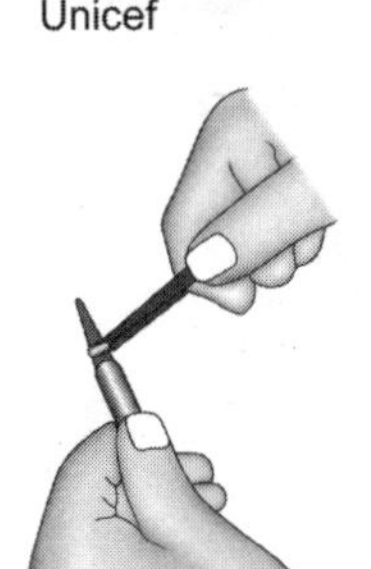

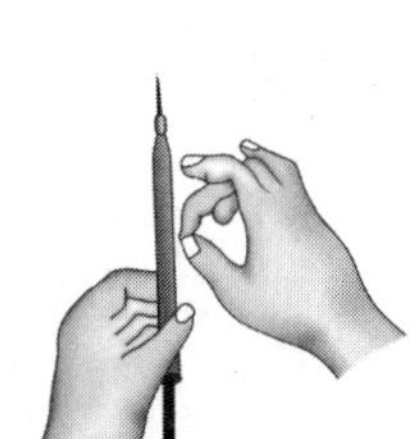

Injection techniques: steps involved

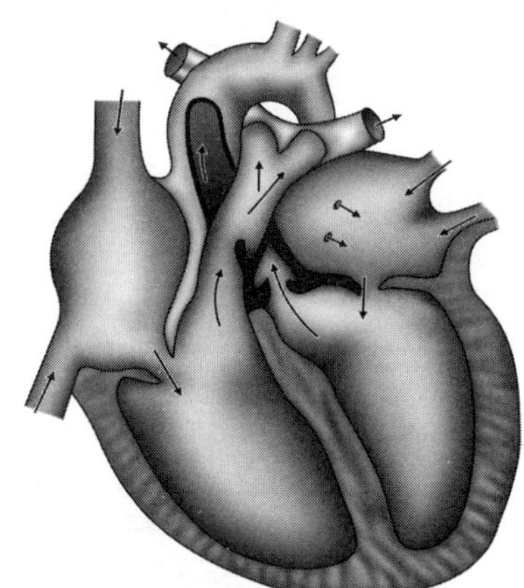

Structure of anatomy of organs

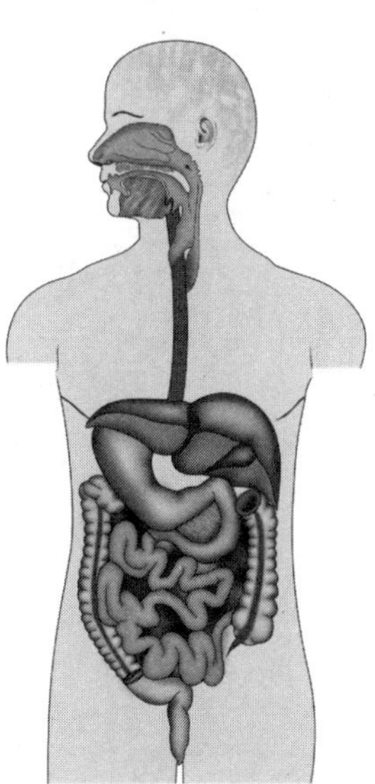

Anatomical structures of different organs

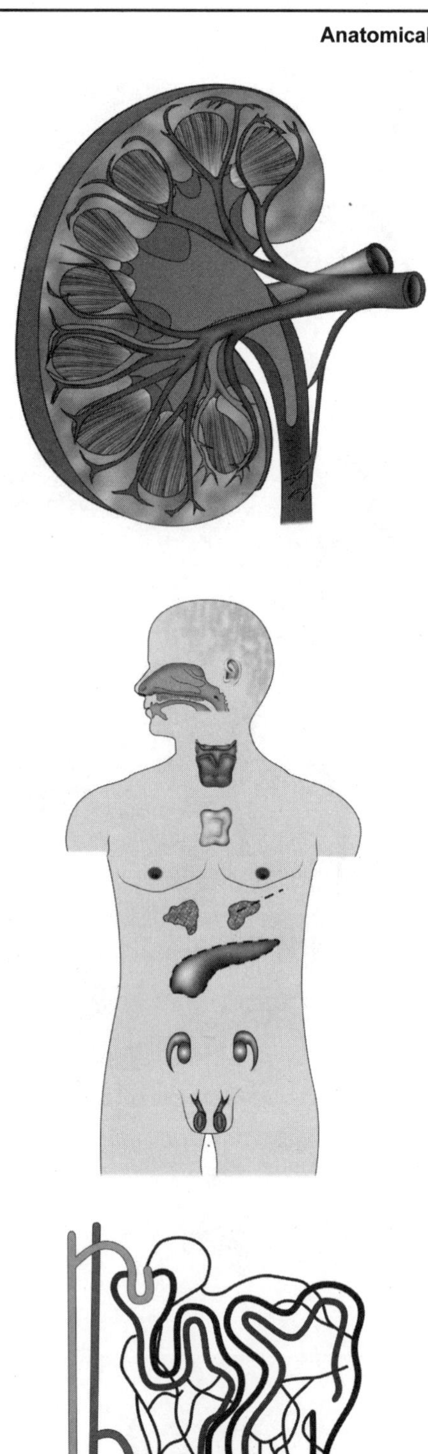

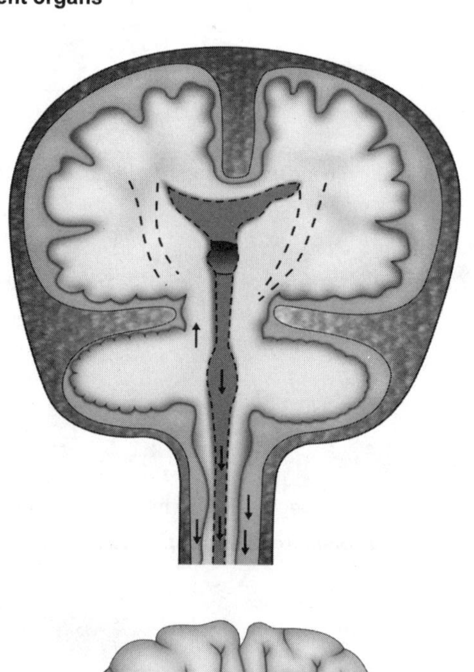

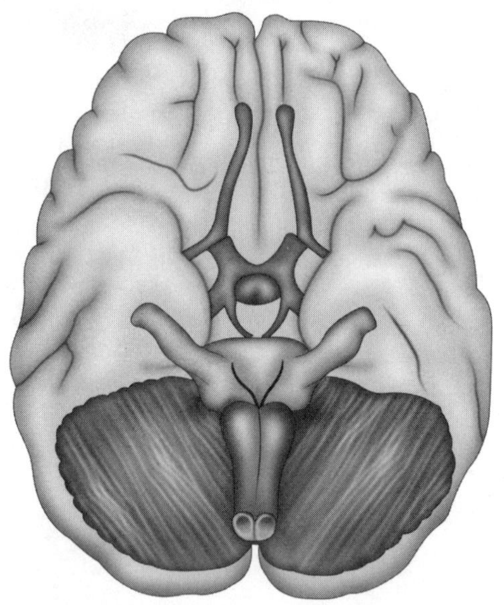

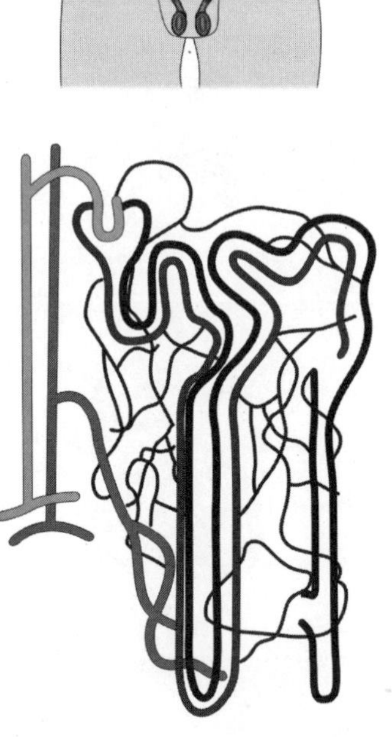

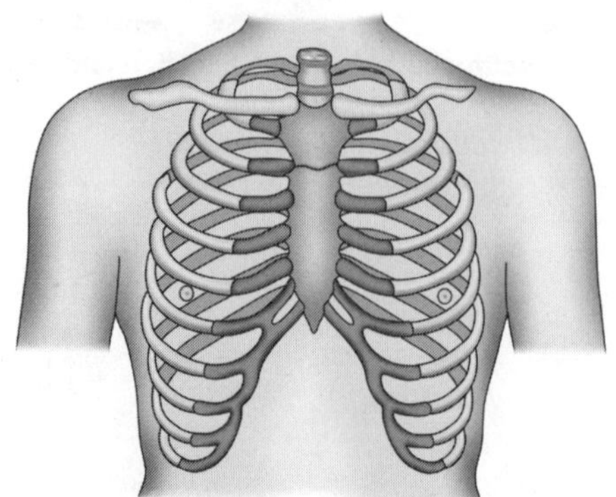

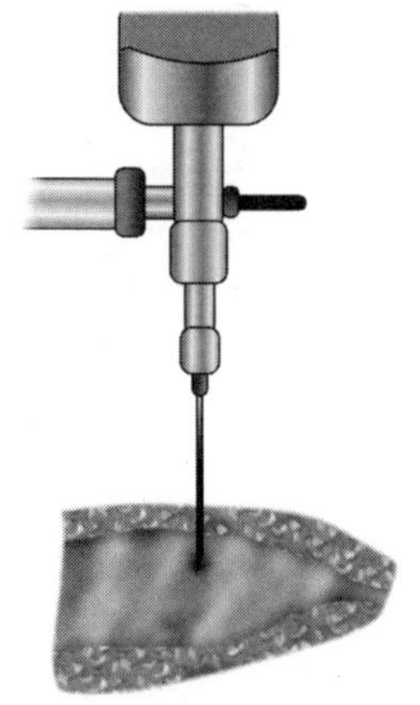

Growth

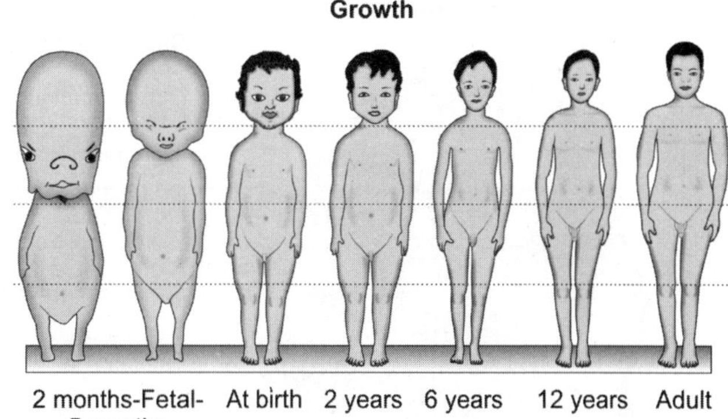

Birth of a baby

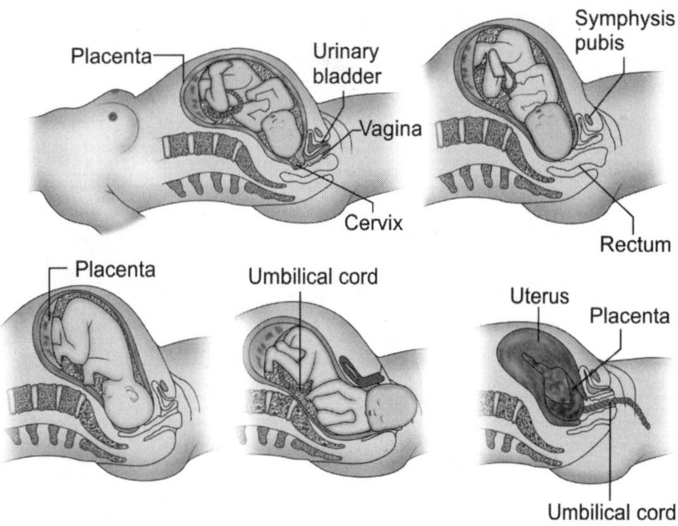

Human respiratory system

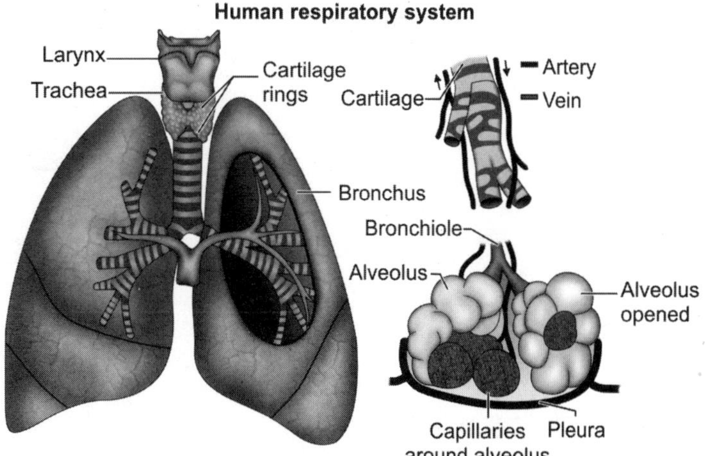

Human heart

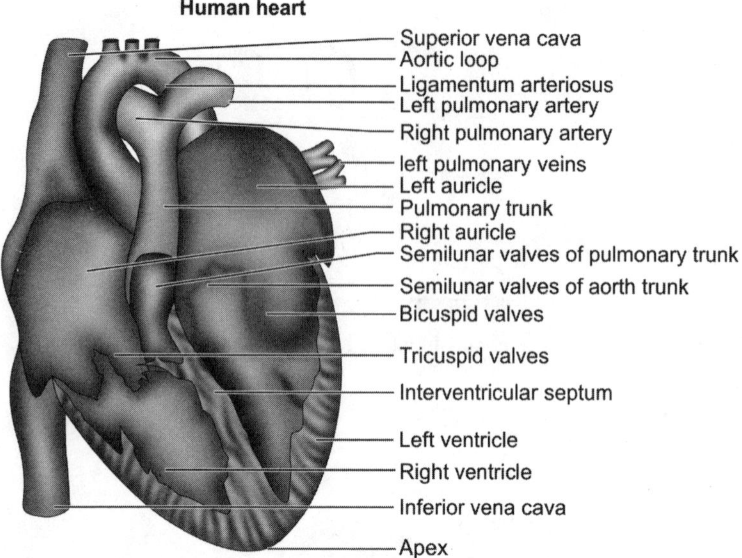

Human endocrine glands

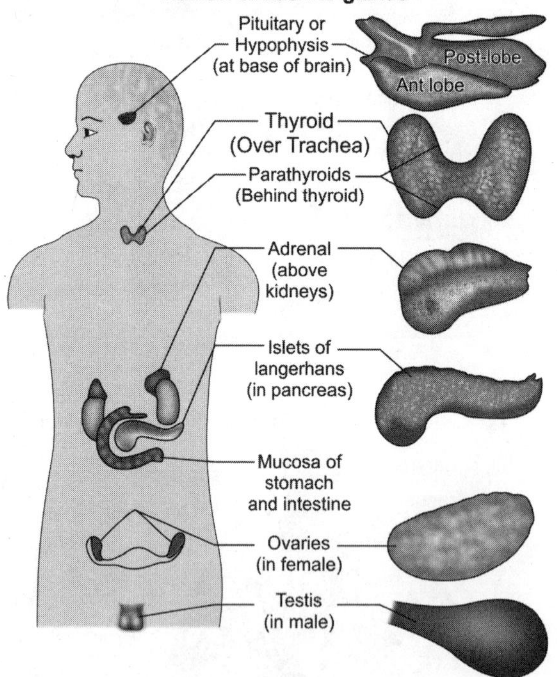

Liver and pancreas

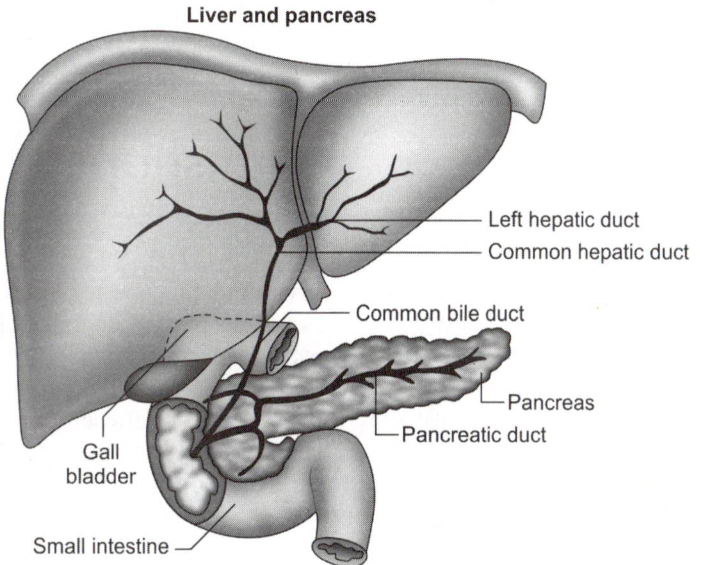

CHAPTER 41

Workshops and Field Trips

Abstract

Workshop is a meeting at which a group of people are engaged in intensive discussion and activity on a particular subject or project. A brief intensive educational program for a relatively small group of students that focuses especially on techniques and skill in a particular field.

Field trip: Field trip is a trip by students to gain first-hand knowledge away from the classroom, as to a museum, factory, geological area, or environment of certain plants and animals.

FIELD TRIP IN URBAN AND RURAL AREAS

In field trip students have group activities for report writing such as they have to know the physical layout of the village, administrative pattern, population, culture, custom and food habits of the people, facilities available, e.g. market, temple, well, roads, transportation, school etc. health problems identified, areas of improvement could be made among the villagers, merits and demerits on their stay in village, point to be improved about total program. They have to submit and give the health talks, fill family folders, health assessment, home procedures, clinical evaluation, etc.

At the end of this trips experience the student will be helped to develop realistic view of existing rural/urban health care service to the community and will help to identify the major health problems in the field.

In urban field posting they have to identify the community health needs and problems through house visits in their respective families. They have to also develop an ability to set a priority according to the health needs of the community. Develop a skill in planning or organizing nursing activities in a given community. Acquire ability to communicate with the group through health education in prevention of health problems. Develop an ability to assess the health problem of various age groups by conducting health program in market places, in community gathering halls, near the place where usually people gather, according to their time and connivance. To make it interesting use multi dimensional creative audio-visual aids to capture there attention and keep them listening.

In rural field area they can gain the knowledge about the function of public health centers and know the administrative set up. Acquire knowledge about various rural developmental schemes that require for the uplifting villages. They have to take active part in programs like ICDS, Anganwadi, mahila mandal, gram panchayat. They can do home visits, survey the community for specific purpose, do assessment, treat minor illness, give health education, visit schools, do exhibitions, have awareness and motivational program through role play and skits, fork dance, awareness songs and live with the people to understand the lifestyles of people and why they act in certain way or why they do not act on certain ways they will come to know, teach good habits, teach personal and environmental hygiene.

Usually any Indian villages you visit you will see this scenario—people have pucca and kacha houses. All cast and religion stay together. Some have toilets in the house and others go open defecation. Animal like goats, buffalos, and poultry is either side of the house or close to the house; some have still inside the house part and parcel of home. They grow rice crop and some seasonal vegetables. Some are educated still majority are ignorant. There are small shops in and around village. Poverty is visible, still poor personal and environmental hygiene.

Once they find out the observation they have to prepare an action plan for the identification of problem.

Power to the people. The decision makers fail to realize that more than subsidies, it is round the clock and quality power supply that holds the potential to completely transform life in rural India. There is urgent need to evolve national consensus in this direction within the political class and among policymakers.

Field trips bring the students into direct contact with a real life situation which is more concrete and most real of visual technique. Objects, materials, cultures can thus be studied first hand in their natural environment. They blend and correlate theory into practical providing direct touch with community situation, help to develop observation and keenness and help to verify what is learnt.

Field trip gives direct experience with reality and provides an excellent opportunity to give first hand information in learning experience in natural setting. It is a kind of audio-visual media of learning for students. As teachers cannot do an effective teaching in a classroom alone, the exposure to the world around is also vital in learning. it is a concrete real down to earth experience of educational procedure. Here students are enriched with their observation, social skills, lifestyles of people and culture where new ideas and knowledge is acquired. They can correlate personal level with direct touch with the community's sanitation, economic condition etc. where they can develop their leadership and decision making qualities.

There are many types of field trips such as local school trip, community trip, inter school visits, individual trips etc field trips needs to be well planned and organized with educational purpose so that with proper knowledge, objectives in mind, preparation of students, taking time of transportation concept and under the guidance and supervision of the teacher, keeping in mind responsibilities of teachers and students responsibility. As it is costly, and needs maintaining the planed schedule, it is time consuming, it has advantages and limitation too. It can be a enriching and fruitful experience that students can treasure.

Field practice and experience is provided through arrangements with a variety of health agencies, community facilities and hospitals to the students during their training period where they get exposed to different set ups and learn appropriate experience. They are provided residential facilities and accommodation, they are provided supervised practical training; where guidance is provided as how to go about, what exactly they are suppose to do during this field experience. By this they are able to improve basic skills in the practical field, it is useful learning experience for developing confidence, improving competencies where they have experience of an intensive nature. They are provided transport facility where the school is affiliated where arrangements are made. Here a careful and continuous assessment of a student's knowledge, abilities and attitudes are formed and supervised. This helps to provide a balance education where a student becomes self directed responsible professional nurse. Develops understanding of the application of principles, ability to work collaboratively and appreciates various factors affecting the society.

A workshop is a series of educational and work sessions. Small groups of people meet together over a short period of time to concentrate on a defined area of concern. Purposes for workshops may vary typically, a workshop has two components.

WORKSHOP

Workshop consists of a series of meetings. A workshop is a meeting during which experienced people and resources people come together with expert and consultants to find solution to problem which they have faced during the course of their task and they have difficulty in dealing with it on their own. It is a meeting to deal with educational problem faced by them.

The total workshop is divided into small groups, and each group will choose a chairman and a recorder. Each group solves a part of the problem with the help of consultants and resource personnel. The emphasis is on individual work within the group. Learning takes place in a friendly happy and democratic atmosphere under expert guidance.

In workshop there are 10 to 12 persons who share a common interest. They meet together to improve their skill. Experts are invited to provide awareness and understanding of the topic and a suitable illustration done. The groups are formed on basis of subject where the supervision of work done. After individual sharing in the group reports are prepared, participant can give comment suggestions for improvement, the expert also adds suggestions.

In a workshop certain principles are to be followed like:

- Allow the participant to select the objective to help get more participation
- They themselves take active role in sharing to make it more effective
- Helps to improve the skill and quality of work when problems and doubts and resolved with correct knowledge
- It improves relation and attitudes with each other
- Clarifications and doubts and current concern and problems are resolved
- We come to know that every person in the work place is worth and can give valuable contribution for common good
- Increases cooperation
- Barriers are broken and better communication becomes possible
- Working towards the common goal
- Students and teacher will improve and understand each other better.

Each group solves a pat of the problem with the help of consultants and resources personnel and the emphasis in on individual work within the group.

Conclusion

It is important feature of workshop to have complete active involvement of every participant of the group. It gives each one the opportunity to make his valuable contribution. When each one shares at the conclusion one comes to know the different point of views; and how the selected topic becomes enriched with sharing of all the view. It helps to improve knowledge, participants exchange ideas freely, and they reflect, think and speak which at the end improves and enhances their active learning. It can have preliminary reading, clarifying sessions, practical exercises, group presentation, individual consultations, etc.

Group Discussion

Group discussion is considered a very effective method of health teaching. People learn by exchanging their views and experiences. The group is not less than 6 and not more than 12 people. There should be a group leader, who initiates the subject, helps the discussion in the proper manner, encourage everyone to participate and sum up the discussion at the end. The proceedings of the group discussion are recorded by a "recorder" who prepares a report on the subject a well conducted group discussion is usually effective.

Discussion involves a group; it is oral; it involves interaction; it is purposeful; systematic; realistic goals. It can be individual conference, seminar, and clinical conference, case analyzing etc. multiple discussion groups, symposium, and panel discussion.

Explanation—a field trip and examples of workshop and discussions are shown in the figures for students to understand the concept.

Keywords

Field trip, principles, work shop, conclusions.

Workshop

Workshop is virtual interactive world of creative educators connected in cyberspace. Workshop that allow them to express their creative ideas by sharing files and applications in a collaborative effort to unveil the possibilities of what can do for your program.

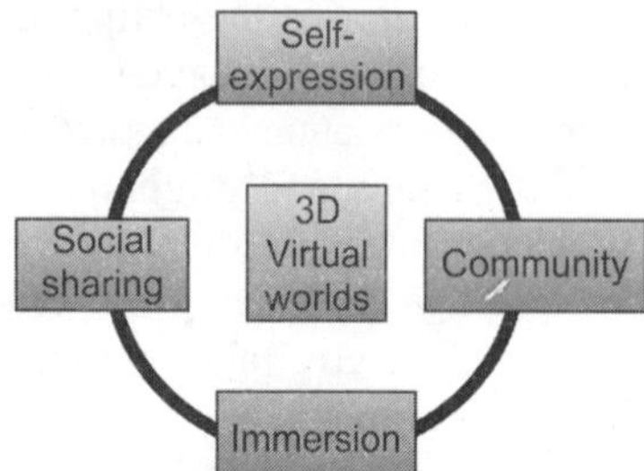

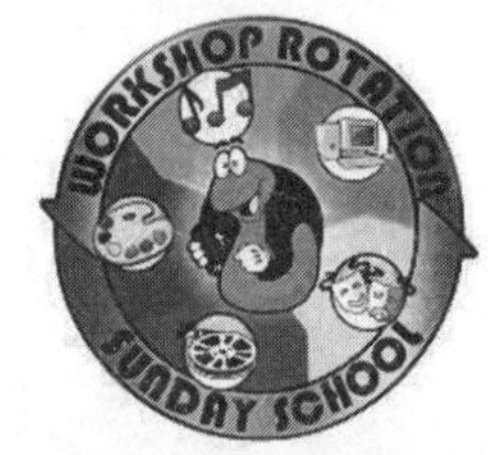

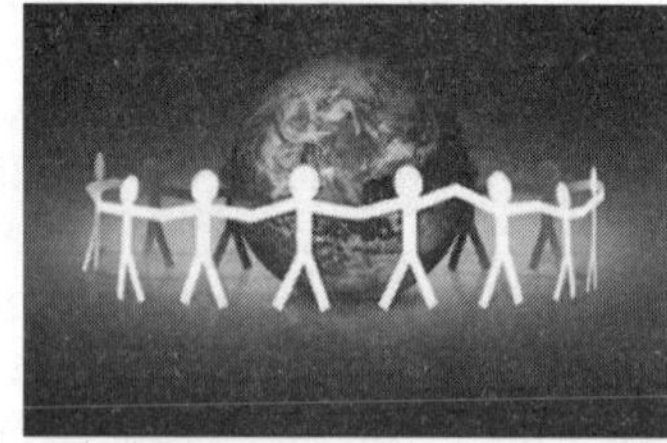

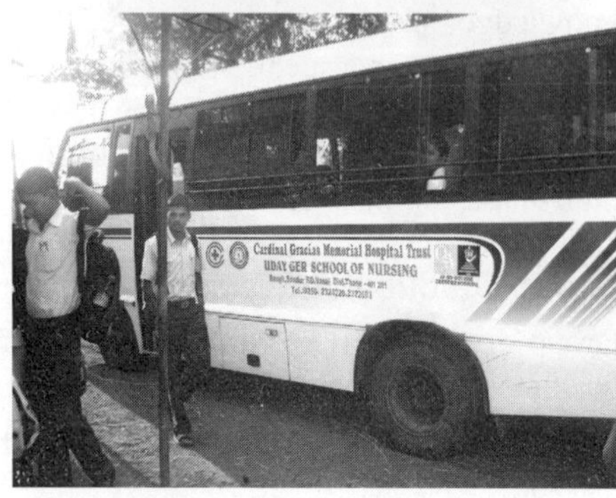

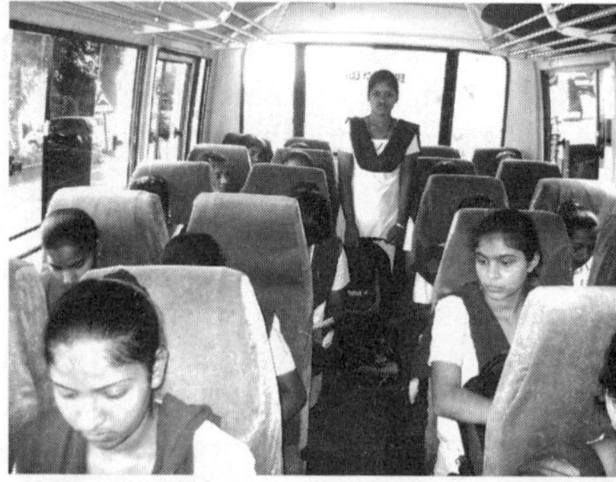

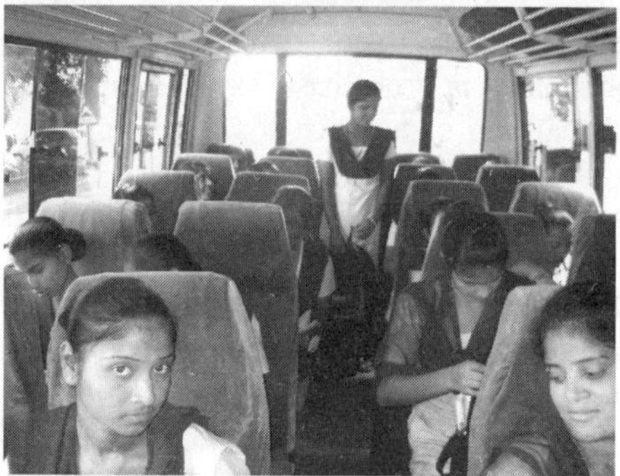

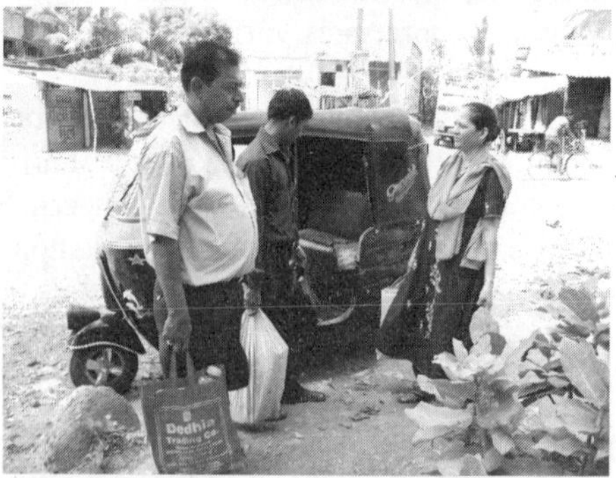

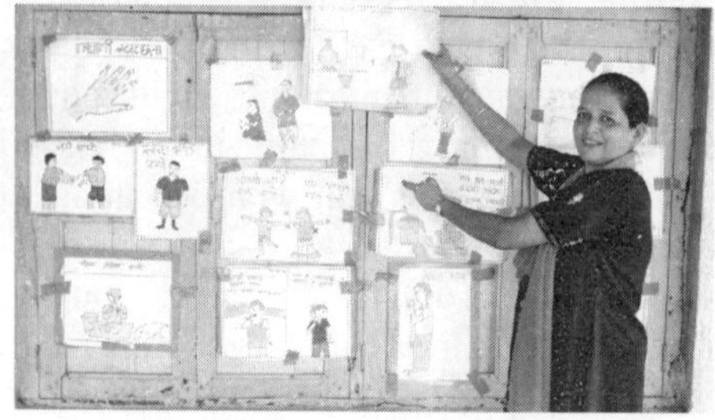

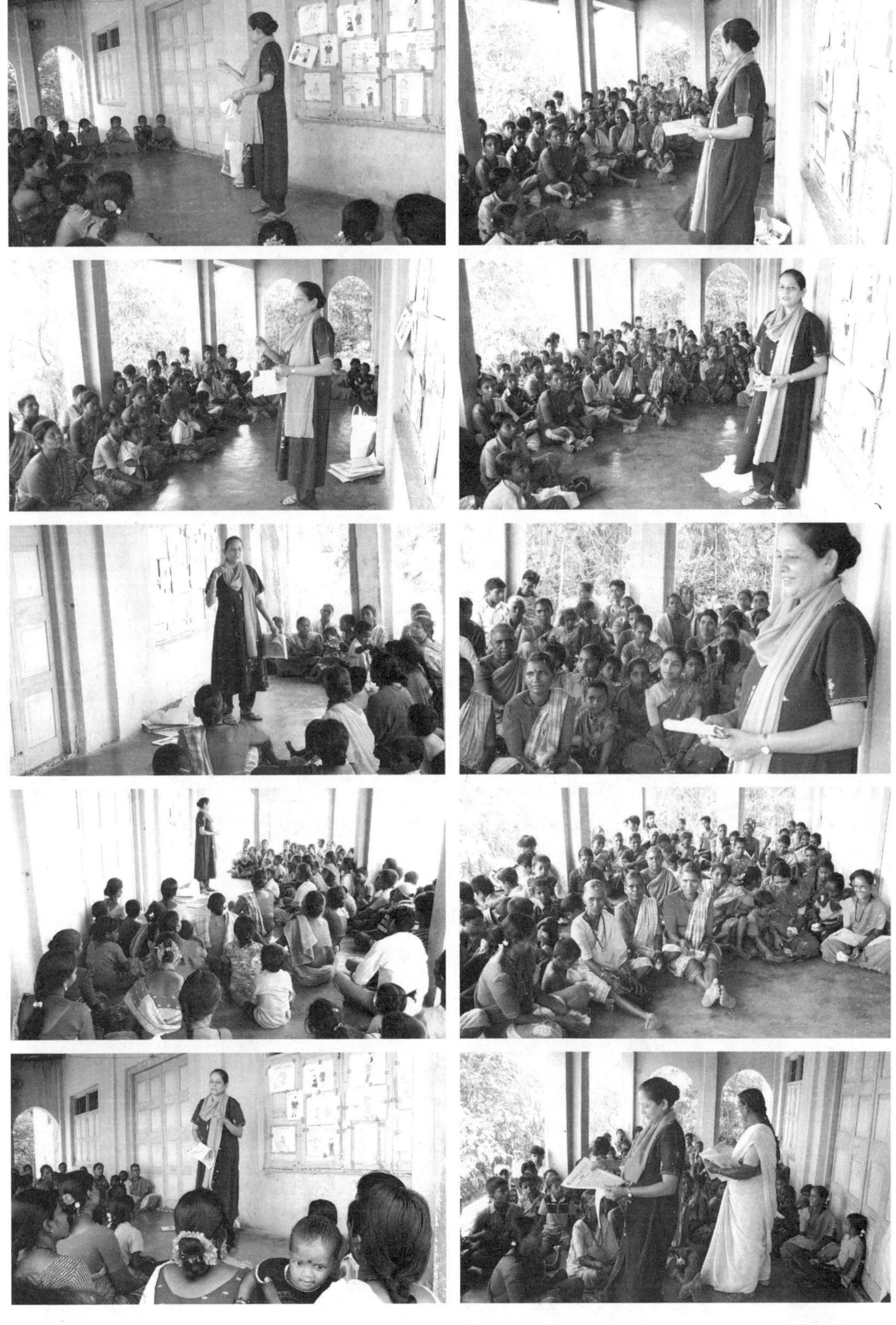

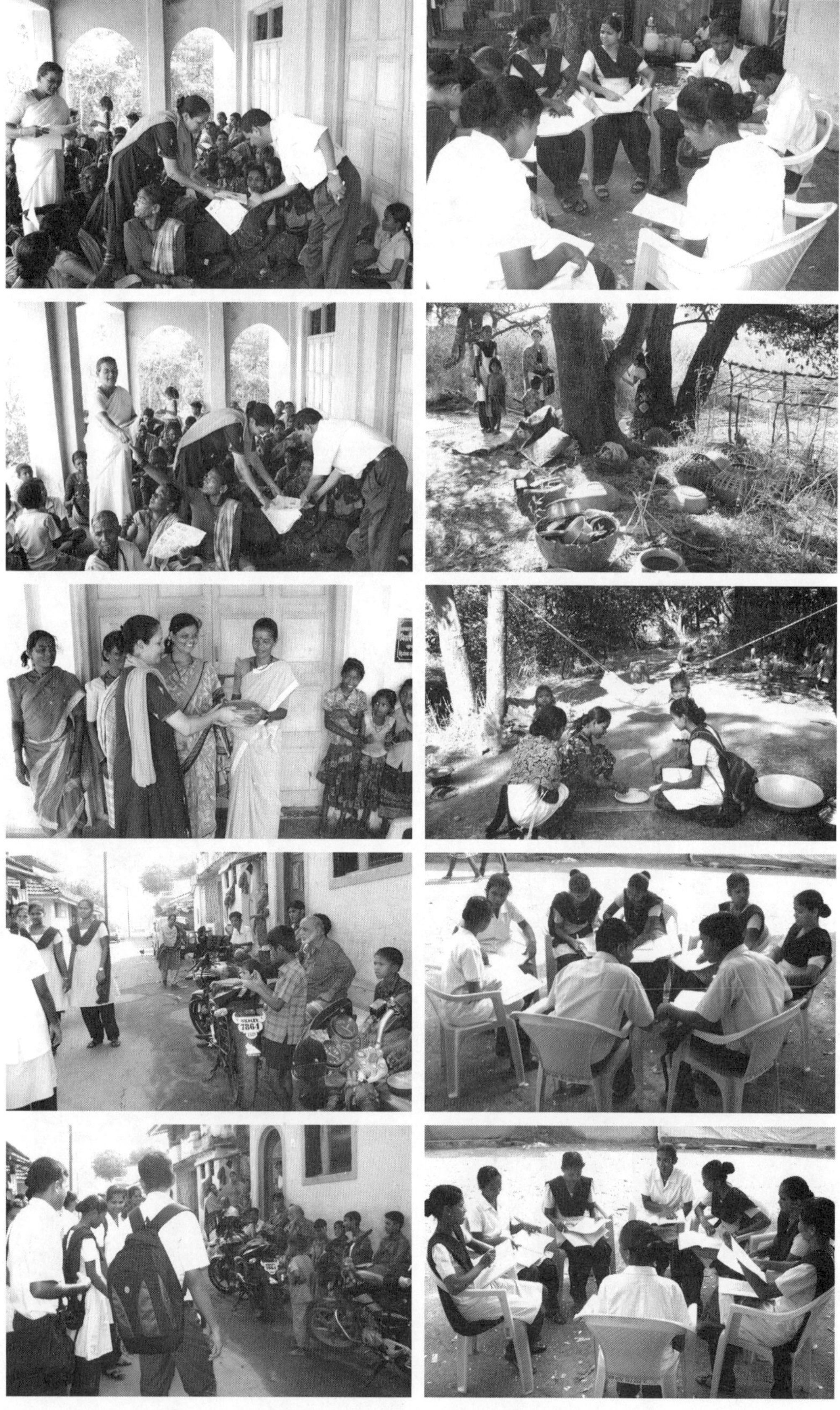

CHAPTER

42

Art and Craft

Abstract

Art and craft: Describes a wild variety of activities involving making things with one's own hand.

LEARNING THROUGH ART AND CRAFT

Man has great cognitive powers. The journey of man from stone age to jet age has been facilitated by development in sciences and technology.

Art and craft exhibition to enable the students display their artistic outlook. The students displayed art and craft projects, where each group was given different categories or topics. The students prepared different projects. The students were given about a month to prepare the selected topic which helped them to gain practice, knowledge and learning. The students were found sharing their colors and other craft material. This helped them to work as a team ands learn good values.

The visual image is created in the minds of the public when they do something practically rather than learning from the books (best out of waste materials). Organic paper, match box, scrap and waste material were made, models of fire brigade, ambulance, police jeep, public transport busses were on display. The exhibition has story telling charts, sock puppets and beautiful drawings. The students too eared the lesson for life. Providing students with a platform to build self confidence and give them the chance to showcase talent, to tap hidden talents and help them to identify their skills, help them in their holistic development.

It is not just a place where you get to learn Newton's Laws of Relativity. It is also place where you can think beyond the classroom. What is taught in class helps us think to the best of our abilities. But if you really broaden your horizon, you've got to do something out of the box 83 million fake accounts on Facebook—the most popular networking.

Limit salt intake is no less than 1.500 mg or about three-fourths of a teaspoon each day. Limited salt intake would significantly reduce the risk of high blood pressure, heart diseases and stroke. Most of the sodium consumed is hidden in processed and prepared foods.

Learning and teaching ideas through shadow play.

The National Museum of Health and Medicine, a division of the Armed Forces Institute of Pathology, was founded as the Army Medical Museum in 1862 to study and improve medical conditions during the American Civil War. The Museum houses a collection of over 24 million items including archival materials, anatomical and pathological specimens, medical instruments and artifacts, and microscope slide-based medical research collections. The collections focus particularly on the history and practice of American medicine, military medicine, and current medical research issues. Today the Museum floor features exhibits on Civil War medicine including artifacts documenting the death of Abraham Lincoln; evolution of the microscope and medical instruments; a hologram of the human body and a computer interactive station of the anatomy allowing visitors to view the human body from a 3-D perspective.

Explanation—different Indian popular art and craft figures are displayed for students to understand the concept. Indian culture is the most complex and colorful, you will see the way of dressing, music, dance, art, craft everything is different every 50 or 100 km in the country. The variety of people is incredible diverse culture of great India.

Keywords

Learning, Explanation.

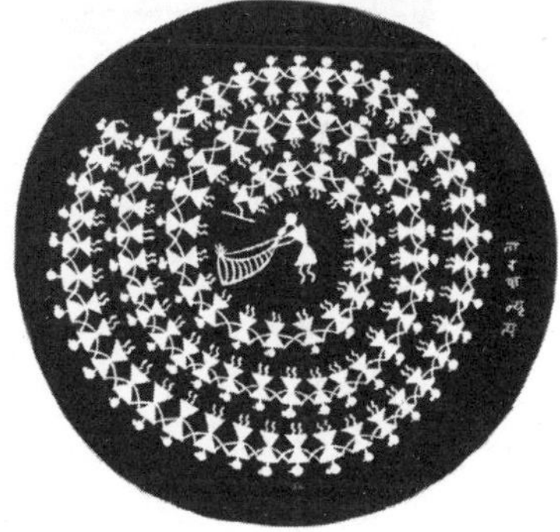

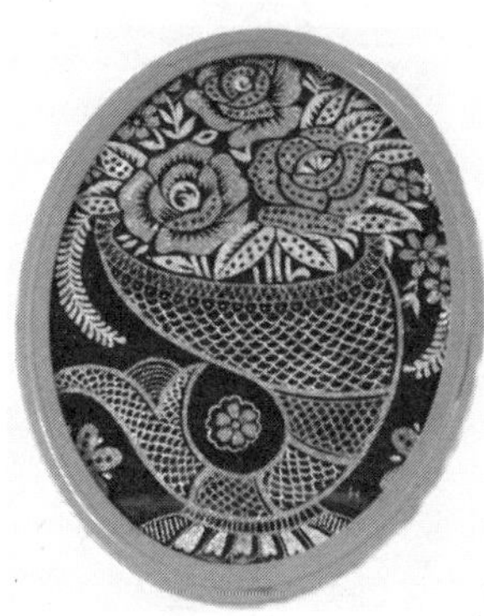

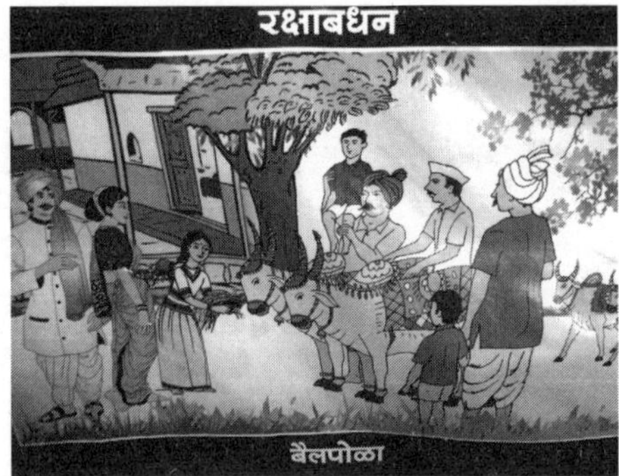
रक्षाबधन
बैलपोळा

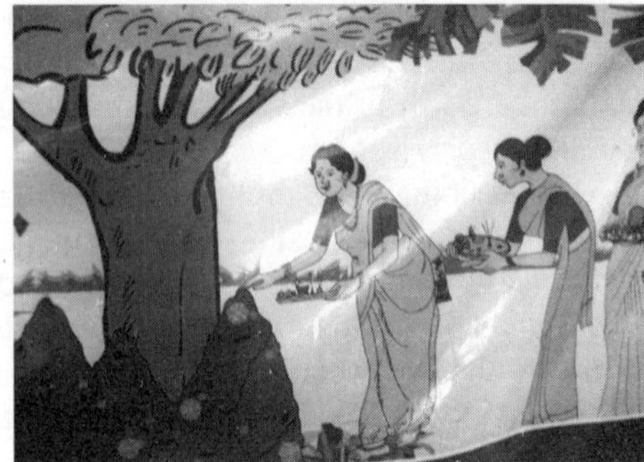

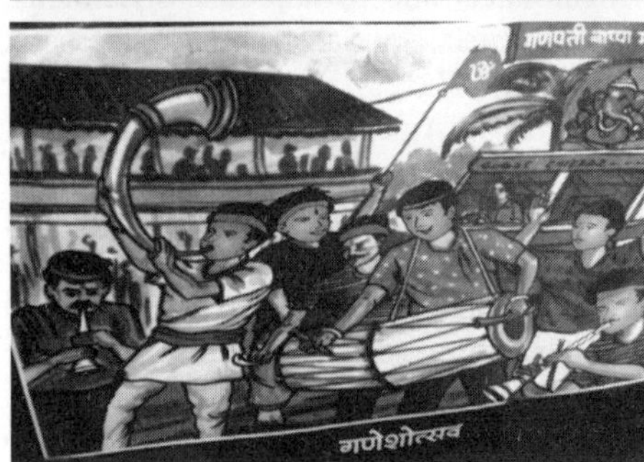
गणेशोत्सव

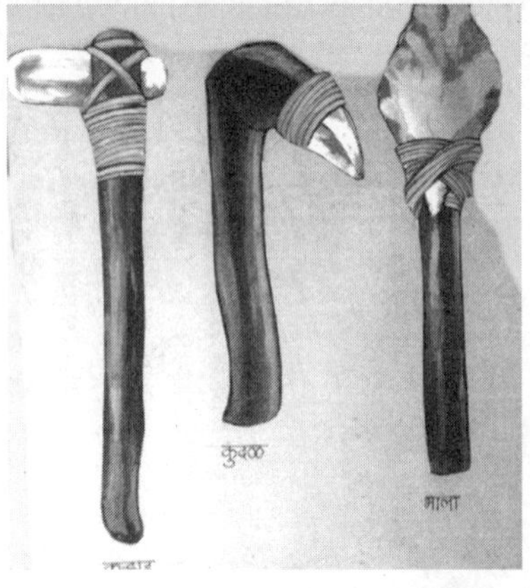
कुदळ

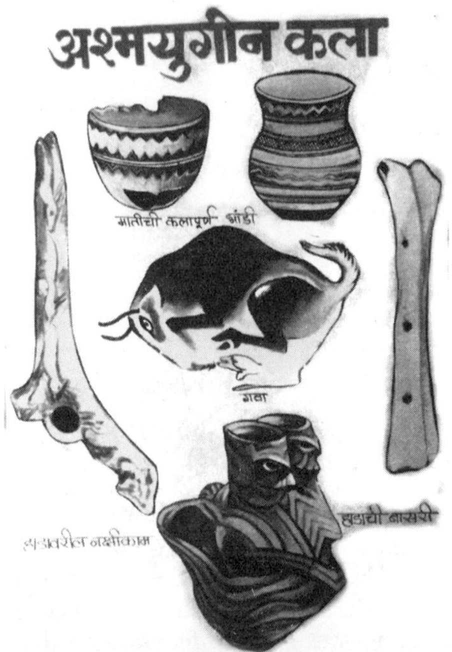
अश्मयुगीन कला
मातीची कलापूर्ण भांडी
हाडाची बासरी

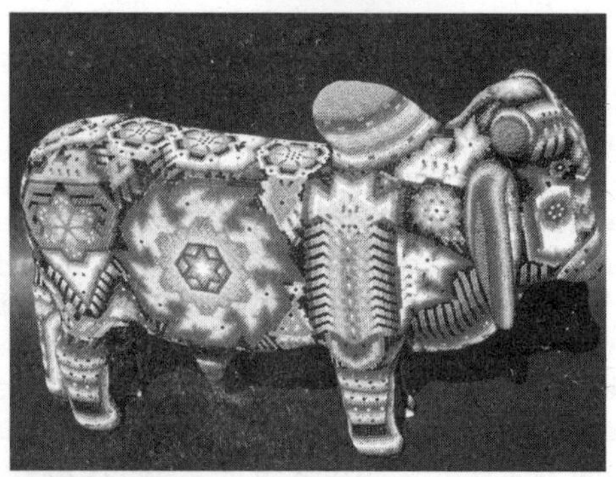

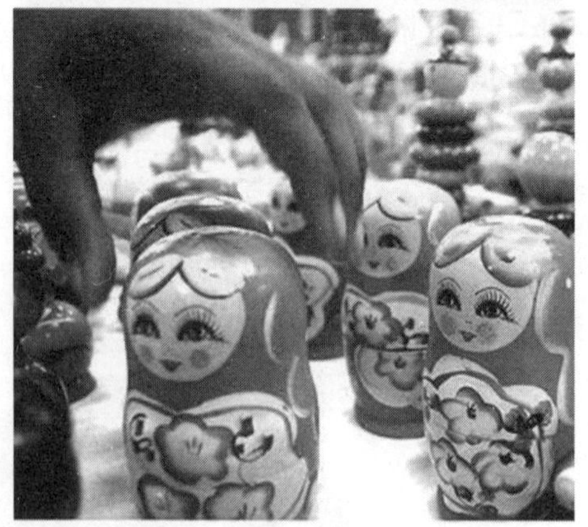

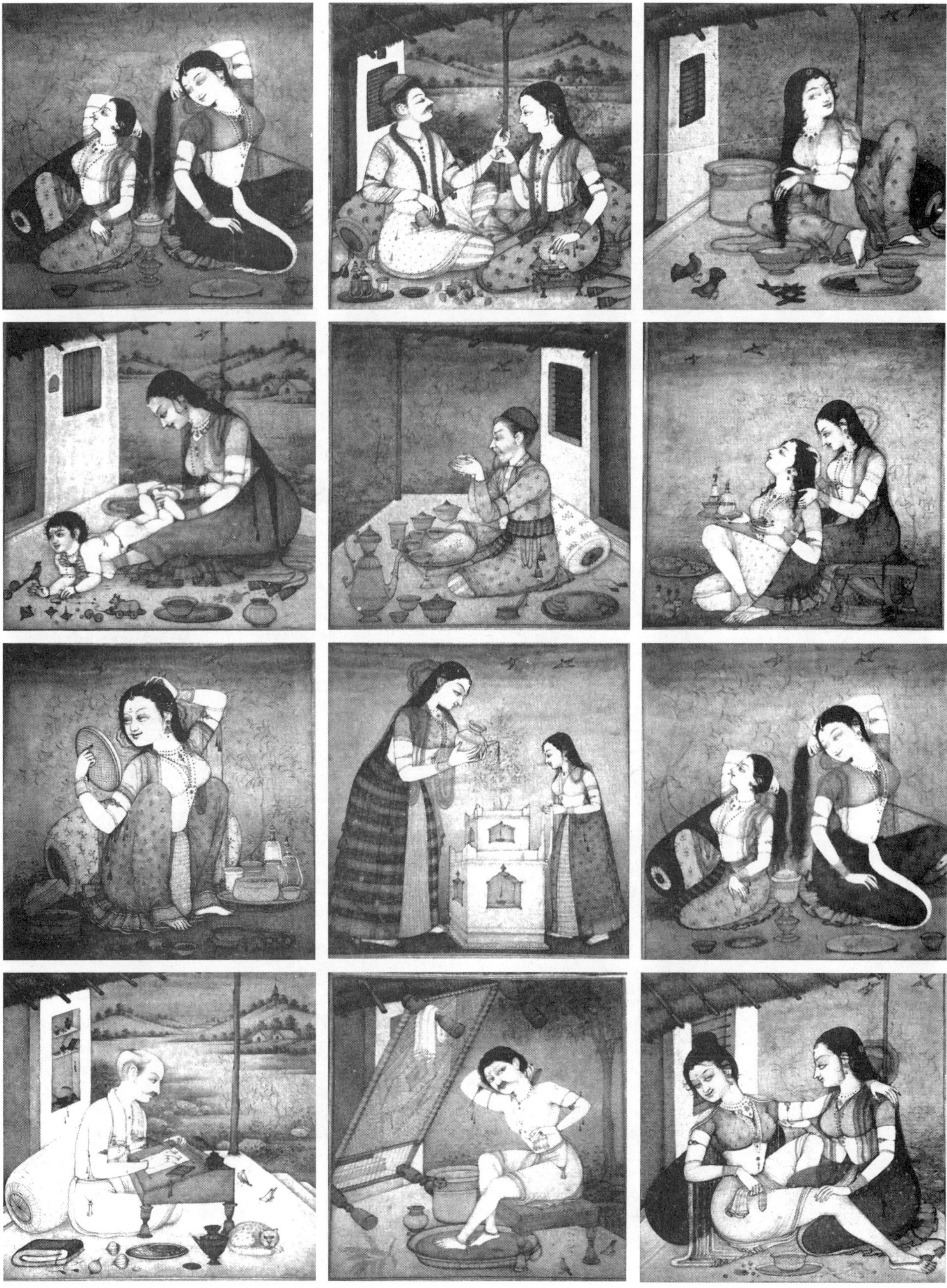

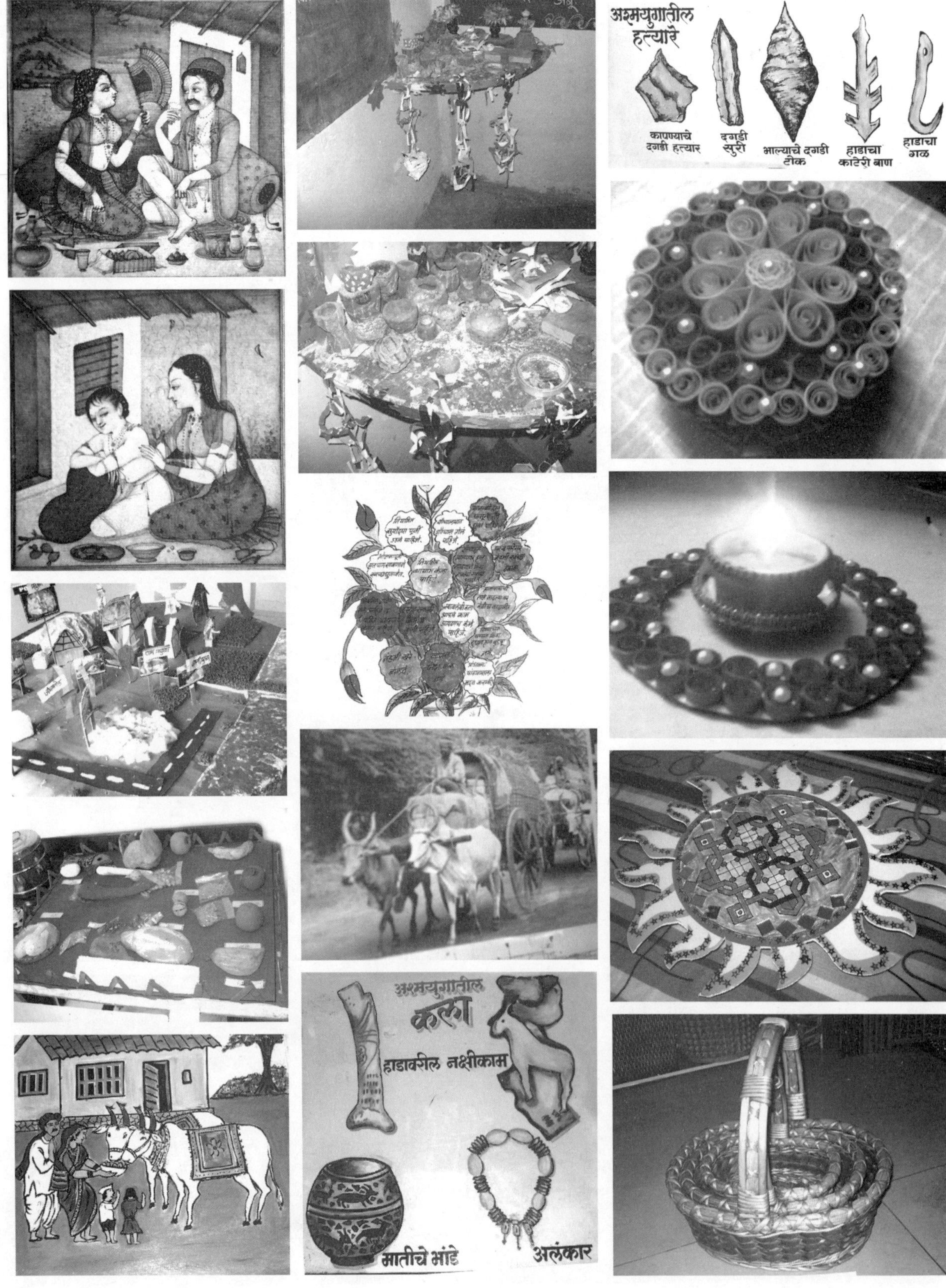
अश्मयुगातील हत्यारे
कापण्याचे दगडी हत्यार
दगडी सुरी
भाल्याचे दगडी टोक
हाडाचा काटेरी बाण
हाडाचा गळ
अश्मयुगातील कला
हाडावरील नक्षीकाम
मातीचे भांडे
अलंकार

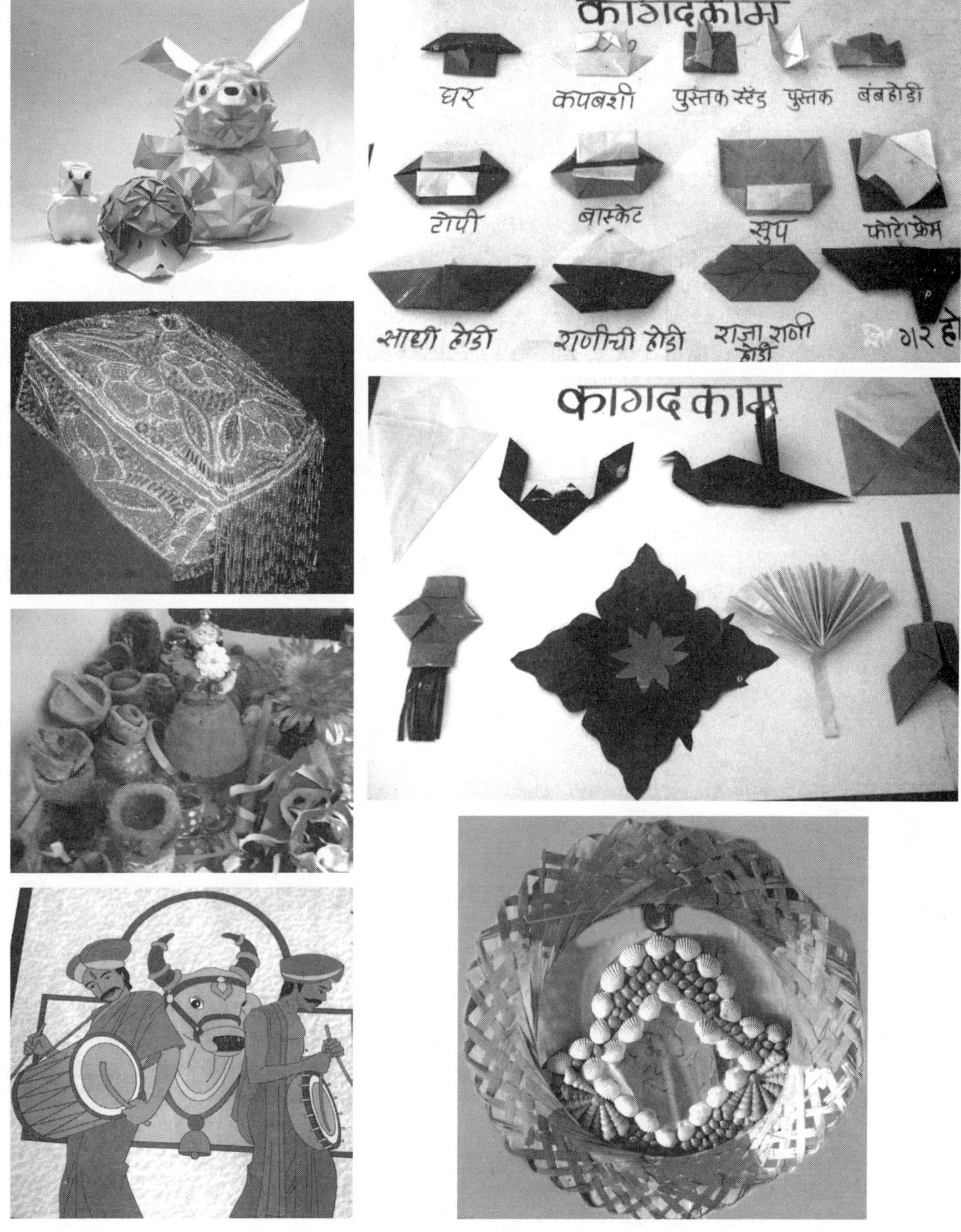
कागदकाम
घर
कपबशी
पुस्तक स्टँड
पुस्तक
बंबहोडी
टोपी
बास्केट
सुप
फोटोफ्रेम
साधी होडी
राणीची होडी
राजा राणी होडी
कागदकाम

CHAPTER

43

Physical Assessment

Abstract

Physical assessment: physical examination is the process of evaluating objective anatomic findings through the use of observation, palpation, percussion, and occultation.

INTRODUCTION

Students have to do physical health assessment in the rural and urban field of there posting period. They do assessment of infant, toddler, pre-schooled, schooled, adolescent, adult, old age and antenatal mother. They have a prepared format to follow and extra sheet in case of more information they find. They can ask the guidance of the supervisor while they are doing the assessment.

They have following points to get the information such as:

- Identification date
- Anthrometric measurements-assessment of growth "nutritional anthropometry" weight, height, circumference etc.
- Developmental assessment
- History of illness/medical history-birth history, past medical history, immunization, illness etc, chief complaints and present illness if any
- General examination—routine examination; any specific observation checklist in that
- Physical assessment—appearance of a person who is thin, medium or fat
- Wearing clothes neat, tidy or untidy, etc.
- Clinical examination—Physical examination involves a detailed clinical examination of all the systems of the body from head to foot dandruff, lice, hair fall, vision, Biltot's spot, dark circle around the eyes, failure to hear, earache, wax in the ear, discharge from ear, nose, nose bleeding, sore throat, excessive salivation, coughing, sneezing, tonsils, adenoids, bowel habits, worms, knock knee, bow leg, gaits, spoon shape nails, rough skin, itching, boils, pimples, patches, nails biting, bed wetting, thumb sucking, tongue ulceration, dirty teeth, caries in the teeth, bleeding gums, pigeon chest, etc.
- Health teaching given for the health need identified and plan of action
- For aged persons five dimensions are taken into consideration—such as activities of daily living; physical health; mental health; social health, economic functioning
- The child's health card provides checklist for examination, which are used in all ICDS projects
- Physical examination of under five-example part of the body skin see color where there are any depigmented areas, bluishness, pallor, rough skin, bois, pimples, etc. look for rash, sores or blisters with crusting round itchy, scaly patches and bruised areas. Test for the elasticity of the skin. Test for edema, look for BCG vaccine taken scar. It is important to examine the skin in detail because it can give clues to the presence of diseases. It will help a nurse to see deviations from normal. Reduced sensitivity to touch could be suspected as leprosy, pallor suspected as anemia, malnutrition, round itchy scaly patches can be ringworms; dry inelastic skin could be dehydration. Eyes pull down lower eyelid and inspect conjunctiva and note any discharge or pustules on eye lids, dark circle, vision, squint, Biltots sport etc each part of the body is assessed.
- Growth monitoring is to weigh the child periodically at monthly intervals during the 1st year and every 3 months thereafter up to the age of five to 6 years. The child's weight is plotted on the growth chart (road to health) the curve is obtained which is known as growth curve. This card has two lines. The upper line represents the growth curve of well nourished children; the 2nd line below represents the growth cure of the average child. If the child is growing normally, the growth curve will run parallel between the top two lines. The chart also shows the degree of the malnutrition. Children's whose growth curves fall below the top two lines are stated to be malnourished that is they are not growing properly (growth failure) their nutrition must be improved by providing nutrition supplements and by nutrition education of mothers. She can bring the card whenever she visits the clinic. These charts are used to early detection of growth failure. Nurse has to be familiar with the use of growth charts and maintain them regularly. Growth charts are standardized tools that serve as norms to compare an individuals growth

There are formulas for assessing growth parameters in children. There is also formula calculating BMI.

CLASSIFICATION OF MARASMUS

1. Grade one—loss of fat in the axillae and groins
2. Grade two—loss of fat in the axillae, groins, the abdomen and the spine
3. Grade three—loss of fat in the chest and spine in addition to signs of grade one and two
4. Grade four—in addition to above three grades, the buccal fat is lost.

- How are the anthropometric measurements taken?—this is a system of assessment of body build and nutritional status of children using measurement such as weight, height, wrist circumference, skin fold thickness, upper arm circumference, chest circumference and head circumference. Anthropometric measurements recorded over a period of time reflect the patterns of growth and development and how individuals deviate from the average in body size, build and nutritional status at various ages.

How the height is measured?

Instruct the child above two years to stand against wall without foot wear feet parallel and heels, buttocks, shoulders and back of the head touching the wall with head comfortably erect which will aid in accurate measurement of height. you can make a mark on the wall with the help of the ruler touching the top of the head horizontally. Ask the child after that to move away and measure the length of the wall using the measuring tape. The other way of measuring the height is assist the child to stand on a weight scale with stand meter with head in midline parallel to floor. Make sure that the medial mallets touch each other to get accurate reading.

How the chest, wrist, head and mid-upper arm are measured?

Check the circumference by encircling the specific body parts with a measuring tape and read the result in centimeter. For head circumference place the measuring tape around forehead just above the eyebrows interiorly and around the occipital protuberance posterior. For mid upper arm pinch length wise a double fold of subcutaneous tissue about 1 cm above the mid upper arm with thumb and index finger. Place the teeth of calipers on either side of the tissue fold and note the reading. These measurements are used to assess growth pattern and to identify deviations from normal growth and development. It needs to be recorded on to the growth monitoring charts.

How will you check the weight?

To weight infant place a clean paper or a plastic sheet on the scale and balance it. you can also place the baby on the platform of weighing machine, read the weight and record. The other way you can instruct the mother to take the child weight them both together, then give the child to someone and tell mother to stand alone on weight machine and see the difference minus the weight of the mother that is the weigh of an infant. See that weight scale must be accurate. The baby scale platform must be safe and secure to prevent he baby from falling. The nurse must stay with the baby when she is weighed, baby must wear same amount of clothing each time she is weighed. Emphasize importance of weighing during the growth period. Read the weight by standing in-front of the scale. Measuring adult if food is taken, weight has to be taken after one hour, let him empty bowel and bladder.

How Do You Take Fundal Height and Abdominal Girth?

To do the Examination of a pregnant woman, is to determine the normalcy of fetal growth in relation to the uterus and its relationship to the maternal pelvis. Position woman for examination; place the pillow under her head and upper shoulder. Have her arms sides and expose her abdomen from below to Symphysis pubis. Determine the fundal height using the ulnar side of the palm. Measure fundal height using measuring tape. Measure the abdomen girth by encircling the woman's abdomen with a tape measure at the level of the umbilicus.

Health Assessment of Aged Person

The number of old people is growing and the old have their own special problems of health and they need health care more than younger age group.

Common in elder's problem referred as "5":

1. Immobility mainly caused by pain, stiffness, imbalance, fear of failure
2. Instability-leads to falls and fractures
3. Intellectual impairment like depression, lack of sleep, lack of energy, decreased concentration
4. Incontinence—urinary incontinence needs hospitalization and leads to psychological problems and social isolation
5. Gastrohepatic drug reaction-drug reaction because of change in absorption decreases renal flow, decreases blood flow to the liver leads to drug reaction.

Common in Elders—"5" Dimension

1. Activities of daily living
2. Physical health
3. Mental health
4. Social health
5. Economic functioning

1. **Problems associated with long-term illness**— degenerative diseases of the heart and blood vessels, cancer, diabetes, arthritis, chronic bronchitis, asthma, enlarge prostrate, accidents
2. **Psychological problems in aging process**—associated with various loose of job, income, friends, declining health, death of a spouse, etc.
3. **Common problems are**—depression, delirium, dementia, alzheimer's diseases.

Explanation

Students were asked to do physical assessment of infant, toddler, antenatal, etc. some pictures showing the concept.

Keywords
Introduction, information, classification, measurement of height, fundal height, assessment of aged person,"5" dimensions, checking weight.

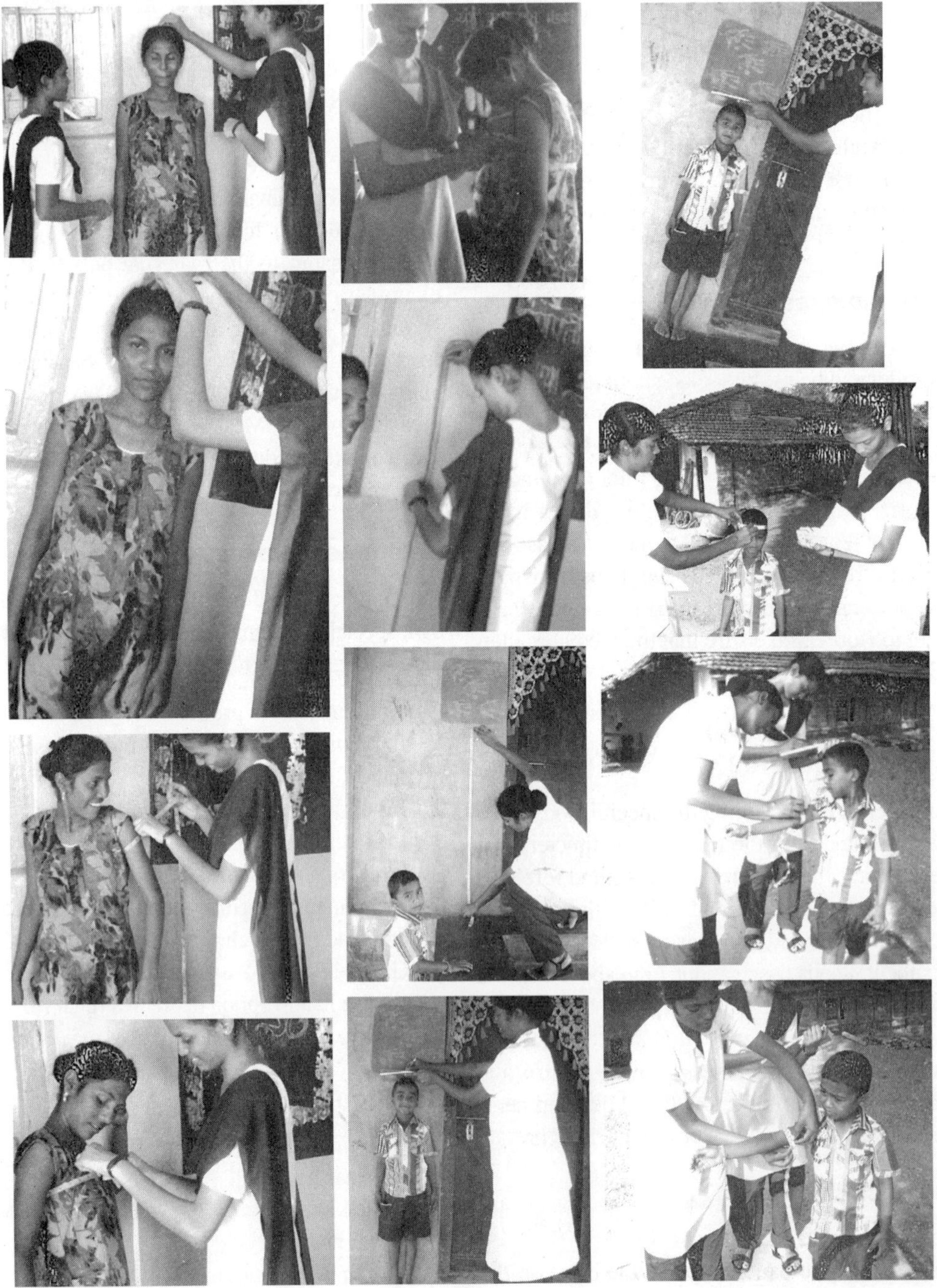

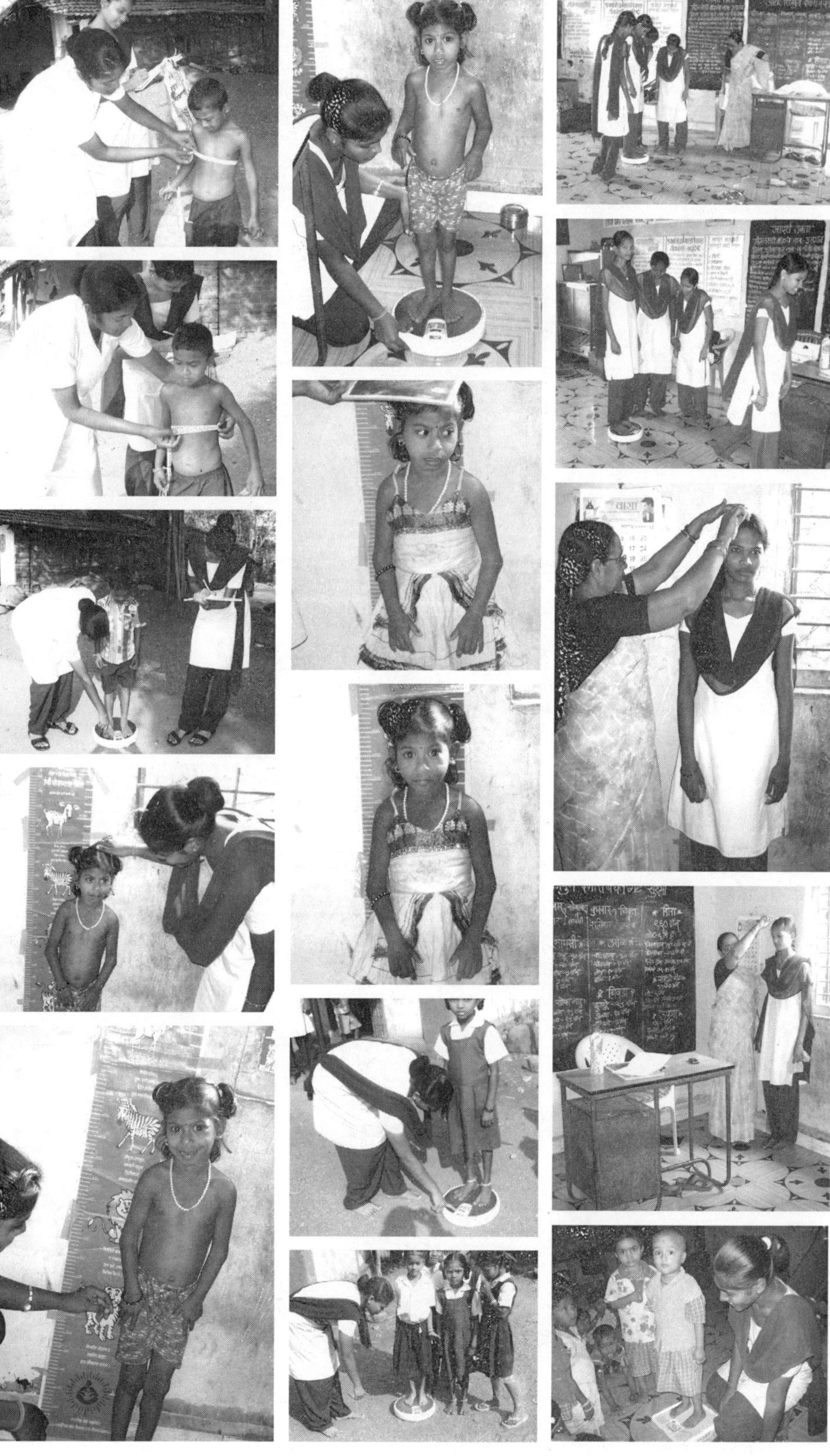

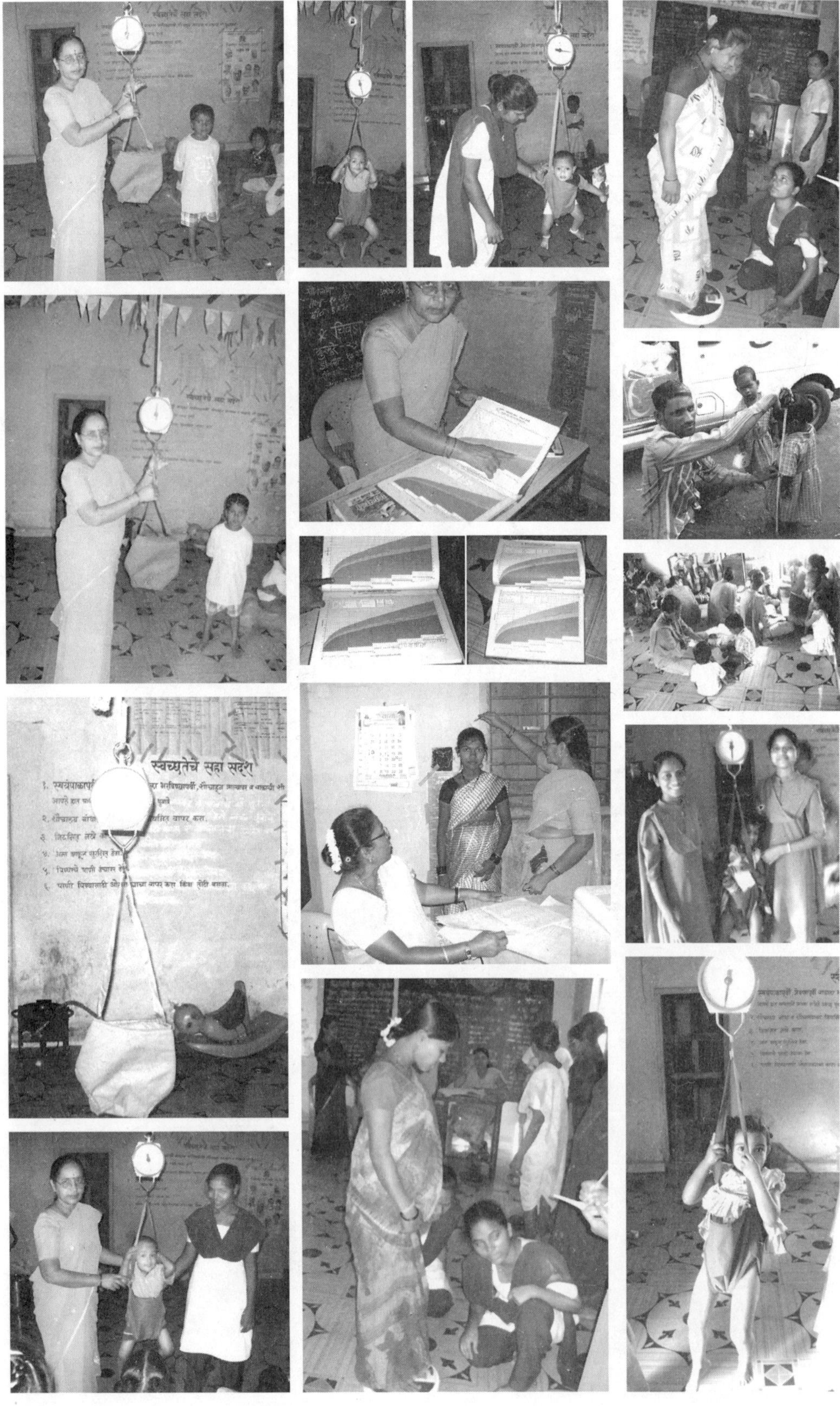
स्वच्छतेचे सहा संदेश

CHAPTER 44

PowerPoint Presentation

Abstract

PowerPoint presentation: It is a computer software created by Microsoft, which allows the user to create slides with recordings, narration, transition and other features in order to present information.

INTRODUCTION

PowerPoint is a complete presentation graphics package. It gives you everything you need to produce a professional-looking presentation. Powerpoint offers word processing, outlining, drawing, graphing, and presentation management tools—all designed to be easy to use and learn. What you can do in Powerpoint is when you create a presentation using Powerpoint; the presentation is made up of a series of slides The slides that you create using Powerpoint can also be presented as overhead transparencies or 35 mm slides. In addition to slides, you can print audience handouts, outlines, and speaker's notes. You can format all the slides in a presentation using the powerful slide Master which will be covered in the tutorial. You can keep your entire presentation in a single file—all your slides, speaker's notes, and audience handouts. You can import what you have created in other Microsoft products, such as Word and Excel into any of your slides. Now that you know what features Powerpoint offers it's time to learn how to work in Powerpoint—how you want to create your new presentation. Powerpoint gives you four views in which you create and organize your presentation. As you create a presentation, you can switch among the four views as you work.

Four PowerPoint Views

Slide View—the Slide view shows a single slide. In Slide view, you work on one slide at a time. Here, you can type your slide title and body, add other text to the slide, draw shapes, add clip art, choose a color scheme, make a graph, etc. In Slide view, you have access to all the tools on the Tool Palette as well as buttons on the Toolbar.

Outline View—the Outline view shows all the titles and body text in your presentation. In Outline view, you can move slides around within your presentation and also edit your text.

Slide Sorter View—the Slide Sorter view shows you a miniature of each slide in your presentation. You can drag slides around on the screen to reposition them in this view. You can also select and copy multiple slides should you want to use them in other presentations.

Notes view—lets you create speaker's notes. Each page corresponds to a slide in your presentation and includes a reduce image of the slide. You can draw and type in Notes view the way you can in Slide View. You now know all of Power Point's views. Now that you know all of Power Point's views it is time to learn how to work within a slide. In general, presentations will be based on a Master Slide it contains objects that you want to appear on each slide in your presentation. With a Slide Master, you only have to create an item once and Power Point will automatically include them on every slide. Some things are set up by Power Point (for example, place for slide title and text) so you don't have to create them each time. If you want to add additional items to a master, you can at any time. The Slide Master has boxes already set up for the slide title and text. They're called the Master Title and the Master Body object. The format of these objects determines the way your text will look on each slide. You can always make slides look different from the Slide Master, but a Slide Master gives you a consistent starting point. The Slide Master is flexible. You can move objects around, add art, add headings or labels, change colors and fonts. As you create a slide, you have the option of using or not using the elements from the Slide Master. To change the entire presentation, you simply change the format of the Slide Master. Power Point will then change all your slides accordingly. Power Point also offers templates. **A template** is a presentation containing Power Point masters and a color scheme. Power Point offers 160 pre-designed templates to help you get started quickly. Applying a template to a presentation you are creating means the design work is already done for you. You can apply a template when you are just starting a presentation, or you can create a presentation and apply the template later. Now that you have learned about Power Point masters and templates it is time to learn create a slide.

In addition to formatting text and bullets you can also format the following: Slide Background Slide Color Scheme, Experiment with these on your own. Power Point also has a number of features you can use to display your slides when you are giving a slide show. When you display your presentation electronically as a slide show, the slides take up the full screen. All the tools, menus, and other screen elements are hidden so as not to detract from your show. Your computer becomes the equivalent of a slide projector. Power Point offers a number of features you can use when you run your slide show: You can use special effects, such as transitions and builds, to add variety. You can practice giving your presentation and set automated timings for your slides to match your rehearsal times. A build slide is a slide that starts with the first major bullet point and shows more major bullet points as the presentation proceeds. You decide whether you want to dim previous points on the slide as new points appear and what effect you want to use when the bullet points appear (for instance, bullet points can fly in from the right, left, top, or bottom). Transudations moves one slide off the screen and brings the next one on. Fading from black and dissolving from one slide to another are two examples of transitions. You have a choice of transitions for each slide, plus you can vary the speed of each transition. A transition refers to the way one slide moves off the screen and the next slide appears. When you set your transitions, you can also set how long you want each slide to appear on the screen. Decide how you want to advance to the next slide and, if need be, set the timing. If you want the slide to advance automatically, you need to decide how long the slide should appear on-screen before advancing to the next slide: Type the number of seconds you want the slide on the screen. During the presentation, the slide advances automatically when the time is up.

A build slide is one that seems to build on itself, showing progressively more information as the presentation proceeds. To create a build slide: To start you must have a slide which contains bullets. What is the definition of animation in Microsoft Power Point?

It is an animation is used in Microsoft power point. It is use to adjust and make lovely your presentation and make your slide better and better then begins and it is the main part of presentation. . In power point, you have one slide or image after another, right? Well, there has to be SOMETHING that comes between each one--that would be a transition.

As modern health care delivery system has become complex and there is a need for updated information. Talking the responsibilities for oneself is the key to successful health promotion. Knowledgeable nursing services are indispensable. She is a pillar on which modern care is based. Where she has diverse roles and responsibilities to fulfill.

Napoleon Hill, the well known motivator-educator said 'whatever a mind can conceive and believe, it can achieve', therefore believe in yourself. Our profession is in no way less then any other profession, it also has wide variety of openings to go ahead.

With profound changes that impose heavier burdens, greater work specialization and high skill growing demand by consumer preferences and new technologies nurse is key drive. How can new and effective educational methods be introduced and strengthened in nursing practice? As the nurses role is in the spotlight more than ever before.

Today curriculum is reviewed, revised and restructured for improving the quality of human life. As a hungry man needs food and water, so the sick man needs nursing care and the nurse is a mediator.

LCD projector is a portable device, subject matter are types in a brief systematic way in Microsoft power point software and stored on a compact disc CD, then the CD is inserted in LCD which has projection mechanism by which information can given to the mass. Follow the manufactures instruction before preparing and operating, adjustment, maintenance, operation technique, preview, presentation, evaluation.

Explanation—some figures explaining the concept of power presentation.

Keywords
Introduction, PowerPoint view, LCD.

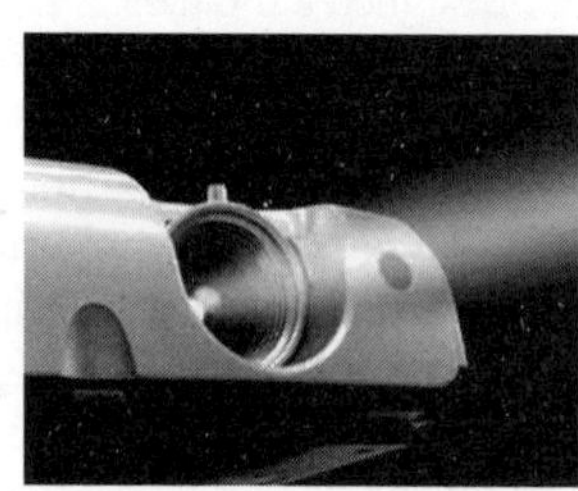

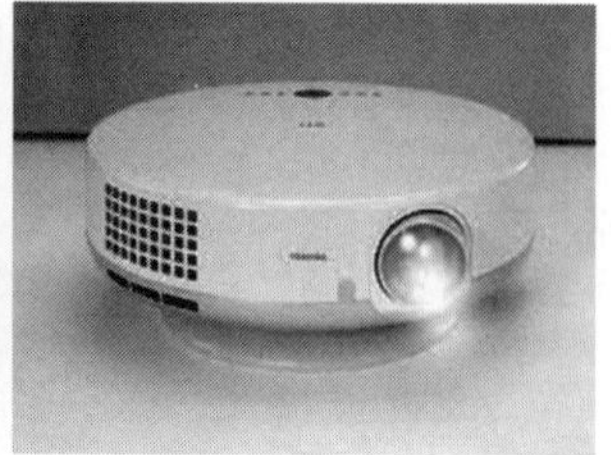

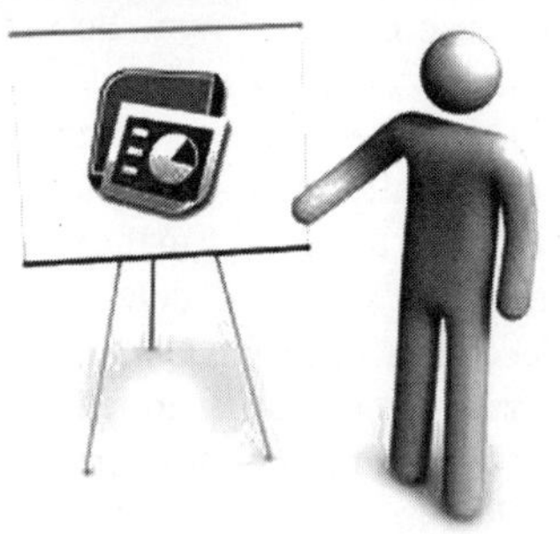

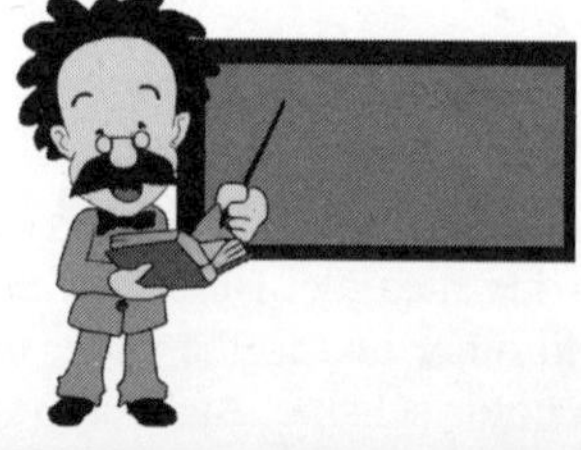

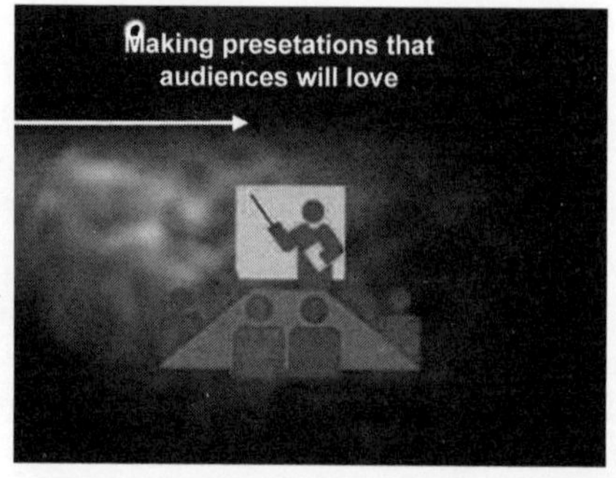

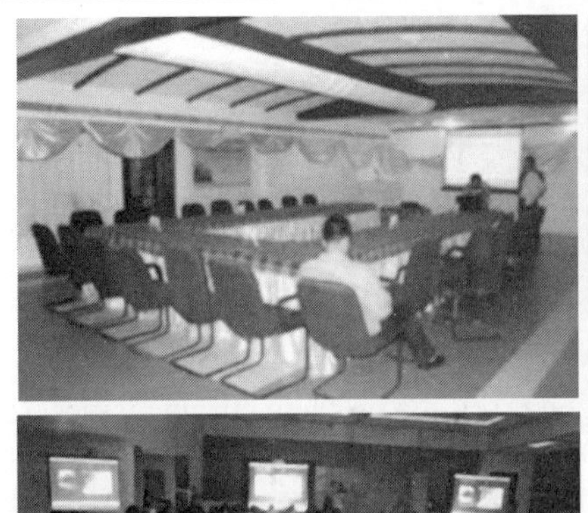
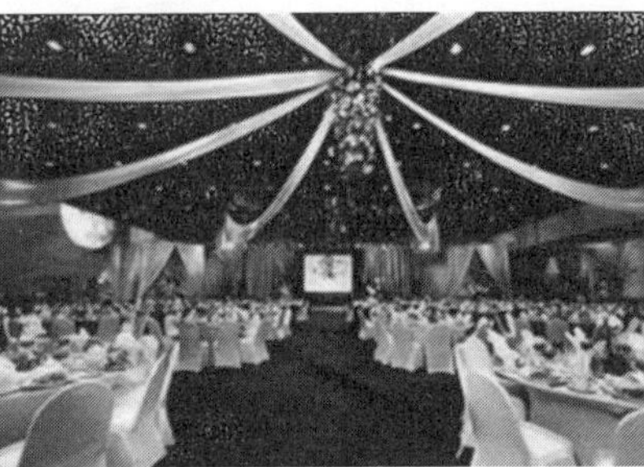
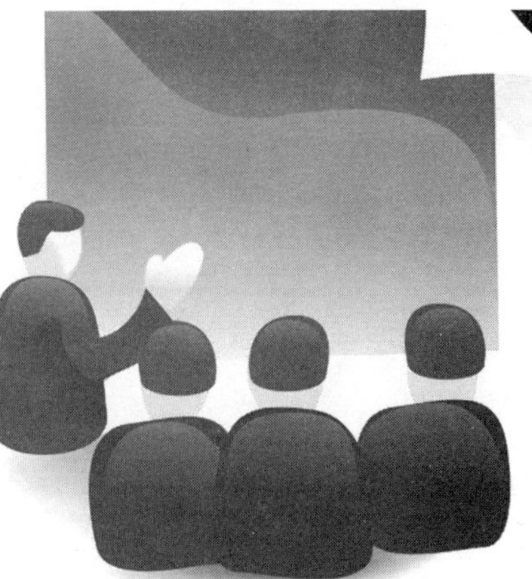
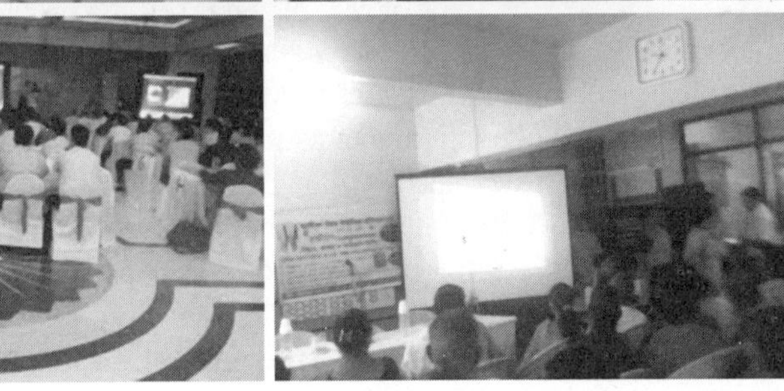

CHAPTER

45

Skits

Abstract

Skit is a short literary piece of a humorous or satirical character, or a short theatrical sketch or act; usually it is comical, and dramatic performance or work.

ROLE-PLAYING

Skits and role play the people small and big enjoy like anything. We were able to draw lot of crowed through acting local social problems and health problems though the small skits and role play. It is powerful media cum entertainment.

Learning the fun way—Telling stories that make a difference- story telling is an internal part of growing up and the fine thread that connects cultures across the world. Story telling is an ancient art. With size of families shrinking and living spaces becoming more and more exclusive many families in the city do not have any more to tell the stories children at home. The digital revolution has filled this gap to some extent. There are DVD and animated video of children's stories, which after all are mechanical so ancient story telling is worth and we have to review this art.

Role-playing refers to the changing of one's behaviour to assume a role, either unconsciously to fill a social role, or consciously to act out an adopted role. Offers a definition of role-playing as "the changing of one's behavior to fulfill a social role" refer to the playing of roles generally such as in a theatre, or educational setting; or person and acting it out with a partner taking someone else's role.

Role playing is an educational technique in which people spontaneously act out problems of human relation through acting, it involves more than one person and deals with majority proems. Audiences identify with the roles in role playing or critical observations, brought about much greater learning than passive watching.

Here the actor really tries to feel the part of the character he is portraying and puts himself in the person's situation. The audience gets into some kind of emotional involvement. it is used to arouse interest in a problem, make the problem seem real and solution seem attainable. Develops leadership skills in students who act out in public, where he lives the problem by acting out and develops sensitivity to another's feelings by having the opportunity to put oneself in another's place.

Steps of role playing- select a problem burning issues; set up the role playing scene.

Amusement—Many children participate in a form of role-playing known as make believe, wherein they adopt certain roles such as doctor and act out those roles in character. Sometimes make believe adopts an oppositional nature, resulting in games such as cops and robbers.

Adults for millennia have practiced entertainment-Historical reenactment. The ancient Romans, Han Chinese, and medieval Europeans all enjoyed occasionally organizing events in which everyone pretended to be from an earlier age, and entertainment appears to have been the primary purpose of these activities. Within the 20th century historical re-enactment has often been pursued as a hobby.

Role-playing games—A role-playing game is a game in which the participants assume the roles of characters and collaboratively create stories. Participants determine the actions of their characters based on their characterization, and the actions succeed or fail according to a formal system of rules and guidelines. Role-playing takes years to master, but it does not take too long to learn the basics. Training where people rehearse situations in preparation for a future performance and to improve their abilities within a role. The most common examples are occupational training role-plays, educational role-play exercises.

Socio-drama scene can deal with real problem enact scene.

Skit—A short, usually comic dramatic performance or work; a theatrical sketch. A short humorous or satirical piece of writing.

Conclusion—it is a spontaneous acting out of definite situation or issues with time allotted, characters assigned on particular theme where the students can dramatize along with verbalization. They learn communication skills, they learn to cooperate as a team, develop insight in to problem and get in to character emotionally in creative manner. When taken from real life situation the audiences participate very actively. The dialogue should be well written with the message and possibly peoples language. it is used as an educational technique where acting is done of concrete burning issues.

Keywords

Role-playing, learning, amusement, games, skit, conclusion.

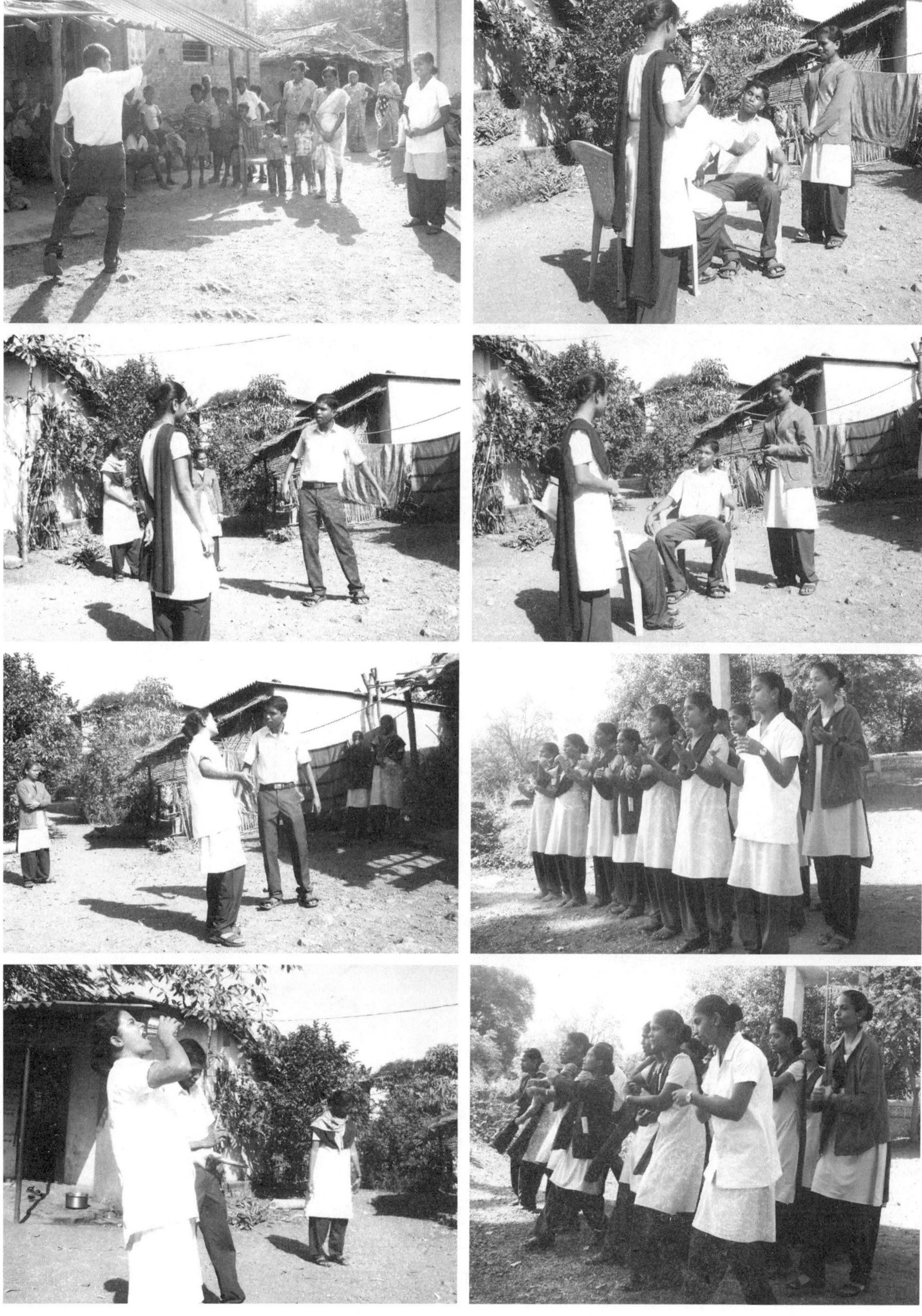

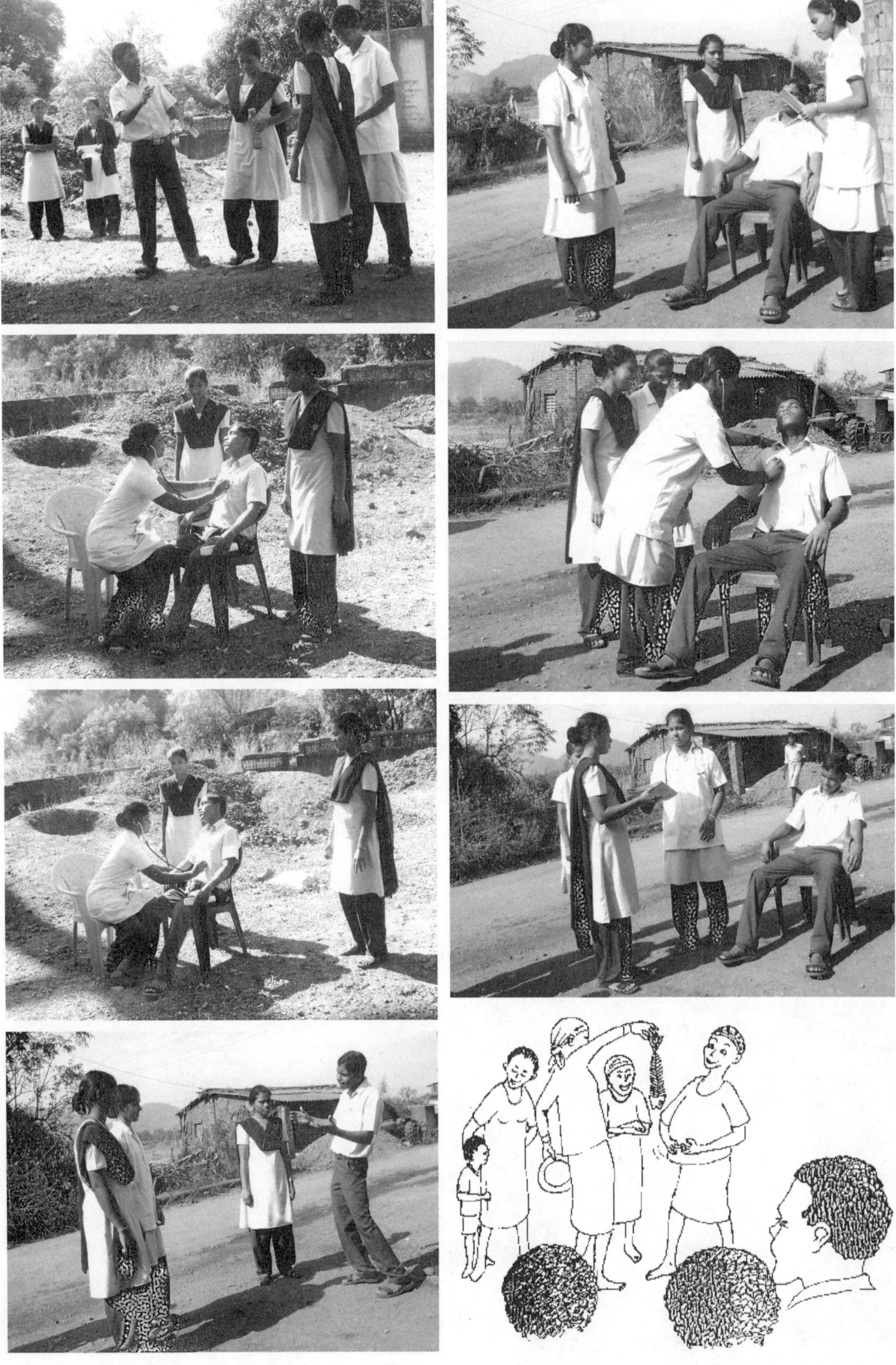

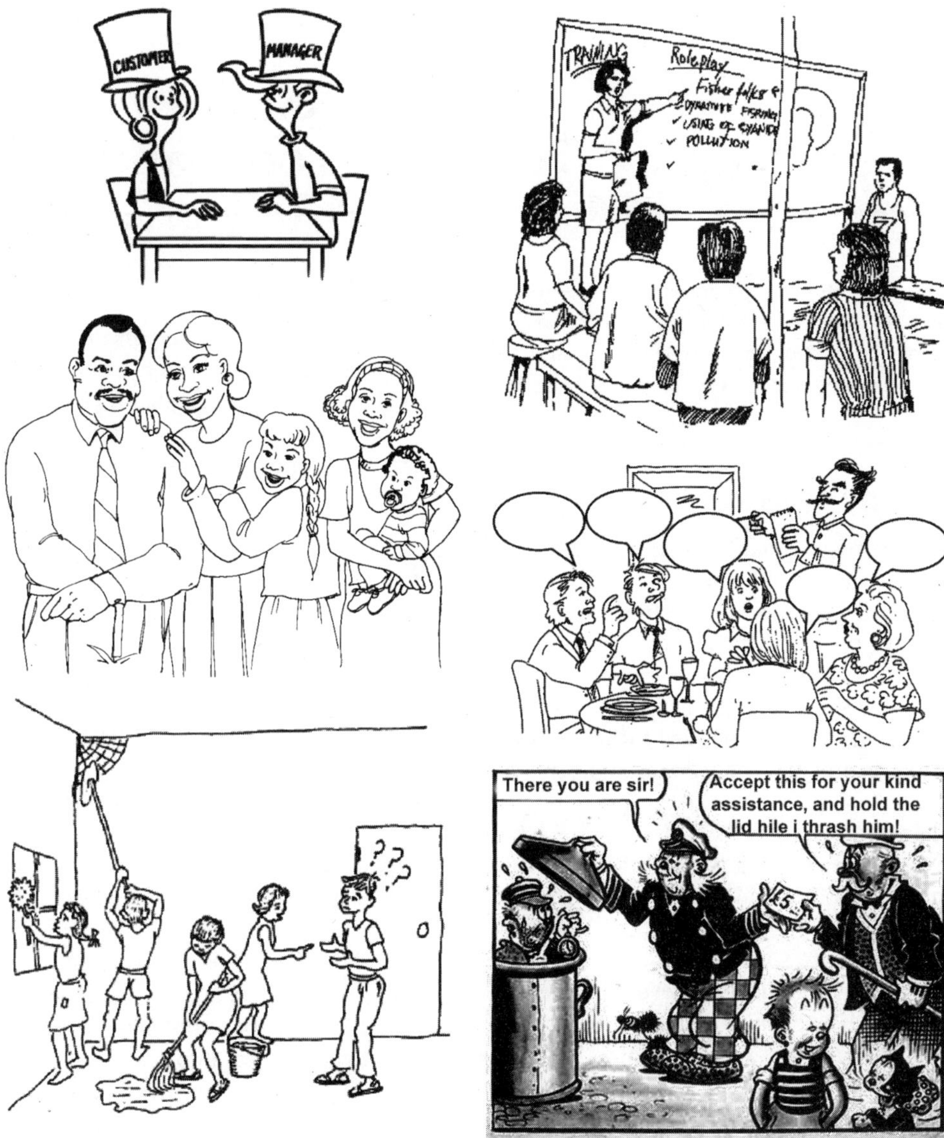
CUSTOMER
MANAGER
TRAINING
Roleplay
There you are sir!
Accept this for your kind assistance, and hold the lid hile i thrash him!

CHAPTER 46

Teaching Tools and Techniques

Abstract

Teaching tools and techniques: are a teaching method comprising the principle and methods used for instruction to be implemented by teachers to achieve the desired learning or memorization by the students.

MARK OF GOOD TEACHING

1. Good teaching recognizes individual differences
2. Good teaching is a cause to learn
3. Good teaching provides opportunities for activity
4. Good teaching kindly and sympathetic
5. Good teaching involves in guiding learning
6. Reduces the distance between teachers and students
7. Good teaching is flexible and not tied to any mahouts
8. Good teaching incorporates cooperatives and suggestiveness
9. Good teaching id democratic
10. Good teaching provides desirable and selective information
11. Good teaching helps the child to adjust himself to his environment
12. Good teaching is progressive
13. Good teaching always consider the level of students
14. Good teaching leads to emotional stability
15. Good teaching is diagnostic and remedial
16. Good teaching is stimulating
17. Good teaching should be on the basis of previous knowledge of the students
18. Good teaching will develop initiative independence in thinking and dealing, self-reliance and confidence among students
19. Good teaching is carefully planned in advance.

Learning by Doing

The best way to learn is to be actively involved. Books and manuals are valuable, but their use is limited in communities where few people can read and write. Long talks without illustrations can be dull to listen to. Practical activities may be more appropriate ways of teaching and learning. Good health education helps people to work out solutions for themselves.

How to Make an Easel

You will need—Three long tree branches and String; tie the branches together at the top, and allow them to splay outwards. Boards may be rested on protruding twigs.

Using Pictures

Visual images can be a very useful way of conveying health messages. Existing materials, can be used to make posters or wall charts, and may be adapted for local use. Walls can be made into billboards for display. For small groups, a simple easel can be made to carry a blackboard, flipchart or flannel board.

How to Make Use of a Flannel Board

You will need:

- A piece of plywood, fiberboard or strong cardboard
- Soft cloth to cover the board
- Cut-out pictures

Stretch the fabric over the board and fix it at the edges. Pictures for the flannel board may be cut out of magazines, copied or drawn by the participants. To make them stick to the fabric of the board, back them with sandpaper, or smear the backs of the pictures with a paste made of flour and water, and then sprinkle wheat or rice chaff on the paste while it is still wet. Allow this to dry, and the resulting rough surface will hold the pictures in place on the soft cloth. With suitable pictures, a story can be very effectively told using a flannel board. To make your presentation as good as possible:

- Plan your presentation
- Rehearse and pre-test the presentation, preferably with a critical audience
- Use only large, clear pictures
- Do not crowd the board with too many pictures
- Lean the board slightly backwards so that the pictures stick well.

Remember to stand beside the board, not in front of it!

In Flannel board-Display material like the cut outs, pictures, drawings and light objects backed with rough surface like sand paper strips, flannel strips, etc. will stick to the flannel board temporarily. Size 1.5 × 1.5 m is used.

Copying and Adapting Pictures

When you have chosen your picture, you can copy it as illustrated below.

To make a copy the same size as the original, use squares of the same size. To make the copy bigger, use bigger squares.

1. Draw a grid of equal sized
2. Squares over the picture using a soft pencil.

3. On a blank piece of paper to be used for the poster, draw a plain grid with the same number of squares.
4. Copy the picture square by square in pencil.
5. When you have the outline, draw over it in ink.
6. Allow the ink to dry, and rub out the pencil lines.

Fill in the outline with shading and colour as required.

Adapting Pictures

Certain details in a chosen picture can be changed to more appropriate ones, for example, changing hair or clothing or combining two images to create a new picture. It can be useful (and fun) to work in a group to adapt pictures. This can be a good way to involve other people and encourage them to participate in learning activities.

Nutrition Playing Cards

Another way of using visual images is with games. These could be either board games, such as 'snakes and ladders', or picture card games. Games are a good way to involve people in active learning, which is always the most effective kind.

Games

Taking part in a game is far more interesting than listening to a talk, and the messages are more likely to be remembered. The board game illustrated shows how certain practices will result in illness, and other practices in health and growth. The card game is suitable for older children or adults, and can be used to test what knowledge has been gained, for example after a class which used flannel board or chalkboard with discussion or role playing. People can always be involved in making up their own games—they can make the rules, or just the cards and boards, for example.

Using Dolls

Keypoints about dehydrating diarrhea can be effectively illustrated using these two simple teaching aids. Children can be involved in making the 'baby' dolls and quickly learn the signs of dangerous dehydration in infants.

Gloved Baby

Learning the different signs of dehydration.

- This can be made from an old glove or sock, with an egg or stuffed ball for the head.
- Hand held straight—belly wrinkle stays
- Fingers curved—skin springs back
- When the 'belly' is pinched, the wrinkle stays
- Using a doll like this makes the test more realistic. It also turns learning into a game. In this position, wrinkles will not stay after the skin is pinched.

Pinch Here. Wrinkles Disappear

This is like the skin on the belly of a **healthy baby**.
But in this position, the pinched skin stays wrinkled for a moment—just as on the belly of a dehydrated child.

Wrinkles Stay

This is like the skin on the belly of a **dehydrated baby**.

When you show the belly wrinkle test to children, make sure they realize that the test should be done on the belly of a baby, not on the hand. You can have the children make a doll like this, out of an old glove or stocking and an egg.

Roller board or magnetic board
Easy to carry and roll and can store.

Display board is the visual teaching aid in the form of a flat surface on which information to be communicated is written or arranged in an attractive fashion the display board available are:

1. blackboard or chalkboard
2. bulletin board
3. flannel board
4. magnetic board

Black board or chalkboard may be made of wood ply hardboard. It is most common used AV aid. It can be either fixed on the wall or may be a portable. There are types which can be rolled and carried

Types of chalkboard—the ordinary adjustable, the roller types, the magnetic, black ceramic unbreakable, black or green glass, lobby stand, exhibition, double side stand, reception, tariff, paging, pressing graph perforated, write and wipe off white, information notice board, etc.

How to Make a Chalkboard

You will need:

- a sheet of plywood or fiberboard (about 5.5 × 57 cm)
- matt black paint

If possible, roughen the surface of the board before painting the first coat. Allow to dry, roughen the surface again, and apply a second coat of paint. When the paint is dry, rub the board with a cloth covered in chalk dust. This will make it easier to rub out chalk marks later.

Using chalkboard—write clearly, do not over crowed the information. Size of the letter should be large enough to be seen properly. Rub off information already discussed. Use color chalks. Use a soft cloth, duster to rub off the chalkboard. Stand on one side of the board while explaining and use a pointer while explaining.

It is convenient and economical. Only it makes chalk powder to spread and inhaled by teacher and students. It makes dull routine and makes students unable to hold the attention for long time.

Magnetic chalkboard—can combine the functions of chalkboard and flannel board both. It can be used to write with chalk sticks display pictures cut out and light objects with magnets.

Bulletin board—is the display board which shows the visual learning material on a specific subject. Relevant material related to the topic are put on the display board on the top center a time is fixed. Below the title a brief descriptions of the subject displayed. The bulletin boards must be at a good height of at least from the ground. It is a good supplementary aid. They arouse interest in specific subject. It will be used for both informational and education purposes. It can motivate, supplement and enrich learning, and stimulate thoughts. It is simple device placed either indoor or outdoor, kept in a suitable place, it can provide a suitable place for the display of all kinds of creative work. It is a soft board, which will hold pins. You use for photographs, cutout illustrations, publications, drawings, specimens, posters, newspapers and pasting important announcements. There are different types of bulletin boards, e.g. flannel board/felt board, magnetic, fixed, movable, folded type.

Laminated black or green **boards:**

1. Most durable and smooth and hard surface.
2. Unbreakable, complete with metal frame and hooks for hanging.
3. BB indicates black board.
4. GB indicates green board.
5. Size 80 cm × 60 cm or 32 inch × 24 inch.

Notice board—Typed or handwritten notices with the help of drawing pins. Size 80 × 60 cm or 32 inch × 24 inch.

White boards use of chalk on the black board, used in conference rooms and lecture room. 60 × 30 cm or 24 inch × 12 inch up to 240 × 120 cm or 96 inch × 48 inch.

Blackboard makes instruction more concrete and understandable. If used properly, it can set standards of neatness, accuracy and speed. It can restore the attention of the group. Many vague statements ca be clarified by drawing sketches, outlines, diagrams, directions and summaries. It initiates aural, visual sensation, helps in learning. It can be a means of motivation and interest. We can present facts and abstract statements can be clarified and the teacher can erase writing and drawings and start a fresh.

It should be clean and letters and drawing should be legible, avoid spelling mistakes on board, write in strait rows, do not talk as you write, face the group after writing, do not fill the board, do not stand in front of the board, can use colored chalks.

Diagram or drawing can be shown by, e.g. stick figures, science figures, geometry diagrams, facial expressions. It can be drawing which is neatly drawn in proper proportion and well labeled and explained so that it can be moved and seen from all angels.

Puppets

Old and popular art in India aid in effective aid in learning.

Specimens

Part of real object from natural settings, e.g. section of the uterus.

Objects brought from natural setting into the classroom to provide sensory experience to make instruction understandable and meaningful, vivid and impressive. It makes direct appeal to the senses, e.g. splints, forceps, and thermometers.

Diorama is a three dimensional scene in depth incorporating a group of modeled objects and figures in a natural setting. It can be set up on a small stage with a group of modeled objects kept on the foreground, which is blended into a painted realistic background. It is a 3-dimensional scene in depth incorporated a group of objects and figures in a natural setting like an harvest scene, scene from freedom struggle, an stage diorama in religious festivals like crib.

Leaflet is a single sheet of paper folded to make a full page of printed matter on single side.

Pamphlets—paper can be folded into two or three or five, the matter will be printed either single side or both sides.

Hand outs are the briefing of a session in a single sheet. It supposes to have simple, clear language with short sentences. It needs sketches, graphs that is to be drawn and labeled. You have to give title and sub-title to it, you can under line the words and use suitable colors. It can be given before or after the presentation to leave a record as well as to do follow-up.

Activity Aids

Role play/enacting is a relatively new education technique in which spontaneously act out problems. It helps in understanding others point of view.

Sketching—nature has provided us sand, material, soil and mud which can be very effective, inexpensive and are readily available which ill be used to prepare some models or illustrations and present different ideas.

Field Trips

Brings into direct contact with a real life situation, is most concrete and most real of visual technique. It co-relates and blend studies to real life outside world providing different touch with person and with community situation, help to develop observation and keenness, gives opportunity to apply that which has been taught and help to verify what has been learned. They provide actual material for study effective means of supplementing he subject of the curriculum.

Demonstrations

Co-relating theory with practice an opportunity to evaluate knowledge, used as a stronger motivational force concrete illustration. It activates several sense and increase learning.

Method of **clinical teaching** where clients care is observed, studied, discussed demonstrated and directed towards further better care by the further expert clinical guidance the skill is learnt on dummy or doll, and then the students will practice in real field under supervision which is planned, allotted and guided. After acquiring knowledge students are allowed to practice skills, discussion of problem experienced in actual client care and by applying theory in practical situation provide opportunity to gain deeper knowledge and skill where they understand entire procedure before attempting to perform.

Audio Aids Like Radio

Has emotional impact, authenticity conquest of time and space, audition, one way communication. It develops increased skill in listening provides interest and varied sources of new knowledge.

Discs

Are computer assisted devices with the help of computer use can copy either audio or videos material and display on the commuter or can take the print outs.

Tape/Cassette

Enables one to listen and hear recording previously made. Language learning is facilitating by the use of tape, the class can tape their own sings, discussions and listen in order to improve them later.

Projected Skill Slides

They are still pictures on positive film which you can process. It results in colorful, realistic, reproduction of original subject, easy to revise and update it requires skilled photography color processing is costly.

Opaque Projection

Which can project a variety of materials e.g. coins, post cards, stamps, give a large screen image in the color simple operation.

Mock-up emphasizes the functional relationship between the device reality and its workability. For example, an artificial kidney to demonstrate dialysis.

Moulage—mould can be made up of plastic material to stimulate some life object, e.g. body which shows evidence of trauma, infection, disease, surgical intervention.

Film Strips

Are sequence of transparent still pictures with individual frames on 35 mm films, they are closely related to slides are compact easily handled an always in proper sequence, inexpensive, high storage capacity, provides the multi-dimensional learning though words, graphic and problems solving. Study materials relevant to a specific topic can be stored in the computer memory and retrieved for reference. It is expensive device, produces mental and physical fatigue.

Radio played an important role in creating awareness about many new methods and techniques of agricultural practical, there by contributing to green revolution, new high yielding variety of seeds came to know. Radio is truly a mass media. A large segment of population can be reached through radio. It has the advantage of being affordable, portable and convenient. In rural areas where frequent power failure is normal, it has the tremendous advantage as it is battery operated. It can be vary effective not only in creating mass awareness and interest in new innovations or practices but also in motivating and initiating action.

TV—was 1st introduced in 1959 with objectives to facilitate the process of education and development in rural area. Color TV 1970 was introduced to see better demonstration. Today the cost of TVA has come down and is affordable. Government has planned extension services to use variety of AV aids in their efforts too reach various messages. TV is very powerful effective medium as it uses both audio visual signals. It can play an important role for its being a very visible and popular medium of mass communication.

Video and film show—very effective and have visual appeal the audience can see exactly what you are talking about, e.g. farming techniques, sanitation and health, low cost housing, immunization. It is effective tool of communication with any given target audience.

Outdoor publicity, hoardings and wall writing—common sight in villages. It can be on immunization, FP, water and sanitation or Aids. The messages are put in short and simple phrases in the form of slogans and are easy to comprehend and remember. And these stay for log period exposure for the local people.

Discussion

It is a thoughtful consideration of relationship involved in the topic or problem under study. These are analyzed, compared and evaluated for drawing conclusions.

Formal discussion pre-planned and guided, informal is free, verbal exchanges between participants. Discussion under the leadership will help to interpret and apply in suitable areas of work. In discussion pros and cons of an opinion is critically analyzed by the group members in order to decided its validity.

It gives opportunity for further clarification. Exchange of views and ideas and the conclusions ultimately results in sharing of information, it helps to defend there own view points assertively, optimum utilization of skills and knowledge is possible only in the presence of right attitude.

Discussion is the best method to draw group involvement in solving a problem will help to find a solution through polling the expertise of group members and consolidating their thinking process. It facilitates expression of ideas and interaction gives opportunities for expressing themselves, helps them to clarify the doubts in more democratic and authentic way. It is a collective effort.

Discussion involves group, it is oral, it is purposeful, systematically formed question where exchange of information, which leads to a understanding a concept to find best solution. In study group discussion students study some subject of common interest. So different purpose different types of discussions take place, e.g. work shop, staff meeting, briefing sessions, round table, decision making, public discussion, e.g. panel discussion, dialogue, symposium, forum. The individual conference, the seminar, clinical conference, role play, case analysis are the techniques of small group discussions.

Technique

Teacher can open its session with a key note address give brief introduction on topic and dictate the objectives and guidelines. Leader or facilitators role is assessment, active participation of all, motivating passive ones, allowing and inviting opinion of passive ones leading guiding clarifying different or controversial statement, avoid minister confusion, close supervision and provide adequate guidance. So that discussion proceeds in the desired manner. If any deviation she has to redirect discussion as intended. Leader summarizes the view points and ends with concluding note, if it is properly conducted, it is excellent method. Active participation results better learning and promote retention and recalling ability. It can enhance their self esteem. They learn critical thinking self confident ability and get deep knowledge.

Panel Discussion

Panel discussion is a novel method of health education. In panel discussion there is a moderator, and 4 to 8 speakers. The panel sits and discusses a given problem in front of a group or audience. The moderator opens the meeting, welcomes the group and introduces the panel speakers who are experts on the subject.

He introduces the topic briefly and invites the panel speakers to present their points of view. The discussion should be spontaneous and natural, after the panel discussion the audience are invited to talk part. When properly planed and guided panel discussion is an effective method of health education.

The chairman opens the meeting. Welcomes the group and introduces the panel speakers who are experts on the subject. He introduces the topic briefly and invites the panel speakers to present their points of view. There are no set speeches, but only informal discussion among the panel speakers. The discussion should be natural and spontaneous. The success of the panel depends upon the chairman. After the subject has been discussed by the panel speakers, the audience is invited to take part. If properly planned and guided, panel discussion can be effective methods of health education.

Symposium

A symposium is a series of speeches on the selected subject by experts. There is no discussion on the subject by the experts. At the end the audience may raise questions and contribute to the symposium.

Symposium serves as an excellent device informing an audience, crystallizing opinion and provides understanding on various aspects of theme and problems. Provides broad understanding on topic, a chairman introduces the topic, and the speakers, topic is presented and at the end brief summary given, it gives deeper insight into the topic.

In symposium two or more persons under the direction of a chairman present separate speeches, which gives several aspects of one question, followed by audience discussion. it has broad consideration of the topic, a series of related papers are presented.

Seminar

It is a form of class organization-analysis of a problem chosen for discussion. It is a organized guided discussion. In this teacher is a leader, in this 10–15 members are participating, duration is 1–2 hours, all members take part, in this role of a student is active when they have background knowledge and seminar gives training for self-learning and ability to see and solve our own problems is developed. It promotes group sprit and cooperation.

Projected Aids

In projected aids, a bright light is shown through a transparent picture, and by means of a lens, an enlarged picture is thrown, or projected, on to a screen. The viewer's attention is compelled towards a bight picture in a darker room. Interest is created, destructions avoided. A large number of people can see the illustration. Advance technology in photography, and film processing have put into the hands of the educator a powerful new medium.

The epidiascope—projects the image of a solid object. Bight light is concentrated upon an solid object and the brilliant illuminated image is reflected by a mirror through a very large lens on to a screen. An epidiascope can project a wide variety of material and makes the teacher independent of standard transparent material. He can project flat pictures, postcard and photographs, book illustrations, tables of statistics, handwork diagrams, pupils work, watches, coin, nature study samples, maps, etc. This ability to compel attention, materials can be updated. It can project images or printed matter or small opaque objects on a screen. Any diagram or picture can be projected on a screen without tearing it off from the book. It works on the principle of horizontal straight line projection with a lamp, plane mirror placed at 45 degree angle over the projects so that it passes through the projection lens forming a magnificent image on the screen.

OHP—overhead projection—Still pictures can be projected on a screen to supplement teaching, e.g. slid, film straps. OHP is a versatile visual aid using a system of lean, mirror and lamp; transparencies are projected on to a screen in a way that enables teacher to face the students while teaching. Teachers can maintain eye contact while teaching. The OHP can be used in daylight allowing students to take notes. OHP is user friendly.

The overhead projector (OHP) is visuals teaching aids. It needs low voltage, light weight, metal body and single Halogen lamp. OHP transparencies, accessories projection screen. It projects transparencies with brilliant screen images suitable for use in a lighted room. The teacher faces the class as she uses OHP, and the class views the projections. It is used as aid and tool in teaching-learning situation. It offers a very flexible tool for teaching as wide varity of materials can be used for many different teaching purposes. Materials projected can be changed easily and quickly, shape can be presented and compared.

1. **There are teacher made transparencies**- which permits the teacher to stand in front of the class while using the projector by pointing to the material at the project and at the same time she can observe the reactions to her teaching. To make marginal notes on the transparences for the use of the teacher that can be carried without exposing them to the class, when projected. To give the illusion of motion in the transparency, e.g. Circulation of blood through the heart, through the use of a special device attached to the OHP, this termed as "technimation".
2. Commercial made transparencies.
3. Xeroxed transparencies made from copper.

Computer may also be used for teaching. This is effective in class room education eg power point programmed prepared and displayed LCD, etc.

Powerpoint LCD/laptop display—becoming common in workshops, seminars, conferences, CME. It is very quick, clear and informative, interesting, holds and captures attention, vast pictures and data can be stressed, easy to show and highlight point with anew as it displaced on a screen and becomes easy for a person to explain as points are on the screen and students too can make note of important matter.

TV is a powerful medium for mass education; these are found nearly every home. They are potent instruments of education. Many talented, specialized brain acts, talk, display, depict and many good messages communicated. You have to choose the programs. TV gives entertainment, relaxation, multichannel, multi stationed, multilanguages available. If you use for good purpose of learning and educating purpose and see with critical thinking and evaluate and filter through your mind. Do not get addicted to it. Television because it is a visual as well as an aural medium it has a far greater impact than radio, and far more absorbing, claiming the child's whole attention. As it is a transmitted aid.

Television is the electronic means by which sound and light energy are transmitted from one place to another. It offers vitality and newness, which attracts attention, creates interest and stimulates a desire to learn. It is a multi dimensional and general medium of communication. Instructional television broadcasts designed to aid instruction that is planned in relation to educational objectives and enrichment TV designed towards learning. Educational TV combines sight and sound together and offers opportunities of seeing and listening to the scenes and events.

Radio talks to be of 15 minutes. Radio can describe events as they happen. Through the combined effect of voice, environmental sound and music can be captured and the imagination stirred. Student's knowledge can be enriched by listening to an good topic and radio can bring outside world into the class room. She can increase skill of listening and feed back what she has heard, can take into discussion, get new knowledge and students gets well informed, they acquaint the student with the social effects of scientific discoveries. It is one of the mass-media that can be used to inform the public of the objectives and need for nursing education. Develops critical thinking. Broadcasts are effective means of presenting music, drama for study. Concentrate on the programme, thinking about what is said and what it really means. Helps her to listen with open mind another person's point of view, problem arise when concentration and attention breaks, it is only one way communication.

Tape recording—Is two-way communication, it can be made to play at desire and teaching need. It can be used for introducing a lesson, for illustrating some facts or skills, for summing up a topic. A gramophone record inculcates a love of good music, to teach songs, famous speech, languages and good pronunciation. Tape records are not easily damaged and can be played many more times. You can hear your own voice; students can tape their own singing, classroom programme and listen to it later on.

Videotapes played through TV—films on educational topics shown through TV in the classroom.

Video cassettes can be used as AV aids easy, useful and students understand more easily.

Films are very expensive to produce, and they out dated very quickly, Film show attracts large gathering and is mass communication media.

Motion-pictures—communicating through sound and sight simultaneously, the motion pictures blend pictures, words, objects, motion, and even color to make impact on the students mind. The viewer sees motion that can be recreated, objects can be enlarged or reduced, it makes experience fresh and can make distant past the present relieve in the classroom. For example, if you go to Gandhi ashram you are given a chance to see this light and sound programme here you can hear the sound of a train and at the same time you can see how Gandhi was thrown out from the running train at the same time. Also at Christmas time in big ponds the crib is prepared and light and sound aid through the effect is given to see for the public how herod comes how the innocent children are killed, how shepherds, kings visit the Bethlehem etc.

Health Museums

A good health museum is effective mass media education. For example, exhibited important photographs, music instruments, cultural items, peoples lifestyles, utensils, articles etc.

It can attract large number of people.

Slides sets—2 inch × 2 inch colored 35 cm slides each set contains 20 slides.

Museum

It is made up of materials used in the classroom teaching which in many cases are collected, classified and exhibited. They may be incorporated into a scientific experimental method of teaching

- Permit visual instruction actual museum specimen
- Stimulate enthusiasm for study
- Stimulate interest, cooperation and participation
- Records and record player.

A new digital learning system uses the classic children game to bring interactivity and exercise to education. It can also be used for physical therapy in adults. Researchers have developed a learning system that can motivate the user to move. They have combined a sensor mat with an activity monitor. Children and adults can use the system to stay fit and learn at the same time.

Technological change is now so rapid and so unpredictable that no one can say how we will be communicating in 20 years time. However the SMS messages have been defining texts of the past two decade.

Digital marketing one of the most popular and upcoming career option social media marketing is the new age technique used by corporates to reach out to consumers to reach out to consumers. Digital and social media marketing deals with promoting beands, products and service on digital platform like facebook, twitter, linked In etc. it needs a high level of expertise and can pave way for a bright career.

Therefore, nurse should be quick in making decisions and should be enough knowledgeable, because delay may cause the life of the client, nurse herself should be aware of the linkage system, She should be aware of the categories of the clients, so she can make the priorities. She should discuss their difficulties, review her work plans, exchange experience; To take initiative and interest, to communicate ideas clearly, to develop good rapport, to show interest in learning, Life is a "do-it yourself project". It is safe to look within; change can begin in this moment. Expect future obstacles and difficulties. Do not pretend they do not exist. Remember, there is a good side to every situation. Have the courage to be your own constructive critic. Do your best and hope for the best outcome Because, It will help us to improve the skills or levels of knowledge so that wee can be better equipped.

Explanation—Education is a progressive discovery of our own ignorance.

Keywords

Good teaching, learning by doing, Easel, pictures, flannel board, copying and adapting, nutrition playing cards, games, display board, using dolls, glove baby, chalkboard, magnetic board, bulletin board, specimens, puppets, activity aids, field trip, demonstration, audio aids, TV, projected slides, cassettes, discussion, symposium, technique, seminars, panel discussion, projected aids, OHP, LCD, radio, tape recorder, health museum.

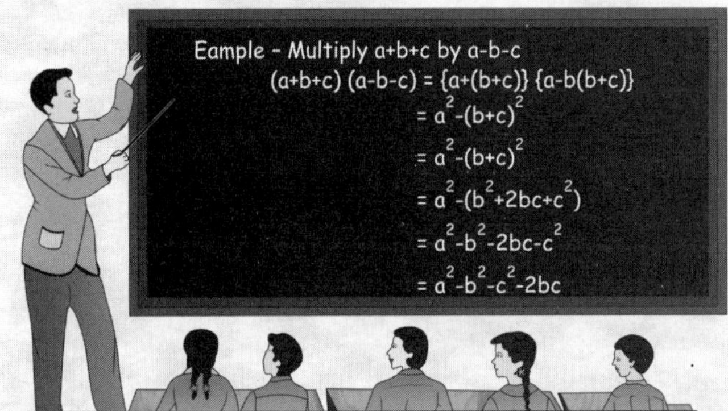

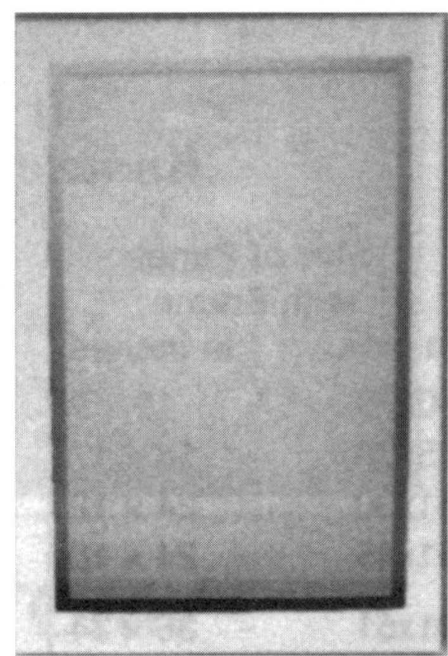

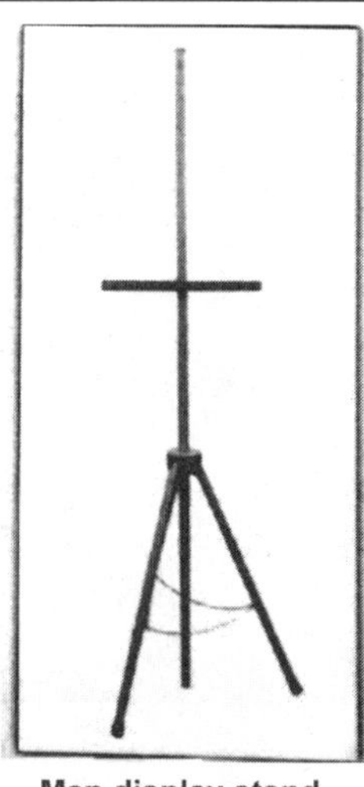

Map display stand

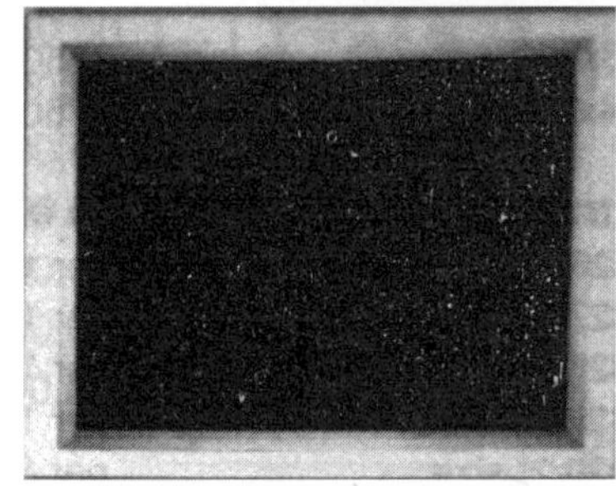

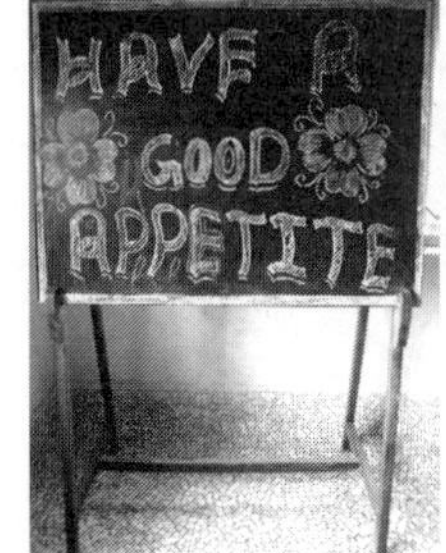

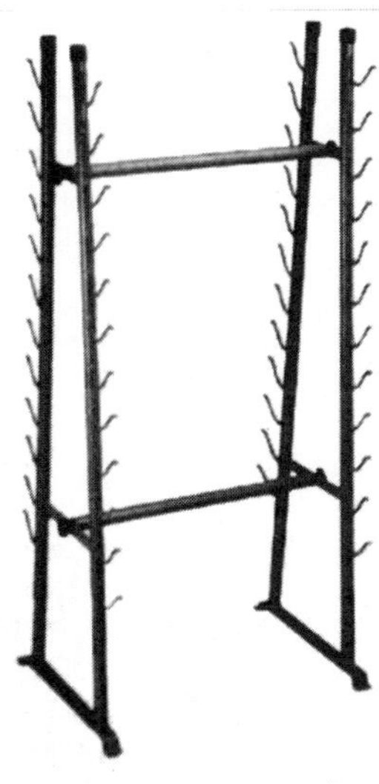

Map storage stand

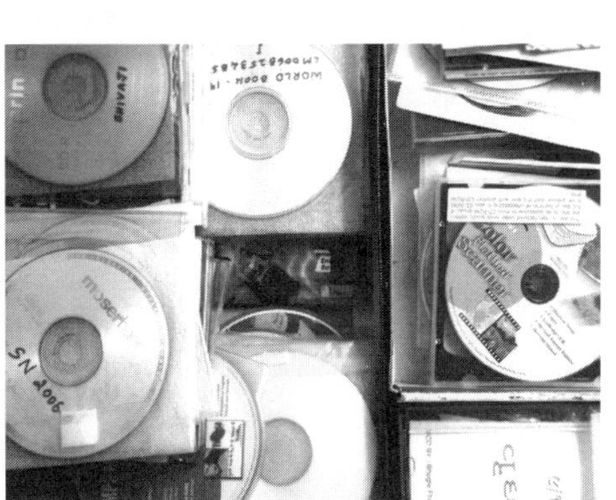

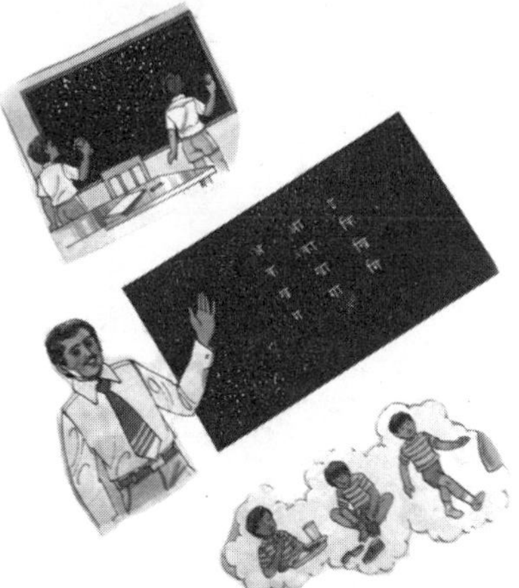

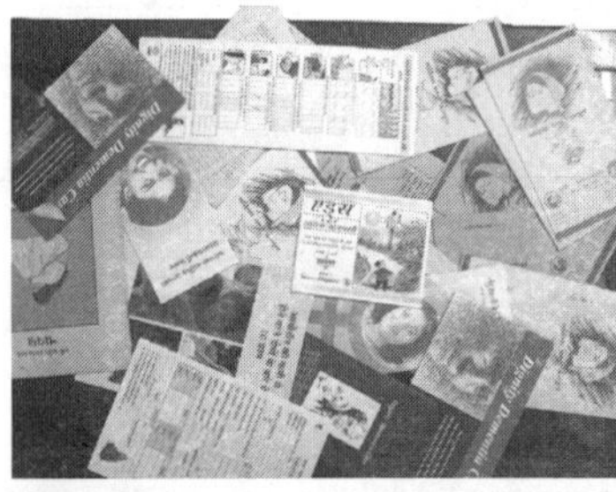

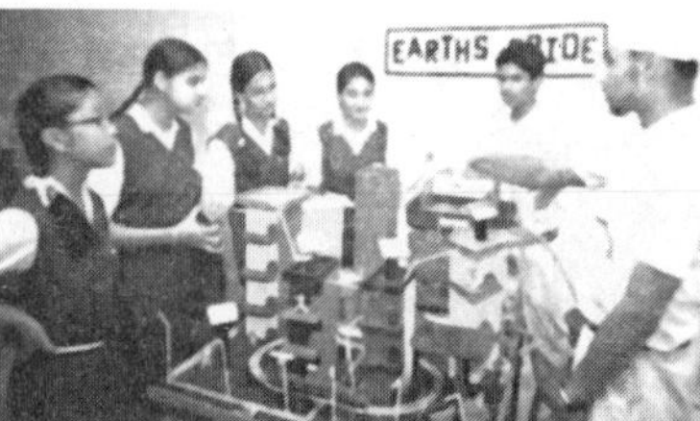
EARTHS PRIDE

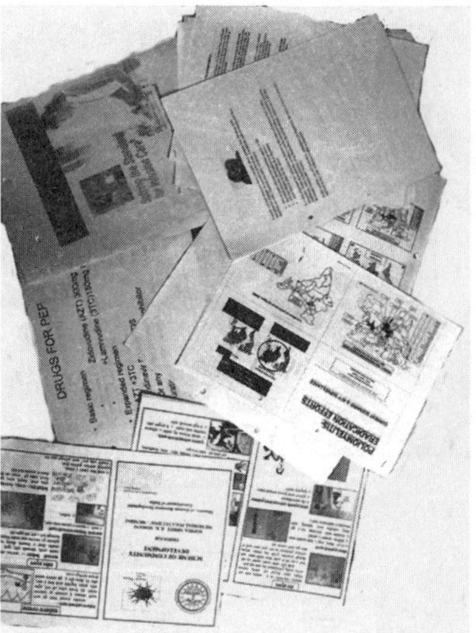
DRUGS FOR PEF

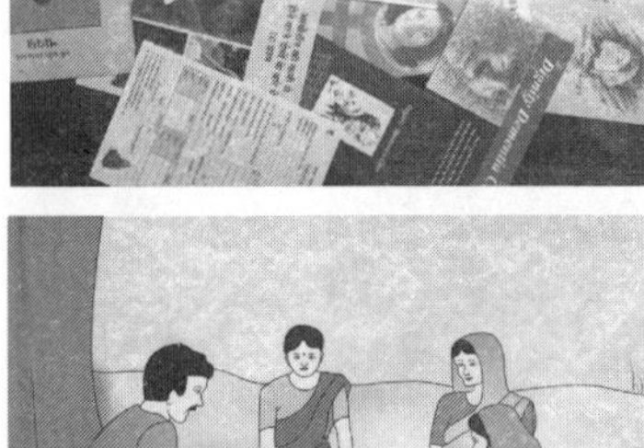

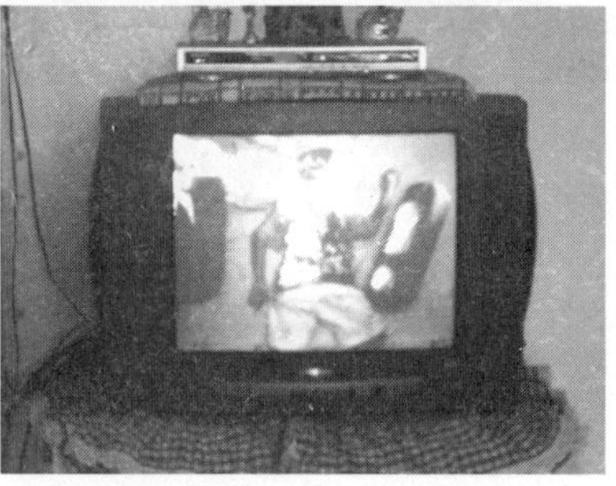

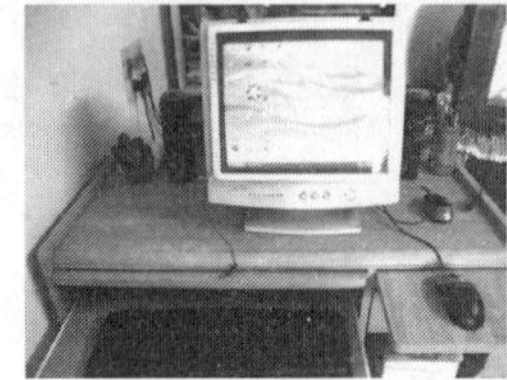

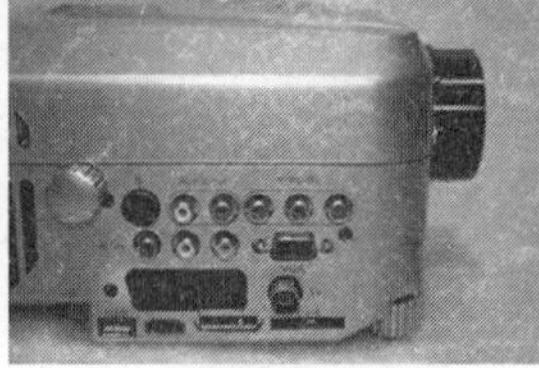

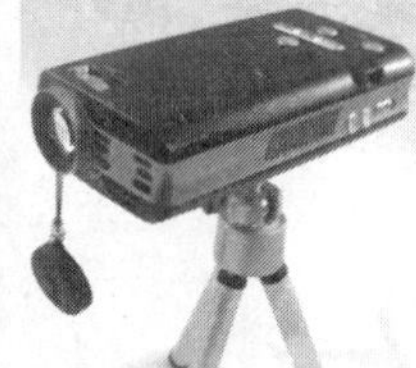

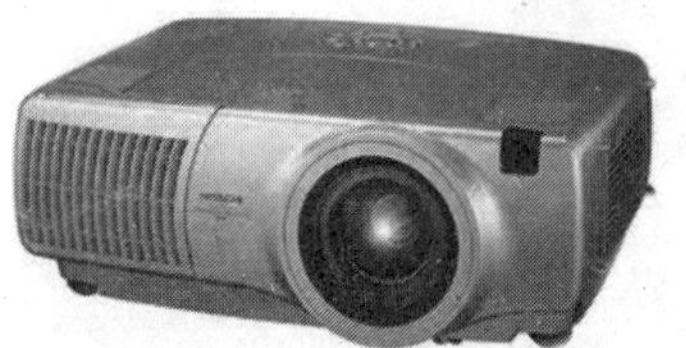

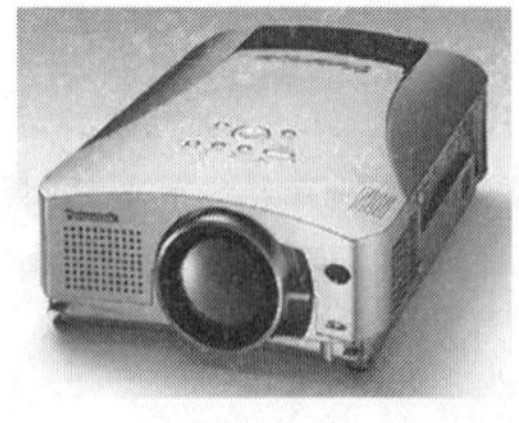

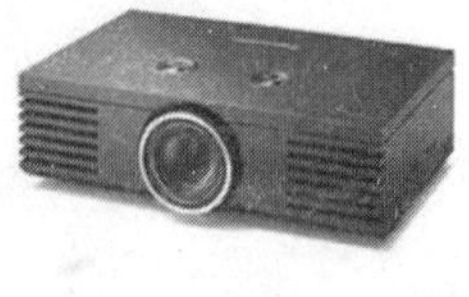

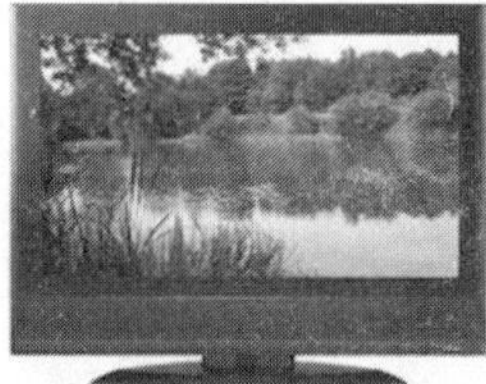

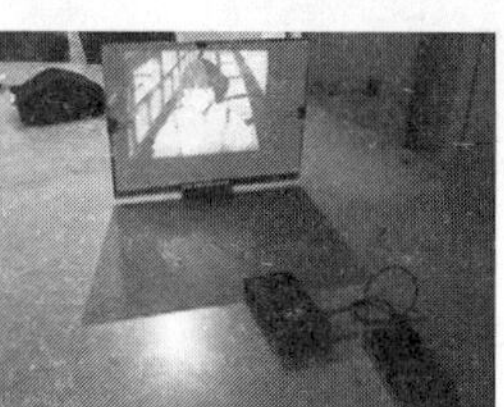

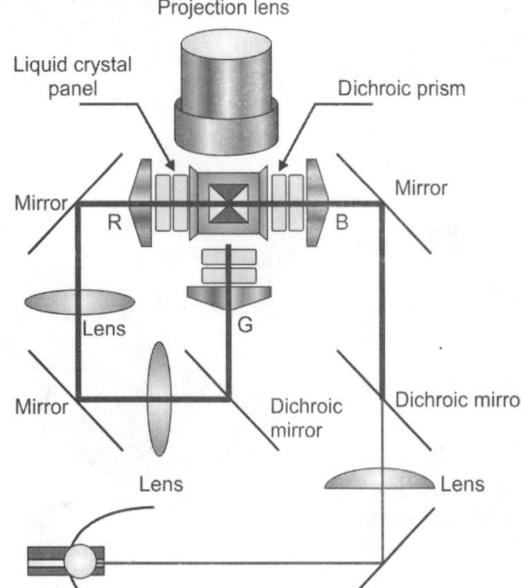
Projection lens
Liquid crystal panel
Dichroic prism
Mirror
Mirror
R
B
Lens
G
Mirror
Dichroic mirror
Dichroic mirror
Lens
Lens
Lamp

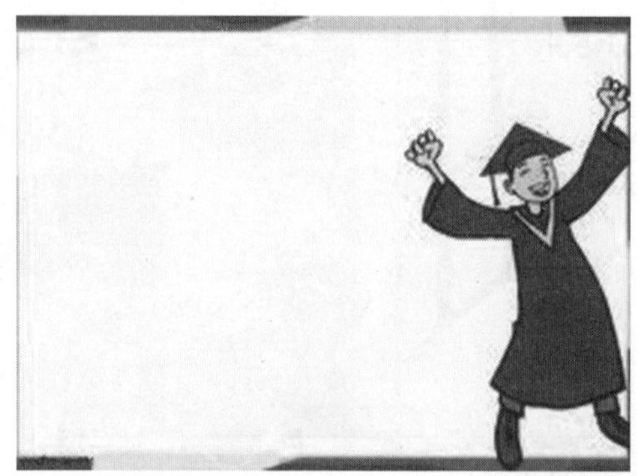

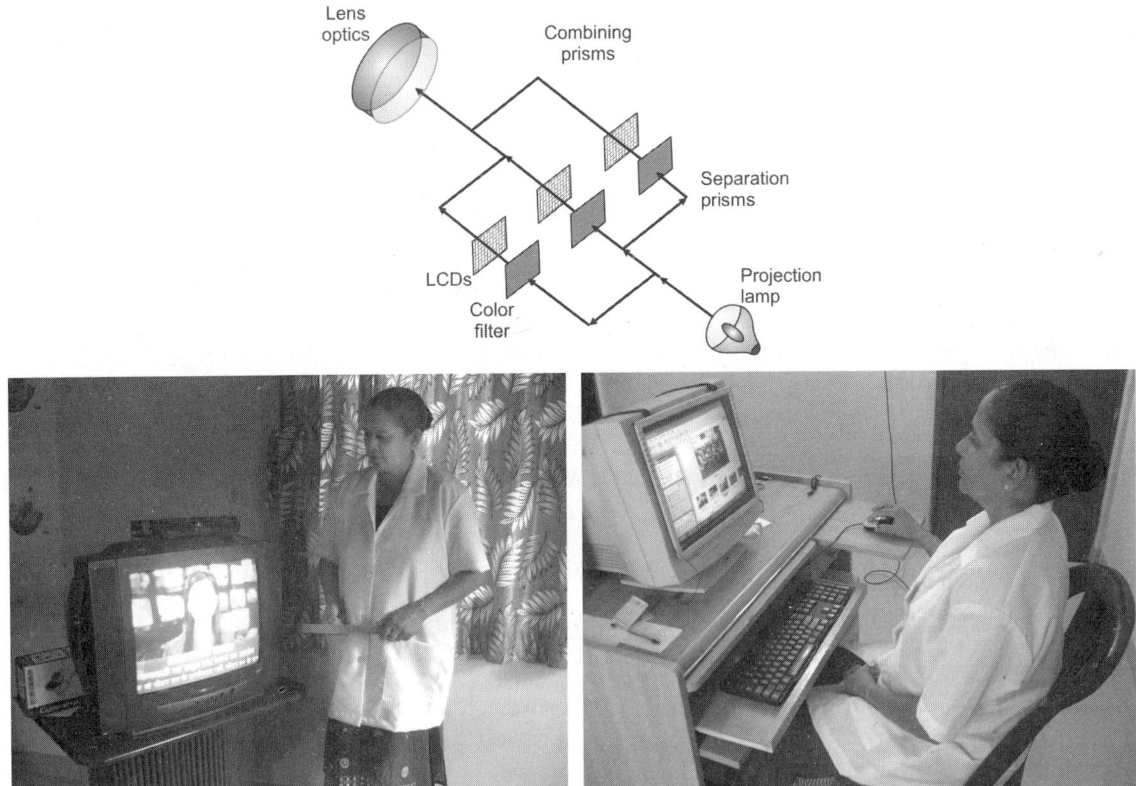
Lens optics
Combining prisms
Separation prisms
LCDs
Color filter
Projection lamp

CHAPTER

47

Health Guidance on HIV/AIDS

Abstract

HIV/AIDS (Acquired Immunodeficiency Syndrome) is a chronic, potentially life-threatening condition caused by the human immunodeficiency virus. By damaging your immune system, HIV interferes with your body's ability to fight the organisms that cause disease.

INTRODUCTION

In giving health education the nurse has to refer many more books, magazines and other sources to get complete subject matter that she needs to teach a lesson plan on the selected topic. She has to think first what AV aids she is going to use to explain the concept clearly and distinctively. What topic she has selected has to be clear and people should understand the matter in a simple manner. She can give lecture cum hold discussions and question answer session. She can conclude the topic and give summary of it. The topic to be interesting she can use different communication skills, awareness songs can be sung, power point programme can be done, can use over head projector, charts and posters or flannel graph, skits, role play etc.

She will have the following format to be followed with specific objectives, introduction of the self and the topic, definition, causes, sign symptoms, investigations, treatment and most important prevention and control part has to be covered.

Format

Specific objective	Subject matter	Method of teaching	AV aids	Evaluation

Aim—to make the public understand the growing magnitude of problem of HIV/AIDS.

Students have to be clear the group of people she is going to address, the place, time and the AV aids she is going to use it.

The problem of AIDS is increasing in magnitude every year. According to new estimates about 2.5 million cases are seropositive for HIV in the country. HIV—the global scenario if we see we find 33 million people are with it in that we find 2.7 million became infected with HIV virus, 2 million died of HIV related cause. We had first case 1986 reported in Chennai (prevalence in antenatal women an high risk group) HIV infected 1.2 lakh in India in 2009—33.3 million across the world were living with HIV. In 2009—One in four AIDS deaths was caused by TB. In 2009, there were 2.6 million new HIV infections, down for 3.1 million in 1999. Ten million till do not have access to ART-AIDS related deaths among children declined from 18.000 in 2004 to 15,000 in 2009 a 15% drop. An estimated 3.6 lakh were newly infected with HIV in 2009 in Asia as compared to 4.5 lakh in 2001. AIDS killed 1.8 million globally in 2009.

Around 3.7 lakh children were born with HIV in the same year.

OBJECTIVES

1. Explain the magnitude of HIV/AIDS
2. Provide comprehensive and holistic care to the patient utilizing family centered and multidisciplinary team approach.
3. Assessments and patient education and social support.

Specific Objectives

1. To explain the group of people about definition of aids.
2. To explain the group of people about epidemiological factors of aids.
3. To explain the group of people about signs and symptoms of aids.
4. To explain the group of people about control and prevention of aids.
5. To explain the group of people about nursing care of aids and national aids control program.

To explain the group of people about definition of aids

AIDS (Acquired Immunodeficiency Syndrome) is a fatal illness. It is caused by a virus known as human immune deficiency virus (HIV). Once infected, it is probable that a person will be infected for life. AIDS breaks down the body's immune system exposing the individual to numerous life-threatening infections, neurological disorders and malignancies.

To explain the group of people about epidemiological factors of AIDS:

Agent—HIV virus; source of infection HIV cases and carriers; infective material is blood and semen of infected persons, body fluids; age sexually active persons from 20 to 49 years; high risk groups like prostitutes, homosexuals, intravenous drug users, etc. immunity man has no natural immunity, mode of transmit ion is aids is transmitted by sexually that is usual way, transmitted through blood, unsterile materials, injections, prenatal transmission that is by mother to fetus before and during birth, incubation period is 6 years and more.

To explain the group of people about signs and symptoms of AIDS:
Major sings are weight loss, chronic diarrhea for more than one month, prolonged fever more than one month. Minor sings like persistent cough for more than one month, generalized pruritic dermatitis, recurrent herpes zoster, or pharyngeal candidacies, chronic progressive herpes simplex infection, generalized lumphadenopathy

To explain the group of people about control and prevention of AIDS:
Education—until a vaccine or cure is found the only means at present available is health education to enable people to make safe, life-saving choices. Prevention of blood borne HIV transmission, people in high risk group should be urged to refrain from donating blood, body organs, and all blood should be screened for HIV before transmission, strict sterilization practices should be ensured and one should absolutely avoid injections unless they are absolutely necessary. Specific prophylaxis antiviral chemotherapy, primary health care, mother and child health care, family planning education.

To explain the group of people about nursing care of AIDS and National AIDS Control Program:
The numbers of infected people is going to increase greatly over the coming years as the time passes, a great number of nurses will be involved in the care of people with HIV/AIDS. At various stages different problems call for specific services and nursing skills effects must be made to reduce the fear and discrimination towards HIV-infected persons in community. As a nurses can provide supportive and caring response to infected individuals. Educate and counsel on preventing the spread of infection. Counsel the woman who are infected to to have pregnancy and if pregnancy does occur strict antenatal care is desirable and delivery should be conducted in hospital. During delivery full infection control precautions must be observed. The over all goal of care is to prevent relieve physical symptoms and maximize level of functioning. Nursing intervention in diarrhea, nausea and vomiting, fever, dysentery, pain, fatigue and weakness, skin problems depression etc. the focus of nursing care at the end of life is concentrated on palliative care, physical emotional comfort, counseling and spiritual care to both family and person. Following the guidelines of safety of nurses is precautions in handling infected blood and other body fluids. Precautions in relation to injections and skin piercing, and effective use of sterilization and disinfection. Hand washing is a single most important procedure for the prevention of infection. Nurses should wear gloves for all direct contact with blood and body fluids.

In family center approach—Assisting them in managing their own care, helping them in adhering to lifelong ART. Increasing their capacity for home-based care of the PLHAS. The family plays an important role in an individual life in terms of support and Providing care.

Nurses role in patient education and counseling—pre-test and post-test counseling, HIV testing, transmission and disease progression, diet and nutrition, discuss issues in confidence, educate them on transmission, prevention and ART etc. **Every person has the right to live with dignity and confidentiality**. Screening for safety purpose, safe blood supply, if husband and wife both positive, discuss family planning options, explain about the consequences of having child, need to practice safe sex, unwanted disclosure should be prohibited, allow disclosure to sexual or needle sharing partner, motivate for partner notification and testing, empowerment of individual to become responsible for their health and well-being, Prevent of parent to child HIV transmission. Educate PLHAS to preserve human life, not to infect deliberately. Nurses could play a vital role in handling networking, to meet legal and ethical issues related to person with HIV/AIDS. Motivate the patients for following conditions testing—STI, TB, chronic diarrhea, weight loss, chronic fever, chronic cough, herpes zoster, oral candidacies, recurrent oral ulcers and lymphadenopathy, pregnant women. BMW management regulation should be imposed.

Explain what is the immune system?

1. Immune system protects and defends the body from infections
2. WBCs is the most important part of the immune system.
3. WBCs fights and destroys bacteria, fungi and viruses that enter the body.
4. CD4 cells, it is also known as helper T cell or CD4 lymphocyte.
5. It is types of blood cell that caries CD4 receptor on its surface and fights infection.
6. It signals other cells in the body's immune system to perform their special functions and coordinates immune response.
7. The number of CD4 cells is a sample of blood is an indicator of the health of immune system. HIV infects and kills CD4 cells, leading to a weakened immune system
8. HIV is the virus that weakens the immune system.
9. The collective presence of different opportunistic infections, as a result of immune deficiency is known as AIDS. CD4 count in an HIV infected individual is less than 200.

How HIV causes AIDS?

Viral replication leads to decrease CD4 cell reducing the body's capacity to fight infection. The individual becomes more susceptible to opportunistic infection. AIDS is characterized by the presence of opportunistic infection

What is the difference between HIV and AIDS?

HIV is a virus and AIDS is a diseases. HIV infection leads to AIDS depending on body's defense mechanism. AIDS is acquired not inherited.

Why are women at higher risk for infection?

Due to large amount of mucosal surface area in the vagina there is a pooling of semen during intercourse. When they have STD, when they undergo menopause due to fragile vaginal tract?

How is HIV diagnosed?

Three tests are done before declaring whether as person is HIV positive or negative. If the person is in the window period the person is advised to return for HIV testing again. The tests are antigen or antibody based tests. HIV antibody based tests are rapid test TriDot, immuncomb, Elisa test.

Progression of AIDS

1. Among individual is variable with some individual it is rapid as within 1–2 years.
2. While others remain healthy for many years.
3. When HIV first enters the body, the immune system recognizes the "antigen" and a cause's flu; like symptoms.
4. During this time, HIV viral load is high and therefore infected person is highly infectious and can easily transmit virus to others during this time.
5. During this "window period" the person although infected, test negative for HIV antibodies.
6. Early immune depletion CD4 > 500 level of virus is low. Advanced immune depletion CD4 > 200, AIDS is having a CD4 count of less than 200.

What is counseling?

1. Counseling services are the back born confidential dialogue between a person and a care provider aimed at enabling the person to cope with stress and make person decision to HIV/AID effective counselor in effective communication. Be positive, focused, make the listener comfortable, ask for a feedback, and emphasize important points. Ensure privacy and comfort. Be sure patient is ready for the information schedule at a convenient time of the patient
2. **Palliative care** in PLHA is the active total care of patients whose diseases does not respond to curative treatment. Freedom from pain, discomfort, functional ability, undue anxiety, fears, feeling of hope, meaning to life, relief of suffering etc.
3. **Pain management**—pain is an unpleasant sensory and emotional experience associated with actual or potential tissue damage; pain is whatever the experiencing says it is, existing whenever the person says it does. During end stage of life, PLHAs can experience tremendous pain and suffering. Providing relief from this pain is a crucial component of palliative care.

Types of Pain

1. Acute—person; looks sick, produces a change in vital signs, diaphoresis, pallor
2. Chronic—pain for more than three months
3. Somatic—soft tissue and bone pain, sharp, throbbing, aching, muscle pain, cramping, gripping, clenching
4. Visceral—direct stimulation of intact receptors, in deep visceral organs like heart, lung, etc. difficult to localized, deep aching, cramping pressure or colicky
5. Neurological—results from disordered function or direct damage to nerves of peripheral, spinal or CNS. Difficult to treat effectively. Peripheral burning shooting, spinal cord, constant dull aching with neurological deficits. CNS changes in vital signs, nausea, vomiting increased intracranial pressure

Assessment of Pain

As experience differs, so greatly from one person to another

1. Assess which part is involve
2. Is it localized or radiating
3. Is it referred
4. What other symptoms are present
5. Anorexia, congestive problems, constipation, diarrhea, difficulty swallowing, dyspnea, fatigue, fever, nausea, neck stiffness, neurological symptoms, seizures, skin problems
6. What increases the pain changing position, lack of medication, fear, lack of support, family problem, lack of care, mood, etc.
7. Why has not the patient done anything about diseases pain
8. Is the patient already on any medication for pain
9. What has been done to reduce pain so far
10. Type of pain
11. Is it burning, sharp, pulsing, tingling, flashes of pain, what is the duration
12. Is the patient chemically dependent on painkillers
13. Level of pain—mild pain, between 1 and 3 on a 10 pain scale
14. Moderate pain—between 2 and 6 on point 10 scale
15. Severe pain—between 7 and 10 on point scale.

Complimentary Pain Control Measures

1. Apart from providing relief with drugs nurses can also provide lot of relief by giving massage, backrubs, cool cloths touch.

2. Keeping patient's room quiet, well-ventilated, addressing any emotional and spiritual concerns that may impact pain and discomfort.
3. Ensuring a comfortable bed and peaceful atmosphere.
4. Teaching breathing exercise.
5. Nurses can address psychological aspects.
6. Majority of people with AIDS are young and it is difficult to watch people in their prime years and children suffer and die of AIDS.
7. Stigma associated with HIV can be towards the patient and their families.

Principles—respect the identity and integrity. Be sensitive and non judgmental. Know when to listen and when to speak. Have the knowledge and skills to intervene in a way that promotes best possible quality of life.

Dimensions

1. Diminished functional status
2. Spending 50% of day in bed
3. Progressive dependencies
4. Dementia
5. When medical treatment is no longer effective
6. Advance diseases
7. CD4 persistently low <50
8. End stage organ diseases
9. Renal, hepatic or cardiac failure
10. Multi drug resistance or failure
11. When the patient decides that he no longer wants aggressive treatment
12. Desire of patient for death
13. Acknowledgment by patient and family of poor prognosis.

Philosophy

1. Affirms life and makes dying a normal process.
2. Neither hasten not postpones death.
3. Provide relief from pain and other symptoms.
4. Takes holistic approach to care.
5. Integrates the clinical with the psychological and spiritual.
6. Provide support to both the family and the patient.

Explain needle stick injury—to asses the incidence of reported and unreported needle stick injuries. To assess the existing knowledge pertaining to it and its prevention

To prepare and validate a protocol related to it. Working in any clinical areas carries a risk and exposure of infectious diseases and needle stick injuries are among the most prevalent routes of infection. It takes place accidentally when disposing conceal in linen, garbage, unexpectedly recapping and improper disposal. Handling potentially infective materials unacceptable way Precautious expose to blood born diseases, hepatitis C&B HIV, blood and body fluids, training universal safety precaution. Research for safer medical devices Due to unreported injury makes it difficult to know how serious the problem is and how well prevention program works. For example, HIV transmission rate of 0.3% injury HCV risk 3–10% HBV 5–40% It means physical harm or wound caused by pointed hollow end of a slender piece of metal, needles, syringes, scalpel, succors, when skin is accidentally punctured. Register, identify safeguarding the health rights of employees and bring standardization of procedure in hospital. Reporting and documentation will help. Condition of work, difficult patient care situation, working at night reduced lighting, inexperienced or new staff, recapping that is single most cause, improper disposal in regular garbage, inappropriate discarding. Lack of basic protective barriers like gloves and mask and absolutely no training for universal precaution.

Nursing alert and precautions while doing following work:

When nurse handles surgical blades, needles left on trolley for staffs to clear up after procedure.

- While administrating injury abrupt movement of patient during and after injection and suddenly get a needle prick.
- Safe working practice and significant elements in the prevention not observed.
- Uniformity in practice incinerated and dumped is not practiced as per protocol.
- When there is unavailability of resources and facilities like counseling. All these above points to be kept in while doing any procedure of HIV/AIDS.

Antiretroviral therapy (ART) a boon to people living with HIV/AIDS

Principles of antiretroviral therapy

1. Limiting the viral replication and protecting injured immune system
2. Monitoring plasma viral load and CD4 count prior to ART and then very 3–6 months on treatment
3. In resource limited setting, ART can be offered to patients with current HIV related complication and high plasma viral load
4. The goal of therapy is maximum achieved suppression
5. Correct combination of effective anti-HIV drugs
6. Correct dosage antiretroviral drugs
7. Women should receive optimal ART irrespective of pregnancy status
8. ART counseling.

Assessment after Starting the Treatment

Once therapy has begun, there should be additional clinical and lab monitoring includes

1. Assessment for signs, symptoms of potential drug toxicities
2. Adherence counseling and assessment of adherence
3. Assessment of response to therapy and signs of treatment failure
4. Weight measurement
5. CD4 testing at last every 6 months
6. Hemoglobin monitoring for patients on AZT

7. At the minimum, monitoring should take place 2, 4, 8, 12 and 24 weeks after treatment begins and then ever 6 months once the patient has stabilized on therapy.

Multidisciplinary Team Effort

ART care—needs physician, social worker, pharmacist, community worker, nurse and patient.

Nurse's Responsibility

1. With physician coordinates patient care and treatment
2. Developing a trusting and supportive relationship with patient
3. A family centered multidisciplinary team approach to care is beneficial; to patient
4. Educating patient on need to strictly adhere to doses. Encouraging him to be regular and educate him on the consequences of missed doses, also encouraging him to discuss freely his reaction to art
5. The nurse recognizes and values each team members contribution
6. The nurse recognizes and values, each team members contribution
7. The nurse is the key resources in referring patients to support from the community and other linkages services
8. Strict monitoring for complication
9. Critical components of the successful treatment of patients in which nurses role is crucial.

The availability of new drugs and drug combination to combat HIV infection has translated into progressive clinical benefits for patients. We have entered an era of improved therapeutic success with reduced rates of opportunistic infections and hospitalization. Nurse's role is crucial.

What is meant by multidisciplinary team approach?

1. A nurse is its member and coordinators the plan of care.
2. She assesses the physical, social and psychological needs of the patient.
3. Provides care and support. Educate and counsel PLHAS on safe sex practice including condom use, facilitate positive living.

National AIDS Control Program—realizing the gravity of epidemiological situation Government of India launched a national control AIDS program in 1987 the components of the program are information, education and communication, blood safety, control of STD, condom promotion, surveillance and clinical management.

An aid is an invisible killer. So, realization of human rights and fundamental freedom for all is essential to reduce vulnerability. Respect for the rights of people living with HIV/AIDS drives an effective response.

Students have to create the creative tools and techniques to prepare there topic. Here I am giving few pictures just to understand the concept of the lesson plan.

Clinical trials on AIDS vaccine-Pune the new AIDS vaccine trial will be in as prime boost regimen, which is a way of combining two different vaccines—ADVAX and TBC-M4—get better response from the body's immune system rather than giving either vaccine alone.

IMPORTANT POINTS

1. Management of needle stick injury- wash with soap and water; allow to bleed; apply antiseptic (70% alcohol); report to clinician.
2. Solid waste that is non infectious put in black bag (e.g. Office waste, wrapping paper, cartons, plastic sheets, newspapers etc.).
3. Solid waste that is infectious put in yellow bag the non sharper, e.g. Tissues (placenta) human organs (amputated part).
4. Red bags put IV tubing, blood bags, casts, gloves, etc.
5. Sharps put in puncture proof container that is used needles, scalpels, blades etc.
6. Magnitude of risk (HIV) depends upon prevalence of infection in the population; frequency of exposure, concentration of the virus, depth of the wound; average risk after percutaneous exposure to HIV infected blood, 0.3% and mucous membrane exposure 0.09%.
7. Disposal of dead body—wash with water; 2:1 sodium hypochlorite solution; nose and mouth are plugged with cotton swab soaked with appropriate dilution, disposal in electric crematorium.
8. Negative impact—lack of education about HIV disease, denial, anxiety, or depression, alcohol or drug use, poor social situation, inadequate health insurance, number of medications/pills, frequency of dosing, stringent dosing requirement and presence of side effects all these are negative impact on adherence.
9. Intervention to improve adherence—take time to educate and explain goals of therapy and need for adherence, develop concrete plan for specific regimen, minimize dosing frequency and number of pills, simplify food requirements, inform patient about potential side effects, and anticipate and treat them, avoid adverse drug interactions, provide written schedule, pictures of medications, pill boxes, and mechanical aids, recruit family and friends to support treatment plan.
10. Pre-testing counseling—provide information on HIV test and its variables, ensure that the test is informed and voluntary, facilitate HIV and other medical risk assessment, HIV infection prevention and appropriate treatment, facilitate the use of social support systems and mechanisms

Selection of protective barriers		
Type of exposure	*Protective barriers*	*Examples*
Low risk—contact skin, no visible blood	Gloves helpful but not essential	Injections, minor wound dressing
Medium risk—probable contact with blood, splashing unlikely	Gloves, gowns and apron be necessary	Vaginal exam, IV cannula insertion or removal, handling lab specimens
High risk—probable contact with blood, splashing, uncontrolled bleeding	Gloves, waterproof gown or apron, eyewear, mask	Major surgical procedures especially orthopedic and oral surgery, vaginal delivery

11. In post test counseling—appropriate disclosure of test result, to facilitate an appropriate emotional response, to reinforce issues discussed in pre-test counseling, to facilitate action plans and to promote continuity in interactions.

Selection of Protective Barriers

Note—this is the topic that is covered here in short, the nurse has to work on it and make according to the group of people she will be addressing, the situation and field of areas she wants to communicate she will have to do the necessary changes and adapt to the situation as per need.

Keywords

Introduction, format, objectives, explain, cause, why, type, diagnosis, progression, assessment counseling, principles, dimensions, philosophy, nurses' responsibility, important points, multidisciplinary team approach.

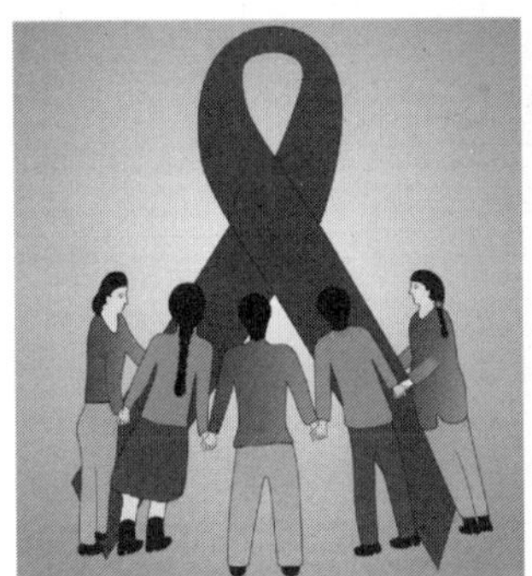

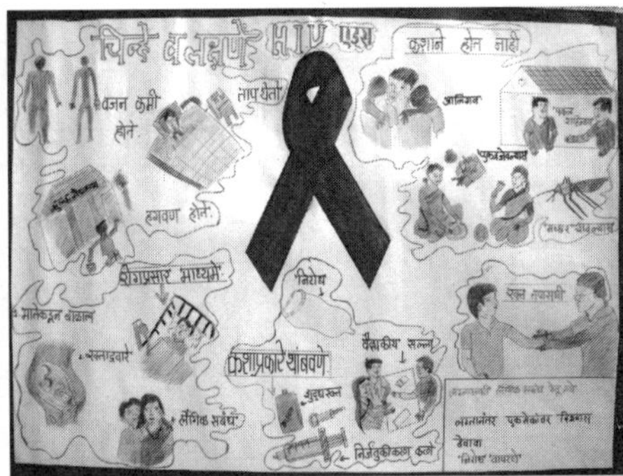

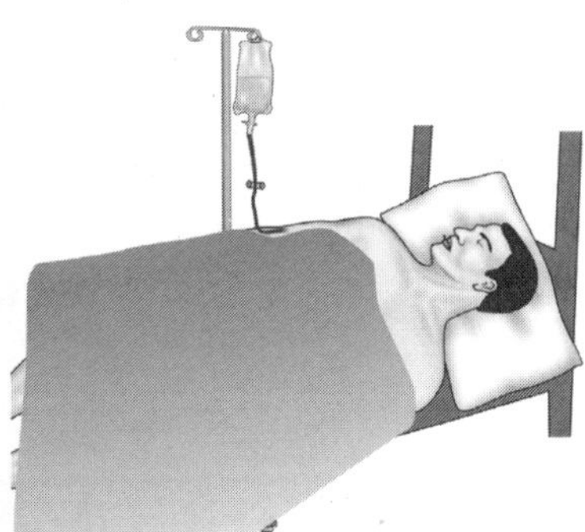

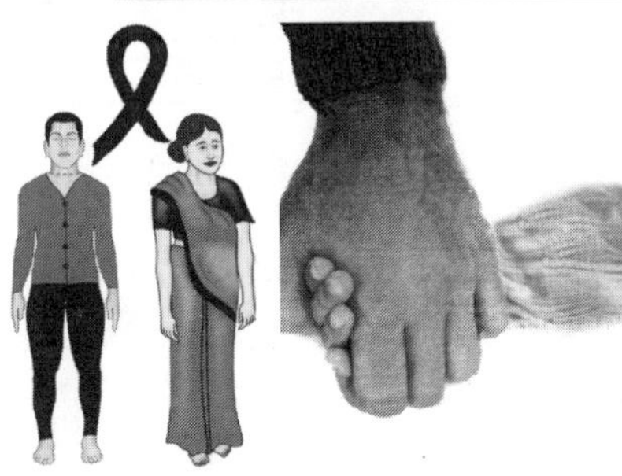

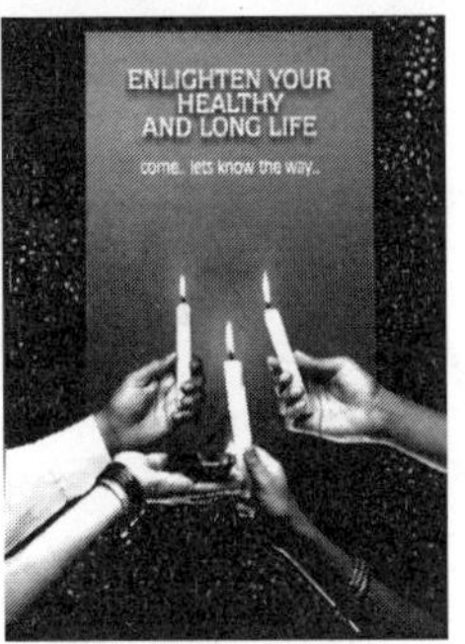

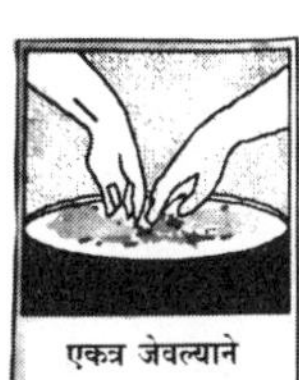

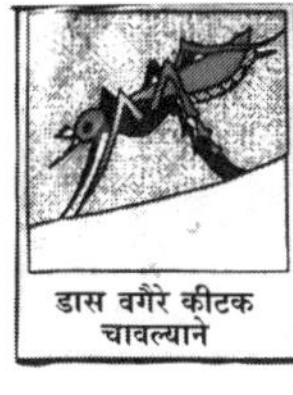

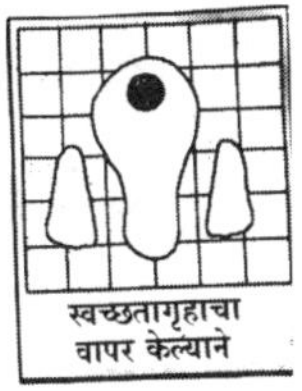

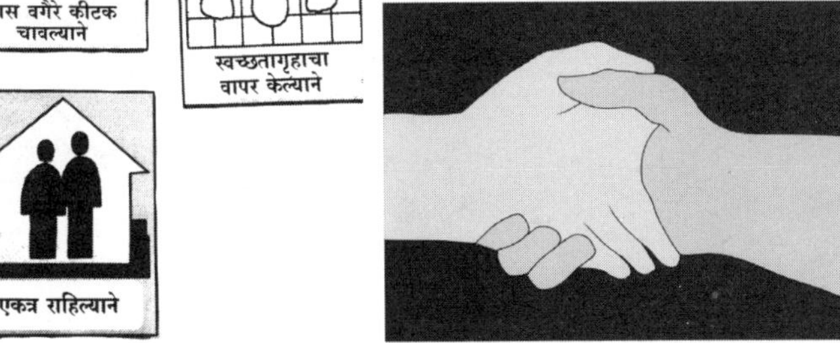

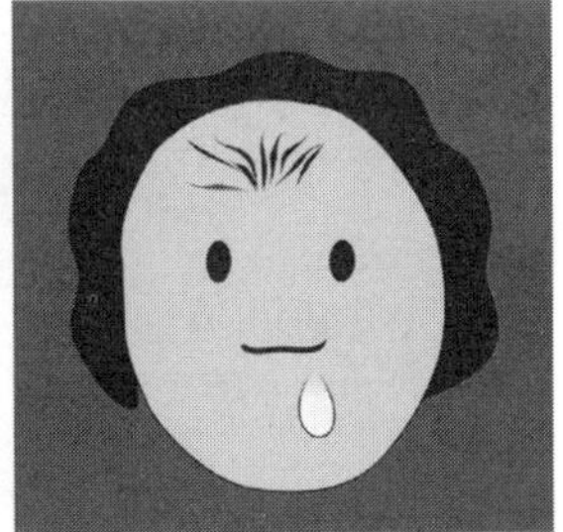

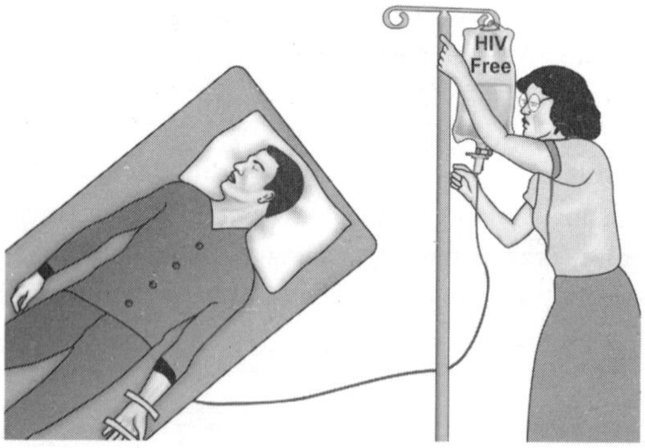

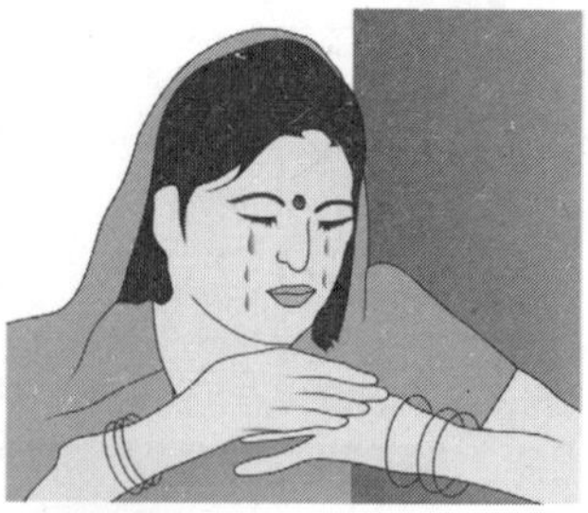

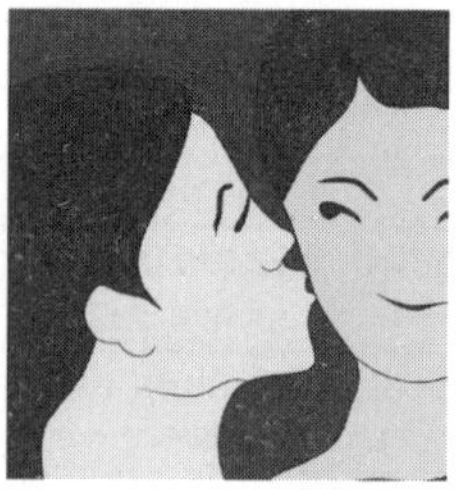

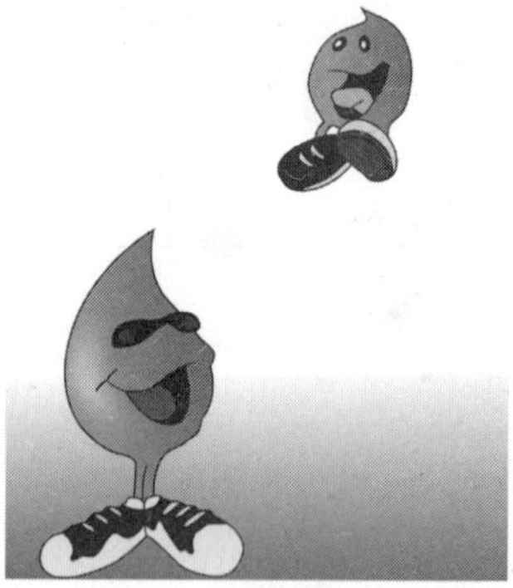

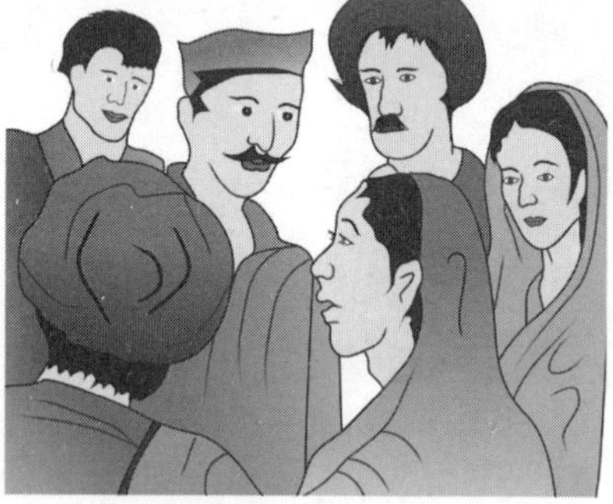

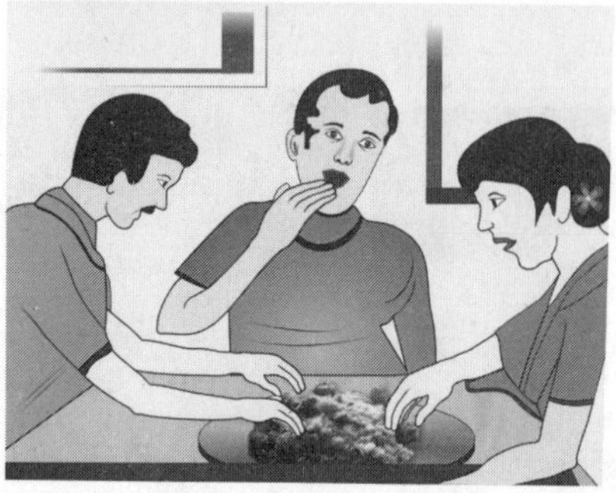

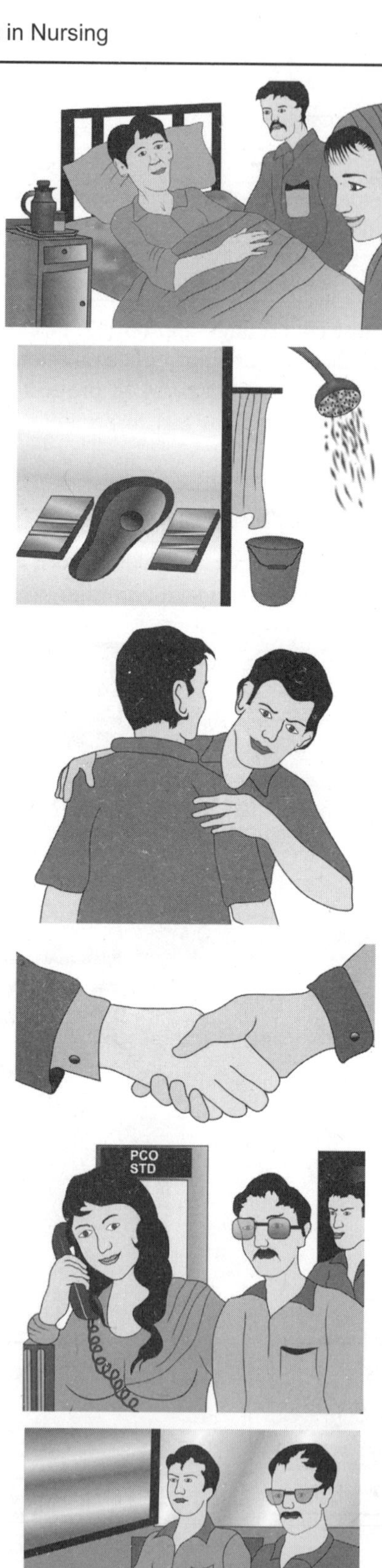
PCO
STD

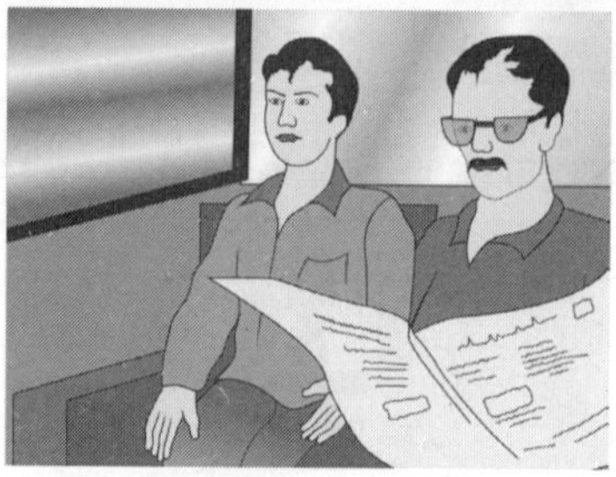

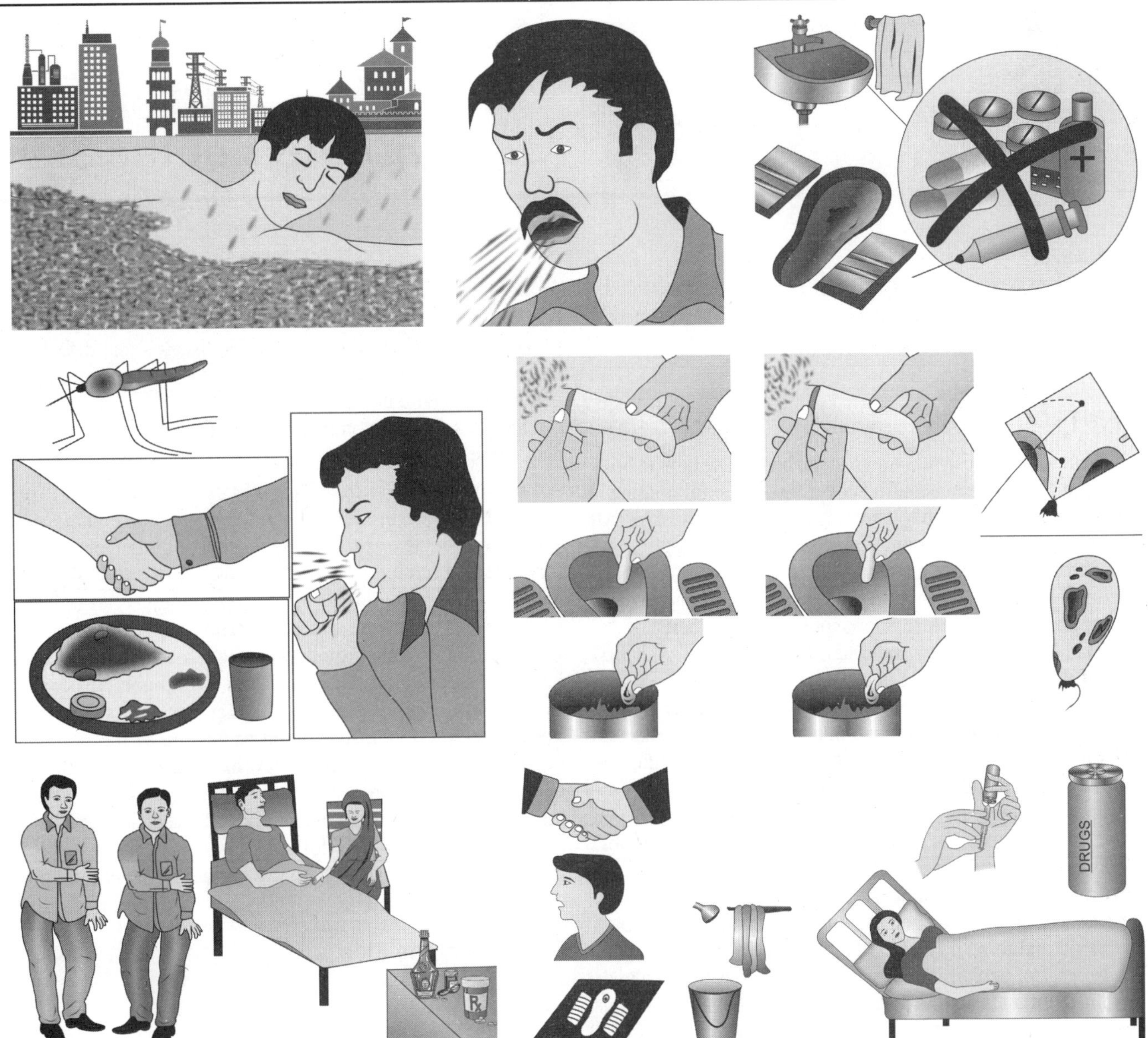
DRUGS

CHAPTER 48

Disorders of the Skin

Abstract

Disorder of the skin is atopic dermatitis—a skin disease characterized by areas of severe itching, redness, scaling, and loss of the surface of the skin.

INTRODUCTION

The skin is the largest vital organ in the body. The human body has been given a most beautiful covering—the skin; nothing is more lovely and attractive than a glowing, healthy skin. All too often, though, one's appearance is marred by ugly scars and chronic eruptions, many of which need never have been occurred had the skin received proper care. Skin trouble often run in families. Therefore know your skin condition.

Skin has several very important functions. It is your first line of defense against the germs that might enter the body. Enzymes on the surface of the skin quickly destroy germs, provided the skin is healthy and intact. But small breaks and tears in the surface of the skin may open the way to infection within the skin, and in the deeper tissues as well.

Skin regulates the temperature of the body. When you exercise vigorously, you produce a lot of heat in the muscles. To keep the temperature of the body as a normal level, this heat must be removed quickly, to cool the body tiny many vessels within the skin open up, allowing much more to pass the blood and to be cooled by the outside air.

Process of perspiration what is it—it is a tiny sweat glands within the skin pour out large quantities of water. As this perspiration evaporates, it carried off large quantities of heat and this helps to cool the body.

When the skin is cut or damaged, it usually heals quickly. This not only seals off the loss of the blood, but also closes the damaged area against the entrance of germs. The healing of the wound is one of the nature's great miracles. Damaged tissues are quickly removed by the WBC, leaving the area clean and ready for the new tissues that will form.

Healthy skin is often an indicator of our holistic wellness. Personal hygiene, unpolluted environment, correct eating habits, mental peace and happiness are important contributors to healthy skin. Bad skin, often, point to the lack of these factors. Beauty is certainly not skin deep. A healthy skin is the results of holistic wellness of body, mind and spirit.

Skin problems can be prevented through fitting food habits. If you require a glowing skin, drink plenty of water in the morning and in between meals.

The skin is the largest organ in the human body. It not only protects the human body by acting as a barrier but also acts as a sense organ; helps in temperature regulation and synthesis of vitamin D. There are over 3,000 diseases that affect the skin. A skin disease may not jeopardize a person's life, but it can interfere with her daily life.

Skin diseases not only cause direct harm to the body but also cause loss of work and revenue.

Anatomy of the skin—The skin is composed of three layers; the epidermis, dermis and the subcutaneous tissue. The Melanocytes are the special cells of the epidermis that are primarily involved in producing the pigment melanin. The hypodermis or the subcutaneous tissue is the innermost layer of the kin. It is primarily adipose tissue, which provides a cushion between the skin layers and such internal structure as the muscles and the bone. It permits skin mobility, molds body contours and insulates the body. Fat is deposited and distributed according to the person's gender, body shape. Overweight results in increased deposition of fat beneath the skin. Hair is an outgrowth of the skin present over the entire body. The sebaceous glands are associated with hair follicles. Sweat glands are found in the skin over most of the body surface. The skin is most visible organ of the body.

Function of the Skin

1. Protection
2. Sensation
3. Water balance
4. Temperature regulation
5. Vitamin production
6. Immune response function.

Major Objectives

1. **Prevent damage to healthy skin**—some skin problems are marked aggravated by soap and water. Deodorant soaps should be avoided.
2. **Prevent secondary infection**—potentially infectious skin lesions should be regarded strictly and proper precaution observed until diagnosis established. Proper disposal of contaminated dressing is carried out according.
3. **Reverse the inflammatory process**—the types of skin lesion (oozing, infected or dry) usually determines which medication or treatment prescribed.

4. Relieve the symptoms
   By direct observation, Family and personal history, Allergic reactions to food, medications, chemicals, Previous skin problems, The name of the cosmetic soap, shampoos and other produced used, The health history-onset, signs, symptoms, location and duration of pain, itching, rashes or other discomforts, will help to know the causes of skin problems.

You can find out skin conditions by following questions

- When did the rash first occur? Was the onset sudden or gradual?
- What site was first affected? Describe the spread and severity
- What was the color and configuration of the rash initially? Has it changed?
- Is there associated itching, burning, tingling, pain or numbness?
- Has it been constant or intermittent?
- What makes the rash worse or better? Is it seasonal? Affected by stress
- What medications are being taken? What topical products have been used?
- What effect did they have?
- What skin products are used? What chemicals have come into contact with the skin, such as insecticides?
- Has there been a pet contact?
- What is the client's occupation? Any hobby as gardening or hiking.

Medical history

- Is there a history of hay fever, asthma, heavies, eczema, or allergies?
- Has the patient had this particular rash or other skin disorders in the past?
- What is the family history of the skin disorder?
- Are there any chronic medical problems?

Diagnostic test

a. Potassium hydroxide examination and fungal culture
b. Tzancks smear
c. Scabies scrapings
d. Wood slight examination
e. Patch testing
f. Biopsy

Patch testing

1. It is done to attempt to identify substances that produce allergic skin responses
2. It is a painless procedure that requires a sill led evaluator to read and interpret the results
3. It is often done to differentiate between an irritant contact dermatitis and an allergic contact dermatitis
4. Small amount of various substances or allergens are applied to the skin using a commercially prepared tape containing the allergens or allergens are placed on aluminum discs placed on a special tape
5. It should not be performed if acute dermatitis is present
6. The tape must be warn for 48 hours without disturbing the patches then it is removed
7. Interpretation are made at 48, 72, or 96 hours and sometimes at one week
8. An eczematous response at the test site with Erythema, papules or small vesicles indicates a positive reaction and confirms an allergic contact sensitivity to the substance on the disc.

Biopsy

1. Skin biopsy is the removal of a skin tissue specimen for histological assessment
2. There are 3 types—shave, dermal punch and surgical excision
3. In all these 3 procedures, local anesthetic is used and small guage needle are recommended to limit trauma to the skin
4. Clean or sterile technique as appropriate should be used in dealing with the biopsy site
5. Depending on size, location and skill of the practitioners, a biopsy is usually a quick and almost painless
6. The specimen is placed in a preservative such as formalin solutions properly, identified and sent for pathologic assessment.

Topical Therapy

1. Skin large surface area allow the absorption, penetration and permeation of topically applied preparation
2. Topical therapy can be used to do the following-
3. Restore hydration
4. Alleviate symptoms
5. Reduce inflammation
6. Protect the skin
7. Reduce scale and callus
8. Cleanse and Debride
9. Gradicate causative organisms.

Topical medications have many different actions and cover a large spectrum of drug categories, including antibacterial, antifungal, and anti parasitic and anti Pruritic.

Explain few conditions as follows:

Pruritus

Pruritus (itching) is one of the most common manifestations of skin problems; It is a symptom not diseases.

Definition—purities has been defined as an unpleasant skin sensation, producing a strong desire to scratch, localized to or generalized over a body area. It can lead to damage if scratching injuries the skin protective barrier possibly with resistance infection and scratching.

Pathology

1. Stimulation of itching can be initiated by almost any chemical or physical substance especially if skin is damaged.
2. Once the itch sensation is established the patient has an almost uncontrollable urge to scratch.
3. Scratching leads to further skin damage and increased inflammation.
4. Purities increases and so does the urge to scratch
5. Thus the itch scratch itch cycle develops.
6. In order to minimize skin trauma caused by scratching, finger nails should be kept short.

Signs and Symptoms

1. Excoriation of skin
2. Secondary skin changes like lichenification
3. Patients description about degree and location of itching.

Rx

1. If dry skin is the source of or contribute to prutitus, then good hydration with topical therapy is helpful
2. One bath or shower per day for 15 to 20 minutes with warm water and a mild soap should be immediately followed by the application of an emollient with or without other topical medications, to prevent evaporation of water from the hydrate epidermis
3. Other topical medications often added to emollients to help alleviate itching include menthol (0.25%–0.5%), camphor (0.25%–0.50%), urea (10%–20%), and lactic acid (12%)
4. Systemic antihistamine's may be prescribed.

Prickly heat—or heat rash is an irritating eruption of the skin to obstruction of the sweat glands over certain areas of the body.

Treatment—avoid scratching, wear cool, light clothing, relieve the itch calamine lotion, keep the skin clean and avoid the use of harsh soaps.

Chafing of the skin—when two skin surface rub together, such as under the breast or between the thighs, one or both surface may become red and irritated.

Apply talcum powder several times a day, cool clothing and avoid strenuous exercise in hot weather.

Dermatitis

1. Usually starts during infancy
2. Red, oozing, crusting rash
3. As child grows the skin tends to show the chronic from of dermatitis with thickened dry texture, brownish gray co lour and scales
4. The rash tends to become to closed to the large folds of the extremities as the client becomes older
5. It is found mainly on elbow bends, bends of knees, the necks eyelids, back of hands and feet
6. Pruritus is major symptoms
7. Urge to scratch may be mild and self-limiting or it may be intense, leading to several excoriated lesions infection and scarring.

Complications

1. Bacterial, viral, fungal, skin infections
2. Most common viral infection is herpes simplex
3. Honey colored crusting extensive serous weeping, folliculitis, pyoderma and furuncolosis indicate bacterial infection by staphylococcus aurous
4. Bath at least once everyday for 15–20 minutes topical immediately after bath
5. Use warm water not hot
6. Use superficial soaps, e.g. Dove of soap for sensitive skin oil of day euchring
7. Avoid bubble bath
8. Apply occlusive topical emollient or prescribed topical preparation two or three per day
9. Explain the itching symptom as it relate to cause (i.e. dryness of the skin) and the principles of the selected therapy (i.e. hydration) and the itch scratch itch cycle)
10. Wash all new clothes before wearing for removal of formaldehyde and other chemicals and avoid us of fabric softness
11. Change to a mildex detergent and add a second rinse cycle to ensure removal of soap
12. Wear open weave, loose fitting cotton blend clothing
13. Avoid over dressings, rough or wool fabrics and tightly woven fabrics
14. Work and sleep in comfortable surroundings with a fairly constant temperature and humilities level
15. Air conditioning in the homes particularly the bedrooms may be beneficial
16. Keep fingernails short, smooth, clean
17. Appropriate use of antihistamines may reduce itching to some degree
18. Use sunscreen on a regular basis
19. Immediately after swimming, take a shower or bath, washing with a mild soap from head to toe and then apply an appropriate moisture.

- Ensures that the patient understands the importance of not self-threading with left-over medication at home
- Emphasize that it is important to take the antibiotic on schedule over the entire course
- Encourage the client to teach others that eczema is not contagious unless severely infected
- Encourage the client and significant others to share feeling with one another and professional counselors
- Reinforce the patients sense of identity and personal competence
- Encourage self-management of eczema and understand that controlling searching will greatly reduce lesions.

Contact Dermatitis

Contact dermatitis is an inflammatory response of the skin to chemical or physical allergens. Irritant contact dermatitis is exposure to a chemical or physical irritant such as cleaning produces, fragrances and topical skin care produces. Allergic contact dermatitis is a delayed hypersensitivity reaction resulting from contact with an allergen. This reaction is an immune mediated response by previously sensitized lymphocytes to a specific allergen, e.g. poisoning and nicked allergy.

Management

1. Determine the causative agent
2. Patch testing is done
3. Pain ad itching may be controlled with topical medication or wet dressings
4. Antihistaminic and steroids may be requested
5. Avoidance of allegiance.

Cellulites—It is an inflammation of the subcutaneous tissue of the skin. Obtain history of trauma to skin, needle stick, insect bite, or wound. Palpate for abscess formation. Comfortable position and immobilization of the affected area. Monitor side effect. Use bed cradle to relieve pressure from bed covers. Teach client with impaired circulation or sensation proper skin care and inspection of skin for trauma.

Nursing management

1. Place client on warmed air fluidized bed to distribute weight with minimal shearing force
2. Handle client with extreme care as skin is very fragile
3. Gently apply warm or wet compresses
4. Apply antiseptic solution to reduce bacteria
5. Watch for new areas to toxic epidermal Necrolysis
6. Isolate client to prevent infection
7. Assess bowel sounds
8. Weight daily
9. Maintain electrolyte
10. Administer analgesic
11. Provide emotional support
12. Avoid suspected medication in the future
13. Maintain input output.

HERPES ZOSTER

Herpes zoster/shingles is an inflammatory condition in which a virus produces a painful vesicular eruption along the distribution of the nerves from one or more dorsal root ganglia. The prevalence increases with age.

Nursing management

1. Relieve pain and inflammation
2. Maintain skin integrity
3. Assess client's level of discomfort
4. Apply wet dressing for soothing effect
5. Teach deep breathing and relaxation
6. Apply wet dressing
7. Apply lotion
8. Apply antibacterial ointments
9. Use proper hand washing
10. Not to open the blister to avoid secondary infection.

Pemphigus

Is a serious autoimmune disease of the skin and mucous membranes characterized by the appurtenance of blisters of various sizes, on apparently normal skin and mucous membranes? Appearing in adult, affecting particularly the axilla and groin. Many variations of it exist.

Nursing management

1. Inspect oral cavity daily and rcport changes
2. Keep oral hygiene and prevent secondary infection
3. Give tropical oral therapy
4. Offer prescribed mouthwash
5. Apply petroleum to lips
6. Keep skin clean and eliminate debris administer cool, dry dressing
7. After bath dry and cover with talcum powder as directed
8. Evaluate fluid electroplate
9. Monitor serum albumin and protein levels
10. Monitor vital sings
11. Give high protein, high-calorie diet
12. Monitor skin/mouth for recurrence of Pemphigus activity.

BENIGN TUMORS

They are common skin growths. Most do not require any treatment but are important to recognize to differentiate malignant lesions.

CANCER OF THE SKIN

Skin cancer is the most common malignancy; basal and Squamous cell carcinoma is easily curable due to early diagnosis and slow progression. These cancers are locally invasive and tend not to metastasize. Conversely, malignant melanomas are less common and metastasize eventually.

Clinical Manifestation

1. Basal cell carcinoma occasionally ulceration and appears sun exposed skin, neglected infection and cosmetic disabilities.
2. Squamous cell carcinoma appears as reddish rough, thickened, scaly lesion with bleeding and soreness. Seen most common on lower lip, rims of ears, head, neck and back of the hands
3. Malignant melanoma circular with irregular outer portion. Has combination of colors.

Nursing management

1. Examinee entire skin surface including scalp, genital areas, gluteal folds, and soles of the feet
2. Examine diameter of mole
3. Inspect all moles
4. Teach client to use sun cream
5. Do not tan skin if skin burns easily
6. Avoid unnecessary exposure to sun especially ultra violet radiations are more intense as 10.00 AM to 3.00 PM
7. Was protective clothing like long sleeves, high color, and long pants.

Patient Education of Skin Cancer

1. Do not try to tan if your skin burns easily
2. Avoid unnecessary exposure to the sun, especially during strong sun light
3. Do not become sunburn
4. Apply protective sun cream, sun cream block the harmful sun rays
5. Reapply water resistant sun cream after swimming
6. Wear appropriate protective clothing.

IMPETIGO

Is superficial inflammation and secondary infection where two skin surfaces are in apposition.

Impetigo is an acute infectious inflammation of the skin caused by *S. aureus* bacteria. It is most common among children face, hands and other regions of the body are usually affected. The disease begins with vesicles, changing very soon into pustules. These pustules burst and a yellowish liquid oozes out, when it dries it forms thick crusts. The rash is infectious. The general hygienic condition, nourishment of pt and his whole constitution are of decisive influence.

Nursing management

1. Teach client to prevent skin maceration by separating opposing skin surfaces with gauze or cotton material
2. Skin surface should be dried thoroughly after bathing with a hair dryer on low setting
3. Talcum powder can be applied lightly to the area after drying
4. Loose, airy clothing should be worn

PARASITIC INFECTIONS

Example—Pediculosis

Treatment involves

- Washing with soap and water and washing all infested clothing and linens with hot water
- Teach client the proper use of medication
- Manual removal of nits
- Re-treatment in 3–7 days
- Petroleum may be applied
- Alternatively apply shampoo
- Use fine toothcomb to remove eggs.

Eczema typically present with dry red and itchy skin. It can also appear with cracks that may or may not bleed, along with eruptions that ooze and swell. This may be limited to one area or can be extensive. Most commonly eczema tends too affect the creases of the knees and elbows, neck, scalp, buttocks, face and chest. A drop in humidity is one of main reasons why it intensifies in winter. Food allergies, contact with allergic substances and environmental factors. A lukewarm bath is better than hot water. Diet balance, 8–10 glasses of water drinking helps toxins to clear out.

SCABIES

Superficial infestation by itch mite; transmitted personal contact.

Scabies is an infectious, parasitic disease caused by sarcoptus scabies with an incidence of 10.30% of total dermatological cases. The disease is characterized by papules, vesicles and pustules, violent itching especially at night and vesicles appear first flowed by pustules and scabs with numerous red patches. The most commonly affected parts are the space between the fingers, the wrists, the armpits and genital organs. Amongst children the disease often starts at the buttocks and legs. The treatment is local as well as constitutional. We must kill the organism and prevent its propagation.

Scabies is a kind of itch, which is not, caused by food, but by a small insect you cannot see it with your eyes alone. Usually it gets on your hand between your fingers and burrows under the skin. Then under the skin, this little creature laid eggs. The eggs hatch out and these in then burrow more tunnels and lay more eggs. It causes your skin to itch and become red and sore. Scratching introduces infection. All the sores become filled with pus and soon the rash spreads al over the body. Under the powerful, glass this tiny insect which censuses the itch looks like lice of head. It is quiet easy to treat the itch and it is also possible to prevent it from re-occurring. The public health nurse gave medicines and explained the important steps are to have bath with plenty of soap and water which helps to soften the scabs. Then it is easy to remove them with a piece of gauze or rough cloth. Dry the body well. The finger nails should be cut short to prevent searching. This prevents the itch from spreading. Rub the medicines over the whole body. Keep on the same clothes on until the next day. Take another bath and repeat the treatment as often as the doctor feels it is necessary. Wash the dirty clothes with soap and water and dry in the sun. Bathe every day and wear clean clothes and you will not have scabies.

Eat mixed food. If everyone in the family not treated they will never get rid of itch as it spreads from one person to another in the family where they have close contact with each other. Sulfur ointment, benzyl benzoate or tetmosal used for three days.

Clinical management

- Itching more intense at night
- Small erythmatous papules and short wavy burrows are seen on skin surface
- Frequent seen between fingers or in groin
- Microscopic examination
- Linens in hot water wash
- Infestation with scabies is a problem in nursing homes, hostels needs good had care
- Teach client use of medication
- Leave medication 8–12 hours then washes thoroughly
- Avoid close contact to prevent transmission
- Itchy may persist to weeks due to allergic reaction to mites.

Patient education

How to have a clear, healthy skin; an adult has about two square meters of skin. The skin has some two million pores which can flush toxins and other excesses out of the body. For it means; that your body is at least able to discharge waste through the skin. You will be deep trouble if all those toxins remain inside.

1. To have a clear, good looking skin, you need to- avoid over polluting your body's internal environment
2. Get rid of waste mater that have accumulated over the years
3. Ensure that the main organs for waste treatment and disposal—the liver, colon and kidneys are in good working order
4. The kidneys and colon should be able to handle a normal level of waste. It is only when too much waste matter builds up that the body has to eliminate them through the skin
5. Kidney trouble can happen to people who eat lots of junk food, including meat, fat and food chemicals. Meat even lean meat, is highly pollutive because it releases uric acid and other toxic substances when it is digested
6. Toxic overload may also occur when the liver is malfunctioning and cannot neutralize toxins effectively. That is why the skin turns yellow when a person has jaundice. It can happen when a person has chronic constipation, or when the kidneys are not working well
7. Skin problems, then, are not skin-deep. They point to deeper problems with our diet or lifestyle
8. Take care of oily and dry skin.

You will find in the chapter lots of different skin conditions which you can draw and prepare charts and posters and other communication methods and explain to the group of people of your targeted.

Dermatological disorders

1. Folliculitis is inflammation of the hair follicle
2. Furunculosis is abscess/boils/carbuncles
3. Parongchias is inflammation of the skin folds surrounding the finger nails
4. Tinea pedis is ringworm of the foot
5. Tinea corporis is ringworm of body
6. Tinea corporis is ringworm of groin
7. Tinea corporis is ringworm of scalp
8. Tinea versicolor is fungal inflammation
9. Parasitic inflammation is pediculosis in head, body lice
10. Scabies itch mite transmitted by close personal contact
11. Contact dermatitis is exposure to irritating or allergenic substance, such as plants, chemicals, cleansing products, soaps and detergents, hair dyes, metals and rubber
12. Acne vulgaris is obstructive and inflammation of sebaceous glands and follicles
13. Burns are traumatic injury caused by thermal, electrical chemical or radioactive agents
14. White patches or vitilliogo is chronic skin disorders characterized by de-pigmented patches or starts with small white sports and spreads.

Keywords

Introduction, anatomy of skin, functions, major objectives, biopsy, tropical therapy, medical history, diagnostic test, patch testing, pruritus, pathology, complications, dermatitis, contact dermatitis, nursing management, cellulitis, cancers, tumors, herpes, parasitic infections, scabies, impetigo.

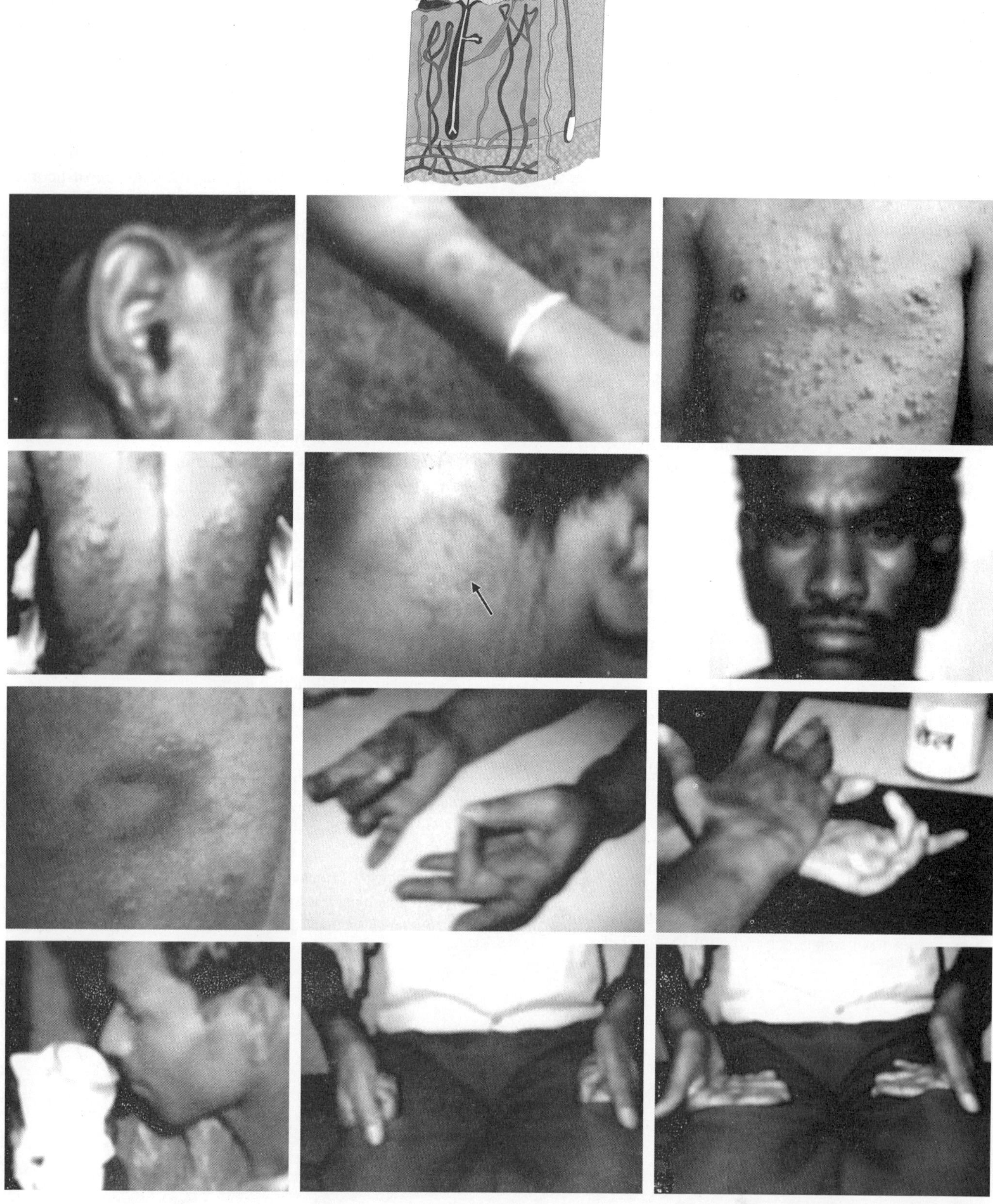

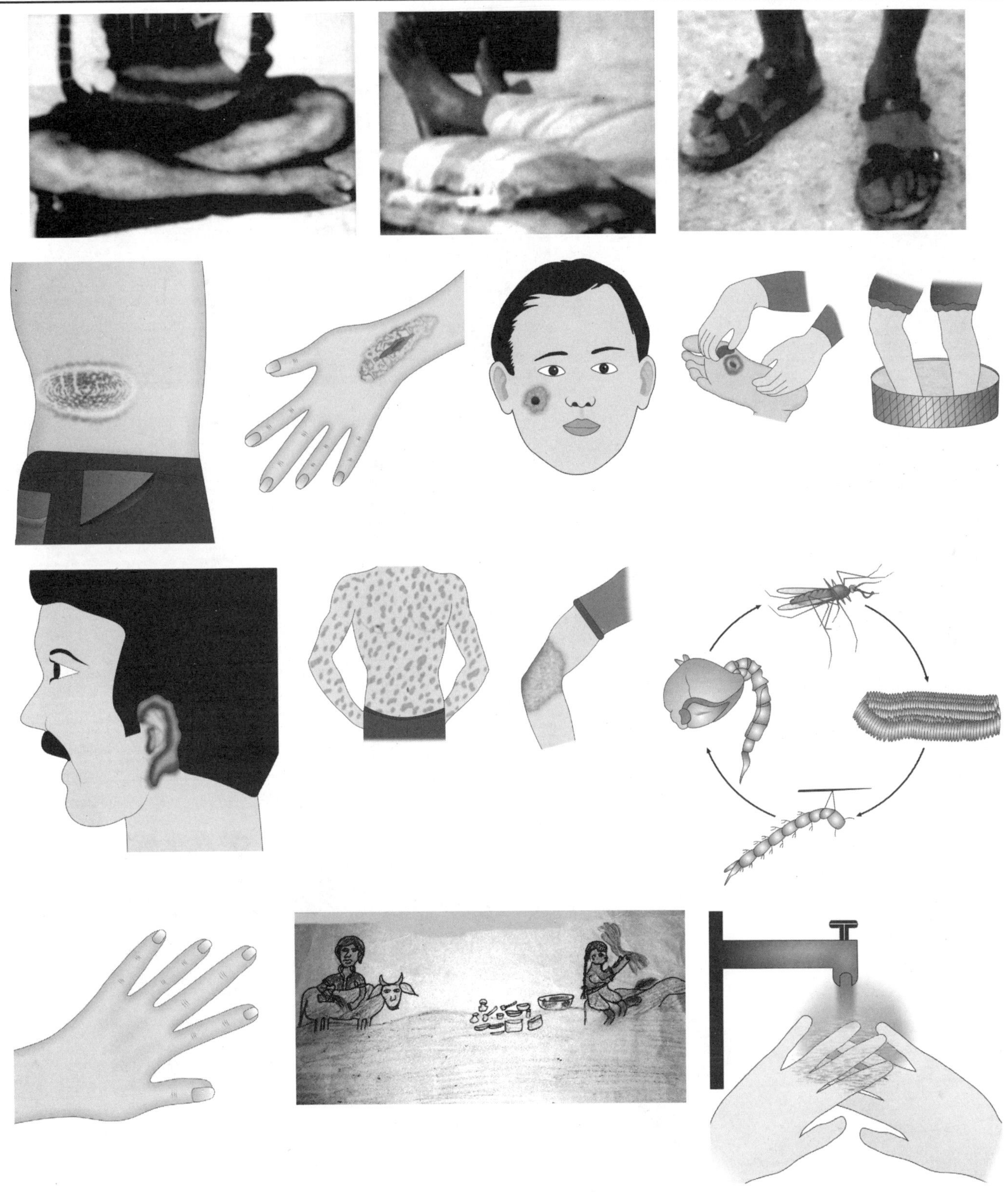

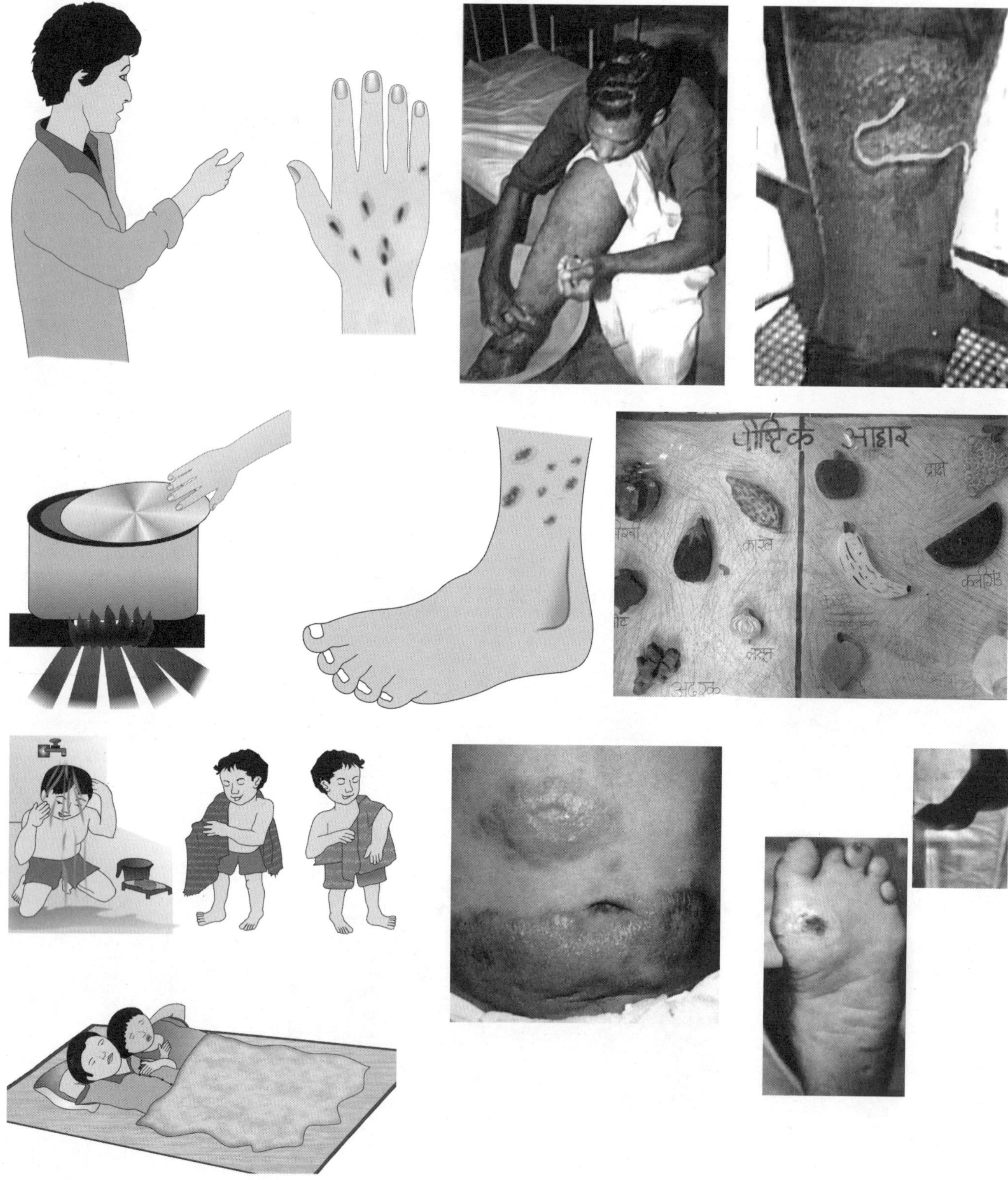
पौष्टिक आहार
द्राक्षे
कारले
कलिंगड
अदरक

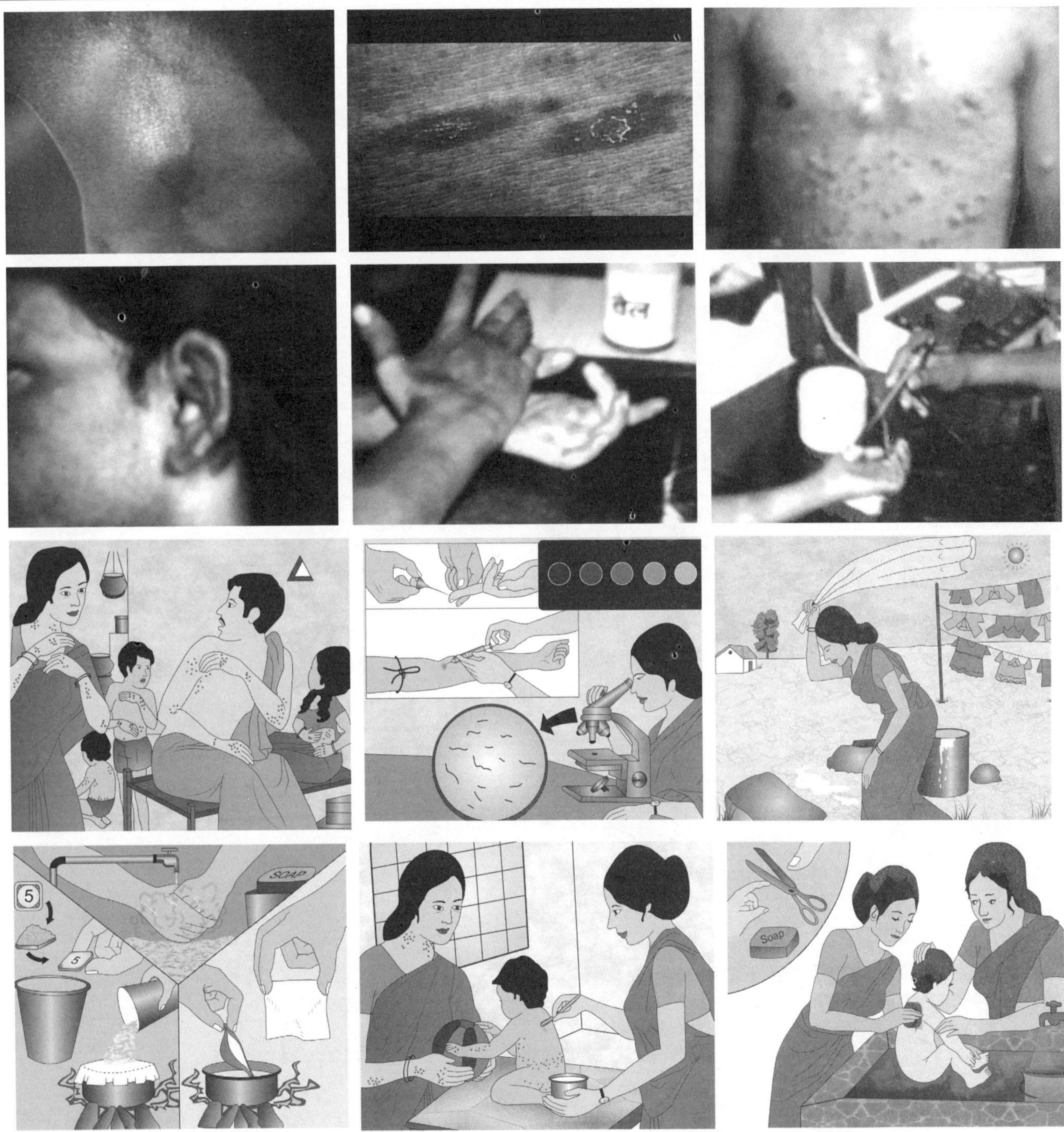
5
5
SOAP
Soap

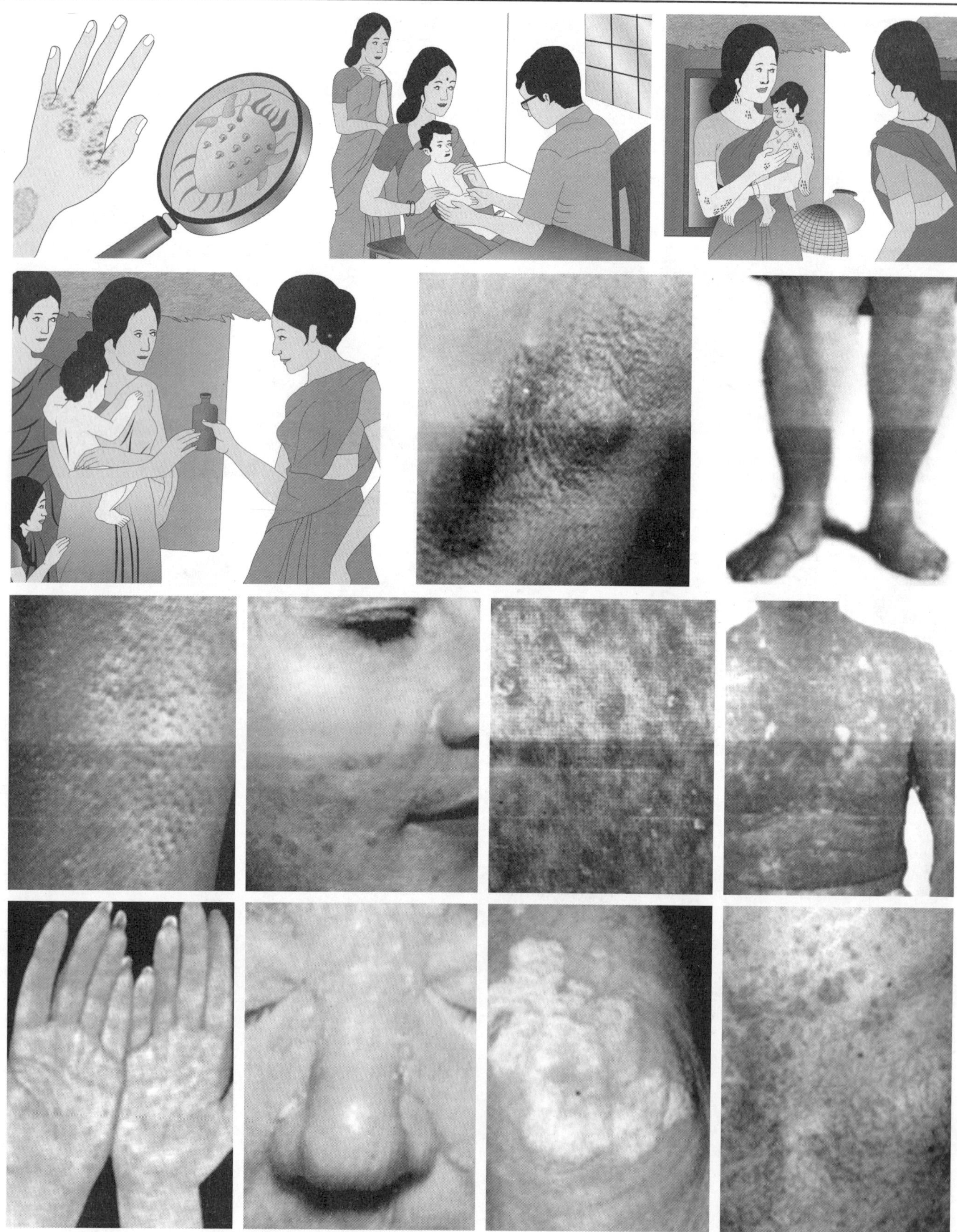

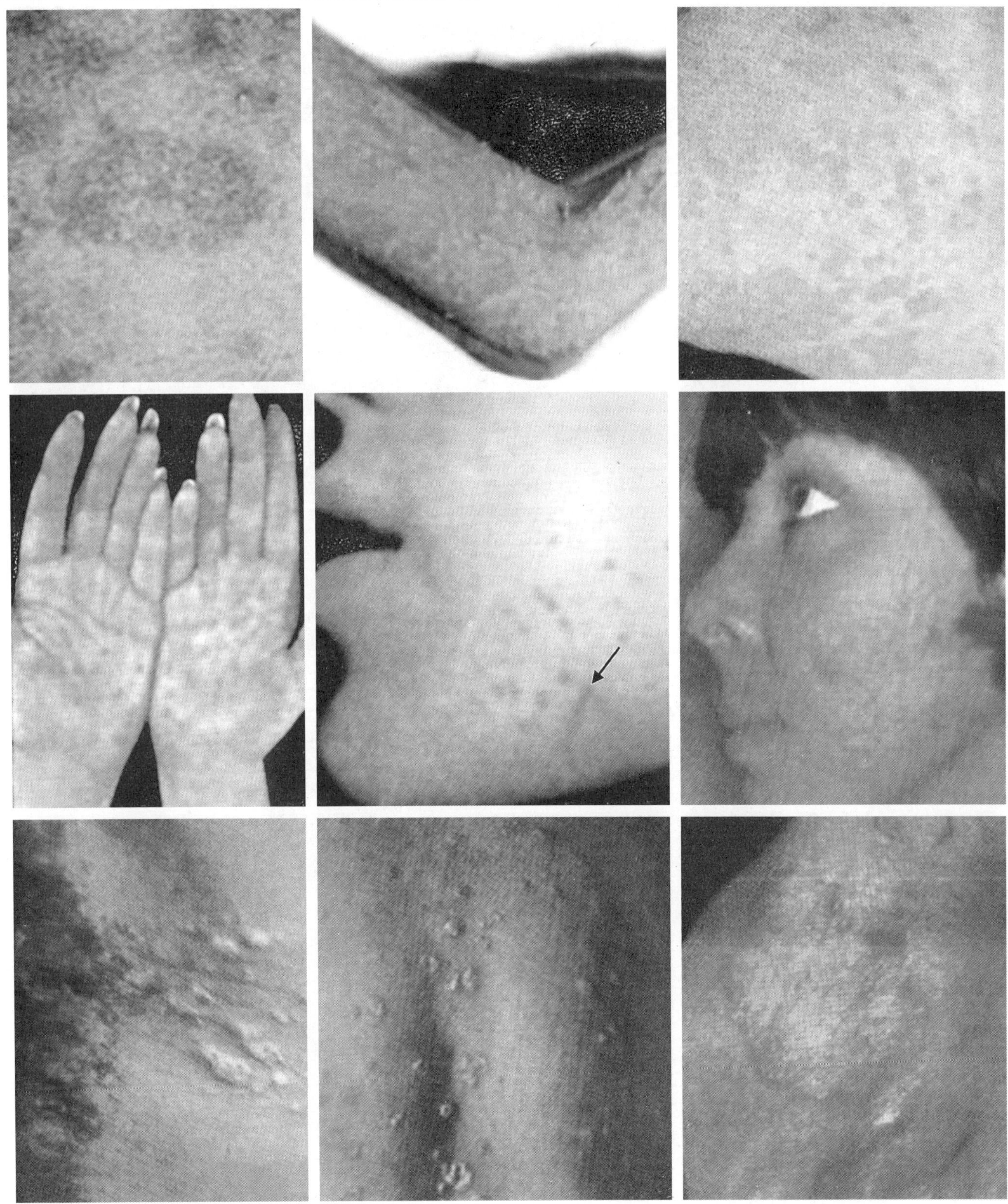

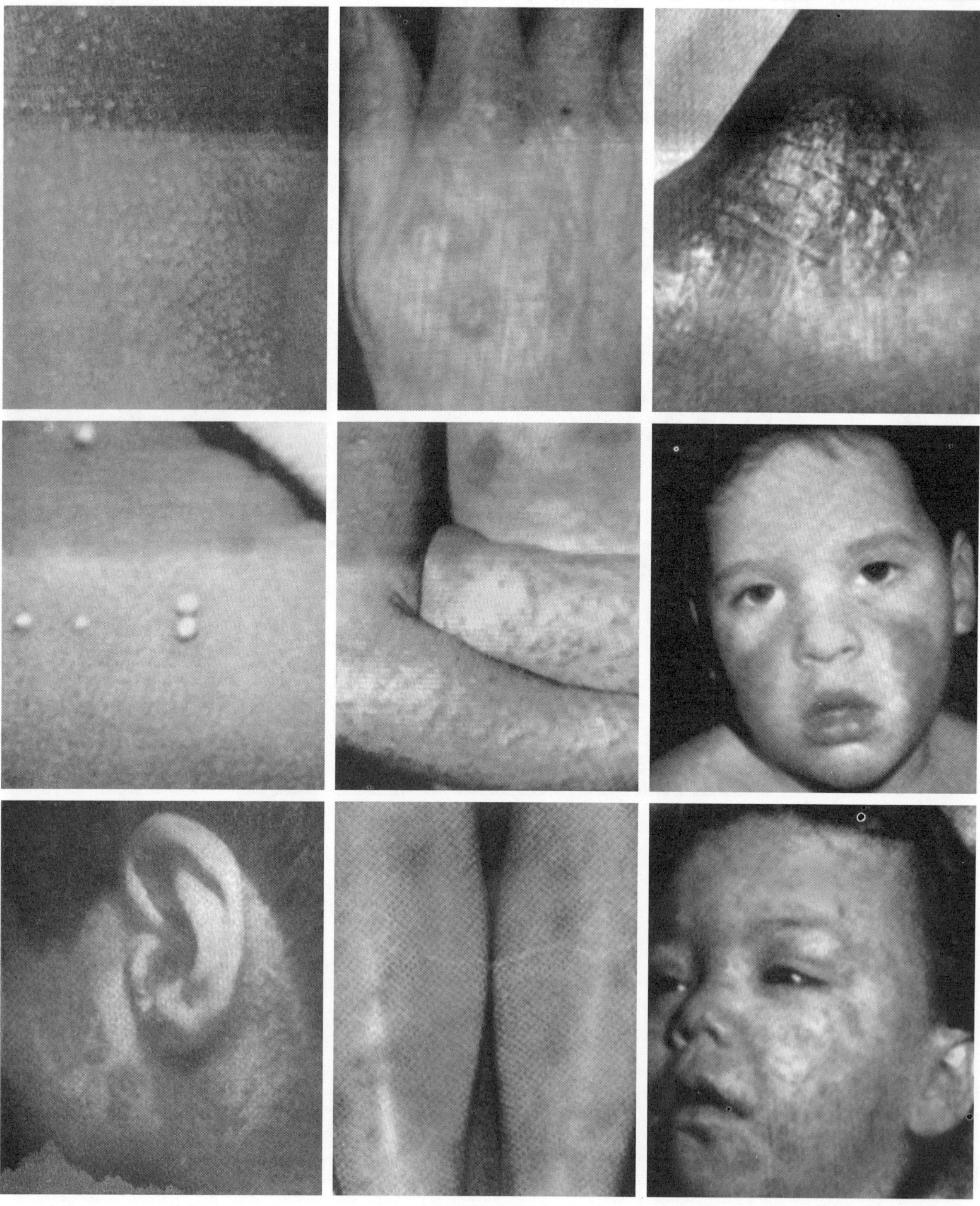

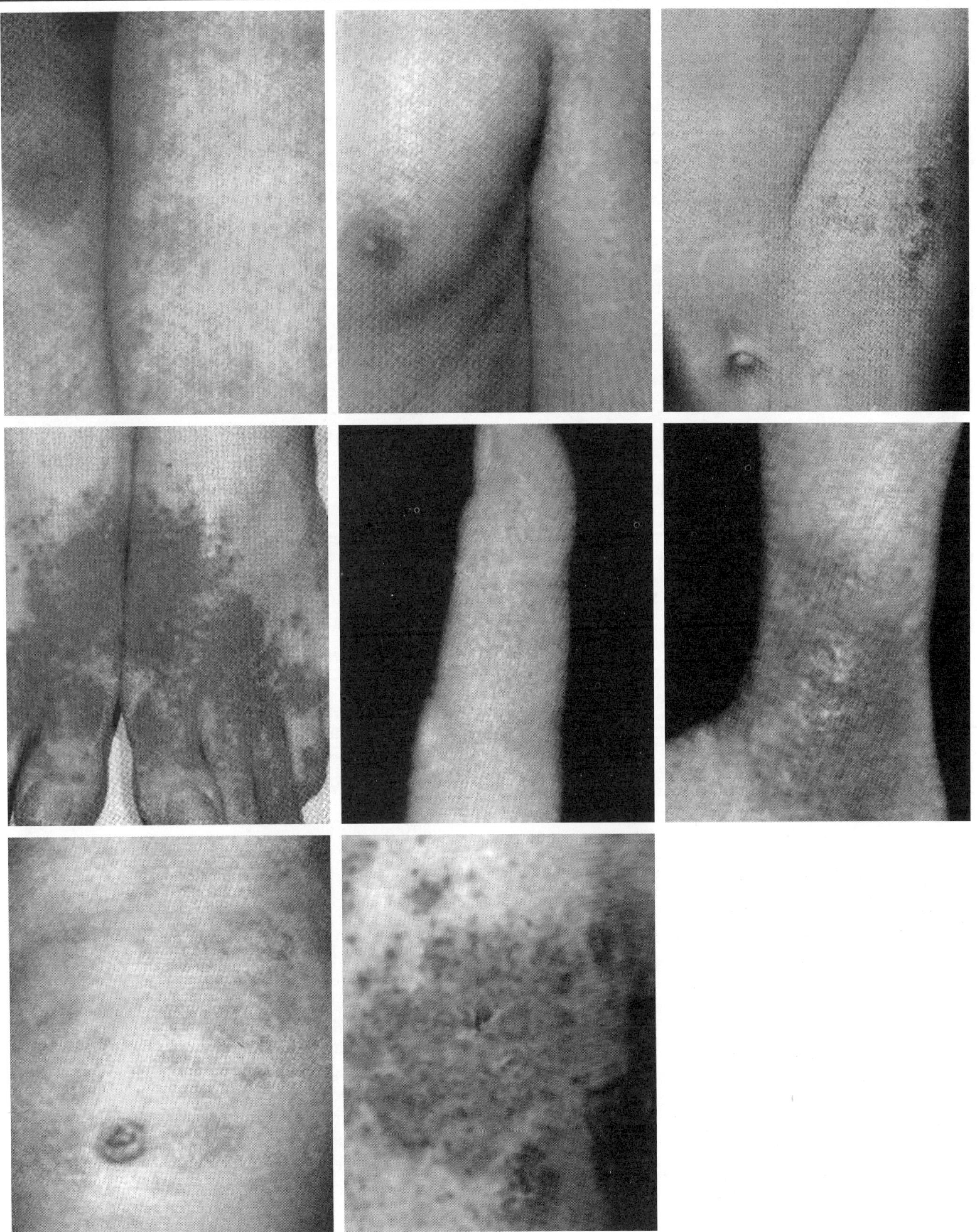

CHAPTER

49

Environmental Sanitation

Abstract

Environmental sanitation means the art and science of applying sanitary-biological and physical science principals and knowledge to improve and control the environment and factors therein for the protection of the health and welfare of the public.

ENVIRONMENTAL HYGIENE/THE SCIENCE OF SAFEGUARDING HEALTH

In health education presentation of topic is important. It should motivate people to listen all through the topic with undivided attention and single minded concentration. Nurse develops voice variation and slowly yet loud enough to listen clearly. In-between introduces humor to become interested avoided irrelevant details. Stress and summarizes key points.

Prepare each session carefully and leave time for answer and discussions. Good facial expressions, friendly atmosphere using simple language. Such information can bring transformation in behaviour and involve thinking, reasoning, and helps in integrated growth by new knowledge. Health education is a life long process from womb to the tomb, from cradle to grave on going.

Know what you wish to teach and what learner hopes to learn. Have a specific goal in mind which you wish to accomplish. Be sure the learner is motivated; you cannot force anyone to learn. Communicate learner at his level. At this stage the people decide that new practice is good and he adopts it. Therefore, ignorance can be removed by helping them to solve their problems by their own ways.

Good and bad influence on health—the key to mans health has largely is in his environment, ill health can be due to water, pollution, soil pollution, air pollution, poor housing which pose constant threat to human health. Often man is responsible for it by urbanization, industrialization and other human activities.

Sanitation is the way of life. It is a quality of living that is expressed in the clean home, the clean farm, the clean business, the clean neighborhood and the clean community.

As it is being way of life must come from people. Faeces deposited near homes, contaminated drinking water (water quality is important), washing hands after defecation and before preparing food (without abundance of water around home personal hygiene becomes difficult,) inadequate water supply increases health hazards, skin, eye infections, guinea worms etc. Healthy lifestyle, water free from pathogenic agents, harmful chemicals we cannot provide health. Disposal of waste, garbage, food, rubbish produces public health problems. Environmental sanitation is the control of all those factors in mans physical surroundings where he lives in.

Environmental hygiene has two aspects domestic and community. Domestic hygiene comprises that of home, use of soap, need for fresh air, light and ventilation, avoid pests, rats, mice and insects.

Environmental consists of basic sanitary services such as water supply, disposable human excreta, vector control, food sanitation and housing which are fundamental to health. To have sanitary wells, latrines and waste collecting facilities.

Environmental health includes:

Physical—water, air, soil, housing, wastes, radiation etc.

Biologic—plant and animal life including bacteria, viruses, insects, rodents and animals.

Social—customs, culture, habits, income, occupation, religion etc.

Much of the ill health is due to poor environmental sanitation in India, such as follows:

1. Use of soap and water
2. Lighting and ventilation
3. Food hygiene
4. Control of rats and mice
5. Safe water
6. Benefits of drainage
7. Good housing.

Unsafe water—If people have safe and wholesome water to drink much of the ill health in the underdeveloped countries could have prevented but it is largely due to lack of safe drinking water is a basic health problem; and lack of safe drinking water is cause of most of ill health. Water must be free from pathogens, harmful chemical substances. Without safe ample drinking water one can not get good health. We have to educate people to prevent impurities of water, to prevent pollution from sewage, proper disposal of industrial wastes, and prevent water related diseases like viral hepatitis A; typhoid, bacillary dysentery, worm infestation etc removal of harness of water and water purification is important.

Polluted soil—Unhygienic disposal of human excreta and refuse—has health hazards—the accumulation of refuse decomposes and favors fly breeding, it attracts rats and vermin, the pathogenic organisms which may be present in refuse may be conveyed back to mans food through flies and dust. This pollutes water and soil too, heaps of refuse are a nuisance. Therefore, refuse should be promptly collected, removed and disposed off in a sanitary manner. It can be done by burning, dumping, controlled tipping, composting. Human excreta are a source of infection which contains pathogenic bacteria, viruses, protozoa, helminthic parasites etc. it must be promptly removed and disposed off in a hygienic manner. Improper disposal of excreta pollutes soil, water, food and fly breeding site, have sanitary latrines.

Poor housing—home gives experience of heaven on earth. Physical structure providing shelter facilities, equipment, storage of food, adequate place for cooking, washing, eating and excretory functions. All this helps to provide protection to the family from harmful hazardous exposure. Family has many needs such as physical needs, psychological needs, health needs, and protective needs- the adverse effect of poor housing has on health people who do not have a well-ventilated house, if they stay in over crowded area, no proper ventilation, light, it has its effect on health condition. More people living in single dwelling space movement restricted, no privacy, lack of hygiene, rest and sleep difficult results in irritability, frustration, anxiety, violence, mental disorders, unhappiness, psychosomatic effects, communicable diseases.

Insects and rodents—mosquitoes, anti-larval measures.

Air pollution—is a basis of all forms of life. Health effects of air pollution are both immediate and delayed. Prevention and control is very vital to have good sound health.

Elimination those factors which are harmful to health such as respiratory infections, irritability, cough, discomfort,

Environmental sanitation causes following health effects:
Water borne diseases—due to pollution and presence of disease causing germs in the water community may get diseases such as

1. Viral—infective hepatitis, poliomyelitis
2. Bacteria—diarrhea, dysentery, cholera, thyroid
3. Protozoal—amoebiasis, giardiasis
4. Helminthic—round worm, whipworm, threadworm, guinea worm
5. Toxic substances—lead, arsenic, mercury, cyanides
6. Deficiency of fluoride—dental caries.

Fly-borne diseases—diarrhea, dysentery, cholera, GI, amoebiasis, typhoid, trachoma, conjunctivitis.

Milk-borne diseases:

1. Through Mitch—cowpox, anthrax, tick-borne
2. Animal—encephalitis, bovine tuberculosis, Bruccosis, streptococcal infections
3. Handlers—diphtheria, viral hepatitis
4. Through Mitch—dysentery, typhoid, cholera.

Family control measures—house flies to eliminate their breeding places. Do not store garbage, kitchen wastes, keep bins with tight lids, disposal of refuse by incineration, composting or sanitary landfill. Stop open air defecation, sanitary disposal of animal excreta, have sanitary latrines and keep house and surrounding clean. Motivate and make people aware as sound environmental sanitation is most effective weapon. So proper storage, collection and disposal of garbage, construction of rat proof buildings, go downs, and warehouses, elimination of rat burrows by blocking with concrete.

Environmental hygiene that we see around
Can you enter a public toilet without covering your nose? Our washroom hygiene is below standard. Public is not protected from the dangerous bacteria. Unclean surrounding, open air defecation, cow dung, animals and dogs in the streets, dustbins and its foul content, not segregated contents dump, roads not swept, open gutters, clogged gutters, garbage and filth openly thrown in the street. So how to create an environment we want to live in. each household can sought its garbage into plastic, aluminum, steel, glass, paper, cloth, combustibles and incombustibles according to detailed classification. Color coded bags put it in. Wash recyclables before putting them into the bags. They system to form will demand time but it can come if we want clean hygienic city and areas. Personal hygiene affects individual comfort, safety and well being. Well people are capable of it, ill people need assistance.

Number of factors influence this such as:

1. During childhood it is influenced by family customs
2. Young age by peer group, personal appearance, make up
3. Hygiene practices may change because of living conditions and a available resources
4. Personal preferences
5. Body image—neatly groomed
6. Affordable—deodorant or cosmetic
7. Health beliefs and motivation
8. Cultural variables
9. Physical condition
10. Perineum care

Surface water bodies can be beneficial as it can supply water for domestic, agriculture, fishing, recreation, it can also be breeding ground of insects, snails, mosquitoes which transmit diseases. Clean environment helps to prevent diseases when home environment is clean.

Find out

1. Is diarrhea common among children?
2. Are worm infestations common?
3. Are respiratory/breathing problems common?
4. Is eye sight common among children?
5. Is malarial fever common among children/people?
6. Do many people have fever?
7. Have there been any out break recently that affected many?

8. Are children undernourished, do they look thin or lack energy? Assessing community perceptions about health is important for a nurse
9. What water sources available in community?
10. Which local water sources do people commonly use?
11. Is the water source protected/treated?
12. How much water is collected by each house hold?
13. Is the water always available?
14. Does every one have the access to water?
15. Does the community know the quality of water?
16. Are there special places for bathing and laundry?
17. What types of sanitation does the community have?
18. Are there separate facilities for women?

The **suffocating smell of a hospital** put you off? Does over powering stench of drugs and disinfectants leave you nauseated? To experience hospitals odor free premises is top priority. The particular smell generally means a threat of infection, dust, humidity; drugs and all kinds of human and medical waste combine to generate the hospital smell. If the smell persists, it clearly means that the hospital is not clean. To have high quality air conditioners to mange the throw in and throw out of the air is the right way. A simple shift from phenyl to modern cleaning agents has worked wonders and cleansing the premises more meticulously.

Gates reinvent toilets—waterless 2.5 billion people around the world without access to modern sanitation. Microwave energy to transform human waste into electricity is being researched. Scientists from around the world have taken up the challenge and it must operate without running water, electricity or a septic system not discharged pollutants, preferably capture energy and operate at a cost of 5 cents a day. Diseases caused by unsafe sanitation results in about half the hospitals in the developing world. Abut 1.5 million children die each year from diarrhea diseases. Most of these are preventable with proper sanitation alone with safe drinking water and improved hygiene. Research expert have to field teats within 3 years the innovation. Many recycle waste into other usable substances such as animal feed, water for irrigation or even just energy and water run their own systems. It looks very low tech but thee is a lot of science behind it. Reinvent of the toilet has the potential to improve lives as well as environment. Gates predicted the result of this project would reach beyond the developing world

Stop pollution—pollution is a serious problem which needs an immediate check. 140 million affected in 70 countries by arsenic pollution. 36.3 billion kg of hazardous pollutants each year generated in industry by USA alone. Fifteen percent of adult's have permanent hearing damage due to noise exposure. 1.5 mn of deaths in the world are the result of indoor air pollution. 250 million of clinical cases of gastro enteritis + respiratory diseases are caused annually by bathing in contaminated water. 10 mn tube wells in Bangladesh contaminated with arsenic. 220 million tons of plastic can contribute to reduce our carbon footprint. Seventy million people in Bangladesh are exposed to water that contains more than the world health organization threshold value of 10 micrograms of arsenic/liter. Two hundred and sixty-seven marian species have been reported entangles in or having ingested marine debris. Fifty percent of packaged goods and bulk cargoes transported by sea today can be regarded as dangerous or hazardous from safety standpoint of harmful to the environment. Sixteen billion the annual global economic cost related to pollution of coastal water. Eighty percent of marine pollution globally contributes by such as agricultural run off pesticides. 2.5 to 3 billion people in the world living without the adequate sanitation system.

Air pollution is perhaps the most common and the most dangerous type of pollution. It involves the direct release of chemicals into the environment. Air pollution caused by burning of fuel that directly releases hazardous chemicals in the air.

Water pollution is caused by the direct incorporation of hazardous pollutants. The source of these pollutants is yet again the large industries and factories that dispose off their waste in lakes and ponds.

Noise pollution can be extremely dangerous. And it is all around us. It penetrates into the human mind and controls it. too much noise leads to severe psychological illness and badly affects the behavior. Noise pollution is caused by the moving vehicles, man made machines and loud music. Other than that noise can be caused by anything, but these three sources are the main reasons for the pollution around us.

How to stop pollution—no plastic bags to curb pollution of our surrounding of our homes. Do not horn unnecessary, use bio-degradable materials etc.

Clean India—cleanliness is next to godliness
Can you enter a public toilet without covering your nose?

Our washroom hygiene is below standard. People are not protected from dangerous bacteria. Due to unclean surrounding, open air defecation, cow dung in front of the house hipped, animals freely in the street roam around eating garbage and plastics, hips of debris in the streets and around the houses, municipality trucks pick up with such a unhygienic way and the odor that is spread all over as the truck passes by, debris and wastage is not segregated and dumped as it is wet and dry wastage and dangerous objects, open gutters, clogged pipes, throw the wastage from window out, from train out. In this way we are far behind the western world that have high standard of cleanliness, cities and towns, villages are well-planned and provided with. Laws are imposed on people if law if broken. Spitting and toileting can not even thin off, the way street dogs and other creatures roaming around freely, no owner, no vaccination, no food arranged, just on the street. Due to ignorance people live in sub human condition and surrounding. Sometimes such a bad habits people practice of spitting in front off you from anywhere which at times splashes on you, they ear tobacco, or brittle leaves and one colorful mouthful spitting splash all over, biting nails, scratches, while eating make funny sounds, shout from one end to another calling out someone, or saying bad words, any how sleep, sit, roam around without combing hair, or well dressed up, loud music, in time of death crying loudly and expressing sorrow, shaking legs, rubbing legs and walk, and many other bad habits needs to be changed 80% of the people in rural areas use open air defecation and this practice is time honored and is considered harmless. Their beliefs that latrines are meant only for city dwellers and they are ignorant that faeces are infectious and pollute water, soil and promote fly free. They are not aware that mosquitoes breed in collections of dirty water causes filarial infestation. The sullage water is permitted to flow into the streets.

Solid waste is invariably thrown in front of the houses where it is permitted to accumulate and decomposed People bath and wash their clothes animals are washed and given drink. These particles lead to the pollution of the well water, tanks ponds used for washing as well as drinking water.

Some rivers considered as holy to have a dip and people drink raw water consider as sacred. Samples of holy water bottled carried for relatives. Live in katcha, thatched, ill-lighted, ill-ventilated houses, human being and animals live under same roof, plaster houses with cow dung chance for tetanus or insect bits.

Branding the skin with iron rod, chewing tobacco, certain food forbidden tin pregnancy, traditional barbers still do the shaving with un-sterile instruments, sleep on the ground, walk on bare foot, menstruating women considered unclean etc.

They have to turn bad habits into good one such as use cow dung for fuel, build separate house in open space, keep animals in common grazing place, white wash house regularly, eat after bath and hand wash, observe fast, oil bath, use neem leaves as a tooth brush etc.

Wastage from market, industries thrown on to the road side where it stagnate and stars rotting with bad smell, so people are advised to re use the wastage for composting into fertilizers.

What is the relationship between environment and health? How are they connected? Environment cleanliness means invite health. What makes environment dirty? What are their adverse effects on health? You are part and parcel of this universe, what good or bad one does affects each other. Water is life, where there is water you can see there is life and vice versa. How many percentages of people do you think get good safe wholesome water? Is it enough what quantity of water we get? Is it clean water? Good enough for the consumption or it contains impurities.

Nurses are responsible and accountable for the care they give. Make decision for yourself that you can justify. Patients whom you care—you are accountable to him, scientific discoveries in medicine advances in medical technology permit intense monitoring of and interventions. The advances have led to increasing specialization within nursing; advances in computer technology, as part of the explosion in scientific knowledge have influenced the delivery of health care. Genetic engineering developments have bought in their wake very complex ethical problems.

Specialist nurses in the community- district nurses, practice nurses, community mental health nurses, community learning disabilities nurses, school nurses, occupational health nurses, PHN/visiting nurses, community matrons (England).

Explanation—the figures show the standard of sanitation. Still open gutters, drainage water running into the street, throwing plastic and wastage on the road and in front of the house, animals and stray dogs, clogged gutters, stagnated water, unhygienic habits, etc. is shown.

Keywords

Environment, unsafe water, polluted soil, poor housing, hygiene, air pollution, milk-borne disease, clean India.

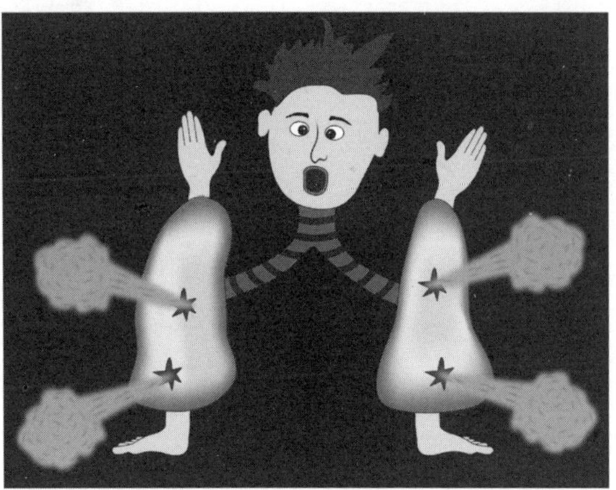

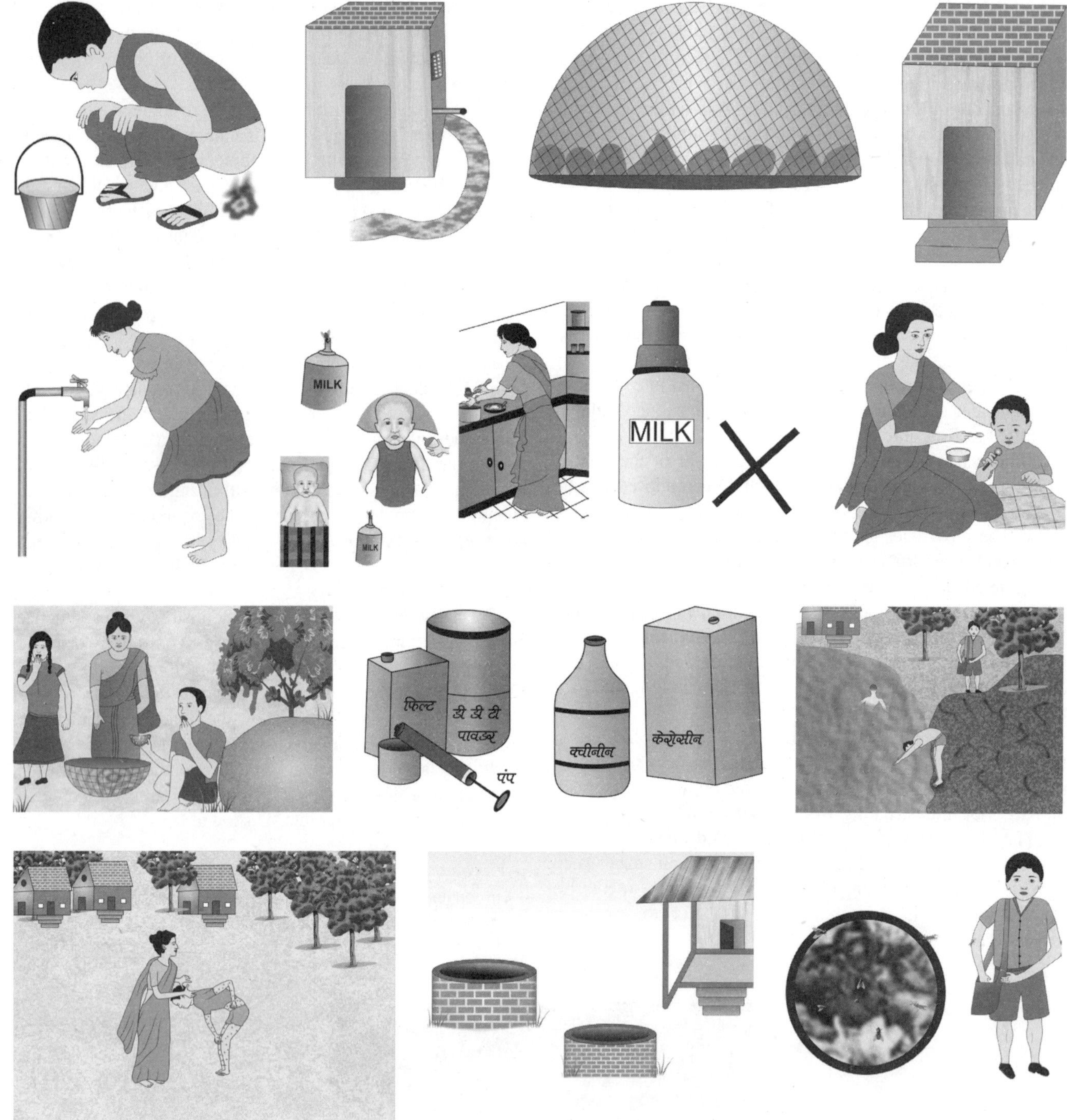
MILK
MILK
MILK
फिल्ट
डी डी टी
पावडर
पंप
क्वीनीन
केरोसीन

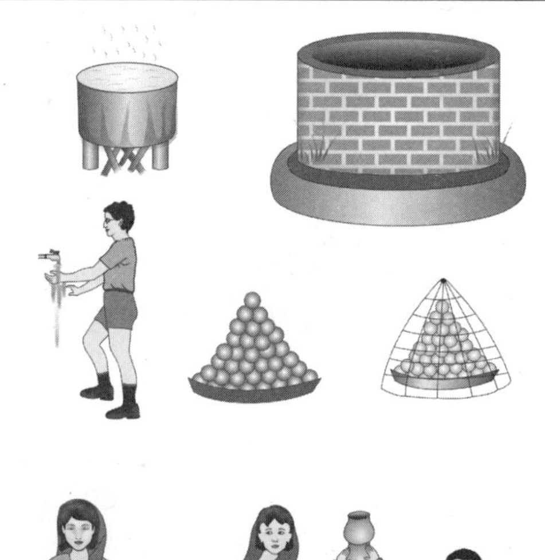

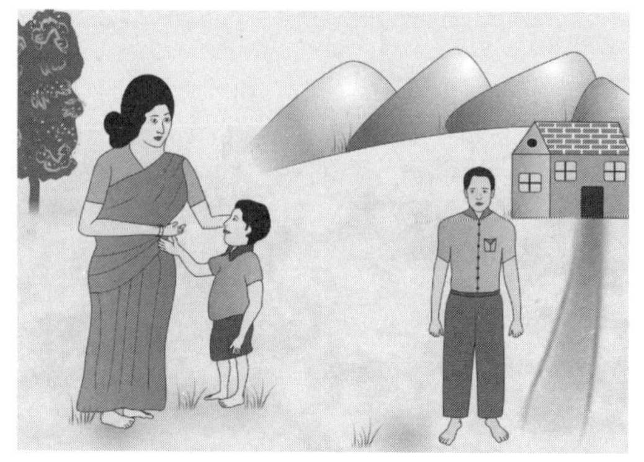

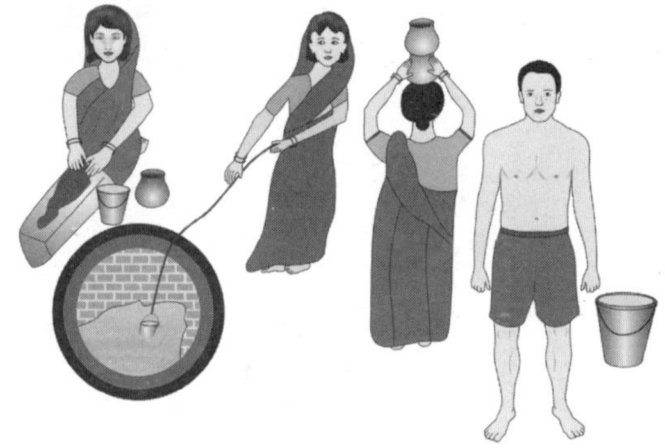

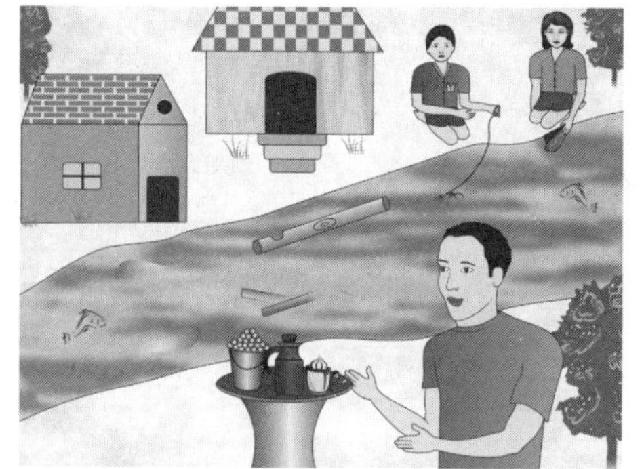

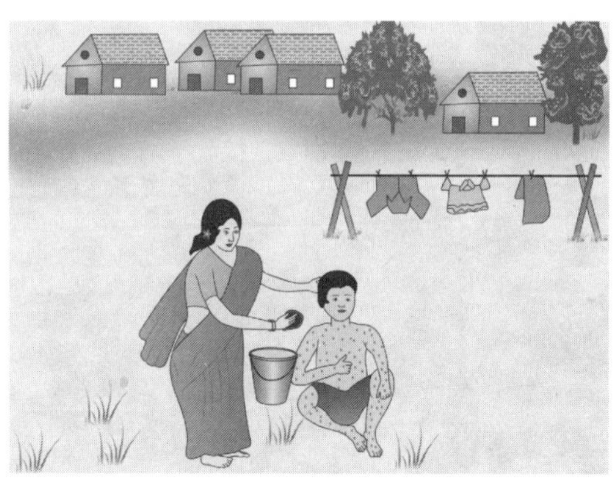

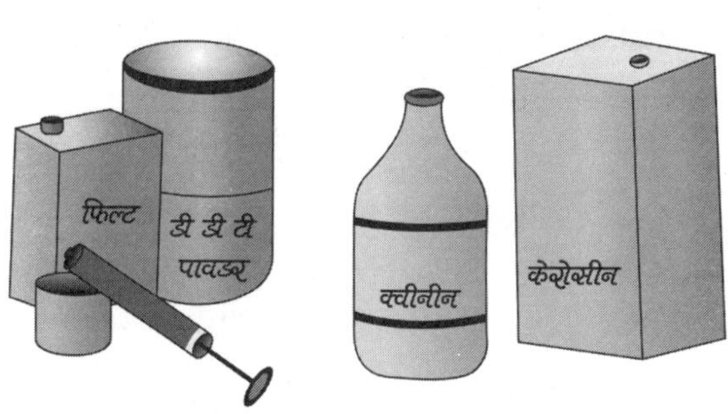
फिल्ट
डी डी टी
पावडर
क्वीनीन
केरोसीन

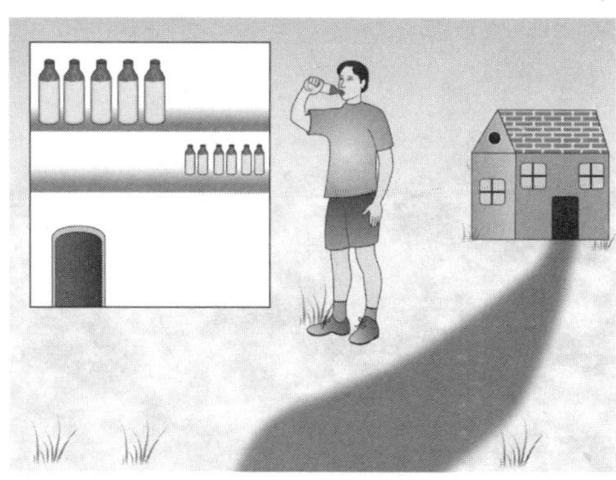

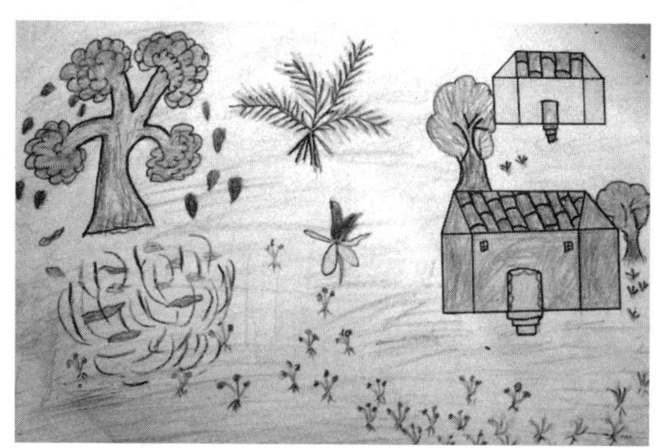

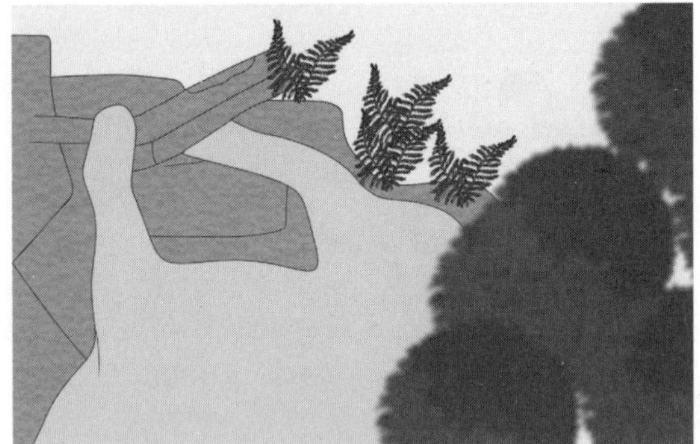

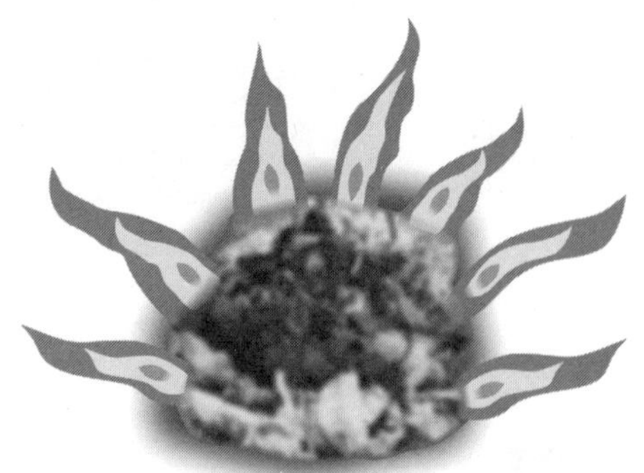

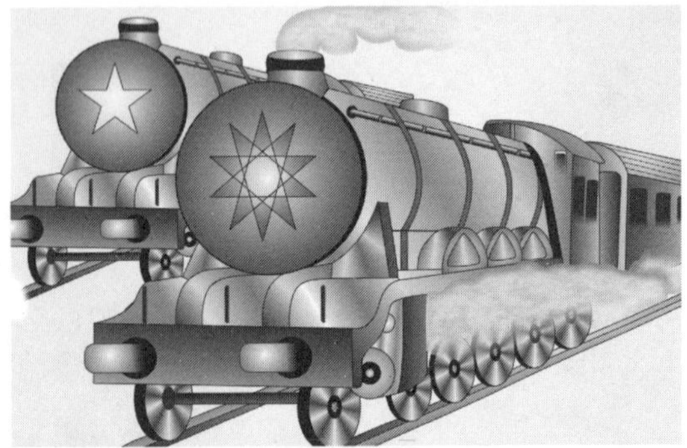

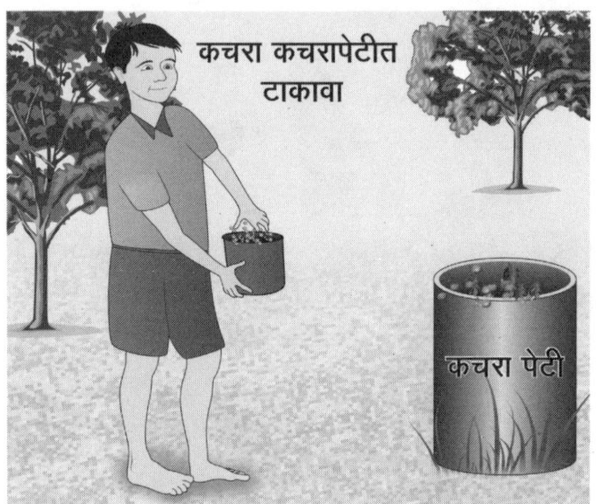
कचरा कचरापेटीत
टाकावा
कचरा पेटी

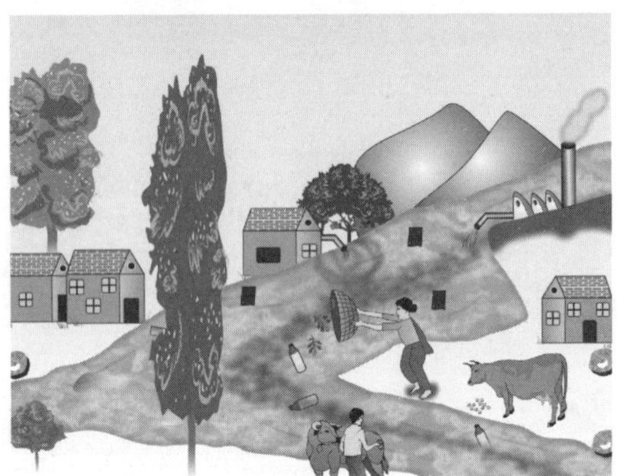

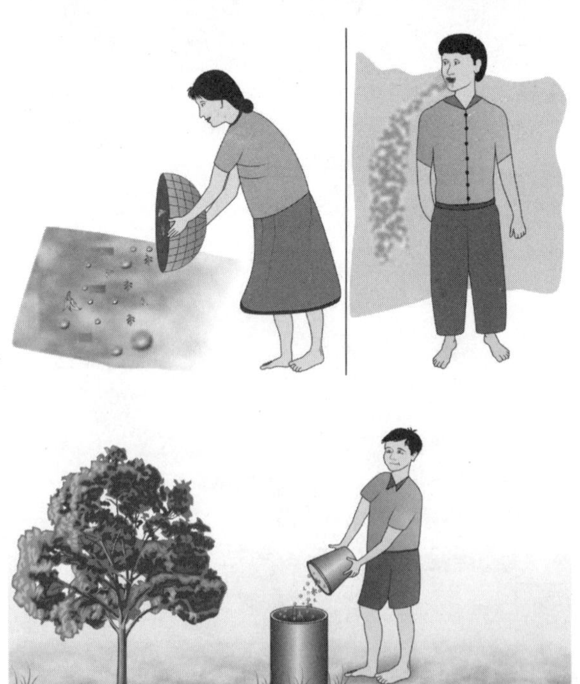

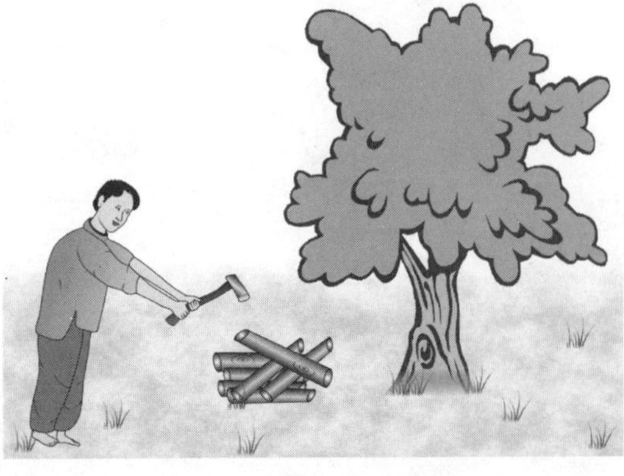

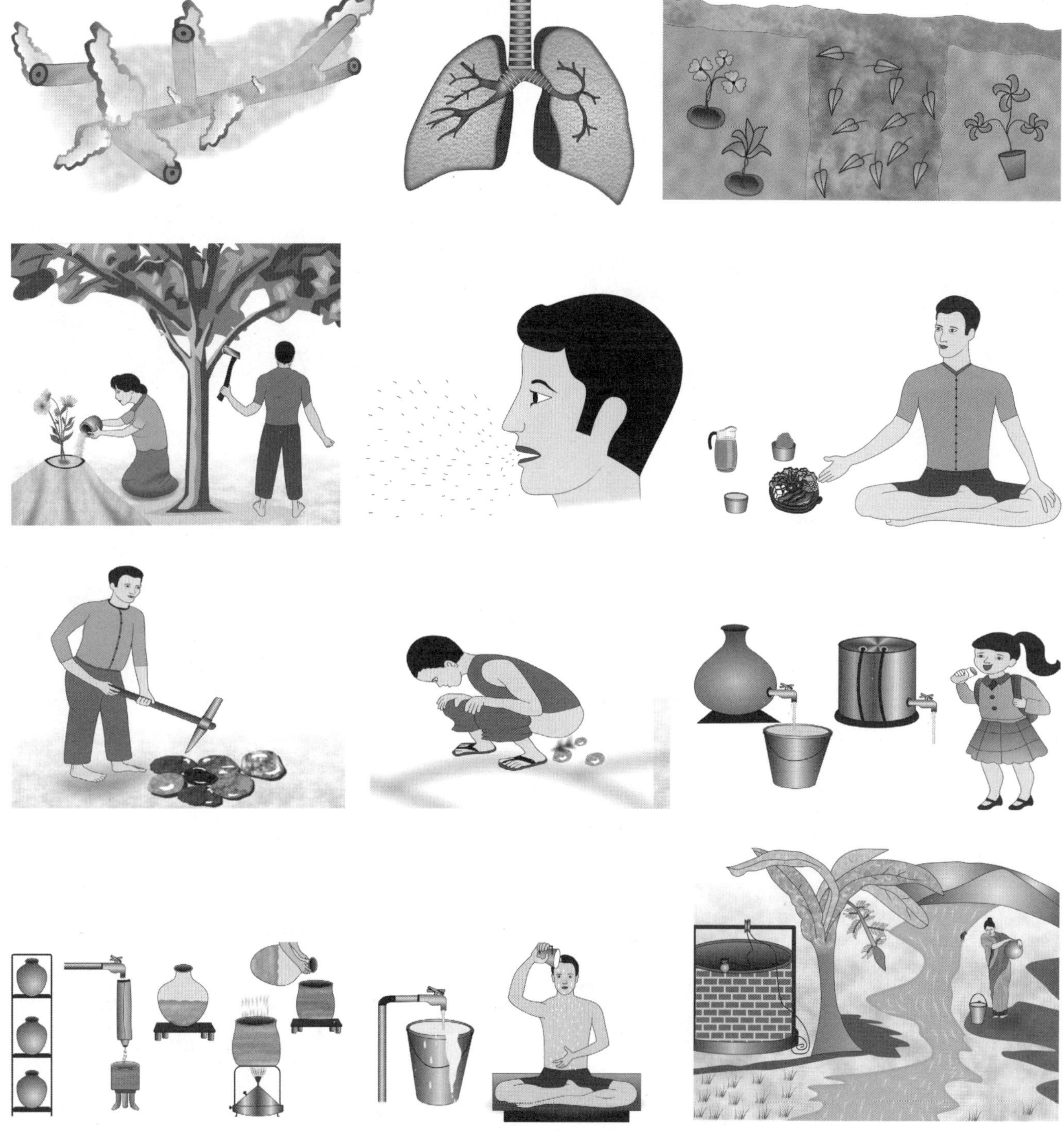

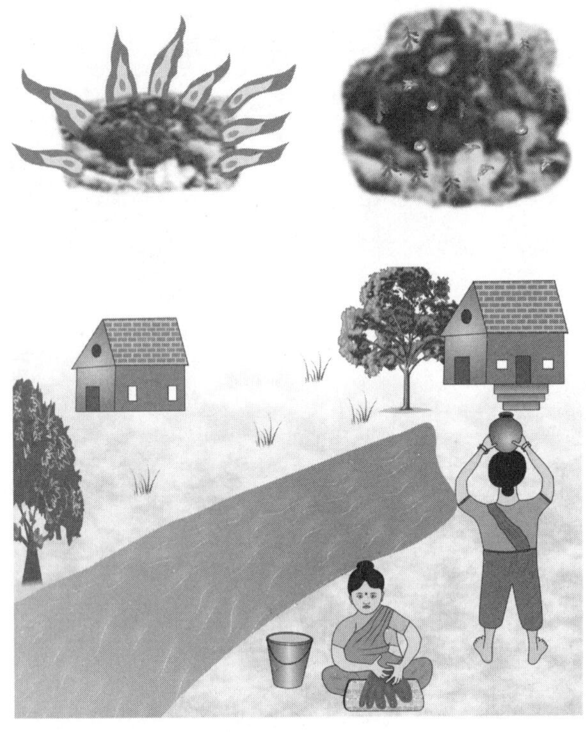

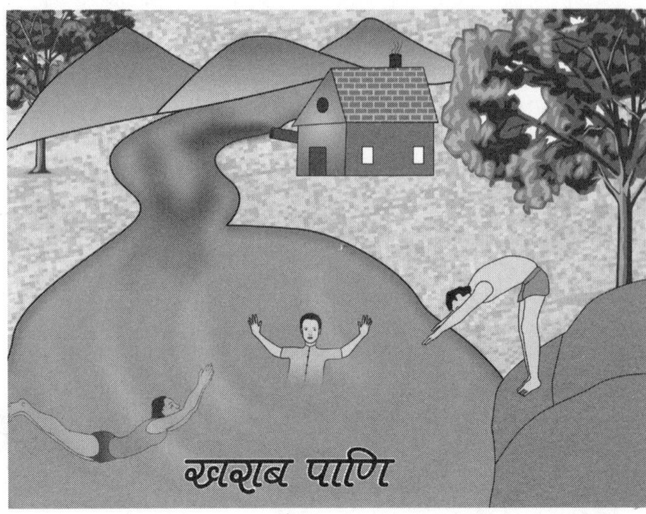
खराब पाणि

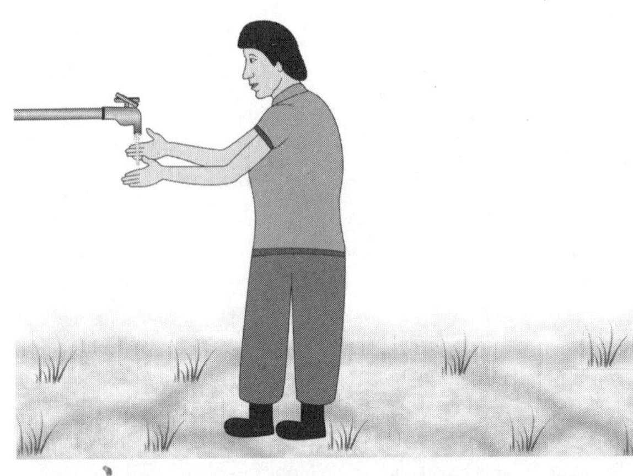

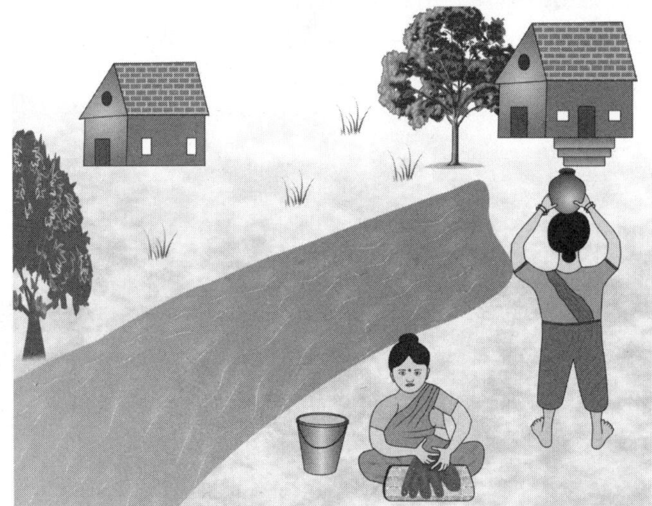

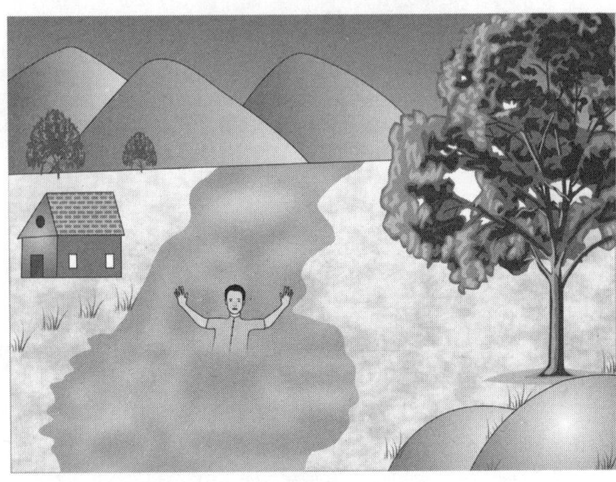

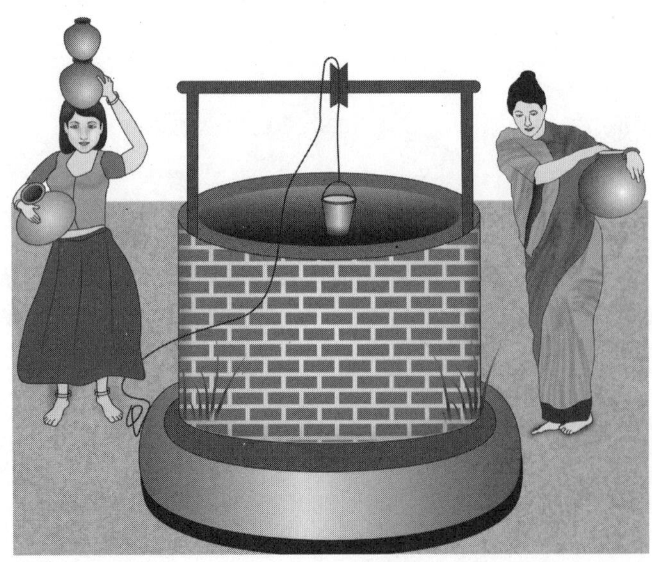

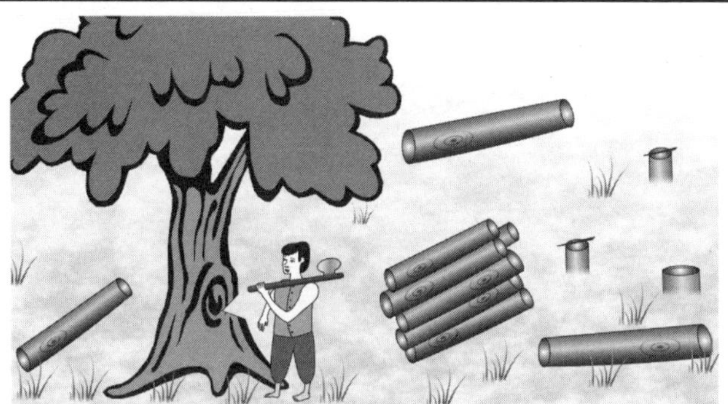
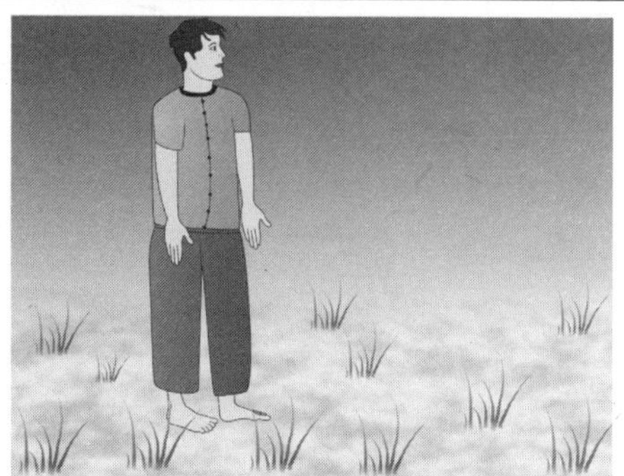
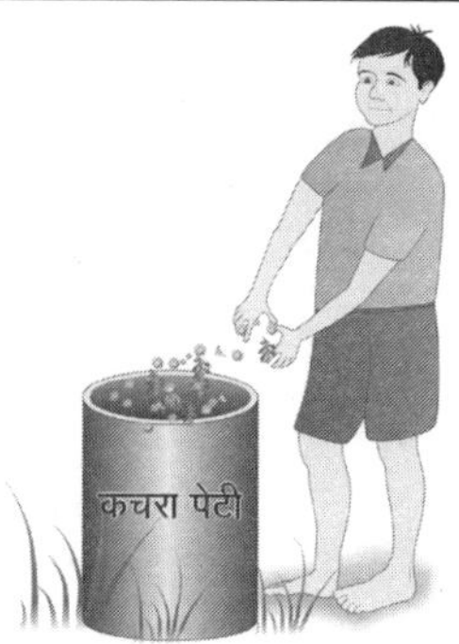
कचरा पेटी
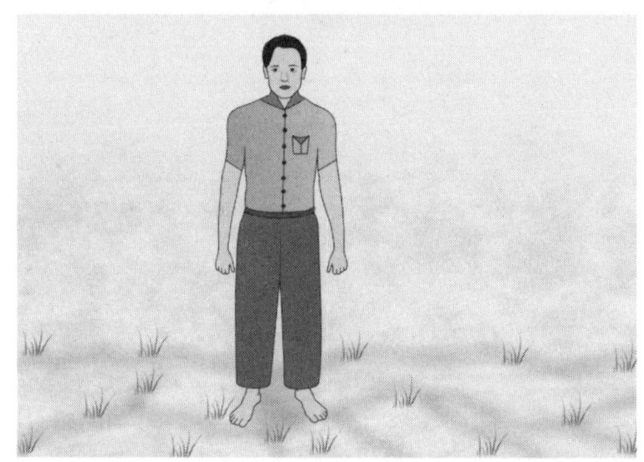
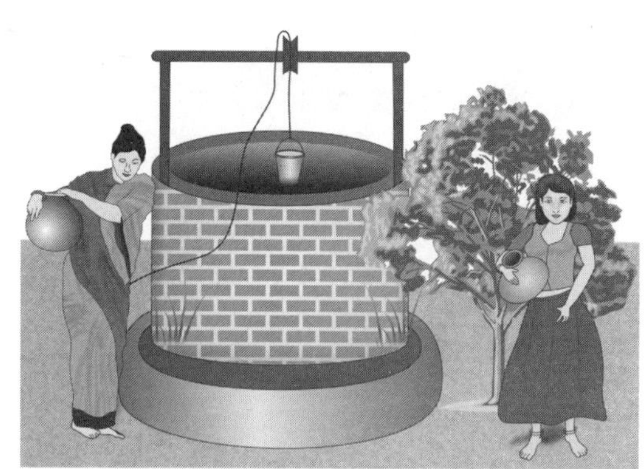
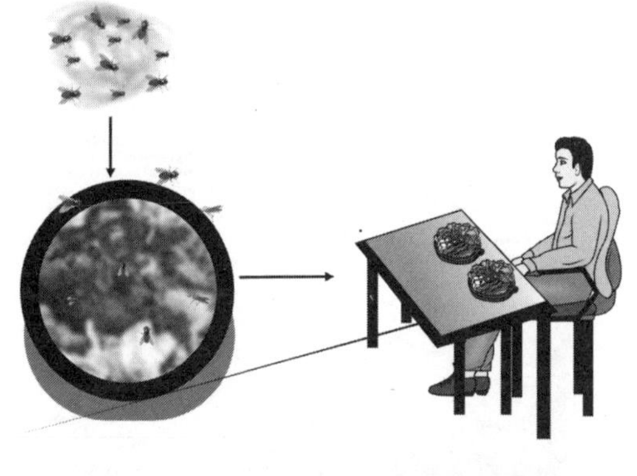
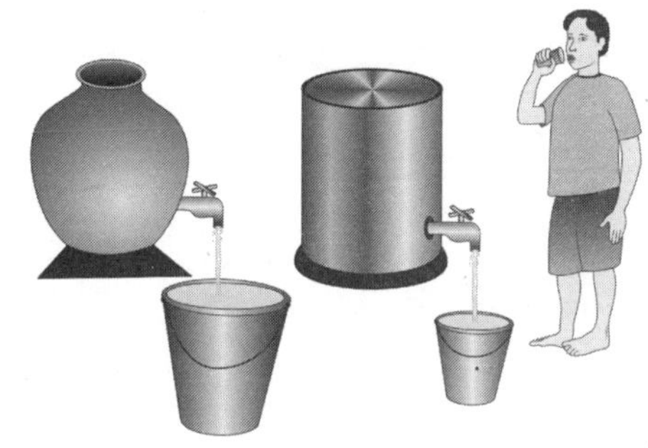
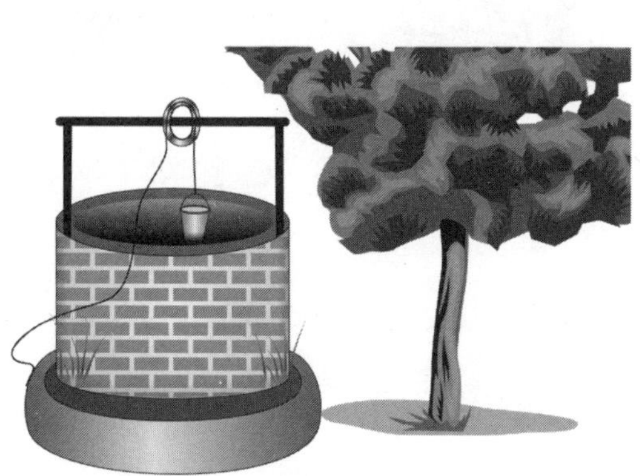
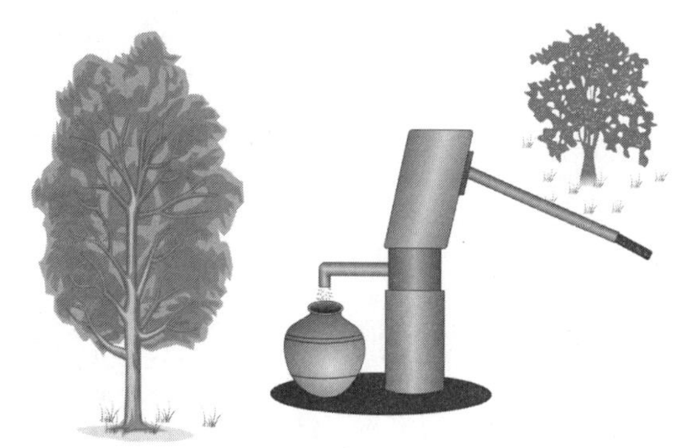

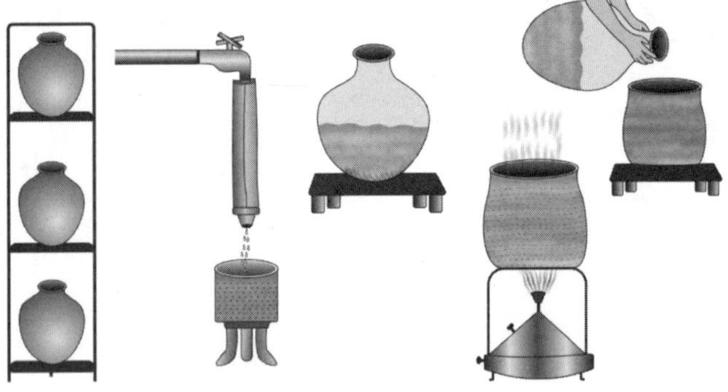

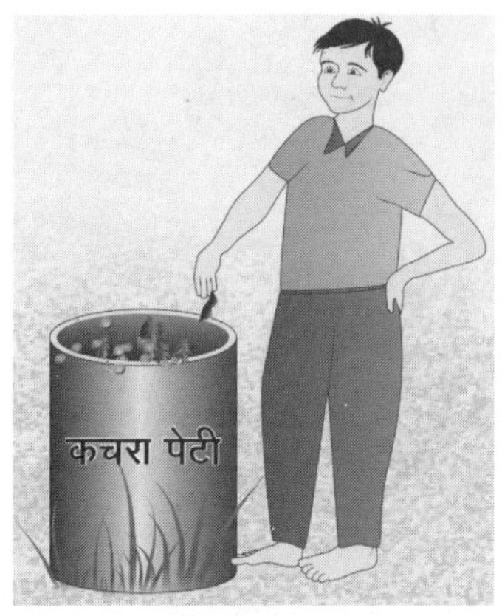

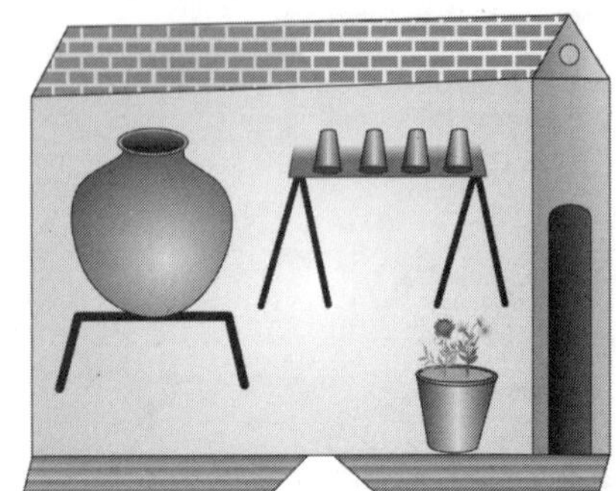

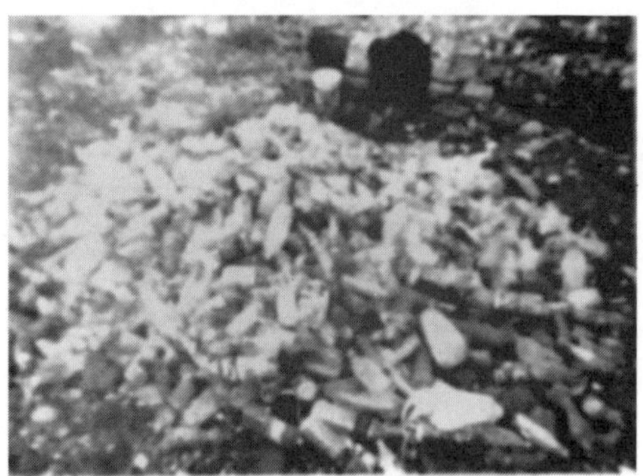

PLASTIC WASTE

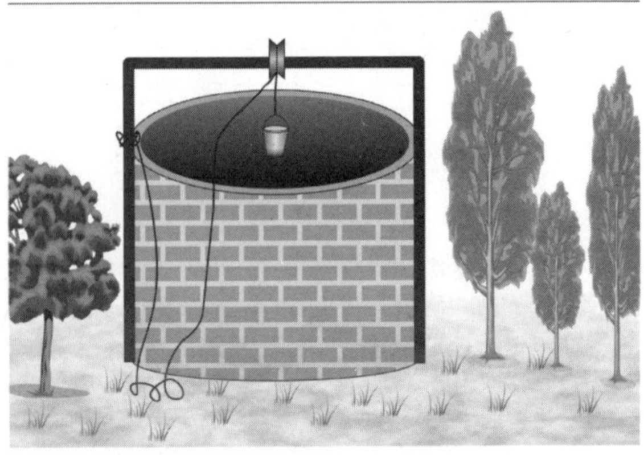

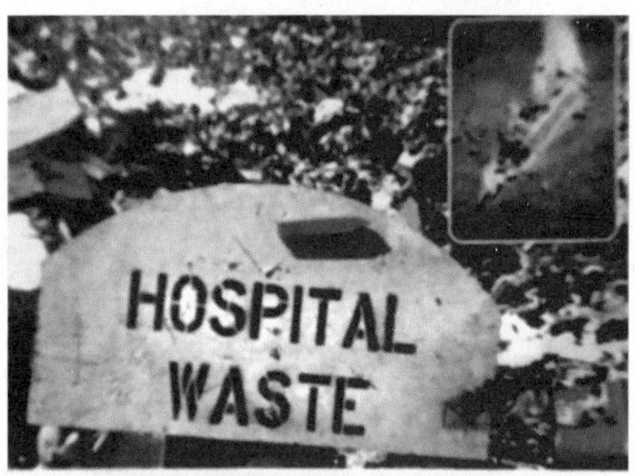

BIO-MEDICAL WASTE

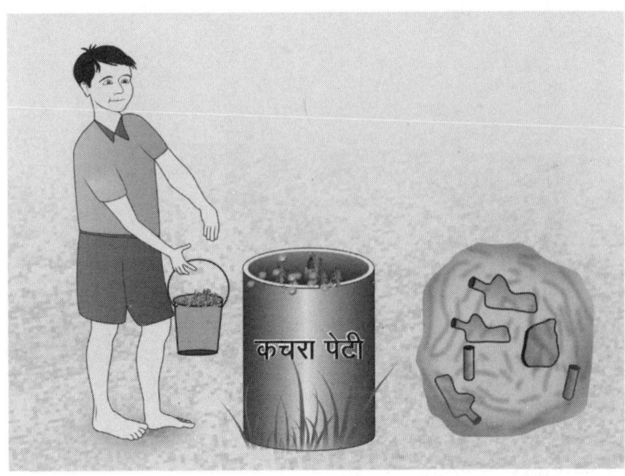

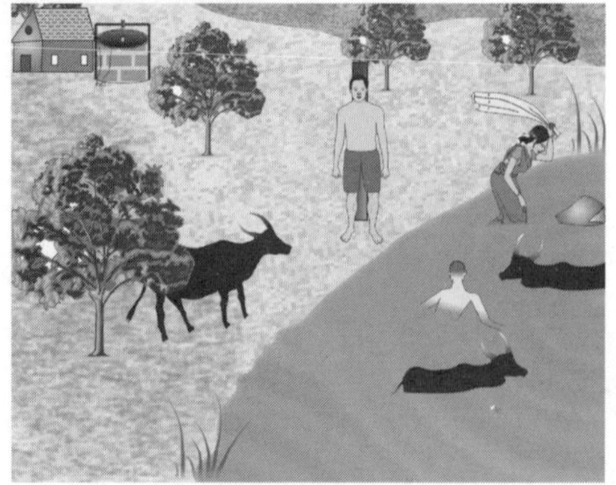

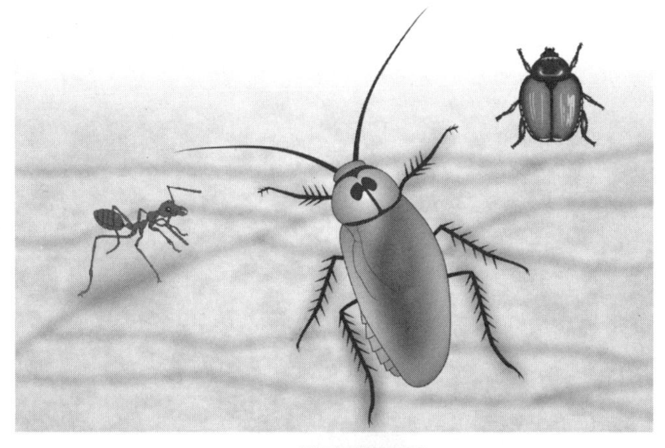

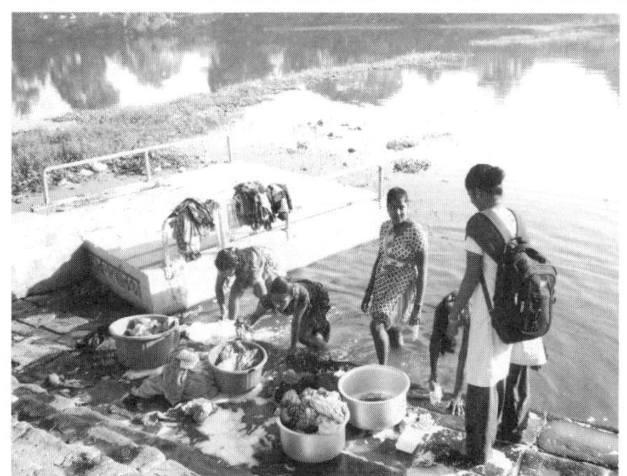

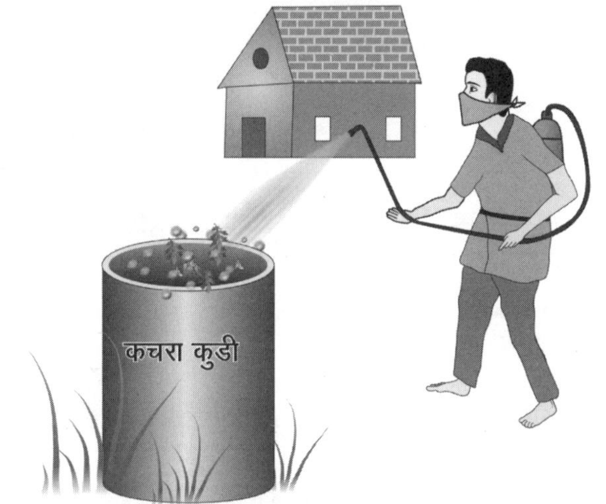
कचरा कुडी

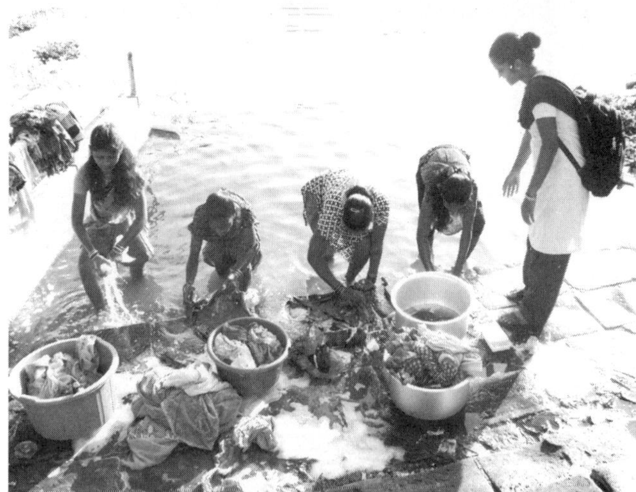

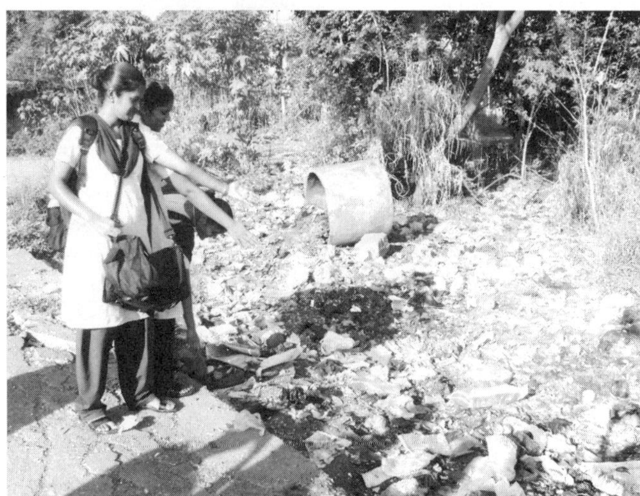

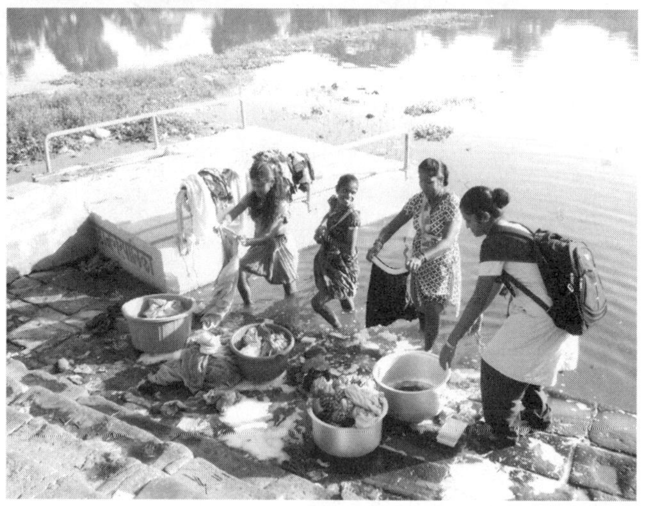

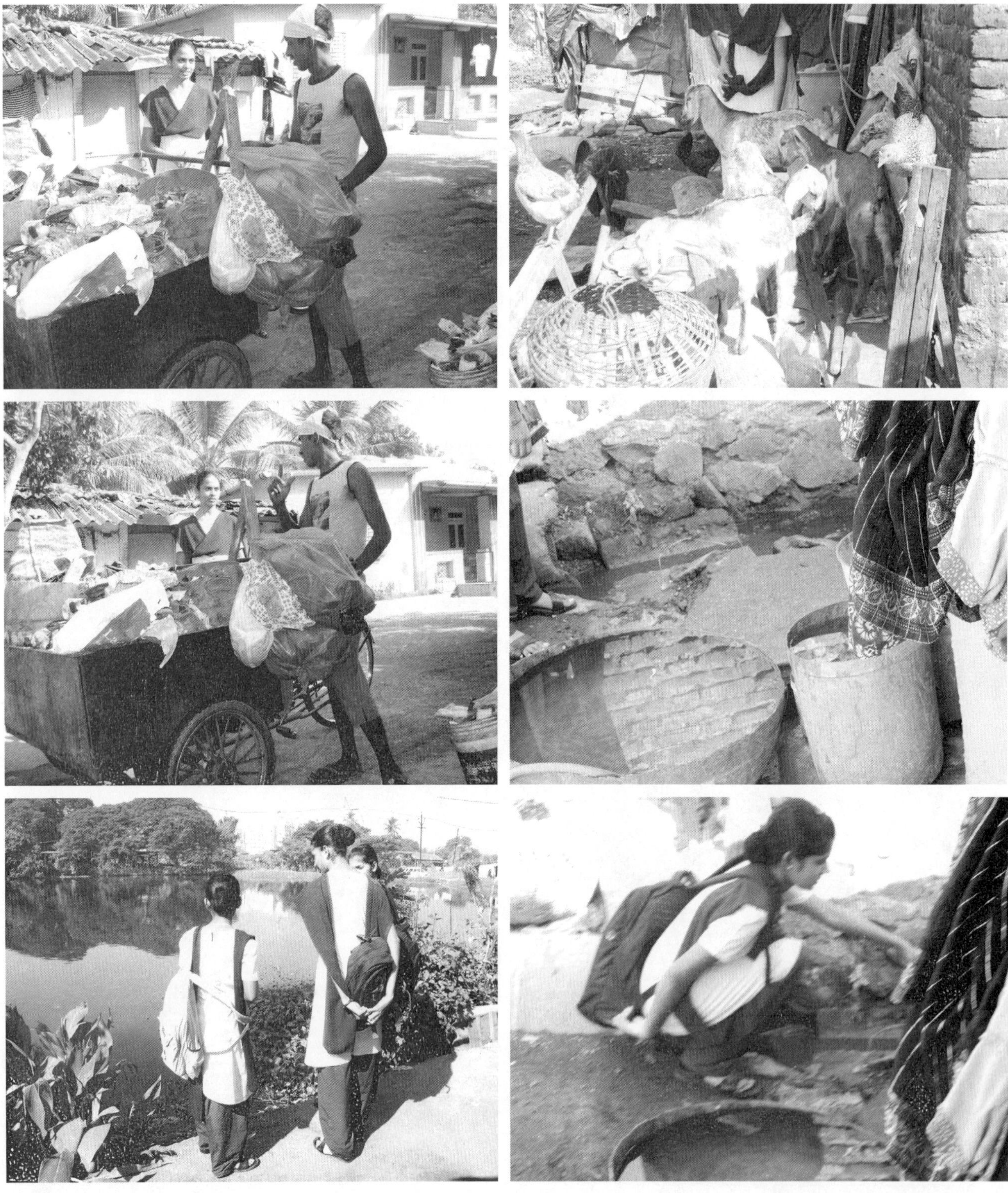

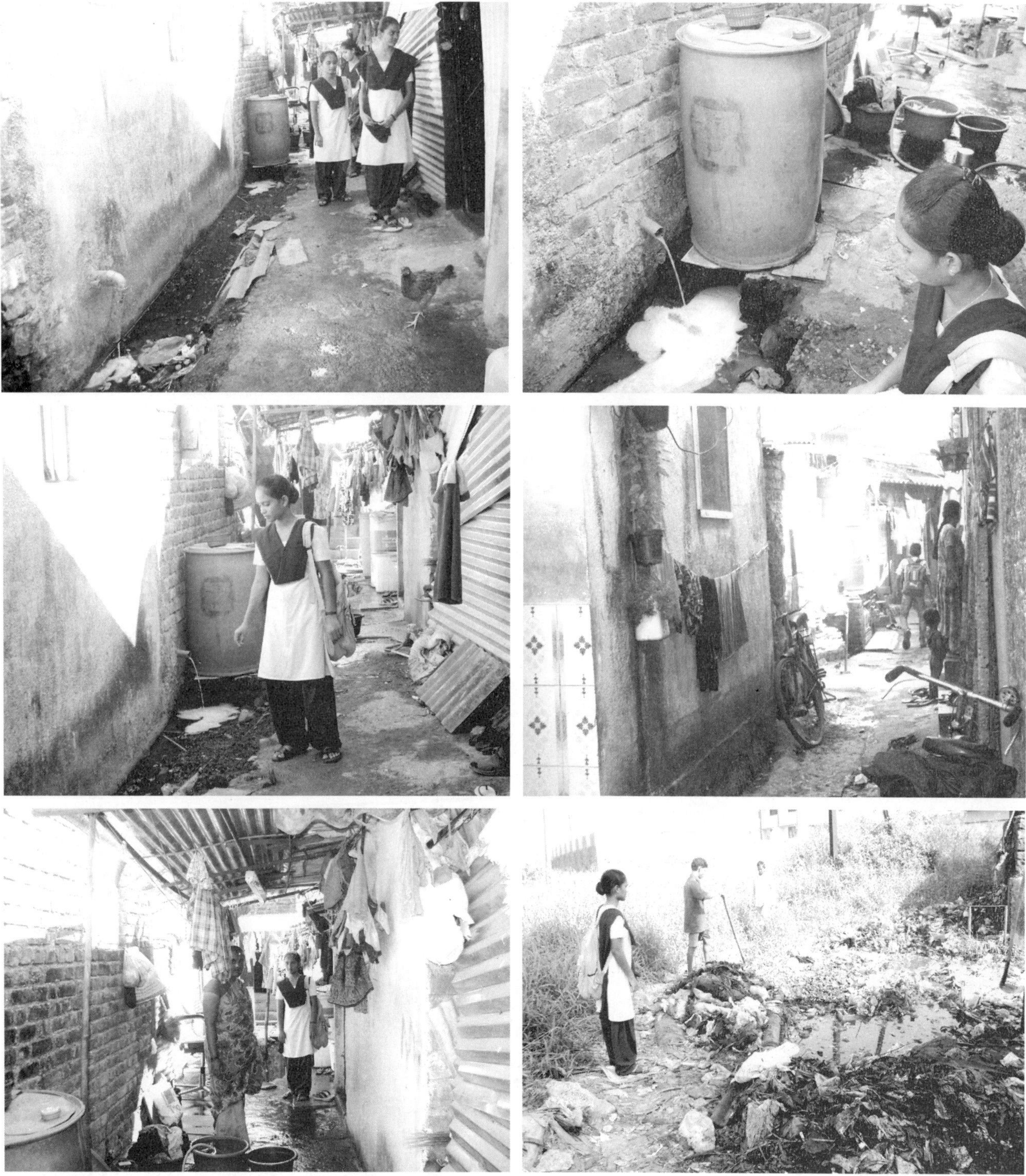

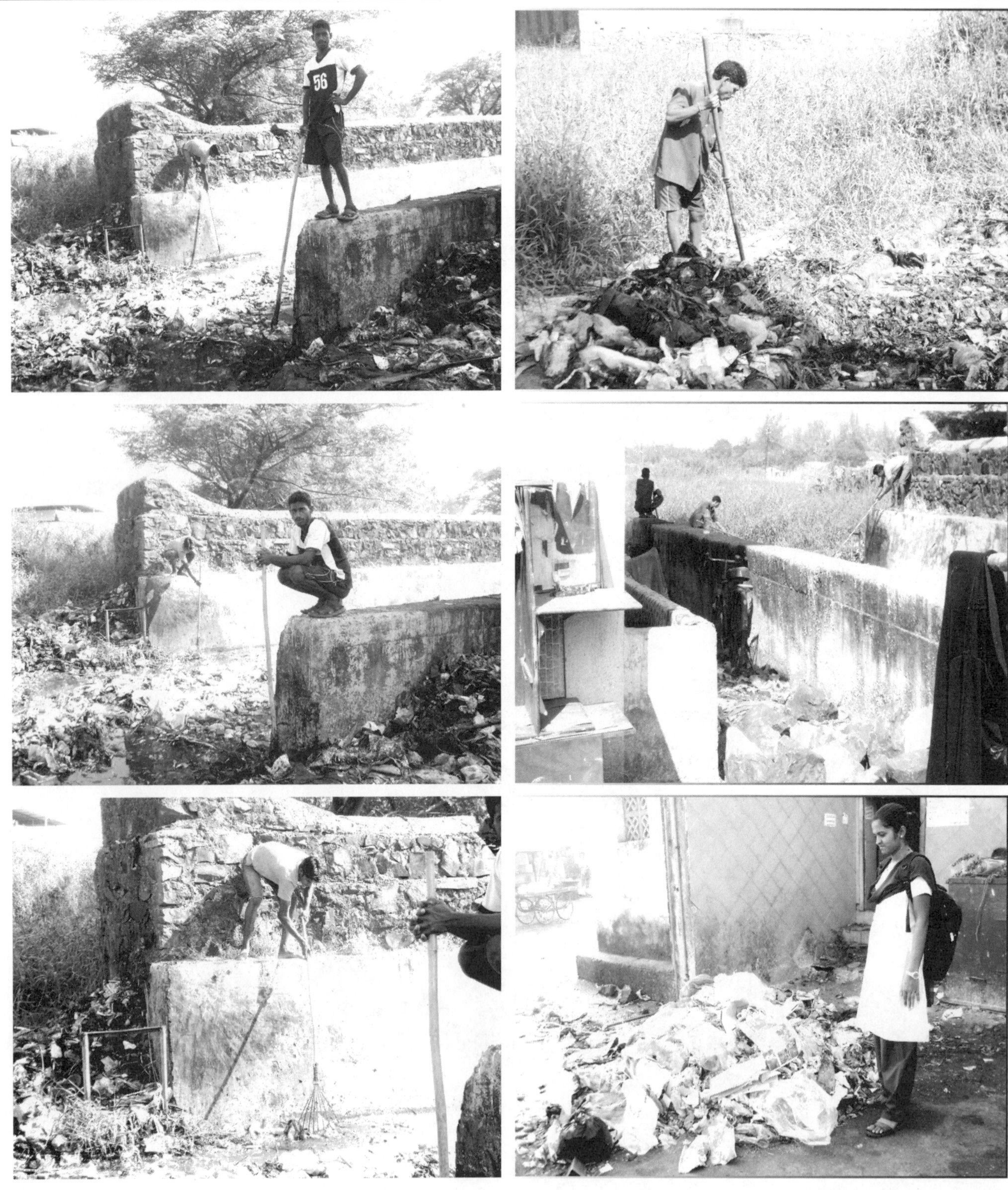
56

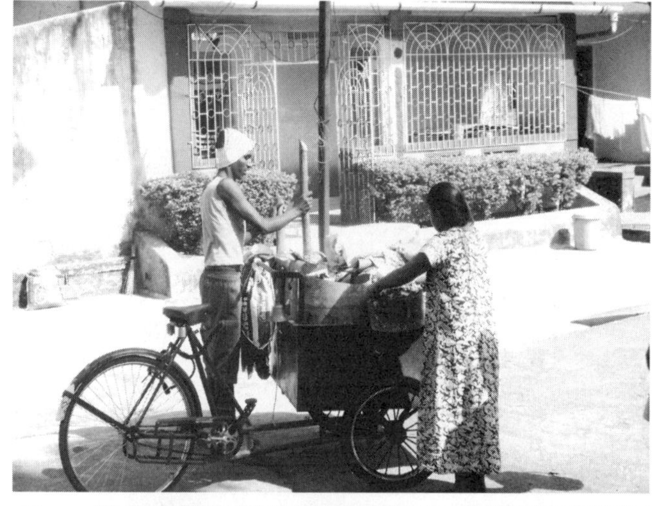

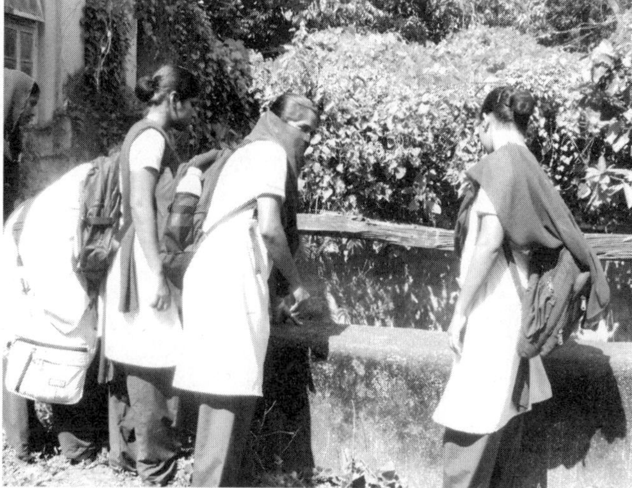

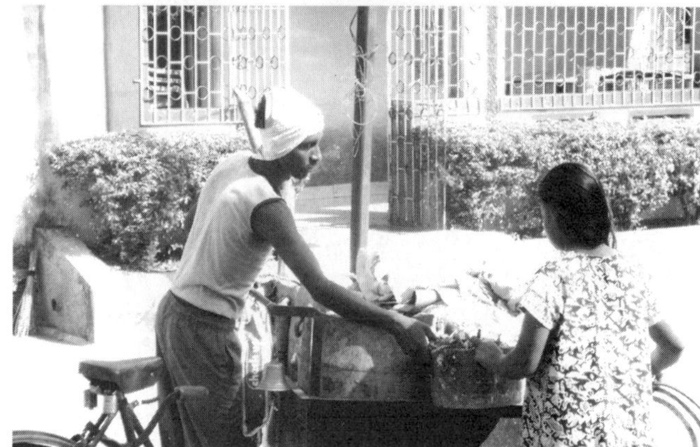

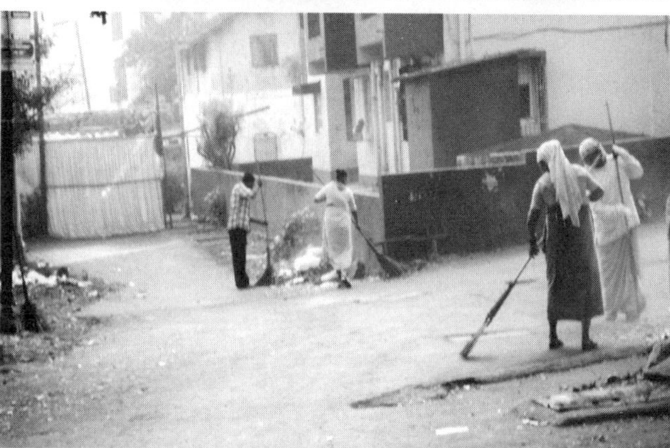

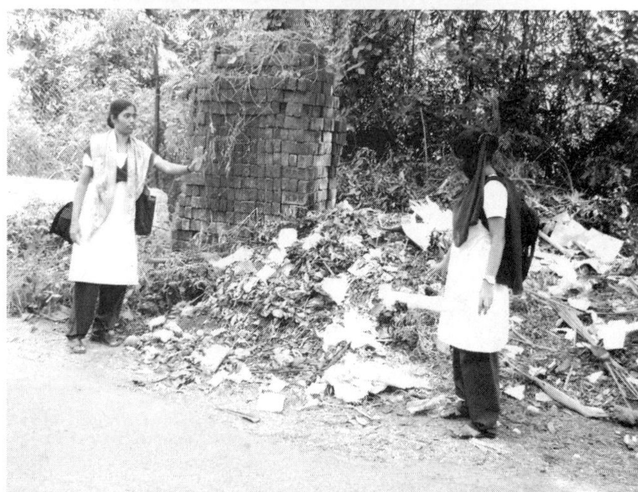

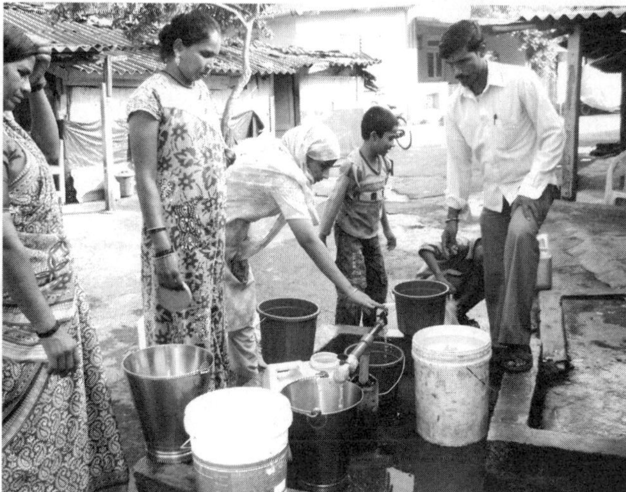

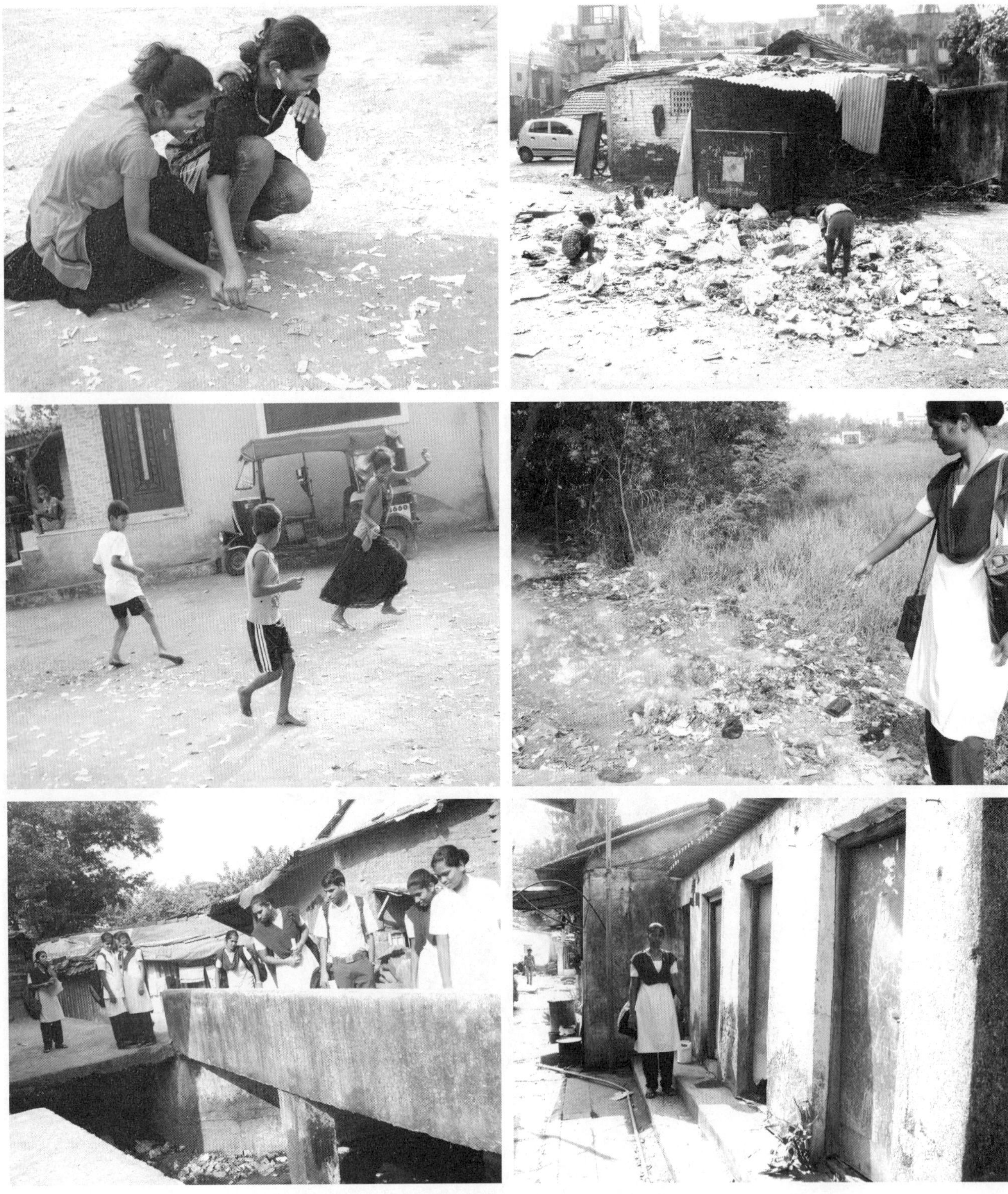

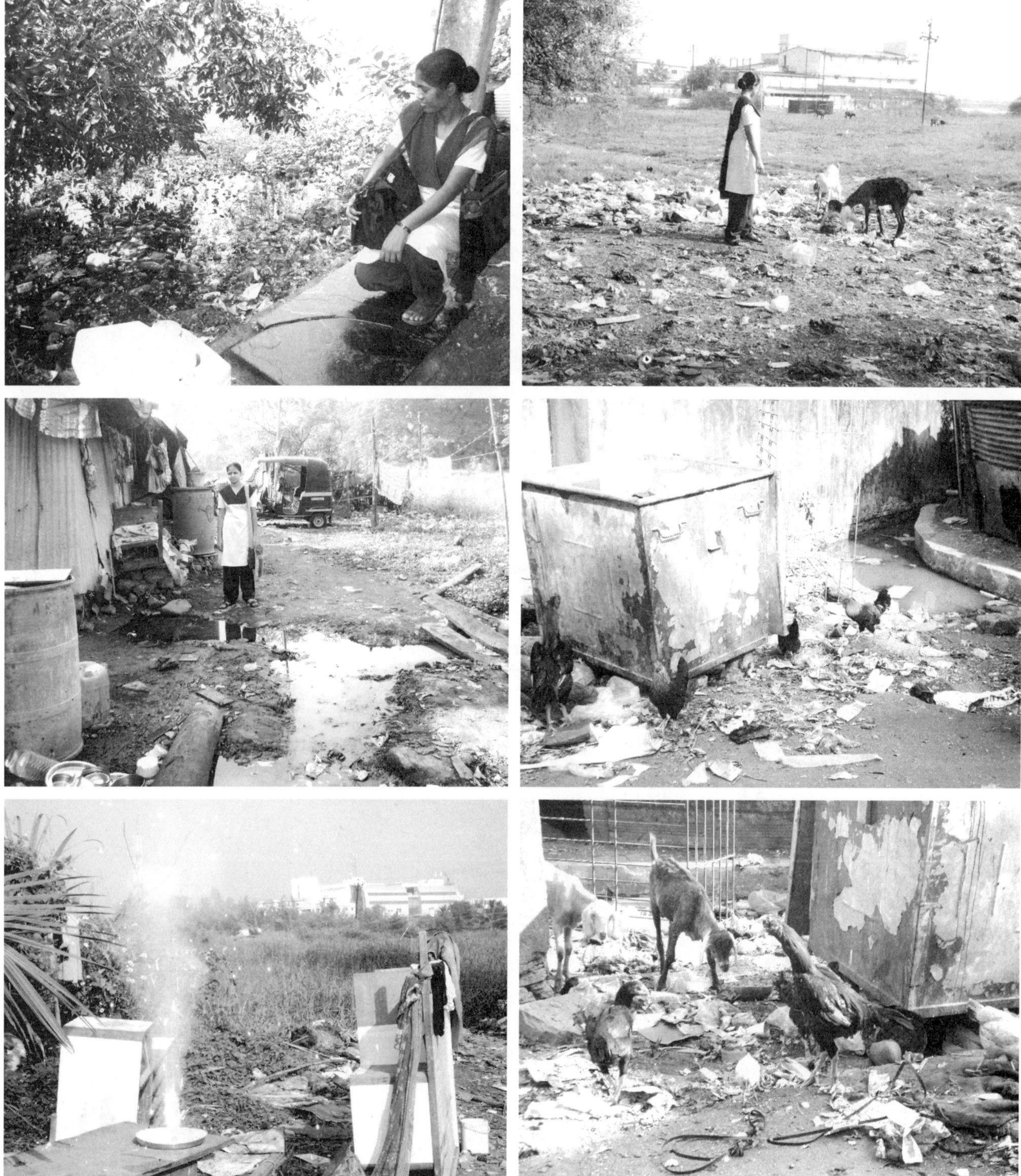

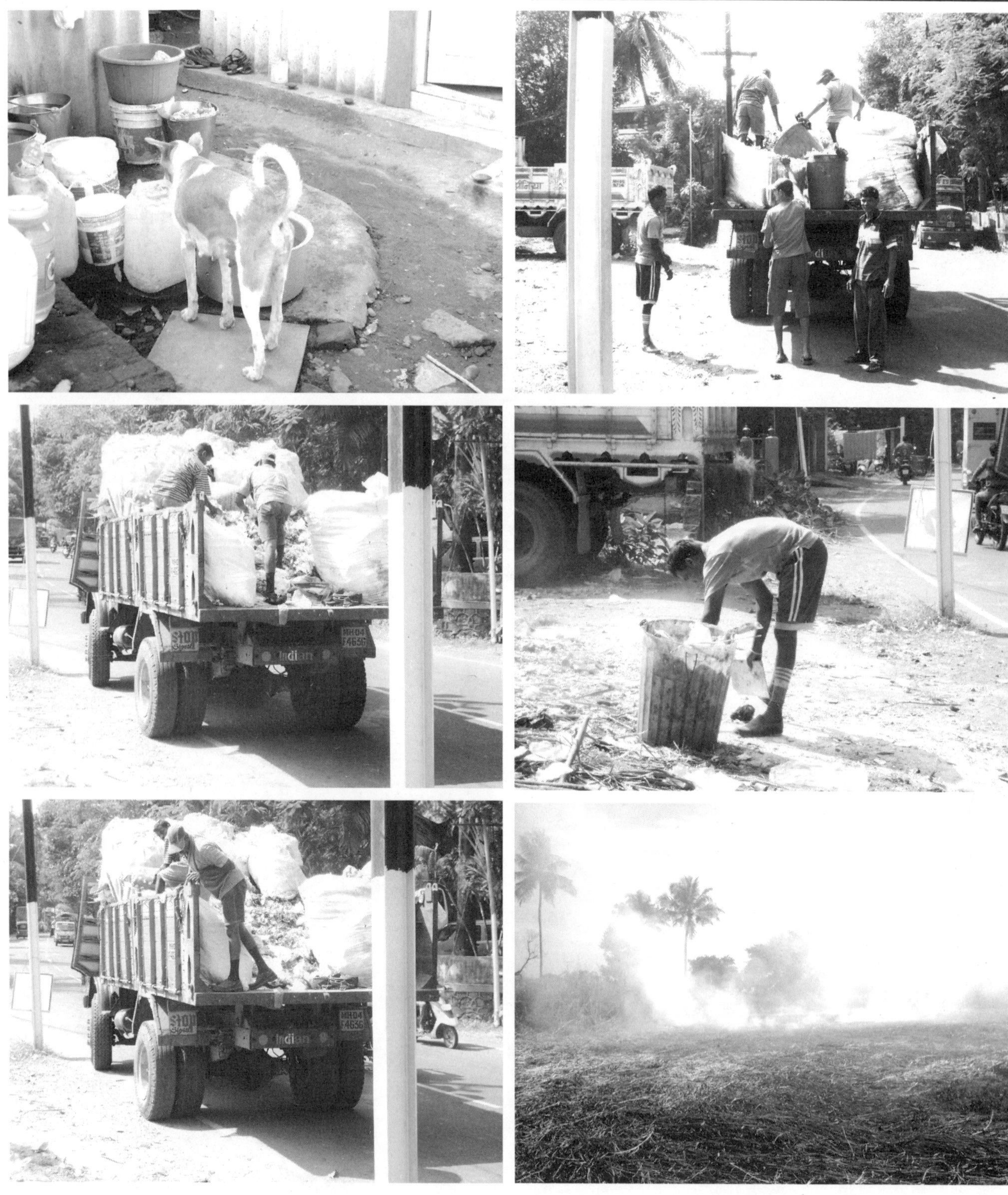

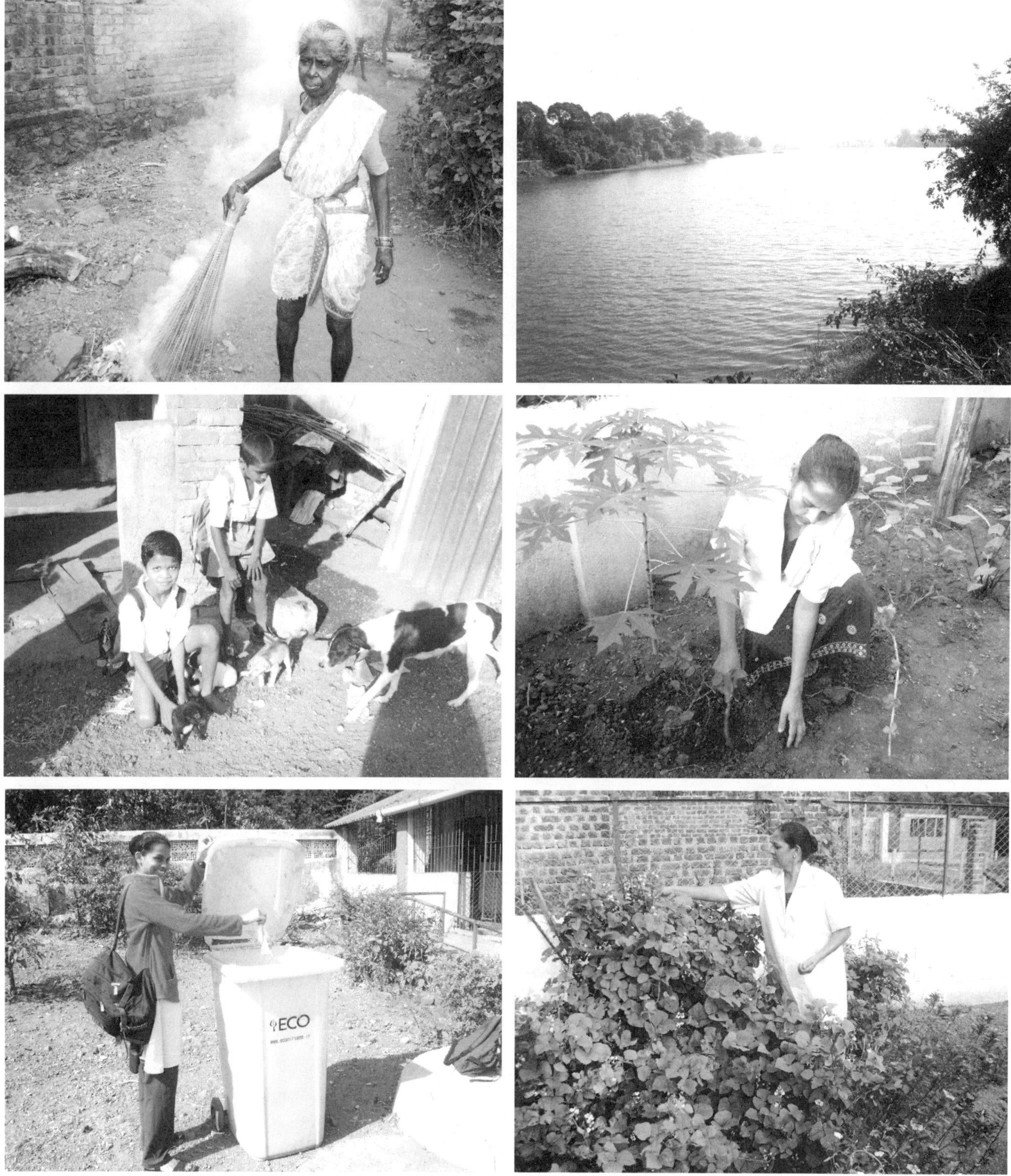
ECO

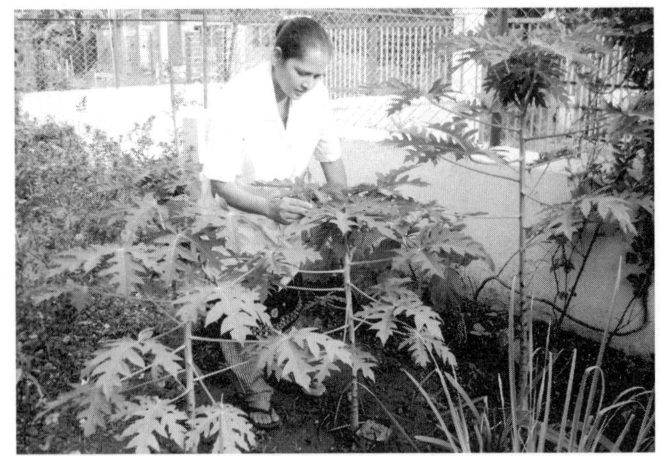

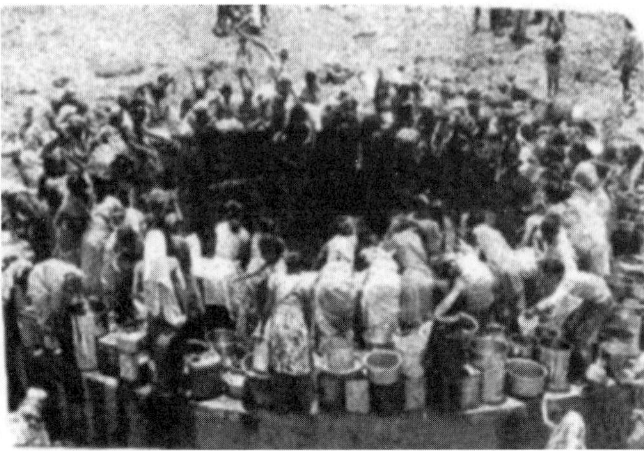

CHAPTER

50

Food Hygiene/Food Poisoning/ Food Adulteration

Abstract

Food hygiene is the practice of properly chilling, cooking, cleaning food and avoiding cross-contamination to prevent the spread of bacteria in food. In proper food hygiene, when handling raw food, may lead to food poisoning. Food poisoning is defined as any diseases of an infectious or toxic nature caused by the consumption of food or drink. The term is most often used to describe the illness, usually diarrhea and/or vomiting caused by bacteria, viruses or parasites. Food adulteration bears or contains an unsafe food additive.

In giving health education on any topic first communication skill is the core which helps towards the development of attitude. Good communication skill is essential tool and it is essence of health education. In rural and urban areas students needs good communication skills. Give people message cum entertainment.

FOOD HYGIENE

1. Food is a good culture medium and a potential carrier of infection
2. Cleanliness and care should be maintained in handling, producing, distributing and serving all types of food
3. Milk is responsible for the spread of cattle bovine TB and typhoid fever and spread by food handlers
4. Milk supplied by the local milkman is potential source of infection than pasteurized milk
5. The milk should be boiled well before consumption, destroying the harmful diseases organism
6. Meat not properly inspected can be a source of multiple infections like tapeworm, TB, anthrax, food poisoning, animals before slaughter are to be examined by veterinary doctors only healthy animals are slaughtered
7. Fish should be fresh to consume unless it has been dried or tinned
8. Vegetables and fruits are contaminated by pesticides, animals and human excreta, especially when they are gown in sewage irrigating land. If they are eaten raw, then they transmitted a wide range of water and food born diseases
9. All food handlers, who cook, serve or distribute food, should be screened for carriers
10. Their personal hygiene, care of hands, fingers nails, hair and clothes should be checked
11. Personal habits like sneezing, coughing, washing hands to be followed before and after touched food

Through using educational method can make the people understand what is the food poisoning and its characteristic and effect on health.

Food poisoning is an acute GI caused by the ingestion of food or drink contaminated with either living bacteria or their toxins or chemicals substances. It can attack many persons at the same time causing similar symptoms in majority of people.

It can be caused by chemicals such as arsenic or certain plant (pesticides) or see food which is non bacterial. And bacterial that is ingestion of food contaminated by their toxins which is infective where toxin production is multiple. Few germs can multiply to millions. Salmonella food poisoning incidence are widely found from prepared food, contaminated meat, milk and milk products, sausages, eggs etc and affects a person within 12 to 24 hours, the onset is sudden with chills, fever, nausea, vomiting and a profuse watery diarrhea which usually last 2 to 3 days. Man gets infection from eating food and the toxins act on the intestine which produces abdominal cramps, diarrhea and dehydration. The organisms are widely distributed in soil, dust and the intestinal tract of the animals and later enter food as spores. Certain food poisonings are fatal where death occurs due to respiratory or cardiac failure.

Person's complete history, lab investigation, stool and vomiting test, environmental study and data analysis needs to be done.

To prevent and control—

1. Meat inspection, animal examination by veterinary staffs before and after slaughtering
2. Personal hygiene among individuals engaged in the handing of preparation of food
3. Food handlers who are suffering from infected wounds should be excluded and medical inspection of food handlers be done
4. Touching food with bare hands be avoided
5. Gap between preparation and consumption of food be short, and food eaten when hot
6. The importance of rapid cooling and cold storage is stressed. Proper temperature control maintained. Food should not be left in warm pantries.
7. Milk and milk products be pasteurized
8. Sanitary improvement and surface, utensils and equipments must be kept free from rates, mice, flies and dust

9. Food handlers should be educated in matters of clean habits
10. Cook and eat on the same day is a golden rule
11. Food samples must be obtained from food establishments periodically and subjected to lab analysis
12. Continuous surveillance is necessary to avoid outbreaks of food born diseases.

Cooking

1. Fresh vegetables contain more vitamin C than stored ones
2. Vegetables must be checked for mould and worm infection, salad vegetables must be fresh, firm and crisp
3 Tomatoes must be examined fore mould
4. Never buy any food in poor condition, over-ripens fruits
5. Vegetables washed properly
6. All food grains should be kept in dry, clean and airtight tins
7. Do not keep food exposed
8. Refrigerated food should be re-heated before consumption.

Few examples of food adulteration

1. **Asafetida/Hing test**—add a sample to water and let it settle, if impure, the solution turns turbid due to presence of starch. Further hing burns like camphor, if pure, but not when adulterated with resins or gum.
2. **Cardamom test**—look for white color on the seeds
3. **Whole turmeric**—place it in beaker of water, if adulterated it will immediately leak color
4. **Chill powder**—when put in water, the sawdust will float on the surface and the color will run. If the sediments at the bottom feel gritty when rubbed, it indicates preference of brick powder
5. **Coriander powder**—immersed in water, the horse dung floats while the coriander powder sinks
6. **Supari**—wood shaving floats in water
7. **Saffron**—pure saffron dissolves easily in water while adulterated saffron does not
8. **Bajara, wheat and other grains**—place the grains in 10 gm of water and add 15 gm of salt, fungus infested grains will loat. To detect datura seeds and karnal bunt observe the grains closely. Datura seeds are fat with edges of blackish brown color, karnal bunt affected wheat, it will have a dull appearance and give off rotten smell
9. **Wheat flour**—sprinkle the flour on water bran will float on the surface
10. **Rawa**—takes 10 gm of raw in a plate and hold a magnet close to it. The iron filling will stick to the magnet
11. **Cinnamon**—mixed with water, adulterated will leak brown color
12. **Black pepper**—when placed in distilled water, papaya seeds get separated since they float
13. **Cloves**—observe closely cloves from which oil has been removed will be shrunken in shape
14. **Coconut oil**—pure coconut oil will freeze when refrigerated, it won't be pure
15. **Sugar**—dissolve a sample in a beaker of water, chalk powder, if present will settle at the bottom, while urea will give a smell of ammonia
16. **Honey**—dip a cotton wick in a sample of honey and light it with matchstick, if the honey is unadulterated, the wick will burn, but if there is water in it, will not burn and will produce cracking sound
17. **Jiggery**—place 10 mg of jiggery in water the chalk powder will settle at the bottom of the container
18. **Sago**—burn 10 mg sago if adulterated, it will leave behind ash
19. **Iodized salt**—cut out a piece of potato, adds salt and wait for minute. Add two drops of lemon juice, if it is iodized salt, there will be blue color on the slice.

Food Safety and Standards Authority of India (FSSAI) monitoring food—established under FSSAI Act, 2006-include prevention of food adulteration act 1954, fruit products order 1955, meat food products order 1973, vegetable oil product order 1947, milk and milk product order 1992 etc.

Regulate their manufacture, storage, distribution, sale and import to ensure availability of safe and wholesome food to human consumption.

The food that we eat is a source of nourishment and nutrition. But it can be also source of diseases and illness. The difference between food and fuel for life and food as a source of ill health depends on the quality and purity of the food consumed.

FSSAI functions

1. Framing of regulations to lay down the standards and guidelines in relation to articles of food and specifying appropriate system of enforcing various standards thus notified
2. Laying down mechanisms and guidelines for a accreditation of certification bodies engaged in certification of food safety management system for food business
3. Laying down procedures and guidelines for laboratories
4. To provide scientific advice and technical support to government for technical matters of framing the policy
5. Collection of data regarding food consumption, incidence and prevalence of biological risk, contamination in food, identification of emerging risks and introduce rapid alert system
6. Creating an information net work to receive rapid and objective information of safety and issues of concerns
7. Provide training for persons who involve in food business
8. Develop international technical standards for food and sanitary standards
9. Promote general awareness about food safety and food standards.

General sanitary parameters

1. All food service premises shall be located in a sanitary place, clean, adequately lighted and ventilated and maintain overall hygiene
2. Windows, doors and other openings shall be fitted with net or screen.
3. The water used in the manufacturing shall be portable.
4. Equipment and machinery that permit easy cleaning shall be chosen.
5. All equipment shall be kept clean, washed, dried and stacked at the end of business.
6. Premises to have efficient drainage system and adequate provisions for disposal of refuse.
7. The workers should use clean aprons, hand gloves and head wears.
8. Persons suffering from infectious diseases shall not be permitted to work. Any cuts or wounds shall remain covered at all time and the person should not be allowed to come in contact with food.
9. All food handlers shall keep their finger nails trimmed, clean and wash their hands with soap before and after any contact with food. Scratching of body parts, hair shall be avoided during food handling process.
10. The habit of washing hands with soap before handling food, whether it is to eat or to cook prevent transfer of bacteria from hands to food.
11. Eating, chewing, smoking, spitting and nose blowing shall be prohibited while handling food.
12. All food stuffs to be covered to avoid contamination.

Food adulteration is a great menace to the public health and economic loss—any substance added to the food something that is not part of it and adversely affects the nature, substance and the quality of food. Know your consumer rights and rewards.

A healthy body is the key to a healthy mind. Select fruit and veggies that are in season—they taste better and are usually cheaper. The body has the power to heal itself. Naturopathy aims to positively catalyses the body's healing process through proper diet and complete rest.

Foods processed commercially like bread, biscuits, cakes, jams, sweets, jellies, ketchups, ice-creams etc. all contains food additives. Additives are non-nutritious substances which are added intentionally in small quantity to the food to improve it appearance, flavor, texture or storage properties (flavoring agents like vanilla essence, strawberry essence) acidic acid, vinegar.

Food additives are considered safe for consumption. But uncontrolled use can lead to toxicity and health hazards.

Food is considered adulterated if the content exceeds the limits

Food adulteration is a malpractice in which the food quality is sub standardized by mixing up of food products with contaminates like ghee with vanaspathi, milk with fat extract of earth worm; addition of water and starch; chilly powder with tamrind seeds powder, black gram husk; cereals wheat rice dals with mud, stone, turmeric powder lead chromate powder. Tea leaves used tea dust, saw dust, butter starch, animal fat, and coriander powder with starch with horse duck.

Giving false labels, putting up decomposed foods for sale, abstraction of nutrients. They are for economic significance and not considered health of community. Food adulteration act in 1954—foods which does not confirm standards, which affects health of community to check and punish under act. ISI Mark (Bureau of Indian standard) it guarantees the quality. There are also PFA standard, Agmark standard. These genuine marks satisfy the consumers demand in respect to health and quality of food.

There are varieties of food commodity in the market. We get some in raw form and other in cooked form. It is very important to take into account its nutritive value, safety and food handling. It prevents risk of infectious diseases on food consumption. Food from manufacturers to consumer is handled by many people in between. Food should be selected, stored in hygienic condition.

Nutrition is a basic need. Nurses must have enough knowledge to educate public and all who come in contact with her profession. To assess the dietary method planning menus, hygiene and solve the problems of mal nutrition at family level. Large number of Indian population depends upon agriculture for food. Malnutrition is widely prevalent, e.g. PEM, vitamin A deficiency, anemia, goiter which needs education to take supplementation.

Science of nutrition is study of food in relation to health. 18th century Liverier the father of nutrition science—1st September nutrition week celebrated.

Food is an substance which is used by body for its growth, development, regulation and repair. Healthy being depends up on healthy eating. Human nutrition is influenced by climate, economic status, culture, age, religion.

In 19th century emphasis was laid on energy yielding food 1950 emphasis was on vitamins and amino acids were discovered. Consumption and utilization of food in the body is through process of ingestion, digestion, metabolism and excretion. Good nutrition leads to healthy living. Eat fresh foods, eat hygienically, cover the food, do adaptation from time to time in seasons changes, eat at proper scheduled time, eat balanced diet and maintain ideal weight. Do not over cook food, avoid excessive salt, sugar and spices. Do not over eat, avoid saturated fat and fried things.

Any nutrition is consumed either in excess or in deficient may alter the metabolism in the body and can cause many abnormalities. Different food groups from different sources have different impact on body. Some food provide calories, other food builds body, others are non-digestible and acts as fiber.

Nutrients are the substances which are consumed in the diet and utilized to promote the body functions. All the nutrients are essential in any balanced diet in appropriate amount. Lower of excessive amounts can disturb the body mechanism. Calorie rich diet is good for a normal person, where as on the other hand it may be harmful for an obese person

Nutrient value varies in different food products. The nutritive value and safety of food depends upon proper selection of foods.

Food poisoning is acute gastroenteritis caused by ingestion of food or drink contaminated with either living bacteria or their toxins or inorganic chemical substances and poisons derived from plants and animals.

It is also caused by non-bacterial by chemicals such as arsenic, certain plants and sea foods, fertilizers, pesticides, mercury.

Salmonella food poisoning is a common form of food poisoning. Widespread use of house hold detergents interfering with sewage treatment, infections from farm animals and poultry through contaminated meat, milk and milk products, sausages, eggs and egg products. Rat and mice get infected and contaminate food stuffs by their urine and faces

The organism found in faeces of humans and animals, in soil, water and air. Food cooked and kept and eaten later, spores survive in cooking etc.

The onset is sudden with chills, fever, nausea, vomiting and a profuse watery diarrhea, which last for 2–3 days. The toxins act directly on CNS. Food poisoning may be mistaken for cholera and acute bacillary dysentery

Watch what you eat—meat that is not cooked. Do not cut meat and vegetables on same board. Sanitation and washing hands done regularly before and after cooking. Follow preservation of food methods.

Assessment of Food Poisoning

1. How soon after eating did the symptoms occur? (immediate onset suggests chemical, plant or animal poisoning)
2. What was eaten in the previous meal?
3. Did the food have an unusual odor or taste? (most foods causing bacterial poisoning do not have unusual odor or taste)
4. Did anyone else become ill from eating the same food?
5. Did vomiting occur? What was the experience of the vomit us?
6. Did diarrhea occur? (diarrhea is usually absent with botulism and with shellfish or other fish poisoning)
7. Are any neurological symptoms present? (these occurs in botulism and in chemical plant and animal poisoning)
8. Does the patient have a fever? (fever is characteristic in salmonella, ingestion of fava beans, and some fish poisoning)

Prevention—meat inspection, personal hygiene, food handles hygiene checked periodically, sterilization of all work surfaces, keep food away from rates, mice, dust etc. proper temperature control of refrigerator, do not leave food in warm pantries, a few germs cam multiply to millions in few hours, cook and eat on same day hot food. Give health education to food handlers, fellow clean habits.

Conclusion—adulteration of food is one of the major threatening problems today. All consumers need high quality foodstuffs in low price. So the supply of food products of low quality. Most of the sellers are doing adulteration because of the large demands of food and shortage without considering public health. It can cause grace problems sometimes even death. For example, adulterant Argemone oil is one, which is mixed with edible oil results in swelling of body due to water retention, rash, puffiness of face and even death. When individual doubt adulteration in food stuffs, they have to inform the food health authority. If persons are found selling adulterated food the persons involved can be convicted.

Keywords

Food hygiene, prevent and control, cooking, FSSAI , food adulteration, sanitary parameters, food poisoning, conclusions.

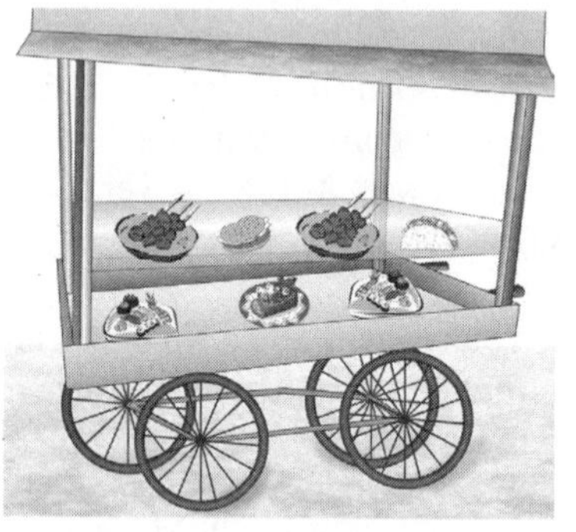

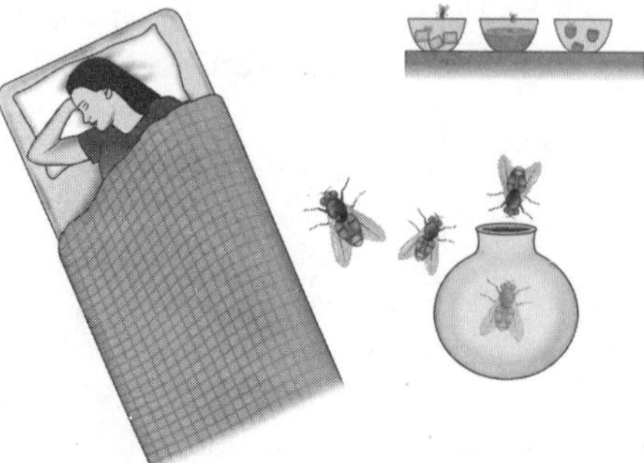

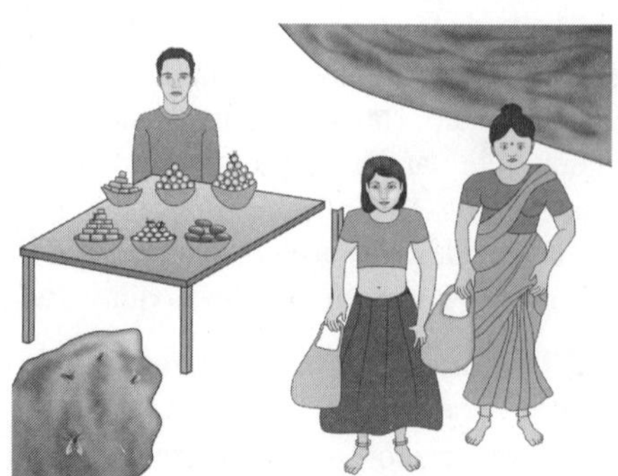

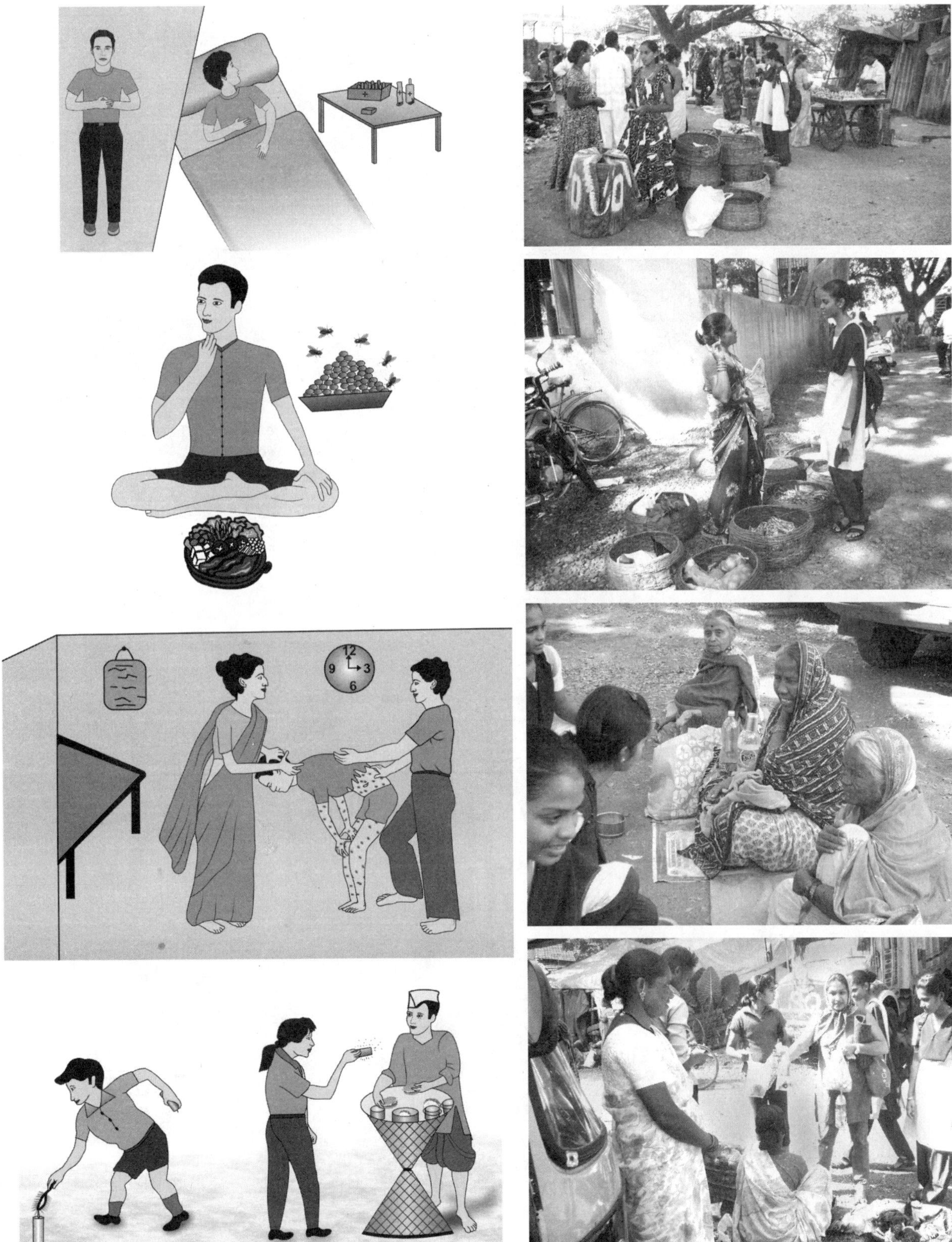

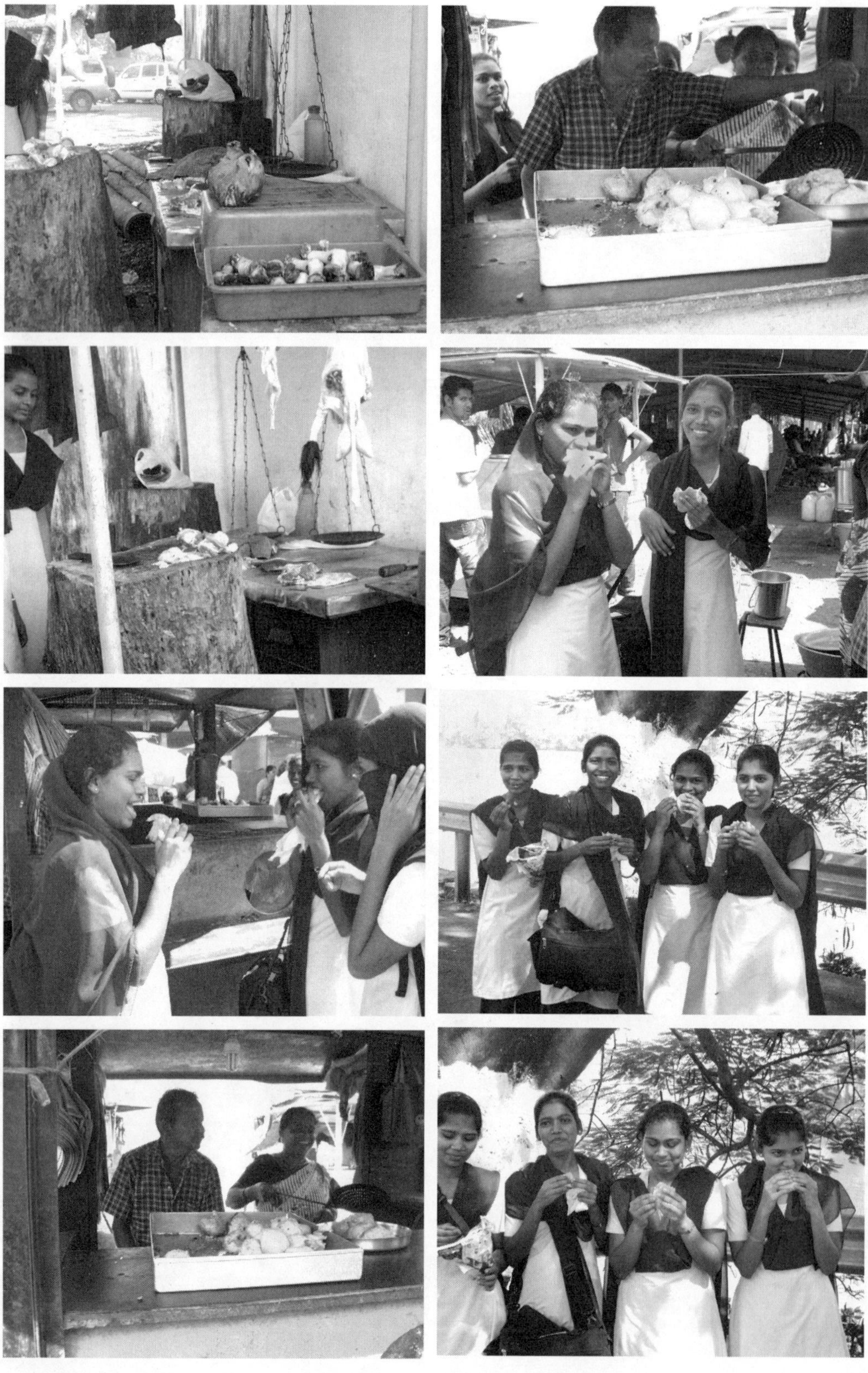

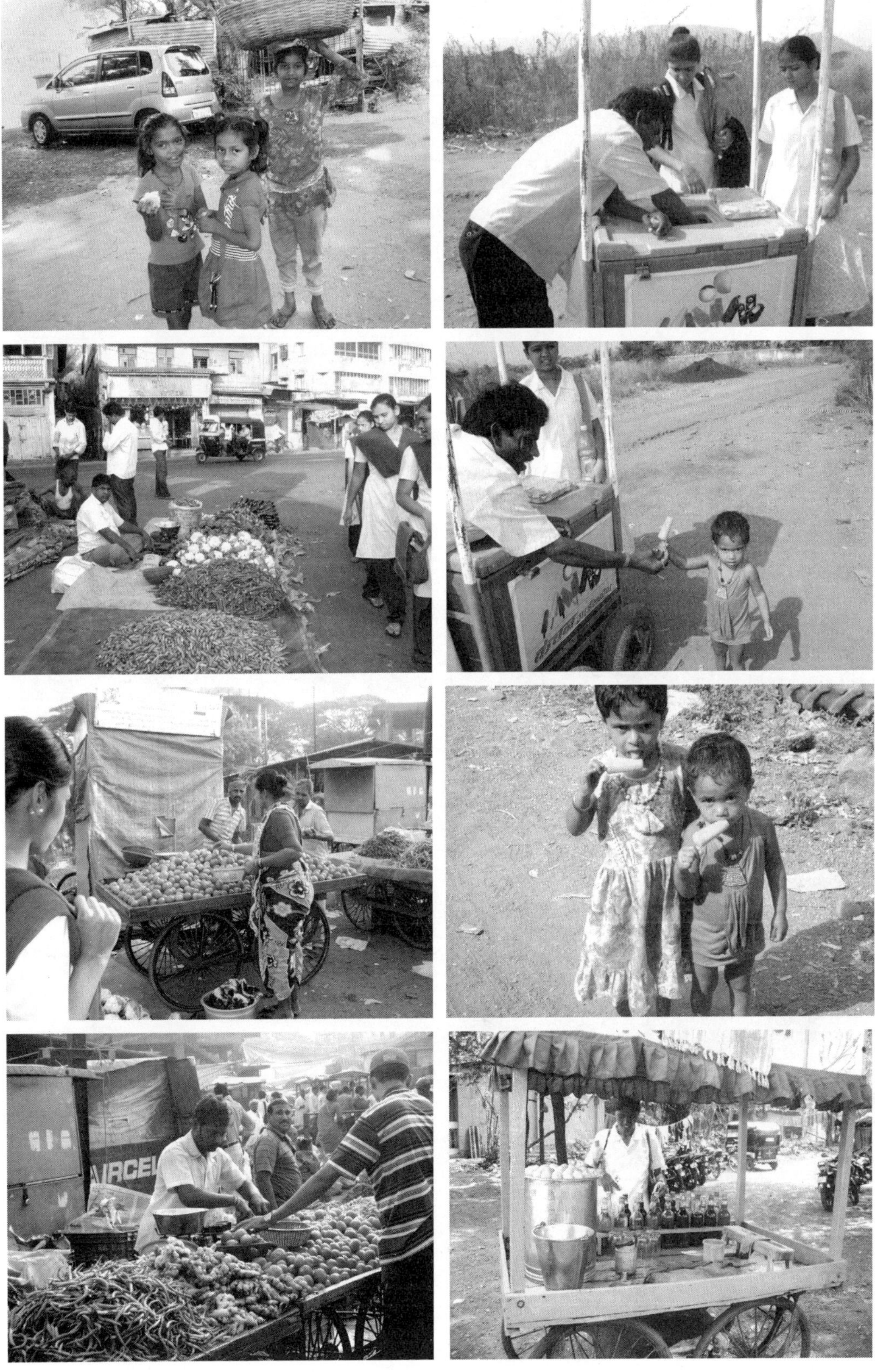

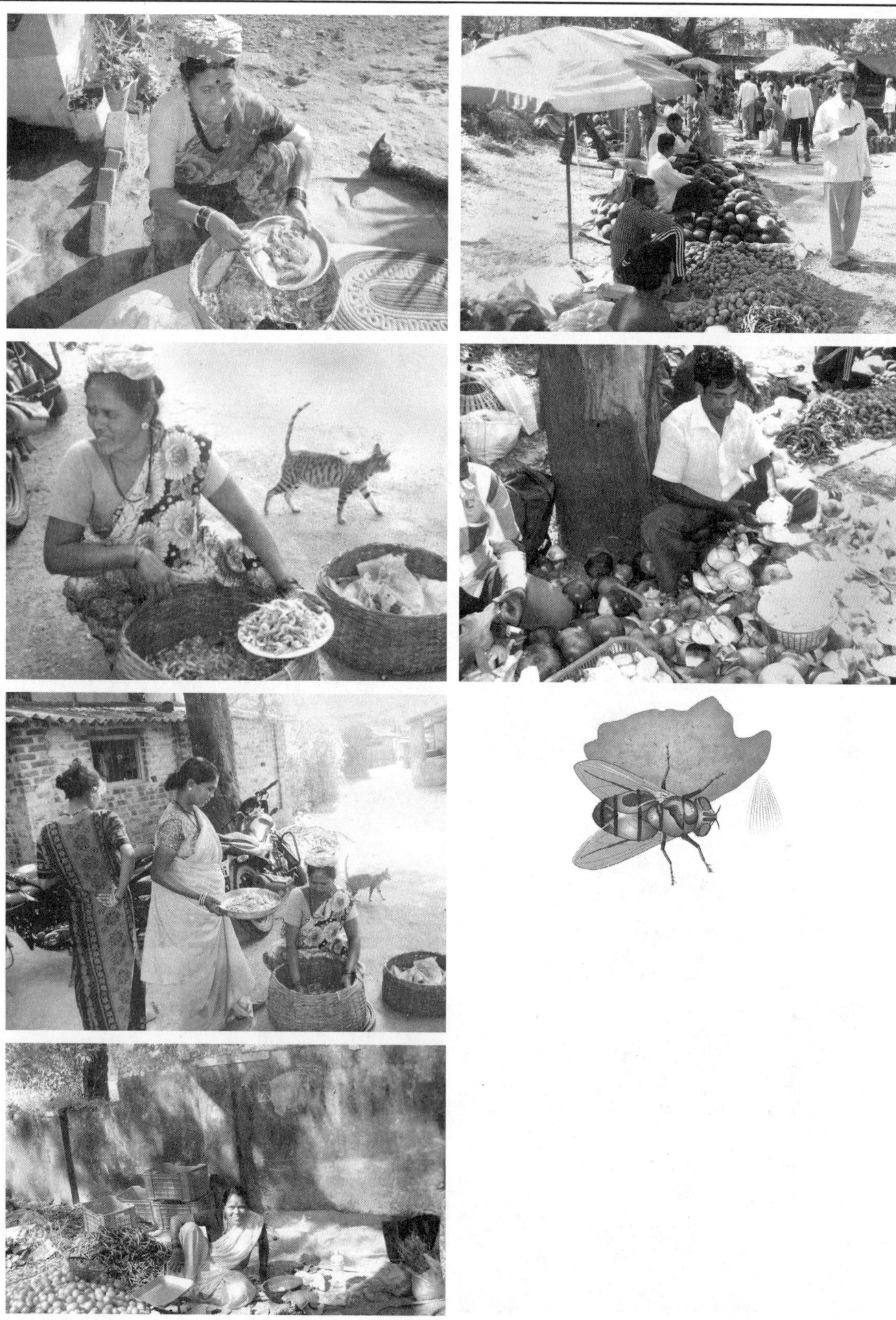

CHAPTER 51

Personal Hygiene

Twenty-first century media is playing major role. Technology has made possible such sweeping advance in communication, AV aids enhances clarity and providing diversity and brings abstract remote events of space or time into the class room.

Human biology is an area of current interest. The structure and functions of the body are always a marvel to the layman. Ignorance in this field can be removed only by health education. The topics can be covered under the areas of education.

Human Body

1. Structures and functions of the body
2. How to keep physically fit
3. The need for exercise, rest and sleep
4. The effects of alcohol, smoking and dugs on the body
5. First aid
6. Reproductive biology—how conception takes place.

We normally **value our body** for its beauty youth, health on usefulness without realizing that it is a walking miracle. From birth to death the body carries out innumerable life sustaining activities. The heart beats 86,4000 times and lung breaths 21,6000 times every day. All this is possible due to the inexhaustible power called the soul that is enshrined in the body which is making life throb around it. When we are aware that we constantly carry this scared energy we will never misuse it to perform actions which are harmful, demonic, criminal or destructive in nature.

Within our bodies—each of us has 96.000 km of blood vessels, a distance greater than two trips around the earth. The surface area of our lungs if stretched out would be equal to the size of a tennis court. We use 200 muscles to take a single step. Three hundred million cells die in our bodies every minute. More than 32 million bacteria almost all harmless and many beneficial—live on our skin, which sheds 6,00,000 particles per hour. A cell from our brain can contain 5 times as much information as the encyclopedia. None these enormously complex republics that we call our bodies function is by and large a mystery to us. We cannot consciously control the way our blood flows or how our nails and hair grow or how sensory messages reach the brain; they just do all these things independently of us.

Cure yourself—There is concrete proof with documentation evidence throughout history that the body has in it the extraordinary power to repair itself spontaneously remissions of illness, people who begin to see or walk again such medial miracles have happened in the past and can definitely occur again in the future. All have power to repair within ourselves we need to trigger this process and stimulate the body to repair itself. To repair ability lies within the genes of the human body, which are constantly on the alert to defend and protect the body. This gift lies within our genetic material, expressed as proteins which are responsible for the way the body expresses and defend by either inflammation like fever, construction like a growth or destruction like an ulcer. Thus all diseases in reality a form of defense by human body.

Hygiene is of Two Types

Personal hygiene—bathing, clothing, washing hands, toilet training, care of feet, care of nails and teeth, spitting, coughing, sneezing, personnel appearance.

Environmental hygiene—clean house, use of soap and water. Light and ventilation, control of rates and mice, safe water, drainage.

Personal hygiene is crucial for health and well being of a person. Several diseases occur due to poor personal hygiene. Personal hygiene includes bathing, clothing, washing hands, care of feet, nails and teeth, spitting, coughing, sneezing, personal appearance clean habits etc. Hygiene is the science of preserving and promoting/improving health. Habit is acquired through repetition, a habitual action is automatic. It requires little attention once it has been acquired. Cultivation of healthy habits and life-styles is vital. Therefore, Maintenance of personal hygiene is necessary for an individuals comfort, safety and well-being.

The science of health embraces all factors which contribute to healthy living. It is the science of preserving a promoting health. The personal hygiene not only helps to preserve health but also to improve it. Personal hygiene cultivates good habits and encourages physical health, the knowledge will promote physical well-being.

Hygiene of the skin—since skin is in contact with external environment it accumulates dirt, this dirt clogs the opening of the sweat glands, and not removed may lead to skin infections such as boils, scabies, ringworms. Daily regular bath with soap and water is essential to remove dirt and free body from bad odor. It will keep the skin clean and prevent infections. The skin is a finely laminated coating, it has 3 layers, that is hypodermis, dermis and epidermis. It weights about 4 kg depending on the size of the body. It is roughly 1.5 square meters.

Good skin care has a great deal to do with your diet, lifestyle, digestion, hormones levels, stress level and the state of your entire nutritional health. Anti-aging skin care means maintaining a properly balanced diet, drinking plenty of water, regular exercise, developing a positive attitude to maintain the body immune system. Protect your skin from the exposure to the sun is the number one cause of skin damage, including wrinkles, use protective sun cream, hats and clothing to limit skin exposure to the suns harmful rays. Hormone manifests as irregular periods, thick facial hair, acne and weight gain needs hormone correction. Natural supplements sun shine vitamins to keep skin glowing. Keep skin moisturized, learn the type of skin one has. Diet rich in cucumbers, papaya will provide soothing relief for puffiness, swelling, lines and wrinkles.

Therapies—skin polishing is a freshening technique that helps repair facial skin to remove the dead, outer layer of the skin. Chemical peels, wrinkle fillers, lesser skin towing remove fine hair and increases skin glow. Damaged skin found in elderly persons, diabetics and skin infections. When you take bath you will notice dead skin coming out, it is said that every seven years we get totally new cells. Makeup's block the skin openings and difficulties that it becomes skin to breath less freely. Looses its natural glow and fast becomes lifeless where people opt for skin lifting. Boils on body shows that, your body is trying to throw away the toxins that is blocked and accumulated under the skin. Young people leave no stone unturned in their anxiety to look good and feel better. Self-image, prestige, confidence and personality development goes along way with skin care. Discoloration of skin, nodule, blisters, flushed skin, cyst, scale, crust, fissures, ulcers, burns, rashes, itching, burning, tingling, numbness, allergies, etc. can be very worrisome. Cellulites is a diffuse inflammation of the deep dermal and sub coetaneous tissues that results from an infectious process. Gas gangrene increasing infection of the soft tissues that spread rapidly along fascias. Toxic epidermal necrolysis is fatal skin diseases associated with erythma, blistering and epidermal sloughing. herpes zoster a condition in which reactivation of the chickenpox virus varicella zoster may be life threatening condition to patient who is immune suppressed. Psoriasis is chronic T-cell inflammatory disorders.

Be beautiful from within is to revitalize skin. Use natural ingredients to keep skin healthy and beautiful. Honey, lime juice, yoghurt cleansing pack having anti bacterial properties. Coconut is great skin nursing that moisture and hydrate the skin in unique manner.

When one has skin problem persons looses meaning in life, stops socializing, dreaded to met people, low self-assurance, uncertainty develops, depression and social withdrawal, psychological stress and distress.

There is unique creation of God to be dark or fair skin one finds in the world. Looking at face we can guess ones age. You can see how the child's skin is and how is the elderly person's skin is.

Skin-care Tips

1. Have cool showers twice a day.
2. Wear loose cotton clothes.
3. Dust talcum/anti-fungal powder in the body folds after bath.
4. Use medicated soap in body folds.
5. Wear open sandals.
6. Reduce caffeine intake.
7. Increase water intake.
8. Rubbing ice piece on face makes you refreshment
9. Sunburn rashes can apply calamite lotion.
10. Take anti-allergic tablet.
11. Apply mud-pack weekly.
12. Take supplement of vitamin A, zinc and antioxidants.

During winter our skin dries and after that our skin is exposed to intense heat it becomes itchy and irritant. The salt in your own sweat irritates the skin and worsens it. The sticky feeling on the skin due to humidity should not be mistaken for hydration. Skin drying in summer needs to be hydration, which makes the skin smooth, glowing and baby soft.

Age of skin is judged on biological factors rather than your date of birth. Our skin is the largest organ and the skin provides an honest mirror of our inner health and well-being. Facial rejuvenation, a skin treatment—effectively reduces wrinkles, treat sun sports, tightens loose skin, improvers skin tone and complexion, remove blotchiness and elimination damaged blood vessels. It provides vitamins and minerals that are essential for skin enrichment.

Laser photo rejuvenation is a treatment that makes skin firmer and smoother. The effect lasts for few years with minimum maintains healthier looking and smoother skin reduces pore size, an even skin tone reduced redness and wrinkles. A face lift usually takes about 45–60 minutes. The facelift cannot stop the aging process. What it can do is set back the clock, improving the most visible signs of aging by removing excess fat, tightening underlying muscles and re-draping the skin of your face and neck. After treatment be gentle with your face and hair since your skin be swelling by 3rd weeks you feel better and can go back to work.

Skin—the human body does not consider the skin a vital organ like the heart, lungs and the brain. So when the body faces a crisis such as dehydration, fatigue due to stress or lack of vitamins in the blood stream—the skin is the first to show symptoms, as it is crisis always gets addressed last.

Hydration—the amount of fluid in your skin is important for its health. The fluids don't come only from the quantity of water you drink during the day but also amount of environments you consume. The ability of the skin to repair and produce new cells depends a lot on dehydration. Well hydrated skin is able to produce fresh cells more efficiently. Lack of sleep interferes with hydration and cells renewal and forms new cells and glow comes.

Wrinkles—are formed when the skin cells die faster than the body can replace them. Lack of hydration over sustained periods often leads to this condition. Indentation occurs where there is constant and repetitive, such as the glabellas frown feet at the corner of the eyes. Crow feet at the corner of the eyes, for head lines and nasal wrinkles. In those who do not wear sun glasses, and have a constant frown, these indentations become pronounced wrinkles. New evidence of wrinkles has been found in young people who do heavy weights in the gym and grimace during workouts. Sensitivity due to genes who get uncomfortable sensation when make up, soap, cleanses to come in contact with it. Pigmentation—human skin colors have been classified into 6 types. Indians have a wide rang of skin tones.

Oral hygiene—the mouth is the portal of entry, for both respiratory tract and for food that is eaten. The process of chewing is the first step in the digestion of food. The mouth is an ideal incubator for germ to grow. Proper care prevents oral diseases and destruction of teeth. Brushing, flossing and irrigation are needed on daily basis. Purpose of oral hygiene is to stimulate appetite; provide sense of well-being, message gums, relieve discomfort from unpleasant odor and taste, and to prevent gum inflammation and infection. Patient under going chemotherapy, radiation therapy gets sores, dryness. Shinning white teeth adds an attraction to an individual's personality.

Teeth whitening—cosmetic dental procedure—it is also known as dental beaching procedure where teeth's are whitened without damaging them. People try to brush harder yellow teeth and thus damaging both, teeth and gums badly and irreversibly. Bleaching tightens the gums, it lefts out the stains from teeth surface which accumulate consumption of alcohol, coffees, tea and smoking. A tooth boost your self-esteem and allows you smile and help you to cut these habits of covering your mouth having white set of teeth and sparking and radiant smile can make you look attractive and boost your confidence

Care of the ears—by keeping the ear clean; removal of excessive wax carefully; by instilling a few drops of glycerin to soften before removing wax; preventing water entering in the ear during bathing, protecting ear from loud noise exposure, teaching good habits and teaching not to put pencils, matches and foreign objects, scratching, avoiding insects entering and treating earaches, ear discharges etc in time. Ear is an important sense organ of the body. It is responsible for hearing and body equilibrium. The ear is liable to infection and injury. Ear aches may be due to inflammation and edema of the tissues. Thin and watery or think discharge due to bacterial or fungal infection needs to be cleaned. Foreign bodies and solid objects, insets and excessive wax are treated.

Care of the eyes—eyes has been the source of wonder to humankind more than any other organ in the body. Using kajal surma instilling in eye should be avoided. Eyes need to be washed frequently flashing with cold water. Eye in susceptible to infection, according to doctor order antibiotic eye drops and eye ointment needs to be instilled. Eye is a delicate and sensitive organ. Any discharge, redness or pain in the eye can be caused by the use of infected clothes, handkerchief, and towels, flies etc. Eye is exposed to injuries use protective glasses caused by fire crackers, bow and arrow small practical of charcoal, sand, foreign bodies. Eye strain by reading in moving trains, lying down, glare and excessive brightness. Deficiency of vitamin "A" green leafy vegetables added to the diet. Regular check ups of watery discharge, soreness and the skin around the eye should be kept clean by washing with soap and clean water.

Menstruation hygiene—it is a normal physiological process is to be explained. Regular bathing and frequent changing of the sanitary pads to keep the hygiene. Using clean clothes have good diet and rest. The subject of menstruation is surrounded by superstitions, taboos, and feeling of shame, embarrassment.

Rest and sleep—body needs it for maintenance of health. We spend a third of our lives in sleeping. During sleep the body and mind are relaxed, repair and re-growth takes place, fatigue disappear. We feel fresh and work better after spell of rest and sleep. The amount of sleep requires varies with age, sex, environment, the nature of work and the temperament of each individual.

Care of the hands—hands and nails pick up dirt and bacteria easily so they should be kept clean before eating food and after defecation or urination by washing with soap and water. Cut short nails, do not bit nails and putting fingers in the nose or ears is unhygienic be discouraged. Disease agents such as typhoid bacilli may be directly enter into the mouth if hands are contaminated since nails collect a good deal of dirt.

Nail care—out fingernails can receive a lot of wear and tear from weather, activity with you hands in our day today life and if your nails are chipping can become brittle. If the body is not receiving certain proper nutrients. Biotin is a vitamin that helps the body process fatty acids and proteins. Vitamin B complex helps if supplemented moisturizing them chipped and peeling finger nails can occur if your finger nails are not receiving enough moisture. Nails are made up of the protein, keratin and its function is to provide protein for the finger tips.

Care of the feet—the human foot is one of the most highly structured parts of the body. It is composed of 26 bones connected by ligaments and muscles, blood vessels and nerves. The bones are so arranged as to balance and support the weight of the body. If the feet are allowed to stay in a wrong position for a long time, the bones are twisted leading to limping, poor posture, an awkward gait and eventually foot deformities.

Foot may be neglected or affected in some diseases such as hookworm which are transmitted through the skin of the foot. The infective larvae penetrate the skin when people walk barefoot in muddy fields contaminated with human excreta. Leprosy causes severe deformities of the foot, fungal infections, corns, club feet, excessive perspirations give offensive smell, proper selection of shoes, sandals, socks and be clean and dry, too tight or constricted, cuts and bruises, crakes to be avoided.

The feet must get same attention as the rest of the body.

- Special foot care in diabetes.
- Inspect foot daily for blisters, open sores, cuts, color changes, in grown toe nails
- Wash with soap and water
- Let not feet get dry and cracked
- Do not wear tight socks or knee highs
- Do not use hot water to wash your feet
- Do not use blades
- Do not wear torn or tight shoes
- Do not use hot water bottles to warm your feet
- Have your feet checked by your doctor.

Care of feet and nails

- Biting nails or trimming them improperly
- Exposure to hard chemicals
- Wearing poorly fitted shoes
- Shape, size and number of toes in feet, dry, cracking, fungus, painful feet, disorders can cause limping or unusual gait.
- In diabetes patient inadequate circulation inadequate flow of blood not reaching.

Can ask following questions

1. How often do you brush your teeth
2. Do you floss? How often?
3. Do you use a mouth wash? When?
4. Do your gums ever bleeding?
5. Do you get sores in your mouth? When? Where?
6. How often do you go to the dentist?
7. How often do you have your teeth professionally cleansed?
8. Do you have any loose teeth?
9. Do you have false teeth, bridges, partial plates?
10. Do you have any problem with mouth drying?
11. What medication do you talk?
12. Can you chew all kinds of foods?
13. Have you notice any change in sense of test?
14. Are you able to do your own mouth care?
15. What type of tooth brush you use, soft, hard your brushing technique?
16. The beauty of natural teeth is tremendous, treatment of teeth is expensive affair, daily message and gargle every meal.

Cultivate good habits

1. Early to bed and early to rise
2. Brush your teeth twice everyday
3. Baths everyday keeps you clean
4. Always go to school on time
5. Do your homework everyday
6. Do not scribble on the wall
7. Trim your nails every week
8. Help those in need
9. Do not sit too close to the TV
10. Wash your hands before every meal
11. Save water and electricity
12. Help your mama at home
13. Do not enter the house weeping and crying
14. Welcome a guest to your house politely
15. Do not play on road
16. Always speak the truth
17. Put your toys back after play time
18. Save some of your pocket money
19. Cross the road only when the signal is green for the pedestrians
20. Do not get down from a moving bus.

Study habit

1. Do you like to study
2. Do you study under pressure
3. Are you physically alert when you study
4. Do you definitely react to what you have read
5. Can you give full alteration to the lesson when it is taught
6. Can you take down short notes from what you have heard in there class
7. Do you take notes in your own words
8. Do you keep a study schedule
9. Are you punctual in your study periods
10. Do you have fix place for study
11. Do you finish all the assignments in time
12. Can you concentrate while reading
13. Do you plan weekly review schedule
14. Do you use library books
15. Can you stand criticism without feeling hurt
16. Do your interests change rapidly
17. Do you often experience periods of loneliness
18. Do you find difficult in making up your mind
19. Do you find difficult to speak in public.

Head Lice/Care of the Hair

Care of the hair—good general health and a balanced diet are reflected by the condition of hair, tension or vitamin deficiency affects the condition of hair. hair reflects nutritional status and general health of the body, falling hair, and breaking shows poor health condition, deficiencies in diet with vitamin deficiency leads to early graying hair. Hair wash with soap and shampoo helps as a cleansing agent. Dandruff is an excessive scaling off the scalp skin can be controlled by keeping hair clean and prevents skin infections such as lice infestation ringworms etc.

Hair has no vital function in humans, but the lack or excess of it may cause endless misery. Minor faults in hair texture, color, spending billions of pounds a year. Each hair on the body goes through a cycle of growth independent of its neighbor. The length of each phase of the cycle, as well as its over all length, various with sight and age. An average scalp contains 1,00,000 hairs and sheds about 100 naturally each day. Diseases of the scalps are infections and infestation, bacterial, viral, fungal, pedoculosis, eczemas. We probably spend more time on our hair than any other features of the body. We frequently cutting, shaving, curling, brushing and cleaning. Message well scalp increases oxygen and blood flow and drains toxins and strengthens it. Hair lost an be re-grow, avoid coloring, ironing which rob hair moistures. Steaming hair after oiling helps take towel, dip into hot water, squeeze the excess water and wrapper around like turben which open hair pores and increased blood flow. So cut right, say no shampoo, wear a head scarf or hair band.

Hair—survey of over 1,000 women in five metros found that over 50% of them had a serious hair fall problem, what is hair fall? When a person finds hair sticks to the comb or strands on the pillow or in the shower while combing. Hair grows at the rate of half an inch in a month. A healthy scalp will have a ratio of 4 hairs in anlagen to 1 in telogen phase. Trauma triggers shedding by sending follicles to the relogen phase.

How to control—avoid food high in sugar and fat. Stay away from chemicals that can damage hair, stress is injurious to long term health and color of hair. Get plenty of rest; tangles in wet hair are best removed with a wide toothed comb.

Causes of hair loss can be—poor scalp condition; dandruff, mineral deficiency, keratin deficiency, hormonal imbalance, commonly seen after pregnancy, during menopause, thyroid disorders, stress, acute illness, medication, including hair loss due to chemotherapy, birth control pills, anemia. Hair loss is individualized and not generalized. So what can be normal hair fall for one may not be normal for the other. Hair loss is a delayed reaction; some internal imbalance pushes hair, which is in the anti-agent phase prematurely into the telogen phase. They rest in this phase for 3 months before falling out. Once the imbalance is rectified, hair loss will automatically stop.

- If it persisting beyond 3–4 months falling, see a trichologist
- It is common amongst children and teenagers but sometimes even adults get affected by it.

What is it?

Head lice or louse are tiny wingless parasites biologically known as pedicel's capitis that inhabit and thrive on hair and the scalp. They feed on very small amount of blood that they draw from the scalp. Head lice problem occurs more in women than men, because women usually have longer hair. Loose long hair is more susceptible to lice. And managing a lice infestation is more difficult on a or haired person, as it is difficult to comb, inspect and treat.

Symptoms

1. Intense itching of the scalp
2. small red bumps on the scalp, neck and shoulder (bumps may become crusty and ooze)
3. Tiny white specks (egg or nits) on the bottom of each hair that are hard to get.

Can they damage the hair of scalp?

Trichologist says—lice are not dangerous and do not spread any particular disorder, but are contagious and cause itching that can be terribly annoying and embarrassing. Lice bite may cause ones scalp to become itchy and inflamed and persistent scratching may lead to skin irritation and even infection. It can lead to a bacterial infection which causes the skin to become red and tender and also involves crusting and oozing of pus along with swollen lymph glands. Some cases lice can occur in other hairy parts of the body like eyebrow, underarm, legs and genital hair. Head lice can also have repercussion on ones social relationships, as this problem can be embarrassing. People tend to avoid coming in close contact with people suffering from head lice. People also tend to question the hygienic habits of one infected with has lice.

Remedies

Wash your hair everyday. You may shampoo it once in 3 days, but be sure to pass water through the hair daily when washing the hair, message at the roots of the hair and not at the tips of the hair as it serves no purpose. Always wash your hair after you return home from long journey where you have been in contact with crowded places. Clothing and bed linen can be washed in hot water and detergents. Objects like combs, brushes, hair bands and clips should be soaked in hot water or medicated shampoo or both or they could simply be replaced.

Hair extension shampoo

Remove all the tangles and knots from hair with a wide toothed comb before shampooing. When you pour water directly on your head the direct pressure of water leads to tangling. Hence wet your hair little to prevent dry hair from swelling and getting entangled.

Wash hair with a gentle cleaning shampoo. Do not pile up all the hair on top of the head and scrub. Wash hair in a downward motion starting from the roots and moving towards the end. Gently massage their shampoo and rinse completely use good moisturizing conditioner as alcohol tends to dry hair. Lay your wet hair on dry towel and squeeze out excessive water. Do not rub vigorously to dry. Do not comb the hair wet as it may lead to breakage and you damage them. When go to bed completely dry and tie them up and avoid walking up with tangled mess. Avoid using a brush, comb hair twice a day, be gentle and do not pull and tug at hair while combing in a downward directly, when go for swim wear a cap to avoid chlorine and other chemicals which can damage them severely. The essential oils that are produced in your scalp and which passed into your hair. You need to hydrate ends regularly applying moistening to look them naturally.

Hair care—Hair holds a remarkable charm. There can be no narrative on ones appearance without a reference to hair allure. So losing hair is no fun. It upsets ones self-worth and self-esteem.

Heroes of ancient Greece used harsh soap and bleaches to lighten and redden their hair to the color that was identified with honor and courage first century Romans preferred dark hair which was made so by a dye concocted from oiled walnuts and leeks.

Things have-not changed over centuries. People who are experimenting with styles, or going blonde or simply curling or straightening hair. The work hit are models, actresses who being under bight light are prone to dandruff. Perming, dying and straightening hair is being popular needs to recognize the risks involved before. Girls with curly hair want it straight and silky vive versa. When it is done, tremendous heat is applied in order to change its natural shape. This converts the protein cycling then manipulated into a certain look, 205 hairs getting destroyed.

Regular streaking and dying can cause cumulative damage, hair breakage. It may also cause an auto immune reaction leading to skin diseases caller dermatitis.

Applying excessive heat to the hair can damage the scalp and cause the hair follicles to weaken. High heat and the time for which it is used on the hair will also impact structure of hair. While hair loses its elasticity damage to the cuticle makes it more breakable. Steam forming inside the hair shaft causes hair breakage. Therefore limit the amount of heat and length of time you dry your hair.

Avoid tight brads and ponytails it may cause breakage and tearing of air shaft. The hair root may be too weak to sustain the pressure of the hair, worrying changes in your hair such as hair loss, itching scalp spilt ends contact archeologist immediately

Hair loss can be due to family history, dandruff, ringworm or eczema, psoriasis of the scalp, some medication like steroids, once unique nature, temperament, personality, poor appetite, individual lifestyle, dietary regimen, likes and dislikes, smoking, alcohol affects the hair fall, hair loss. Pressure at the work place, marital discord, acne, irritable bowel syndrome, headache, stress also reason for hair loss.

Lesser hair reduction for smooth, silk skin—there are many techniques for hair removal—shaving, waxing, epilating and using hair removal creams. All these methods have their drawbacks and none of these methods are a permanent solution in hair problem. Some arte painful, some lead to rashes, some darken your skin due to chemicals involved.

Lesser—is safe methods for hair removal, 80% of whether is gone is gone forever. The balance heir is light and fine.

Process is painless, no infection and rashes. The procedures are fast and hygienic. Wax and shave 10 days before you plan for lesser session. Dermatologist opinion is must. It has no side effect, a qualified doctor is must. Doctor will do first patch test to see weather the laser is suitable for you, each part of the body requires at least 6 or more sessions. If pts are suffering from an underlying hormones disturbance like polycystic ovarian syndrome you need to take simultaneously treatment for that, then only the laser treatment shown result.

If you have dark sin you need to be extra careful. It is extremely important that you go to a qualified dermatologist.

The body is like everything else in life is a mirror of our inner thoughts and beliefs. The body is always talking to you, only if we will take time to listen. Every cell within your body responds to every single thought you think and every word you speak.

Dandruff

Apply bhringraj oil at night to prevent dandruff and shampoo the next day. Before washing hair, comb them with a brush. As a result, dead cells and dandruff disappear, the oil glands become active and oil released from the oil glands can also be cleaned. Wash hair once in a week at least. Apply conditioner without fail. Rinse hair with normal tap water. Hot water opens pores which results in dandruff. So while washing hair during winter use cold water for the last rinsing. Conditioning must during winter seasons. During winter there is more moisture in the hair and conditioning helps to retain the moisture as well as increase the skin of hair. Mix a few drops of ginger juice to olive oil and apply it is the roots of hair for one hour and they wash them with shampoo. Do not comb or brush hair time and again because by doing so the oil glands get activated and extra oil reruns from them resulting into dandruff. Hot oil therapy at hone by applying any warm oil on the scalp and message it. Soak a soft towel in hot water, wring well and reap it around your oiled head. Avoid coconut oil as it can stick to the scalp and closes the pores while in turn can cause many ailments pertaining hair.

Kind of needs

1. Hungry man needs food to eat
2. A thirst one needs water to drink
3. A sick man needs medicines
4. A tired man rest and sleep

5. A lonely man needs company
6. A clever man recognition
7. A poor man needs security
8. Human person needs self respect to live in dignity.

Exercise—test your fitness and stamina—warm up, stretches, running, skipping, swimming, hiking, yoga, cycling, climbing steps.

1. Can you climb up six flights of stairs in a building? Without breaking, if puffing and panting, few rest stops, slow and steady.
2. Any out door exercise like trekking or heavy lifting leave your muscle sore—feel aches and pain
3. Can you jog for two or more kilometer without stopping, without difficulty?
4. Can you touch your toes with your fingers without bending your knees easily?
5. How often do you visit your doctor?
6. Can you run about 100 meters under 15 seconds
7. How many pushup can you do in one go? (over 30 men; 25 for women)
8. How ready are you to participate in a city marathon?
9. What is your level of cardio endurance? more than 20 minutes or less than 5 minutes
10. How often do you currently exercise?

Wrong exercise will do more harm than good. Posture and right workout, young wants to become hard core body builder and get right composition of muscles and fat and to work on to strengthening the bones.

Weight training—push ups, dips and pull ups are good for body, out door sports, karate, foot ball; rock climbing will build your body and build mental stamina. Do not pump muscles on machines.

Quick way to increase ones physical endurance climbing steps—may leave you out of breath a you push gradually you will notice your strong mind for strong body—work on your will power before you work on your muscles.

Pin it to something, imagination is key- close your eyes and imagine what it would be like if you actually manage to achieve what you imagine yourself in a toned body, think how life would be which makes a ego boost right. Imagination has power to motivate. When one actually sees what is in store the desire to acquire it becomes stronger

Self-assurance—constantly reminds yourself that you can stick to your regimen. When your mind is told something regularly, you start believing in it, when ever negative thoughts try to creep in, push then away with self-assurance.

Every day have some undisturbed time to clam the mind. When your mind is cluttered, there is a higher possibility of going wrong. Use this undisturbed time to sort out your thoughts, concerns or simplex relax consider your lifestyle and priorities.

An un-restrained mind alone is the cause of degeneration while a controlled mind causes progress. Restraint of mind is the only means to control it to up root.

The mind is like poisonous snake sitting with its hood raised in the forest of the heart. All want happy peaceful life but unless we learn to control the mind, blissfulness would be impossible to achieve. If you over come your mind, you over come the world.

Nutrition

1. Balanced diets
2. Nutritive value of food
3. Storage, preparation, cooking
4. Serving, eating food, food adulteration, contamination of food
5. Removal of prejudices
6. Importance of good dietary habits

What we learnt today forgotten tomorrow, what remains with us changes us. That is why the famous saying I hear and I forget, I see and I remember and I do and I know. If you can dream it, you can do it. Health education is a vaccine. Higher education is expensive. Good education helps in nation building and improves the quality of life, gives you good position in the society, unlocks the doors of modernization and satisfies the intellectual hunger. You come to know what is good and what is bad, and are able to make the difference between right and wrong. You can give only if you have. Mould your character and make you good human beings. Makes you leaders of tomorrow and gives new direction. Makes you critical thinker, bold and better it shapes you life. As soon as sun rises itself darkness disappears. Dispel the cloud of ignorance. In community people are still illiterate and have not yet seen the world beyond the four walls of village.

Explanation—All the appropriate pictures explaining in simple pictures had shown how personal hygiene can be maintained. Students have to select and also creative way get apt pictures and explain the topic.

Keywords

Human biology, human body, hygiene, care of eye, ear, skin, hands, teeth, nails, feet, hair, dandruff, therapies, remedies, exercise, nutrition.

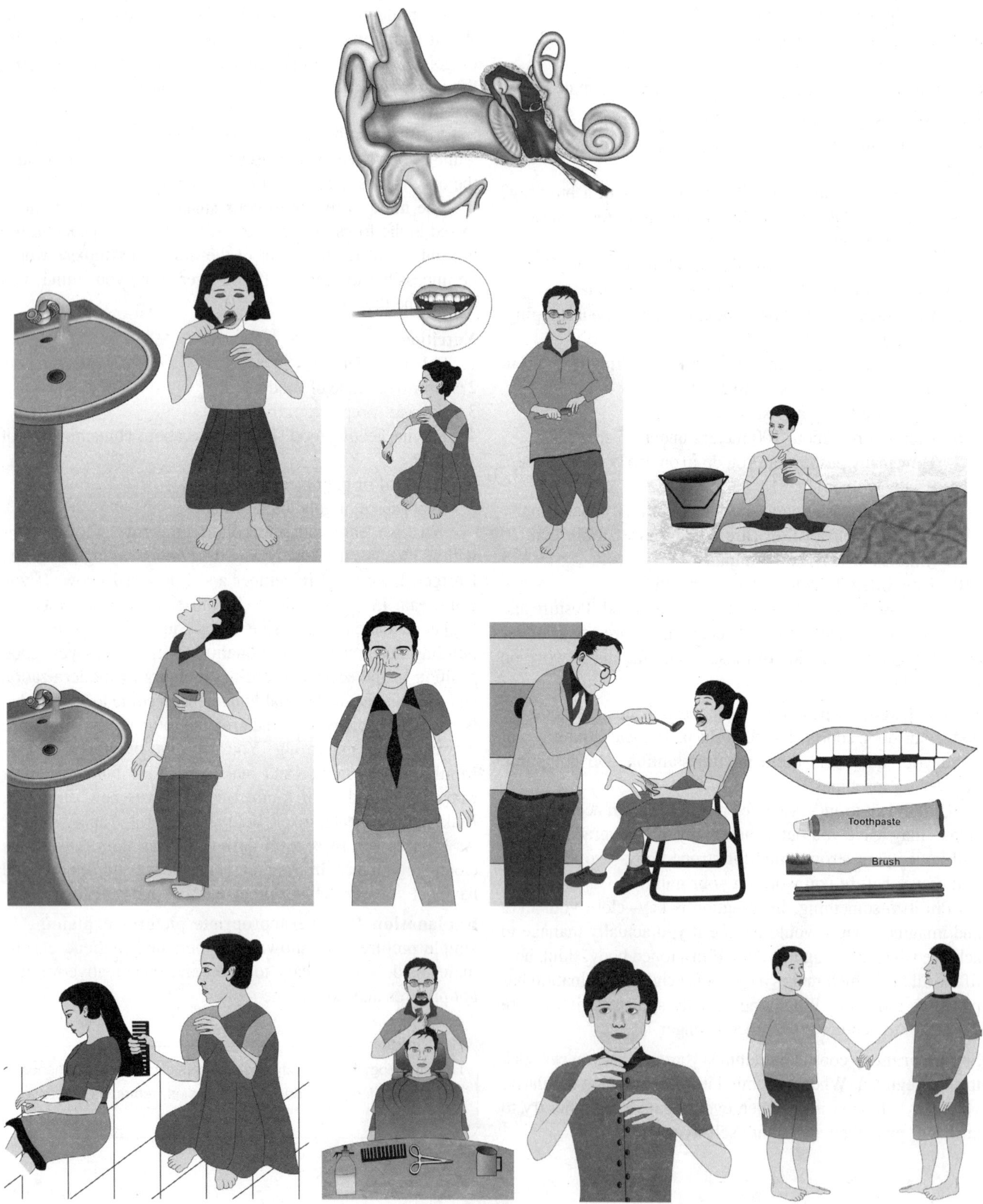
Toothpaste
Brush

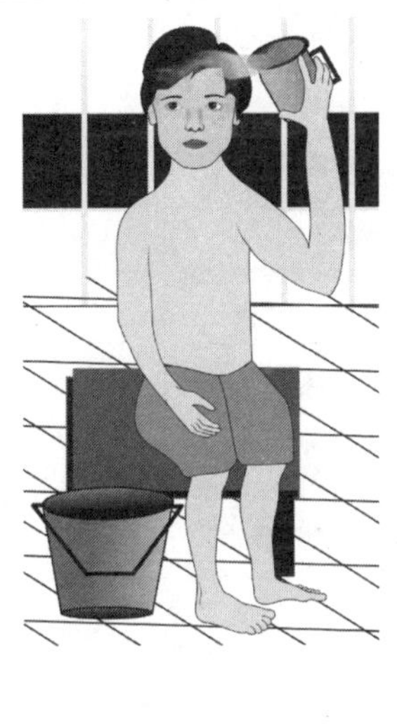

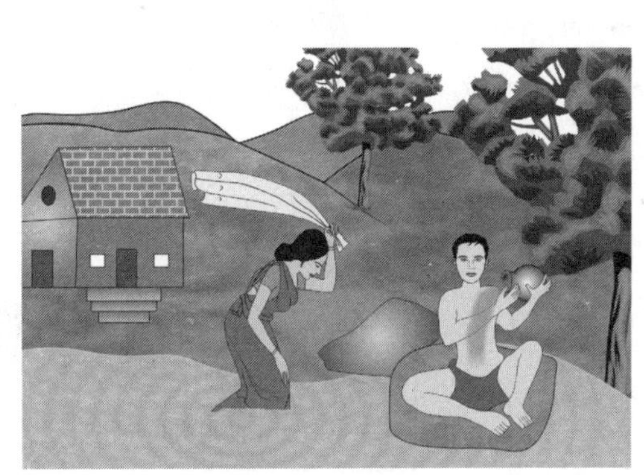

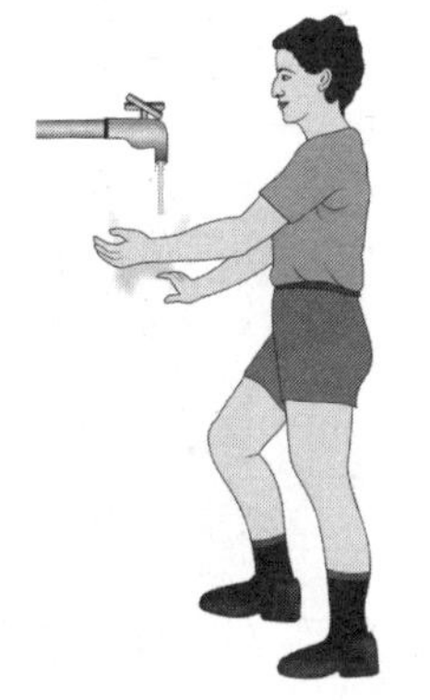

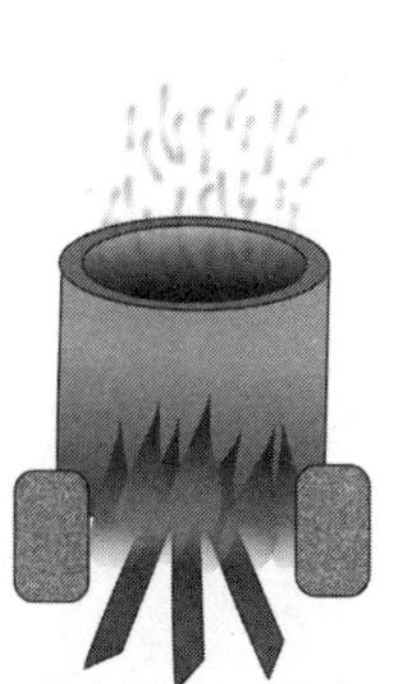

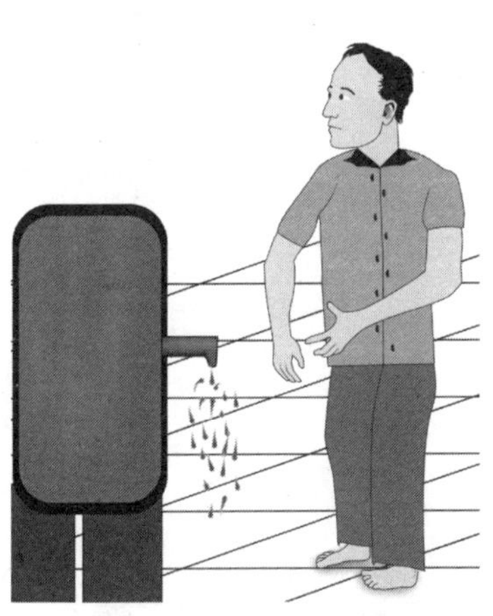

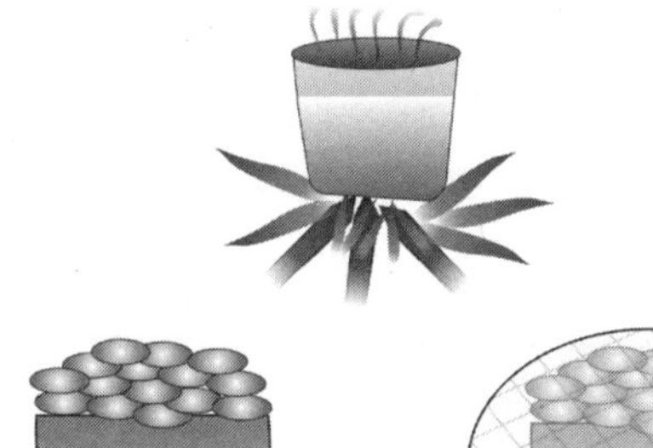

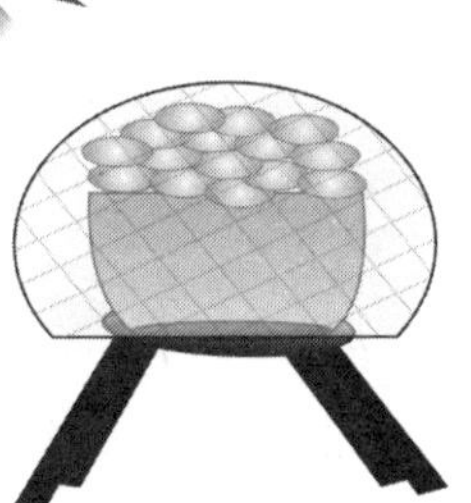

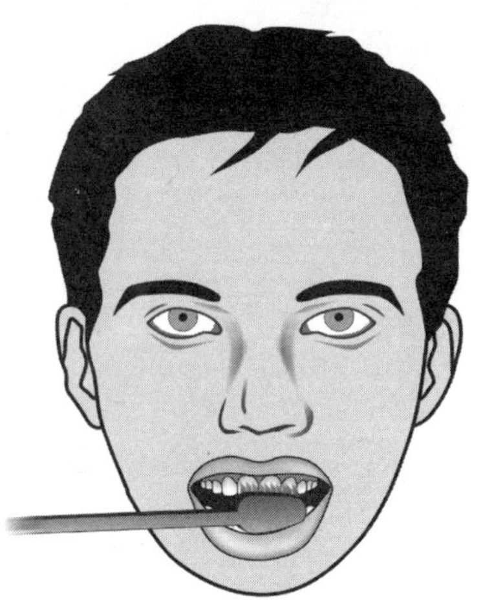

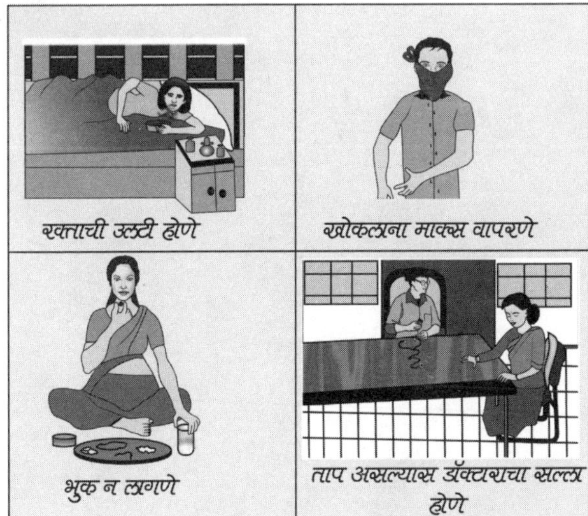
रक्ताची उलटी होणे
खोकलना माक्स वापरणे
भुक न लागणे
ताप असल्यास डॉक्टराचा सल्ला होणे

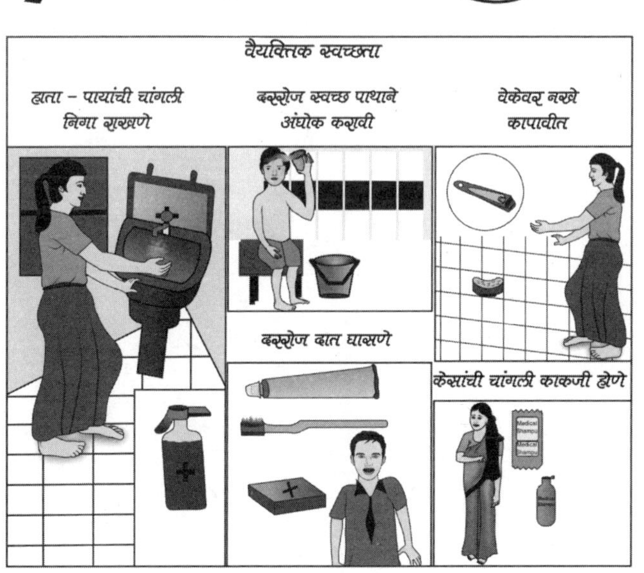
वैयक्तिक स्वच्छता
हात - पायांची चांगली निगा राखणे
दररोज स्वच्छ पाण्याने अंघोळ करावी
वेळेवर नखे कापावीत
दररोज दात घासणे
केसांची चांगली काळजी होणे

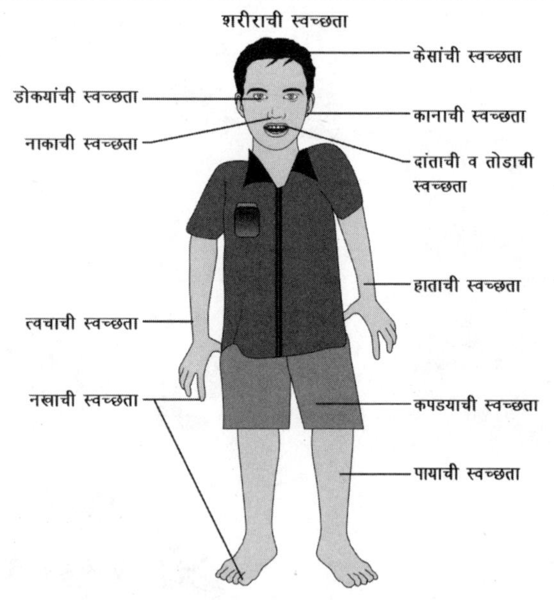
शरीराची स्वच्छता
केसांची स्वच्छता
डोळ्यांची स्वच्छता
कानाची स्वच्छता
नाकाची स्वच्छता
दातांची व तोंडाची स्वच्छता
हाताची स्वच्छता
त्वचाची स्वच्छता
नखाची स्वच्छता
कपडयाची स्वच्छता
पायाची स्वच्छता

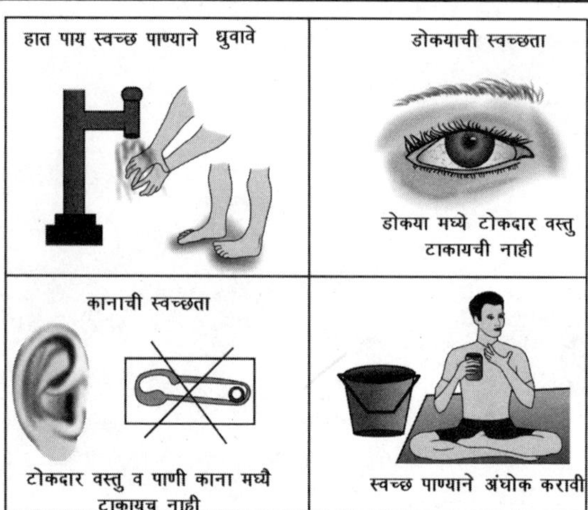
हात पाय स्वच्छ पाण्याने धुवावे
डोळयाची स्वच्छता
डोळया मध्ये टोकदार वस्तु टाकायची नाही
कानाची स्वच्छता
टोकदार वस्तु व पाणी काना मध्ये टाकायच नाही
स्वच्छ पाण्याने अंघोळ करावी

CHAPTER

52

Importance of Nutrition

INTRODUCTION

Balance diet is one which provides sufficient number of calories, adequate amounts of protein, fat and carbohydrate. It also gives adequate amount of vitamins and minerals for maintaining healthy, vitality and general well-being. (Additional allowances needed during pregnancy and lactation period).

Education on nutrition holds an important place in the fight against malnutrition. People are ignorant about balanced diets and optimum nutrition. They should be educated on nutritive value of foods, storage, and preparation, cooking, serving and eating food. Adequate nutrition is the foundation of good health.

Infants, children, pregnant and lactating women's nutritional needs are very important. Special attention must be given to promotion of breast feeding and appropriate weaning with use of local food practices be promoted.

Prevention of anemia, control of vitamins and prevention of nutritional diseases to be taken into account. Proper nutrition is essential for good quality of life. Daily diet should contain all the food factors, like proteins, fats, carbohydrate, vitamins, minerals and water in adequate correct amount. The diet should supply the calories of energy needed by the body. Good nutrition helps in growth and development physical as well as intellectual. There are energy yielding foods, body building foods, protective foods.

Bad diets not only lead to fatigue, but also take a toll on our overall health. Hence it is vital to protect oneself against the damage and nourish the body from within by talking balance healthy diet.

Encourage the villagers to set up **kitchen gardens** which provide fresh fruits and establish poultry and fisheries. It can be done near the house, near the source of water, which is usually waste water from the kitchen. Kitchen garden can help to improve the diet of the family.

They should be taught about correct cooking techniques, preservation of foods, planning a well-balanced meal with locally available cheap foods like combining pulses with cereals to improve the protein quality.

Teach mother proper technique of breastfeeding, weaning methods, dietary requirements and rapidly growing children, pregnant and lactating woman.

Good nutrition helps physical growth, body building and metal growth, building defense mechanism, prevents infection reduction of mortality and morbidity rates. With education comes self-realization and awareness of circumstances. Educated parents know the cost and troubles of binging up a child.

Recommended Daily Allowances of Calories

1. Man 55 kg—work sedentary net calories 2400; moderate 2800 and heavy 3900 calories
2. Woman 45 kg—sedentary 2000; moderate 2300; heavy 3000; pregnancy 2300; lactation 2700 calories
3. Children 0 to 6—months 120/kg
4. Adolescents 13 to 15 years—girls 2100; boys 2500
5. Adolescents 16 to 19 years—girls 2100; boys 3150 calories.

Green leaf vegetables—there is a wide variety of green leafy vegetables. Palak, amaranth sour green, cabbage, methis, etc. they are the cheapest among "protective foods" green leafy vegetables are valuable from the point of human nutrition. They are excellent and inexpensive sources of carotene, B-group vitamins and minerals. They contain cellulose, which acts as "roughage" in the intestine, and helps prevent constipation.

Fruits are prized for their vitamins. Most fruits contain significant amounts of ascorbic acid; fruits contain cellulose which assists in normal bowel movements. Fruits are costly and it may not be within the reach of all to afford them daily. Seasonal fruits are cheaper and easily available if leafy vegetables are included in diet need for fruits are reduced.

Fruits hydrate and rejuvenate your skin; the very smell of it on your face is quite de-stressing. Unlike the chemical beauty treatments, fruits are cost-effective, natural and bring a visible difference. Here are few fruits with their properties, choose what suits you beast.

Banana—this is one fruit that is abundantly available in India all through the year. We know it is good source of iron, magnesium and potassium and helps reduce menstrual cramps. The effect of banana on skin too is not something that can be ignored. Bananas are rich in vitamin A, B, and E and hence works as an anti-aging agent.

Apple—in health benefits are undisputable. Apple antioxidant property prevents cell and tissue damage. Studies by nutritionists have shown that apples collagen that help keep the skin young.

Orange—rich in vitamin C that improves skin texture. Like apple, orange too contains collagen that slows skin-aging process. Rub the insides of orange on your skin to tighten the skin. Orange can be dried, powered, and used as a natural scrub. Like lemon, oranges too help clear skin blemishes.

Papaya—the benefits of this fruit on skin have perhaps been talked about since the time of our ancestors. Papaya is rich in antioxidants and contain a special enzyme called papaya impurities. A glass of papaya milk or just applying the flesh of papaya on your skin can do wonders.

Mango—rightly called the king of fruits for not just its taste but also for health benefits. The soft pulpy fruit has an amazing effect on skin too. Rich in vitamin A and rich antioxidants, it fights again skin aging regenerates skin cells and restores the elasticity of skin.

Adequate Nutrition is Foundation of Good Health

Carbohydrates are composed of carbon, hydrogen and oxygen. They are main sources of energy and also the cheapest source of energy. In balance diet it must provide 50 to 60% of total calories. It provides energy and is essential for oxidation of fats. Daily diet should contain 350 to 400 grams of it, one gm of CHO gives 4 calories.

Protein is very important in human nutrition. Proteins are composed of carbon, hydrogen, oxygen, nitrogen and sulphur in different amounts. The proteins are made up of amino acids. Proteins required building the body, for wear and tear of tissue and their maintenance. The body proteins are constantly being broken down, they have to be replaced for which fresh protein intake is required. For growth and development, for synthesis of hormones antibodies, enzymes body requires producing them. Protein also can be used as a body fuel.

Deficiencies cause during pregnancy still birth, premature babies, small for date's babies, anemic babies. Infancy and early childhood causes kwashiorkor, marasmus, mental retardation, stunned growth and development. In adult underweight, anemia, poor musculature, low resistance, frequent loose stools, general lethargy, incapacity to sustain work, delayed wound healing. Cirrhosis of liver, edema and ascitis.

Fats—are saturated that we get from animal fats and excessive intake are harmful to the body. Unsaturated fats we get from vegetables and fats. They are used as body fuels for the production of heat and energy. A fat provides support to internal organs such as heart, kidney, and intestine.

Excessive consumption of fats results into obesity and diseases of blood vessels that is atherosclerosis. Increased blood cholesterol predisposes to coronary artery diseases. Due to deficiency of essential fatty acids skin becomes rough and dry or toad skin.

Vitamin A—source animal origin foods like ghee, butter, egg, milk, liver, fish etc. all green leafy vegetables such as spinach, coriander, drum stick leaves, carrots, pumpkin and cabbage, ripe fruits like mangoes, papaya, tomatoes. It is essential for normal vision and health of the eyes; it is anti-infective and is required for skeletal growth. Its deficiency causes night blindness, Bitot's spots. Regular intake of green leafy vegetables in the diet is important.

Vitamin C—is required for the metabolism of connective tissues, especially collagen. It is essential for wound healing; it is required for coagulation of blood. It helps in increasing the absorption of iron and is anti infective. We get from all; fresh fruits, vegetables, pulses like green gram etc. its deficiency leads to scurvy, anemia, bad teeth, offensive breath, spongy and swollen gums, loss of weight.

Vitamin D—is essential for the formation of healthy bones and teeth. It stimulates the intestinal absorption and utilization of calcium and phosphorus. Foods like egg yolk, liver, fish, and fish liver oils. Sunlight is an important and cheapest source. it is stored in the body in fatty tissues and in the liver. Excessive intake is harmful.

Iron—has a great importance in human nutrition. It is essential for transport of oxygen, and is required for formation of hemoglobin. Sources are liver, kidney, meat, egg, yolk, green leafy vegetables, and nuts etc iron deficiency causes anemia. Nutritional anemias—include iron, folic acid, vitamin B12 deficiency anemia's which is due to inadequate diet and mal-absorption, worm infestation and infection supplementation with iron, folic acid and de-worming are required.

Niacin maintains healthy condition of the skin and mucous membrane deficiency lads to pellagra with diarrhea, dermatitis, insomnia, mental depression, dementia, erythemia, soreness of mouth.

Folic acid stimulates blood formation. It is essential for the synthesis of DNA. It is essential for the functioning of bone marrow.

Calcium—gives rigidity and strength to born and harness and shining to the teeth. It controls rhythmic activities of heart and contraction muscles. It requires for coagulation of blood. It is essential for regulation of neuromuscular irritability and capillary permeability. Deficiency causes poor development of bones and teeth. Rickets, osteomalacia, delayed blood clotting, hyperplasia of parathyroid glands, low calcium tetany.

Iodine required for the synthesis of thyroxin and its deficiency causes goiter.

Vitamin B12 is an essential; micronutrient, it plays a crucial role in the formation of RBC and maintaining the health of the nerve tissue. It is what the body needs fit must not fall prey to anemia. Efficient functioning of the CNS that is responsible for maintaining alertness and memory recalls also requires healthy doses of B12. it built a reputation for elevating the mood since to helps manufacture neurotransmitters like monoamines that help the regulate the mood and reduce incidence of depression and anxiety. B12 is crucial for nerve nutrition and plays a key role in neuro muscular transmission. It is therefore determines how strong or weak your muscles will be, symptoms like tingling at sole, in the limbs, cramps, giddiness, palpitation, loss of energy.

No single yardstick for measuring health

Egg—keeps you fuller, anything that contains **high protein** gives a stomach filling effect. Eating protein rich eggs reduces hunger and decreases caloric consumption throughout the day. Leucine that is found in eggs plays a unique role in the regulation of muscle protein synthesis and insulin. An egg contains about 121 mg of cholesterol which is present in yolk; recommended amount of cholesterol is about 300 mg/day. So eating too many eggs can increase your cholesterol level. Eat fewer egg yoke each week and eat only the egg white which has no cholesterol. You should not avoid yolk completely as it contains vitamin, minerals and vitamin D.

Why sugar is toxic—sugar makes us fat, rots our teeth—most of us are unaware of the amount of sugar in daily diet. We need sugar to fuel our body and brain but larger amount raises insulin levels, body turns surplus sugar into fat and stores it around the vital organs. Placing us at risk of liver and heart diseases. Sugar can become as addictive as drug and alcohol. Scientists found that chemicals released when we eat sugar travel along the same brain path waves that heroin does. And when we are stressed or sad the foods that can produce this feeling trigger powerful craving, causing us to eat up to 6 times more than our normal intake. Sugar stimulates the release of endorphins which makes you feel good. Cut down sugar when you do you probably will experience headache and feel grumpy and lethargic for few days. After a week you will start feel better. Do it gradually, eat a low glycemic diet which will keep blood sugar levels constant. Reduce sugary sweets, white bread or pasta every day, biscuits and sugar intake in diet.

Nutrition Platter

1. Calcium—milk and milk product
2. Potassium and magnesium—cereals, nuts, dry fruits, broccoli, cabbage, sprouts, cauliflower
3. Protein—milk and dairy products, fish, legume, meat, nuts, dry fruits
4. Iron—fish, cereals, apple, ladies fingers, onions, jiggery,
5. Vitamin 'A'—carrot, broccoli, sweet potatoes, spinach, pumpkin, cheese, egg, papaya, mango, apricot, peas, milk
6. Vitamin 'B'—cereals, meat, liver, lentils, potatoes, banana, chill, pepper, whole grain, beans
7. Vitamin 'C'—citrus fruits like orange, lemon, amla, sweet lime.
8. Vitamin 'D'—cereals, fish, eggs
9. Vitamin 'E'—nuts, dry fruits.

Basics of a Balanced Diet (Table 52.1)

1. **Eggs**—are rich protein, vitamin and mineral content. Eggs improves your concentration, maintains healthy weight, develops the brain, strengthens eyesight as well as prevents birth defects and breast cancers
2. **Quinon**—is a 100% reference protein, which has all essential 9 amino acids.
3. **Yogurt**—good bacteria helps in gastrointestinal conditions like constipation, diarrhea, lactose intolerance, colon cancer and bowel disease as well as prevention of osteoporosis and regulating blood pressure
4. **Oats**—if you want to better chance of fighting high cholesterol, heart disease, regulating your blood sugar, blood pressure and bowel movements, reducing getting risk of cancer or controlling your weight eat more oats.
5. **Spinach** is loaded with iron and host of vitamins, minerals.

Nutrition is fundamental to good health. Much of ill health is due to poor nutrition. The daily diet should contain all the food factors.

Reduce calorie and fat intake in diet will make your body use its reserves of stored fat. Exercise will increase body metabolism and strengthen the core muscles of the abdomen, help you shrink your stomach. Lifestyle and technically advanced society and added stress level have lead to an obesity epidemic. Sit less to live longer which helps the body manage blood sugar and metabolize cholesterol. A flat and shapely abdomen tells a lot about you that you take care of yourself, which your overall health is sound and most importantly

Table 52.1: Basics of a balanced diet

Food groups	*Infants 0–6 mts in gm*	*1–3 years*	*4–6 years*	*7–9 years*	*10–12 years*
Cereals and millets	30	0.5	0.4	06	10
Pulses, milk	30	0.25	01	02	02
Milk products	100	0.4	05	05	05
Roots and tubes	100	0.5	05	01	01
Green leafy vegetables	100	0.25	0.5	0.5	01
Fruits	100	01	01	01	01
Sugar	05	02	03	04	01
Fat/oil	05	04	05	06	04

important benefits of exercise are multifactor. It will not only indicate optimal strength and endurance of the problem but also his nutritional choices and happy lifestyle. If you rest, you rust.

Every junk food meal damages your arteries. The main problem with the obesity time bomb ticking in India is the people's attitude. There is lack of awareness about the biochemistry of fat the peculiar "Indian fat" is different from that found in Caucasians and very difficult to metabolize and its co-relation to serious diseases. Indian fat is dangerous because unlike the westerner's fat, it cannot burn down to form energy. Indians tend to store more fat people do not understand the need to maintain their weight. Obesity is like any other chronic disease that needs lifelong treatment. It is not just enough to lose your excess weight through medicine or exercise, maintenance is most different part

Explanation—different variety of food like pulses, fruits, vegetables etc are shown in the figure. Health education to be given for the use, frequency and health benefits of balanced diet.

Keywords
Calories, bad diets, good nutrition, adequate nutrition, deficiency causes, excessive consumption, nutrition platter, basic balanced diet.

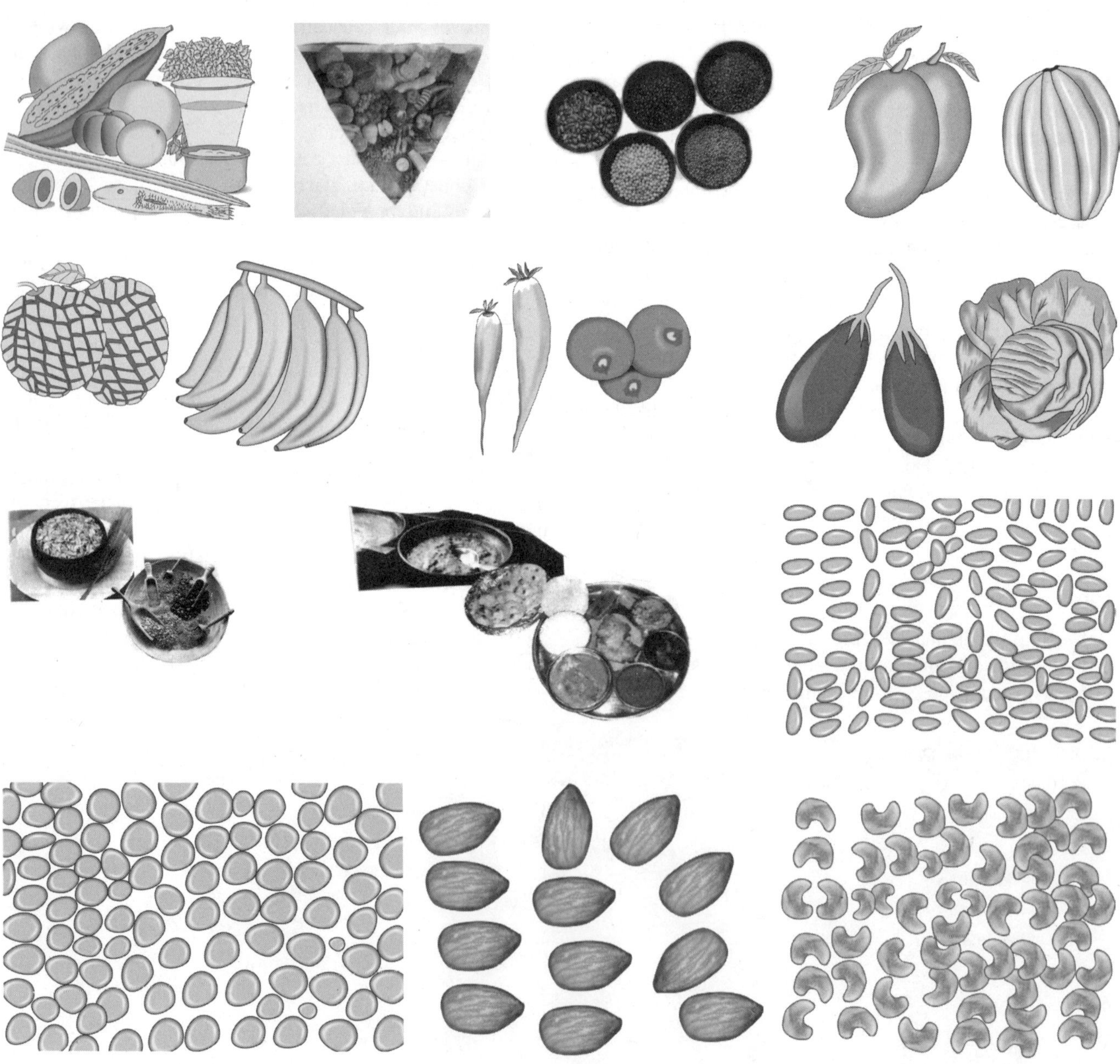

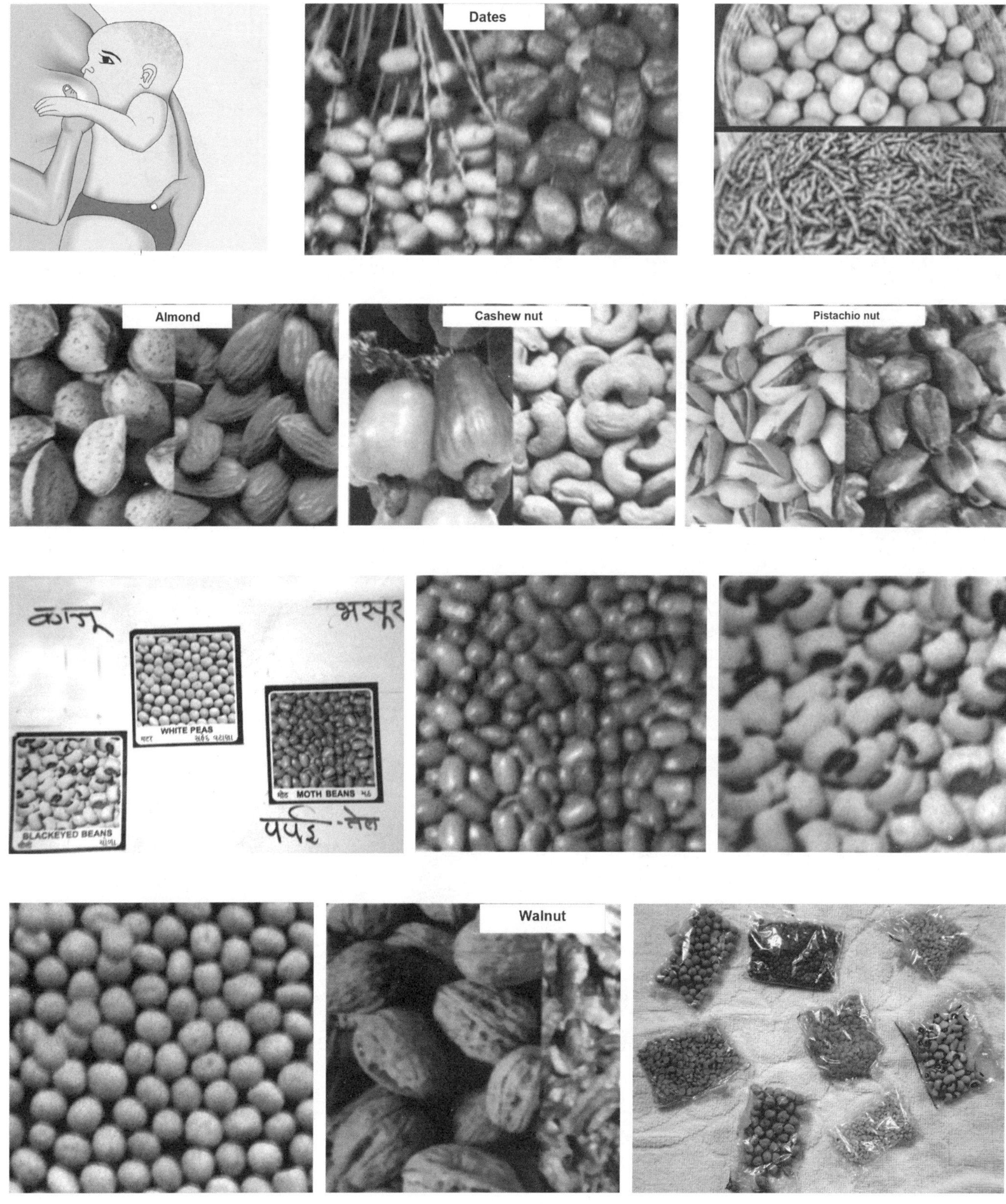
Dates
Almond
Cashew nut
Pistachio nut
WHITE PEAS
MOTH BEANS
BLACKEYED BEANS
Walnut

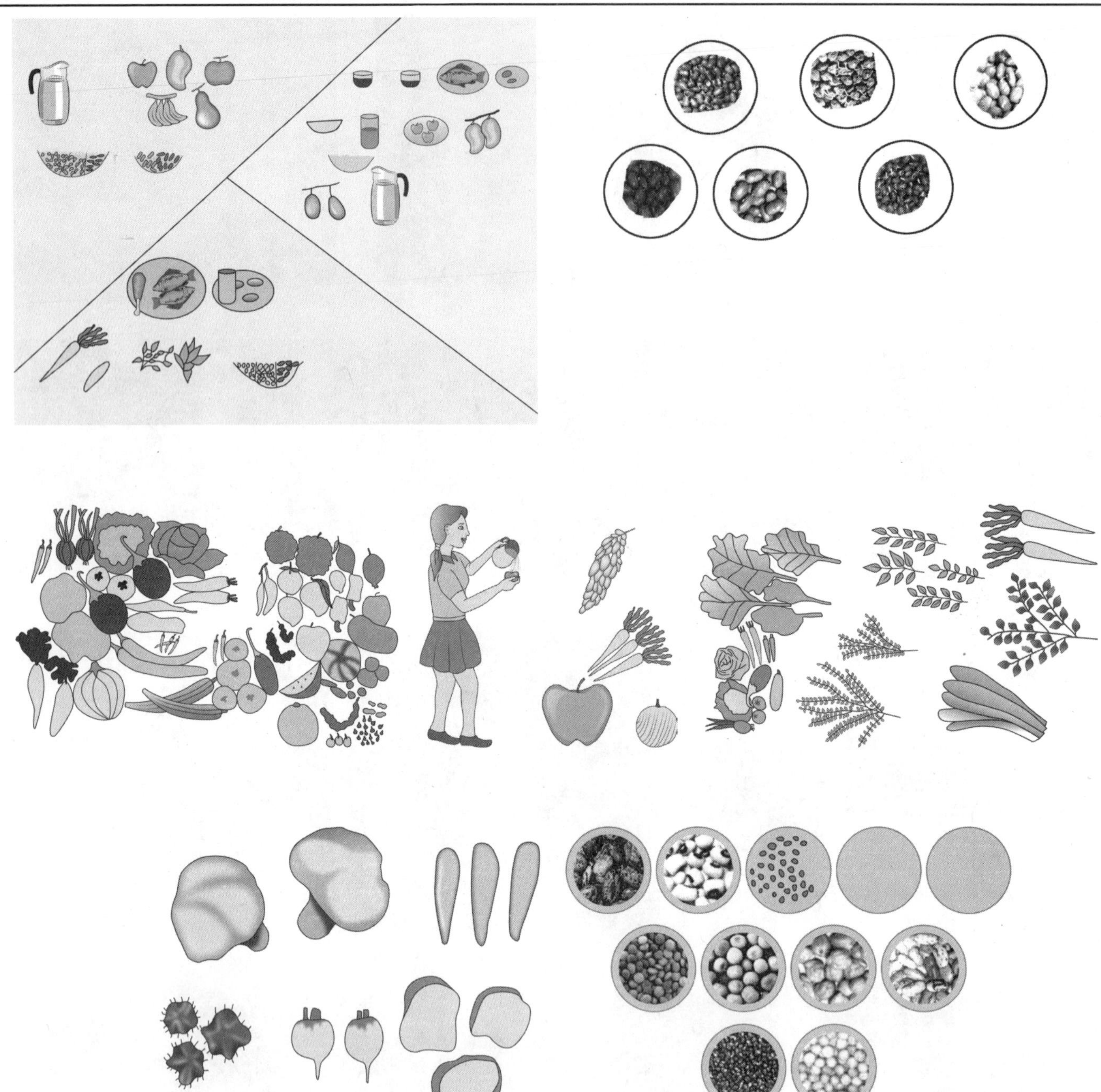

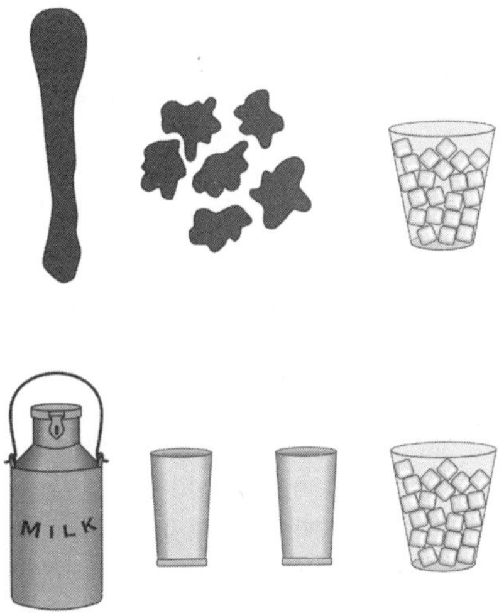

MILK
Apricots 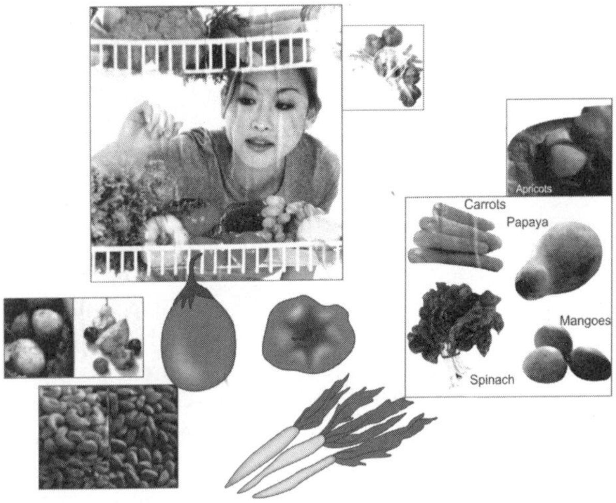
Carrots
Papaya
Mangoes
Spinach 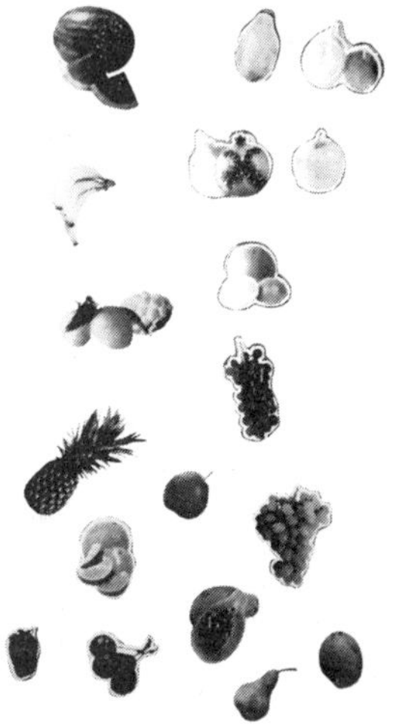 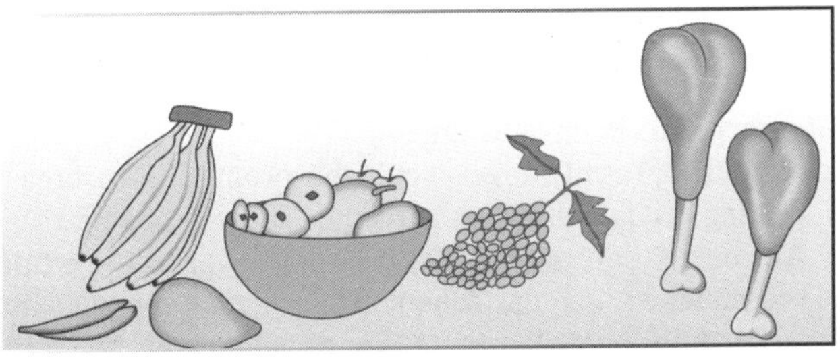 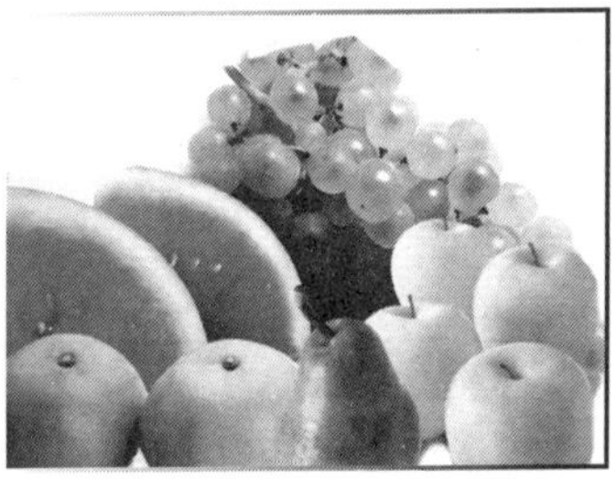
Constituents of food

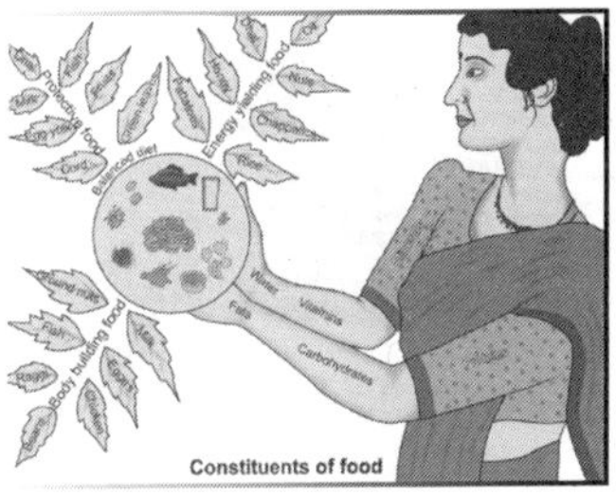

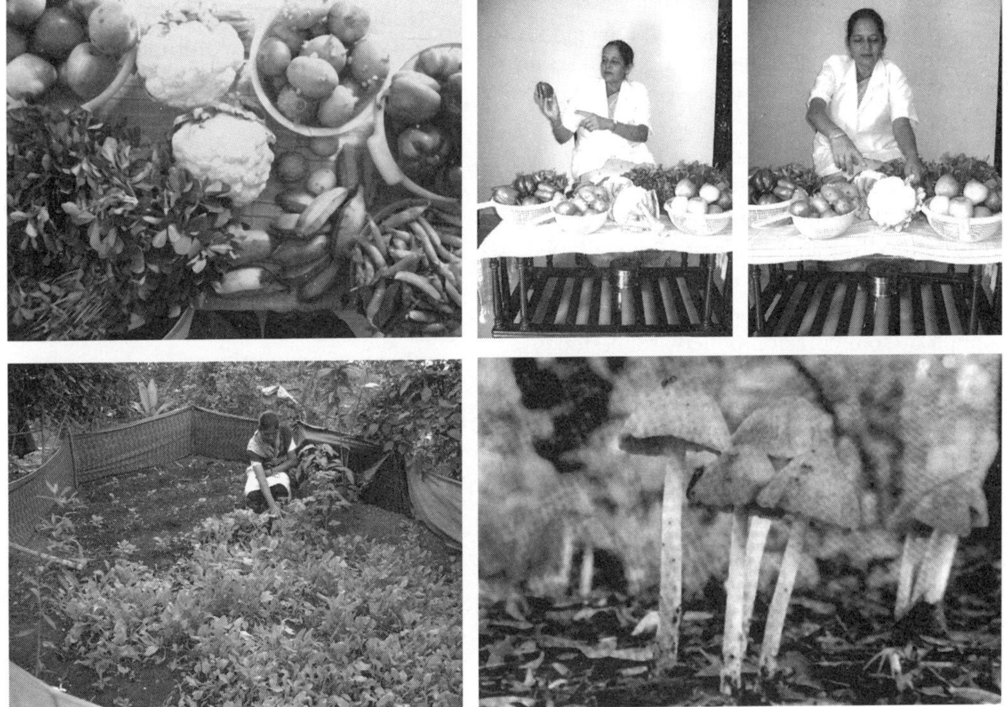

CHAPTER

53

Malnutrition

INTRODUCTION

Malnutrition occurs when the body does not get the proper kind of food in the amount needed to maintaining health. It can occur in any age but mainly found in children, Malnutrition usually occurs between 6 months and 3 years of age.

Causes

1. **Conditioning influences**—diarrhea, intestinal parasites, measles, whooping cough, malaria, tuberculosis all contribute to malnutrition, minor childhood ailments, environmental conditions, infections.
2. **Cultural influences**—lack of foods is not the cause too often there is starvation in the midst of plenty. **Food habits**, customs beliefs, traditional and culture have deep psychological roots and associated with family shaping food habits which are passed from one generation to another. In some communities men eat first and then women eat last in such situation health of a woman adversely get affected which may lead to malnutrition. **Religion** has a powerful influence on the food habits; there are known food taboos which prevent people from consuming nutritious food even when these are easily available. In the selection of foods **personal likes and dislikes** play an important part which can stand in between correcting nutritional deficiency. **Cooking practices** like draining the rice water at the end of cooking prolonged boiling in open pans, peeling vegetables and fruits all influence nutritive value of food. Childs raring practices vary from region to region and influence the nutritional status of infants in that breast feeding, adoption of commercial products, refine foods.
3. **Socioeconomic factors**—it is by product of poverty, ignorance, insufficient education, lack of knowledge regarding nutritive value of food. Inadequate sanitary environment, large families and poor quality of life are the determinants of malnutrition.
4. **Food production**—increased food production should lead to increased consumption. There is uneven distribution within the countries, so equitable distribution in accordance with physiological needs.
5. **Health and services**—properly organized and radical action taken, nutritional surveillance implies continuous monitoring community individual as well as groups and nutritional supplement will help detect malnutrition. Health education will help appropriate action to reinforce elements of health services and its usage.

To detect nurses have to do physical assessment by Screening by talking **height and weight** to identify malnourished children; keep growth monitoring chart and road to health is a simple and inexpensive way to monitor child's nutritional status. **Mid-arm** circumference another technique to measure malnutrition clinical and lab examination protein and mineral deficiencies, estimation of hemoglobin

A problem of malnutrition is kwashiorkor and marasmus is protein energy deficiency, infection like diarrhea, anemia, and vitamin deficiency.

Therefore nurses have to take—

1. **Action at family level** would be promotion of breast feeding, planting kitchen garden or keeping poultry.
2. **Action of community level**—supplementary feeding programmed, mid day school meal, vitamin prophylaxis, ICDS programmed, immunization, periodic health check ups, nutritional education, formal education to school children.
3. **Action on national level**—rural development to improve socioeconomic development. Increase agricultural production, stabilization of population, nutritional policy, nutritional intervention programmed, prevention and control of endemic goiter through iodized common salt, control of anemia through distribution of folic acid to pregnant and nursing mothers. Nutritional related health activities.
4. **Action on international level**—food and nutrition is a global problem just as health and sickness. Several international agencies work together to combat the problem of malnutrition.

Signs and Symptoms of Malnutrition

1. Child looses weight.
2. Eye changes—dryness, night blindness.
3. Hair changes—light color, brittle.
4. Anemia.
5. Apathy, listlessness, soreness of mouth, bowing of legs.
6. Growth failure that is loss of weight in children.
7. Edema.
8. Anemia.
9. Skin changes that is dry and rough, loss of subcutaneous fatty muscles.
10. Night blindness.

Identification of Malnutrition

1. **Height and weight**—take child's height and weight regularly, maintain the growth chart
2. **Mid-arm circumference**—the child 1 to 5 years of age and is malnourished his mid-arm circumference is less than 12.8
3. **Clinical and laboratory examination**—examine the child from head to foot for signs of malnutrition. Find out protein, vitamin and mineral deficiencies. Find out a hemoglobin percentage of the child.

Problems of Malnutrition

Kwashiorkor and marasmus—these are diseases protein energy malnutrition. It develops in children between 1 and 3 years of age. These are due to a diet lacking in proteins and calories and infections such as measles, diarrhea, bronchitis, which lead the child into malnutrition. Kwashiorkor and marasmus affects the physical growth as well as mental development of the child. It can cause death too.

Prevention of Malnutrition

1. Give proper antenatal care to the mothers, because a healthy mother gives birth to a healthy baby.
2. Encourage mothers to breast feeding.
3. Proper weaning of the child. Start supplementary feeding around the age of 4 to 6 months, because breast milk alone is not sufficient to sustain the growth of the child. Proper use of supplements helps in preventing malnutrition during the weaning period.
4. Give nutrition education to the mother.
5. Fully immunization of the child against childhood diseases, e.g. tetanus, diphtheria, measles whooping cough tuberculosis.
6. Practicing food hygiene to prevent infection is important.

India has the highest prevalence (and largest share) of malnourished children, low birth weight babies and anemia levels amongst children and women in the world. Other micronutrient deficiencies (vitamin A and iodine) also constitute serious public health problems. Various government schemes set up to combat these problems have not had the expected impact in reducing malnutrition or micronutrient deficiencies. This is not only due to low utilization or inadequacy of the schemes but also due to the population not adopting appropriate behaviors to improve their health and nutrition.

Providing correct and timely technical advice on nutrition to their patients and their families is often given inadequate emphasis by health team. But when we know that malnutrition contributes to 55% of child mortality which has been stagnating in most states, medical practitioners, whose advice on health matters is very much needed by the population, can play an important role in reversing this trend. India is home to the largest numbers of malnourished children in the world—not only in terms of the number of children but also in terms of the proportion of Children under five years of age. While India has close to 22% of the Developing world's population, our share of malnourished children is almost double at 40%.

In fact, India has the dubious distinction of having the largest proportions of malnutrition at birth (low birth weight rate at over 30%), in early childhood (53.4% undernourished by weight for age criteria and 52 per cent stunted, i.e. by height for age criteria) and during adulthood (47.1% of women and 46.4% of men having chronic energy deficiency according to body mass index criteria). Such unacceptable levels of malnutrition have been persisting for more than twenty years in spite of the country having several good programme such as the public distribution system to distribute food grains at subsidized prices, to provide supplementary nutrition through programme such as the Integrated Child Development Services.

Goals and Objectives: The National Health Policy (1983) aimed at reducing the low birth weight rate from about 30% in 1983 to 25% in 1985, 18% in 1990 and 10 per cent in 2000. The National Plan of Action for Children (1992) and the National Nutrition Policy in its objectives for the 90s expected that India will be able to bring down the malnutrition levels in children below 5 years from nearly 60% in 1990 to 30% in 2000. And yet, progress if any in each of these fronts over the last two decades can be described at best as 'stunted' To understand why not much progress has been made, we have to look at some of the recent data. Prior to the National Family Health Survey (1992–93), data on child malnutrition was invariably analyzed by broader age groups and therefore most recommendations were to focus on children with higher levels of malnutrition, i.e. children aged 3 to 6 years.

Malnutrition and Feeding Patterns: Only 51% of India's children are exclusively fed on breast milk during the first three months of life; less than a-third of children (31.4% in 1992–1993 and 33.5% in 1995-1998) receive complementary feeding on a regular basis during their age 6–9 months. We already know that a growing infant needs about 1,100 kcal of nourishment everyday. Breastmilk even at peak production capacity can meet only part of this need after six months and therefore, it is absolutely essential that solid, mushy foods are introduced as additional feeds on a regular basis to all children at around six months of age.

Studies reveal that a child of 1–4 years has a nutritional deficit of about 400 kcal per day. Such deficits are the real reason for malnutrition setting in. A very young child thus loses out on the very important energy needs early in life.

Much of the deficit is not so much due to a lack of food at household level, but to inadequate feeding practices. Health practitioners are amongst the very few whose advice is sought by parents and other caregivers on matters related to child care. Most practitioners meet parents of young children for immunization during the second, third and fourth months of life and critical advice related to feeding and nourishment are given by doctors.

It appears that we are not able to communicate effectively, the urgency and absolute essentiality of quality feeding for all children in this age group. Medical practitioners therefore must begin early in their interactions with parents and caregivers with advice on feeding the young child with soft, mushy foods on a regular basis from the 6th month of the child. This persistent malnutrition contributes to nearly half of the child mortality which has remained stagnant despite improvement in health care delivery in a number of states.

Malnutrition and Mortality: Another reason for growth faltering usually in the second half of the first year is the habit of children to put every object that they see into their mouths and also the frequent respiratory infections that are seen in the young children. While practitioners almost always treat the infections, we fail to give correct advice on feeding, especially the need to give extra foods in the convalescent stages to allow for catch up of weight that was lost during the course of minor illnesses. An important issue relates to how children are fed within households. While it takes two individuals—the child and the mother or the caregiver to ensure that a very young child of age below three years is fed well, there is not sufficient appreciation of this by both family members and those who give advice. Interfamilial distribution of food should ensure that those who are vulnerable—children and women get adequate amounts of quality foods within the household, for they do not generally eat elsewhere; on the other hand, men and earning members of the family generally tend to eat not only within the household, but also outside their homes. One of the simple ways to determine if the child is growing well is to regularly weigh the child and take the length/height of the child and plot its weight on the growth chart and use the chart to help the mother and caregivers understand the importance of physical growth and the importance of timely complementary feeding and increasing the energy intake of the young child.

Micronutrient Malnutrition: Apart from the protein energy malnutrition, three micronutrient deficiencies are well documented in India—iodine, iron and vitamin A deficiency. They affect not only young children but population of all age groups, some more than others. Iodine deficiency can cause irreversible brain damage before birth and is the main cause of mental retardation and increasing levels of deaf-mutes born in certain parts of the country. Iodine deficiency in countries such as ours is rampant partly because of the extent to which environmental degradation is taking place where iodine from the top soil is continuously washed away and our diets are either deficient in iodine or we take other food items which compete with the available iodine in diet. At present, the Government of India policy is to ensure that all salt consumed in the country is iodized and non-iodized salt is not sold for human consumption. This will not only prevent iodine deficiency disorders but also prevent the invisible forms of mental retardation that are seen in communities in the form of decreased IQ points in the populations feeding on diets deficient in iodine. Studies have repeatedly shown that there is no part of India which is free from iodine deficiency. Medical practitioners as a part of their contribution to preventing the deficiency need to continue to emphasize the need for consumption of iodized salt. At present only 70% of the population have access to iodized salt.

Iodine deficiency in different districts of India: Iron deficiency anemia is another major micronutrient deficiency that affects very large proportions of children, adolescent girls and women in the reproductive age group. The NFHS-2 conducted recently revealed that nearly three out of four children below three years are anemic and over half of women in the child-bearing age group are iron deficient. This has important implications for their work capacity, the learning abilities when they get into school, retards their ability to grow well, cause frequent ailments and further contribute to both morbidity and mortality. India has for years been running a National Nutritional Anemia Prophylaxis programme for preventing anemia in pregnant and lactating women. Under the programme, till 1992, 60 mg. of elemental iron were administered to all women for 100 days. From 1992, the prophylactic dose of iron has been increased to 100 mg of elemental iron. Yet, the levels of anemia are very high and possibly contribute not only to anemia being carried on to the next generation but also have a negative effect on the birth weight of newborns. One of the major reasons for high levels of anemia in this country in spite of a national programme is the poor compliance in terms of women not taking the full course of the prophylactic dose that is given to them. As a practitioner, we have an important responsibility to ensure that children and women are routinely examined for anemia, counseled for increasing iron rich foods in their diet and where necessary give complete treatment for iron deficiency anemia with a special emphasis on follow-up for compliance.

Vitamin A is another micronutrient, the deficiency of which not only contributes to night blindness but also to increased morbidity and poor protection against severer forms of respiratory and skin infections. Studies in certain countries have also demonstrated that they have a role in decreasing childhood and maternal mortality as well. The National Survey of Blindness (1986–89), suggests that prevalence of night blindness in children under six years is around 6% with Bitot's spots having been observed in 0.7% of children through another survey during the same period. While the government programme envisages administration of large doses of vitamin A to children aged 9 months to 3 years, the medical practitioners can contribute to decreasing the vitamin A deficiency states in the community by encouraging their patients and their families to consume adequate amounts of green leafy vegetables and other vitamin A rich foods and ensuring that young children receive 2 lacs of IU of vitamin A every six months (1 lac IU during infancy) from the government health centers or by prescribing vitamin A capsules to children below 5 years and to women immediately after delivery to build adequate body stores of vitamin A for increasing the concentration of vitamin A in their breast milk.

Conclusion—the health team and the he community nurses have a major role to play in reducing the very high levels of malnutrition and micronutrient deficiencies in the country. Specific messages and timely counseling of patients, families and the caregivers of children on breastfeeding, timely complementary feeding of young children, adequate nutrition for pregnant and lactating women, consumption of iodized salts, enriching the diets of families with foods rich in iron and vitamin A as well as diagnosing early the deficiency states and providing the correct treatment can go a long way in decreasing morbidity and mortality of the vulnerable segments of the population.

Under nutrition continue to raise their ugly head, **magnitude of malnutrition** adversely affecting the growth of children under nutrition is one of the most critical challenges despite substantial improvement in health and well being under nutrition remains a silent energy of sorts will about 50% of all children under 3 years remaining the age of three are under weight, silent emergency of sorts with low birth weight and 52% of women and 72% of children being anemic. Thirty percent of new born with low birth weight sizable proportion of children and women suffer from the deficiency of vitamin A and iodine. Household food insecurity uneven food distribution within the household imbalanced diet, poor preventative and curative health services and lack of awareness about proper care and infant feeding practices are the major factors leading to under nutrition.

Among women, malnutrition is the main cause of low birth weight babies and their poor growth that in turn leads to increased infant mortality. The surviving low birth weight babies are also susceptible to growth retardation and illness throughout their childhood, adolescence and adulthood, 1975 Government of India started ICDS to instrumental in improving the health an well being of new mothers and children under 6 years of age by providing health and nutrition educator, health services supplement Tory food and pre school education. The ICDS programme is targeted at over 34 million pregnancy 0–6 years and 7 million pregnant and nursing mothers. Mid day meal, NRHM and PDS (public distribution system).

Explanation—different types of malnutrition cause different types of diseases condition especially in children is shown by pictures.

Keywords
Malnutrition: causes, signs and symptoms, identification, problems, prevention, goals and objectives, feeding pattern, mortality, deficiencies, micronutrient.

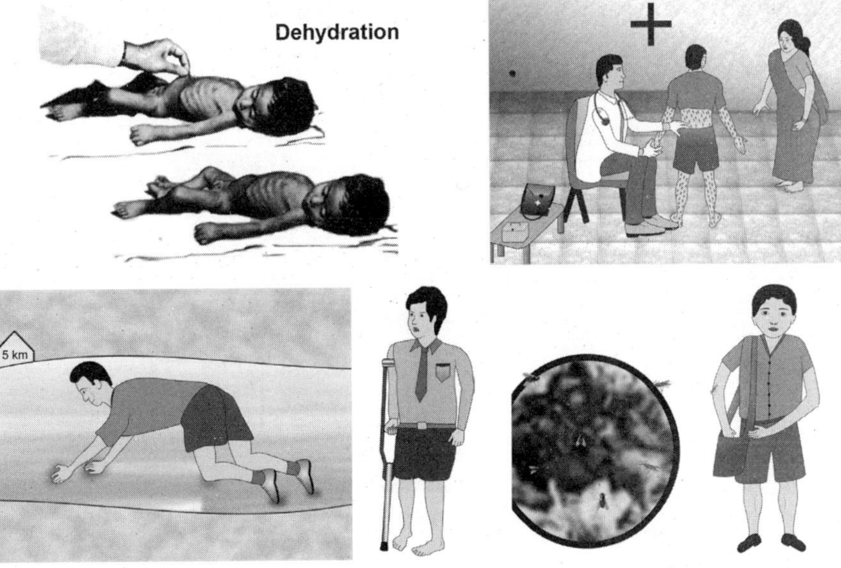

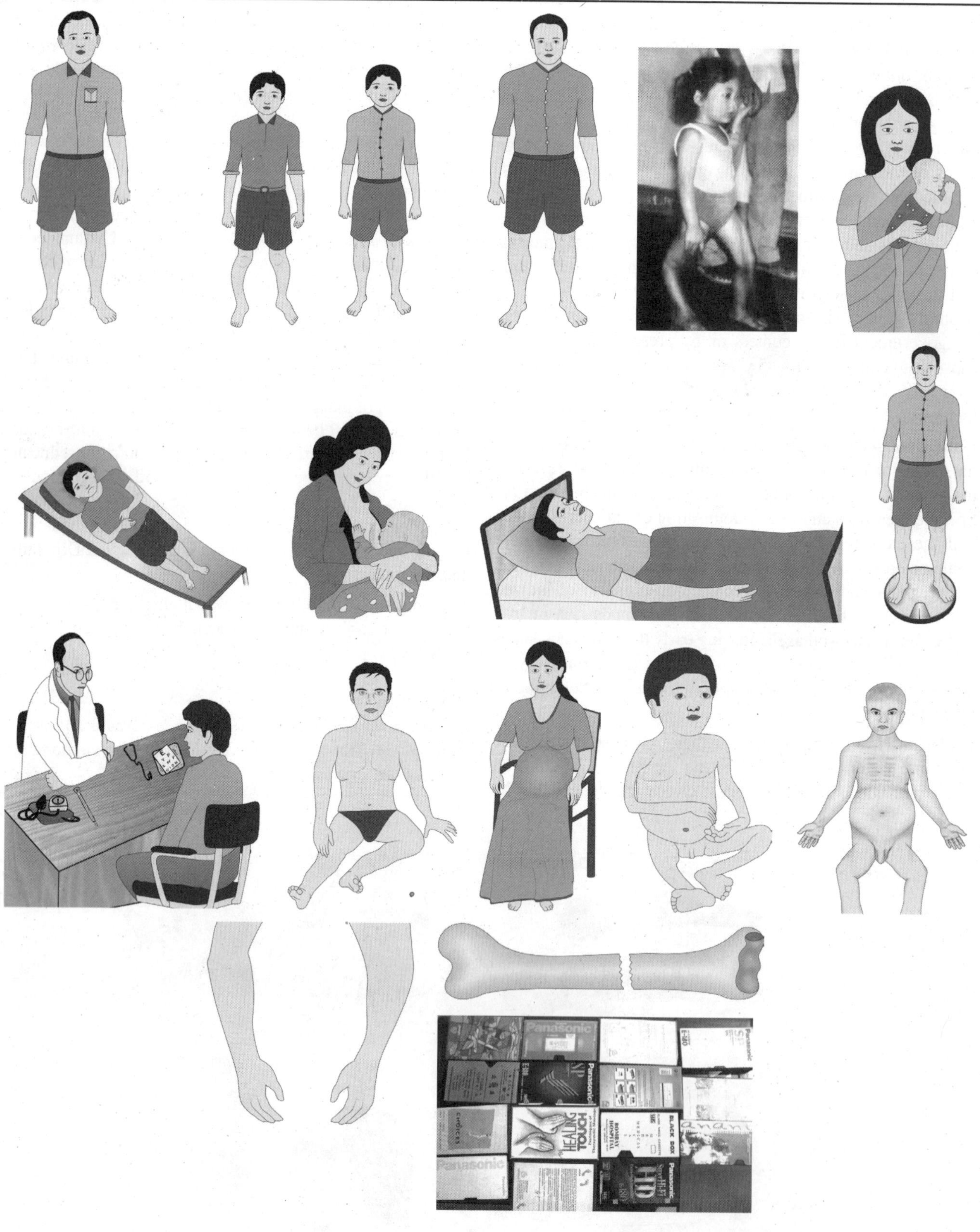
Panasonic
BLACK BOX

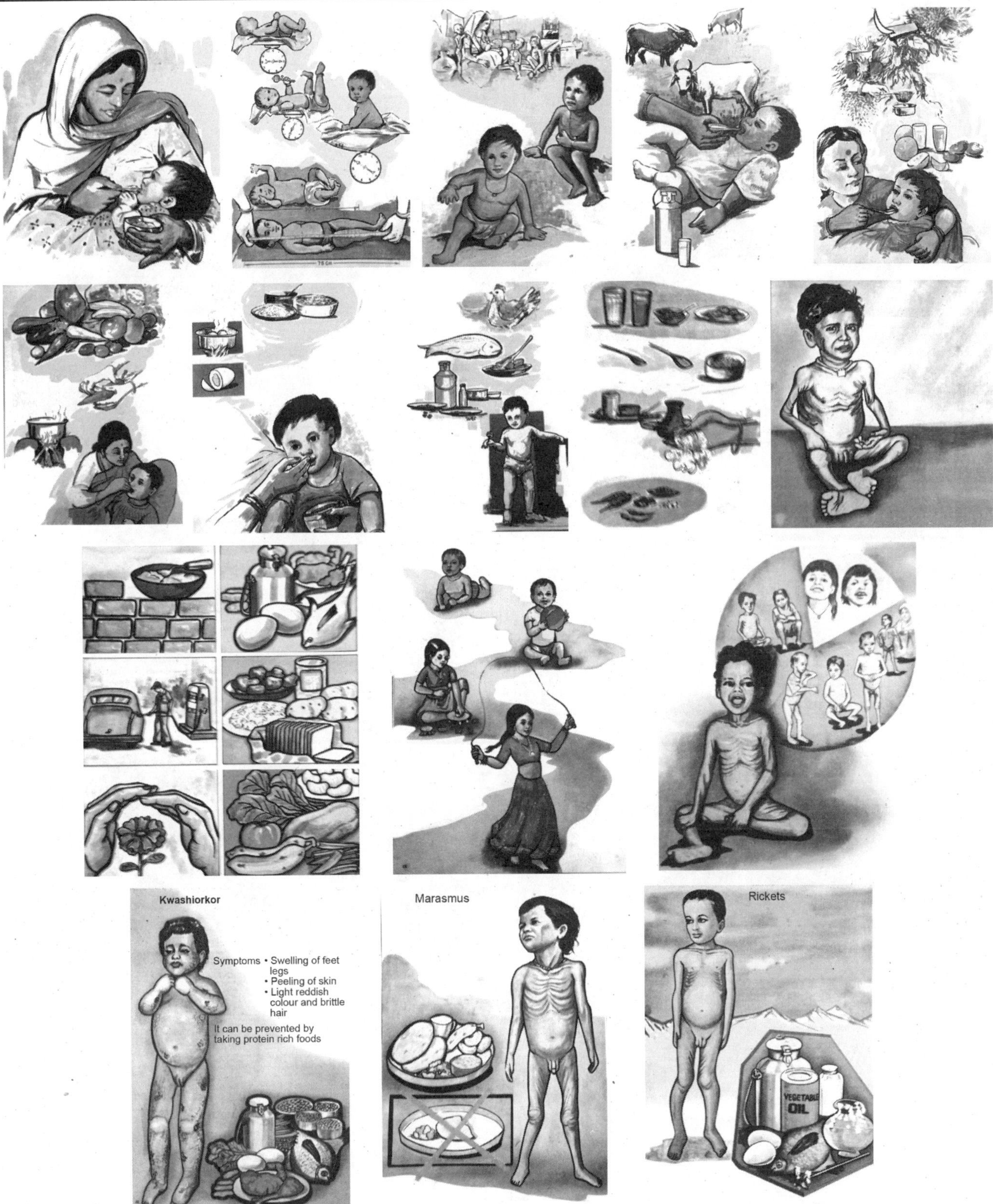
Kwashiorkor
Symptoms • Swelling of feet legs
• Peeling of skin
• Light reddish colour and brittle hair
It can be prevented by taking protein rich foods
Marasmus
Rickets
VEGETABLE OIL

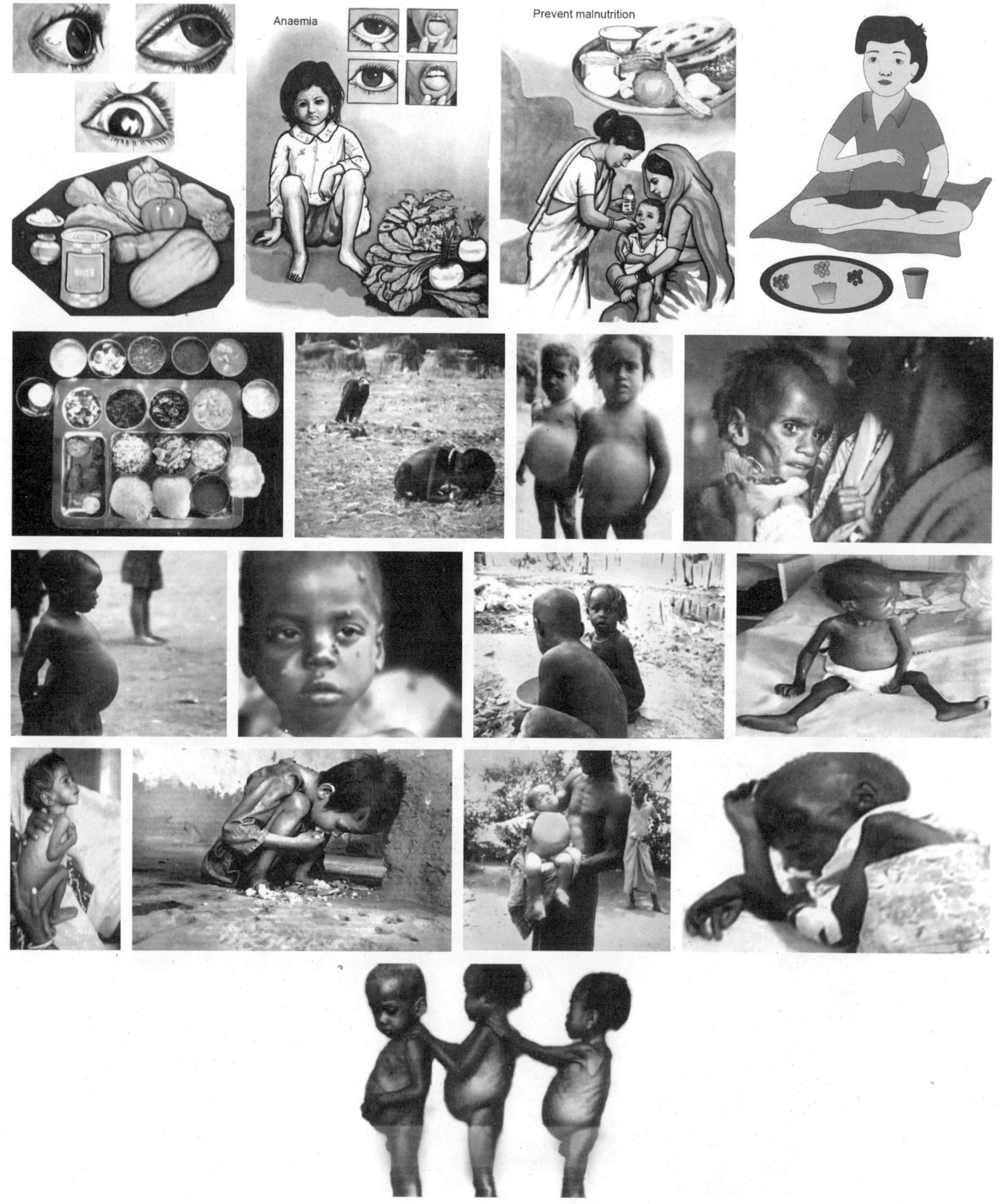
Anaemia
Prevent malnutrition
GHEE

CHAPTER

54

Malaria and Filariasis

The student has to select the topic and get the apt subject matter by referring books. Today malaria has become biggest public health problem. Students have to explain the definition, epidemiological factors, signs and symptoms, causes, diagnosis and investigations, treatment and most important is the prevention and control of malaria and how it spreads. The students have to follow the format and prepare the topic under the guidance of a teacher.

Malaria is one of the oldest recorded diseases in the world. It is most widespread and it is a major public health problem in the tropical developing world. Among all the infectious diseases, malaria continuous to be one of the biggest contributors to diseases burdens in terms of death and suffering.

Malaria is a complex disease and its intensity of distribution vary from place to place. Vaccination against malaria is a burning issue today. Vaccines are designed to arrest the development of parasite and reduce transmission.

Greatest risk of dying are children under the age of 5 years in malaria endemic areas, pregnant women, people moving from non malarias zones for work, migration, refugees, war or tourism, travelers who visit endemic countries and return home with the diseases.

The magnetite of the problem is very great. The ecosystem of the country has been constantly changing due to it the change in epidemiological pattern in malarial history. The economic loss due to not going to work is great to the family.

Malaria is a protozoal disease caused by infection with parasites. Malaria is a mosquito born disease which is caused by malarial parasite (plasmodium) it is transmitted to man by infected:

1. **Female anopheles**—malaria (the female species bites a patient who has malaria, she draws up a small quantity of blood containing the parasites. These parasites are then passed through the several stages of development within the mosquito's body and finally finds their way to its salivary glands. There they lie in wait for an opportunity to enter the blood stream of the next individual the mosquito bites. About 10 days after the mosquito has injected these parasites into a person blood stream many more parasites can be seen under a microscope. Most of them are now within the RBC of the victim. There they grow until they eventually replace all the hemoglobin within the cell. Although probably only one parasite attacks cell. As a cell breaks up, they are released; each tiny parasite then attacks another RBC, thus repeating the cycle every 2–3 days. Many of the parasites are destroyed by the defense system of the boy. But enough of them survive to cause plenty of trouble).
2. **Cules**—filarial, encephalitis.
3. **Aedes**—bite of aedes aegypti mosquito causes also yellow fever, dengue fever, hemorrhagic fever.

MAJOR HEALTH PROBLEM OF INDIA

Incidence rose to a peak of 6.47 million.

Malaria is a serious health problem. Malaria affect all ages, male are more exposed due to out door life get affected more as female are better clothed. It is a public health hazard, tendency to relapse as well as major mortality rate problem.

The clinical features vary from mild to severe and complicated according to the species of parasite present, the patient's state of immunity, the intensity of the infection and the malnutrition. It is clinically characterized by fever which comes on with chills or rigor and leaves with sweating. A typical attack comprises three stages—cold, hot and sweating stage. Enlargement of the spleen and secondary anemia.

Epidemiological factors—agents are species of malarial parasite which causes diseases in man. There is P. vivax which has a cycle of 48 hours fever reoccurs every 48 hours. P. falciparum fever is very irregular there is P. ovale types. Much of the malaria in India is due to plasmodium vivax and plasmodium falciparum.

Life cycle of malaria in man is also known as asexual phase where the parasites develop in the liver of the infected person and then develop and multiples in the red blood cells of the infected person.

In mosquito cycle is also referred as a sexual phase of the life cycle of the malarial parasite. This cycle takes 10–14 days to be completed in the anopheles mosquito, when infective forms of the malaria phase are present in the salivary glands of the mosquito. The healthy person bitten by the mosquito becomes infected.

Source of infection is a person who harbors the sexual forms of the parasite. These are sucked by a female anopheles mosquito when it bites a sick person.

Mode of transmission by the bite of infected, female anopheles.

Incubation period for P. vivax is 14 days; P. falciparum 12 days, the incubation period may be delayed for as long as 6 to 9 months.

Clinical features—cold stage—headache, shivering, fever rising rapidly, cold skin. In hot stage very hot feeling, severe headache, skin flushed, fever starts falling. Sweating stage there is a profuse sweating, temperature normal.

Cases—in early detection of fever cases in the community; door to door or by house to house visits, early administration of drugs, collection of blood films and administration of radical treatment.

Mosquito control measures by anti adults measures, e.g. insecticide spraying, larvicidal operations, protection against mosquito bites by mosquito nets, repellent. In community surveillance measures active and passive, elimination of mosquito breeding places around houses.

Health education is given to the public regarding importance of there cooperation in the spraying of houses and other aspects related to the control of malaria. They are to be provided health facilities and chemoprophylaxis administration of Chiloquin to all fever cases. Prophylaxis to people traveling to malaria zone and desiring to protect them are put on Chiloquin therapy.

Malaria Antigen Test

Sometimes the patient shows symptoms of malaria but in the slide blood test the result is negative. In such cases doctors use the malaria rapid diagnostic kit, a malaria antigen body test which detects the parasite in the blood. Doctors do this test after treatment also, to ensure that there is no malaria parasite in the body.

About 40% of the worlds population estimated is at risk for malaria. An estimated 300 million to 500 million people world wide contract the diseases each year. As many as 1 million of them die each year; a large majority of them are children under five.

Recent reports—anti-malarial drug are beginning to lose their effectiveness as the most virulent malaria stain develops resistance.

Researches are working to develop a process which uses low power microwaves to destroy malaria parasite in the blood minus any medication. There research has been further boosted by a donation from the gates foundation.

The novel methods uses a lower power microwave to heat you the malaria parasite in the blood stream. Microwaves heat the malaria parasite causes it to die without harming normal blood cells.

The parasite has extra iron that enhances the microwave energy absorption by the malaria parasite. As a result, it is postulated that the deadly parasite gets heated preferentially and is killed without affecting any of the normal blood cells. Researchers are on this revolutionary treatment might take time and effect yet unknown.

Objective of national malaria programme is to prevent death, reduce morbidity, reclassification of endemic areas, research, spraying. Management of serious and complicated malarial cases.

Setbacks are technical problem such as resistance to mosquito vectors to insecticides and malarial drugs is a serious obstacle.

Operational failure is inadequate surveillance, inadequate coverage leaving many houses unsprayed, undue reliance of basic workers who are unprepared, experience people leave job etc.

Filariasis is spread through several species of mosquitoes. **Lymphatic filariasis** is a mosquito born disease caused by filarial parasites. It is transmitted by the bite of culex mosquitoes. Two types such as W. baerofit and B. malayi, there are 8 specific filarial parasites. It is manifested as lymphaginites, elephantiasis of genitals, legs and arms, filarial arthritis, though not fatal, the disease is responsible for considerable sufferings, deformity and disability. The adult worms are usually found in the lymphatic system of man, which finds their way into blood circulation via lymphatic. All ages are susceptible to infection. Social factors like migration of people, illiteracy, poverty, poor sanitation and climate is important factors influence breeding in bad drainage, sewage disposal, pools, soakage pits, septic tanks, open ditches, burrow pits etc these carriers are detected usually by night blood examination, they remain hidden or dormant for many years. National Filarial Control Programme launched in 1955 and their main activities are anti-mosquito and anti-larval measures in endemic areas, establishment of filarial clinics for detection and treatment of positive microfilaria cases and provision of underground drainage in hyper endemic cities and towns.

Keywords

Health problem, clinical features, epidemiological factors, female anopheles, mosquito control, health education, antigen test, lymphatic filariasis.

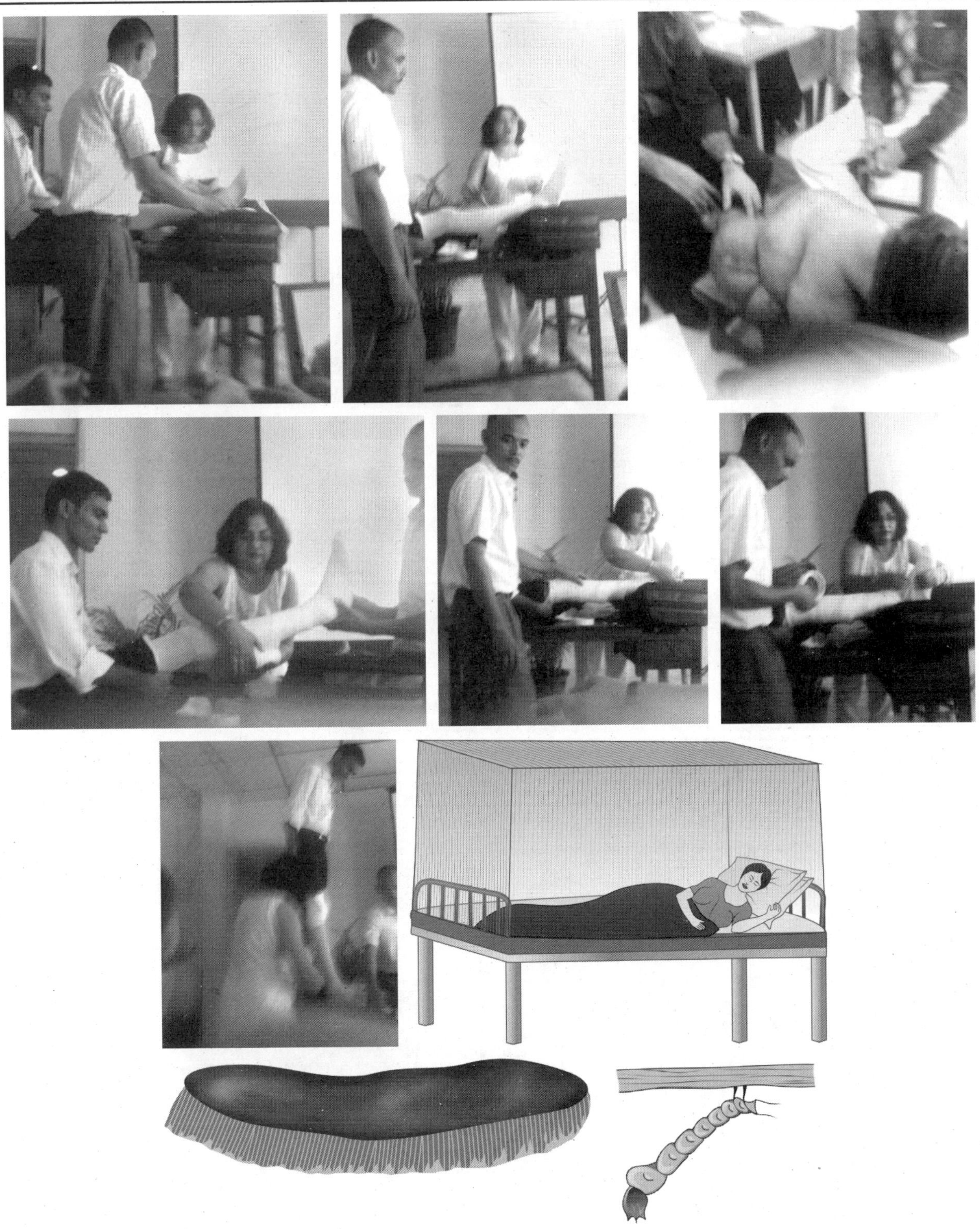

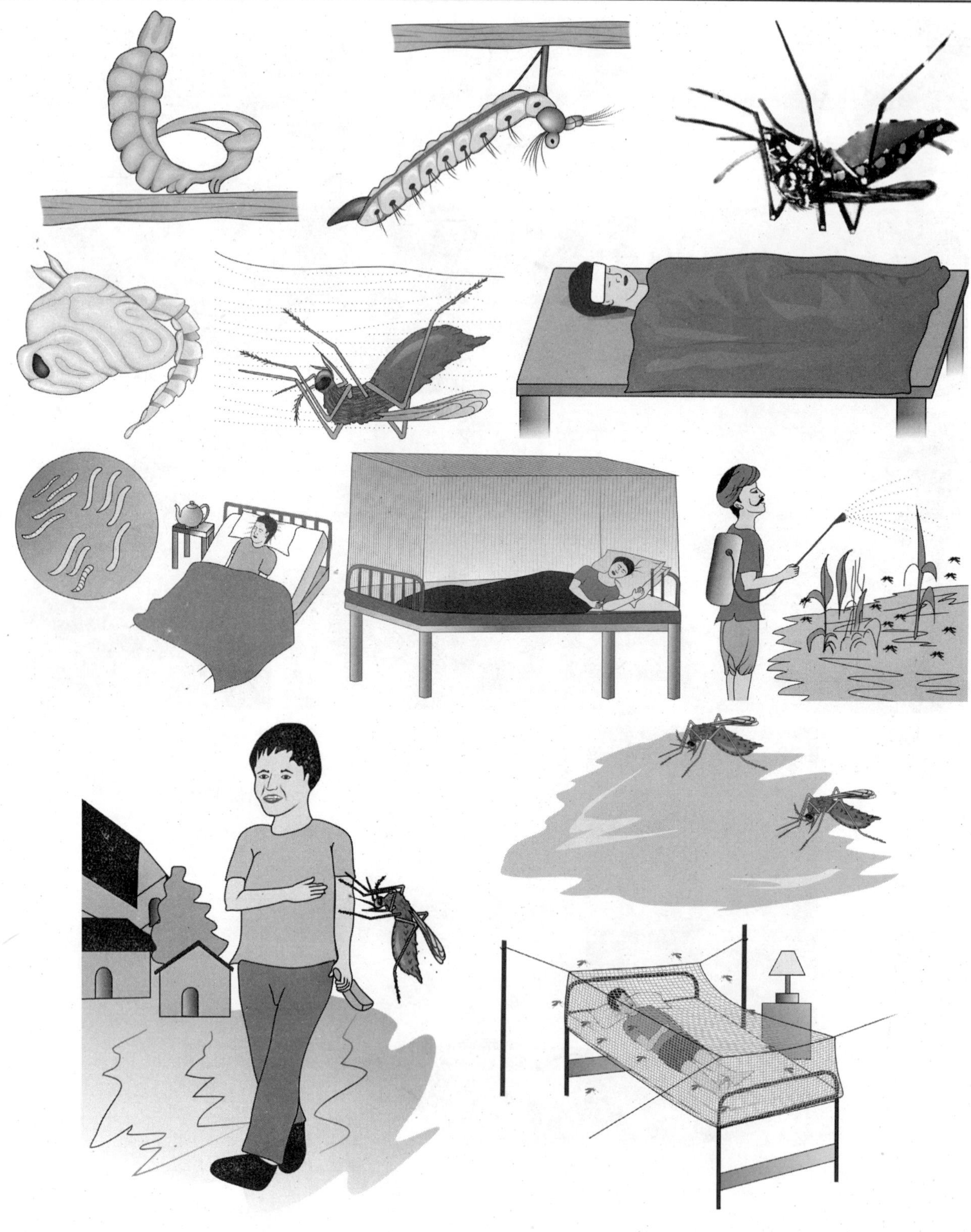

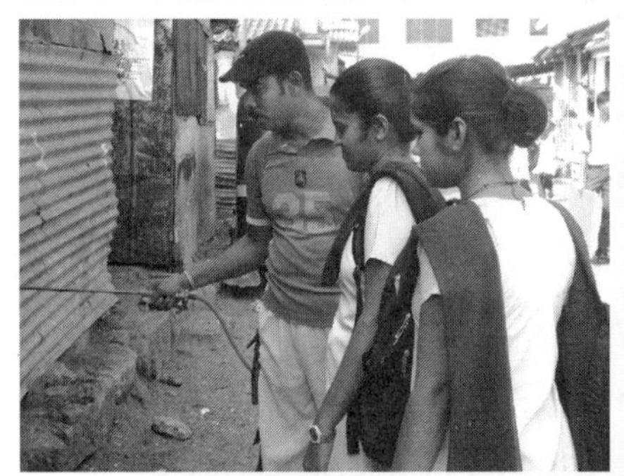

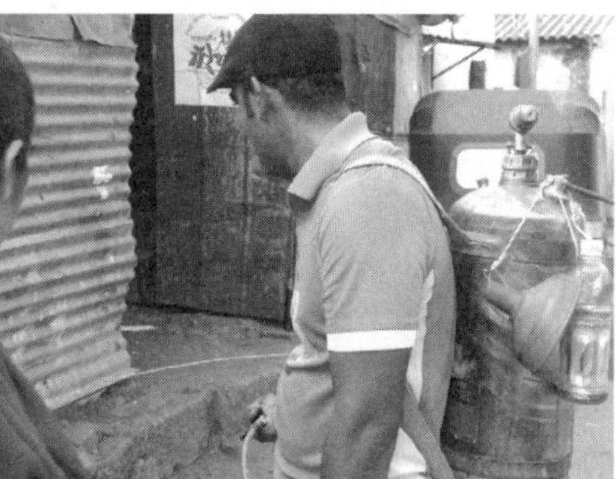

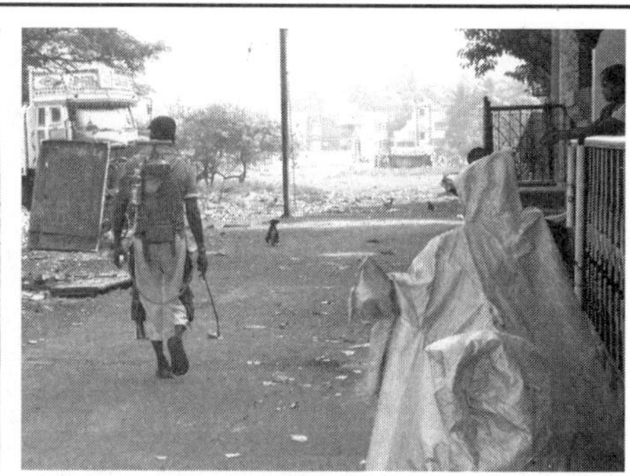

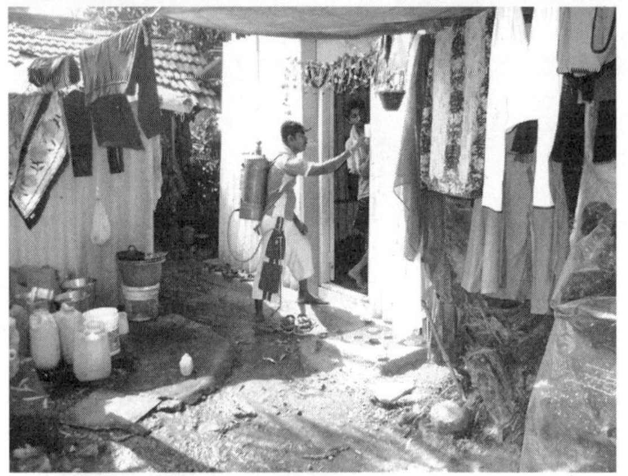

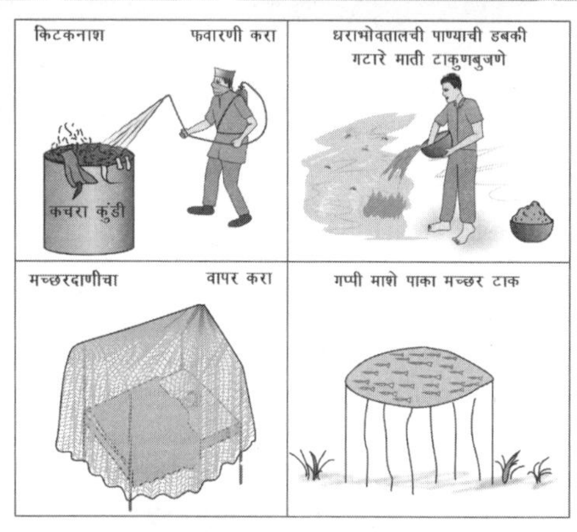
किटकनाश फवारणी करा
कचरा कुंडी
घराभोवतालची पाण्याची डबकी
गटारे माती टाकुणबुजणे
मच्छरदाणीचा वापर करा
गप्पी माशे पाका मच्छर टाक

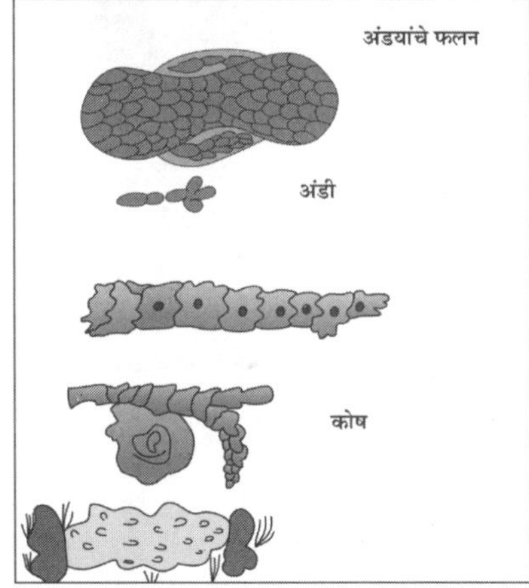
अंडयांचे फलन
अंडी
कोष

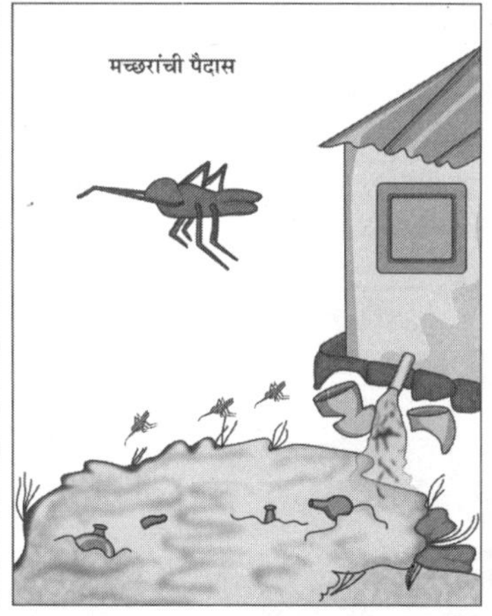
मच्छरांची पैदास

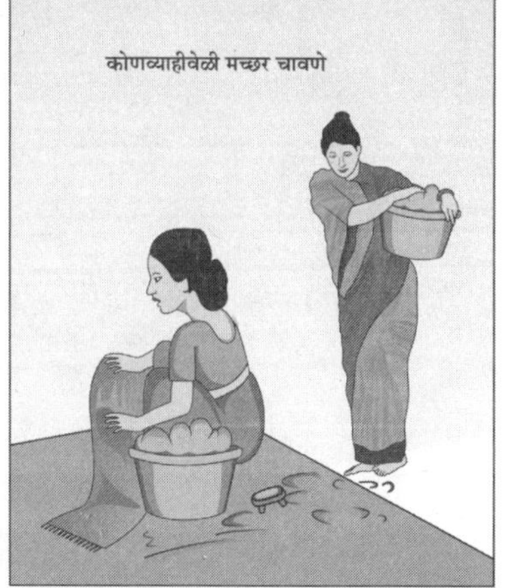
कोणव्याहीवेळी मच्छर चावणे

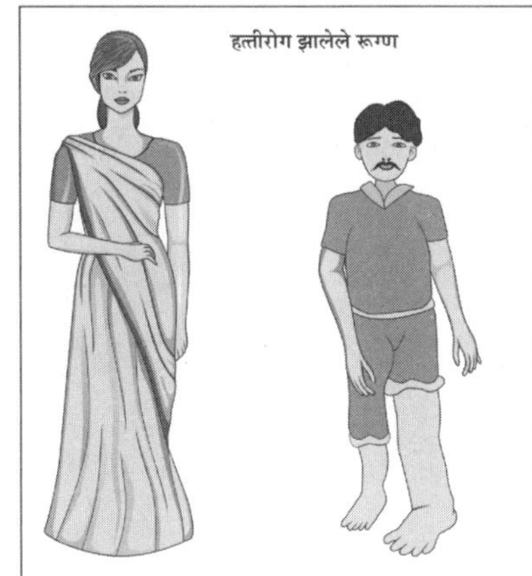
हत्तीरोग झालेले रूग्ण

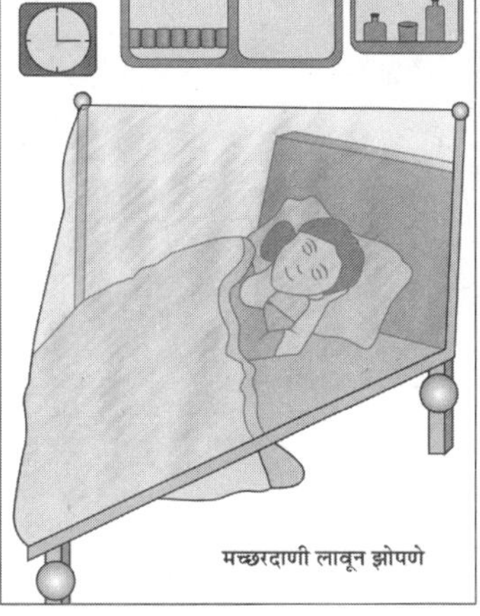
मच्छरदाणी लावून झोपणे

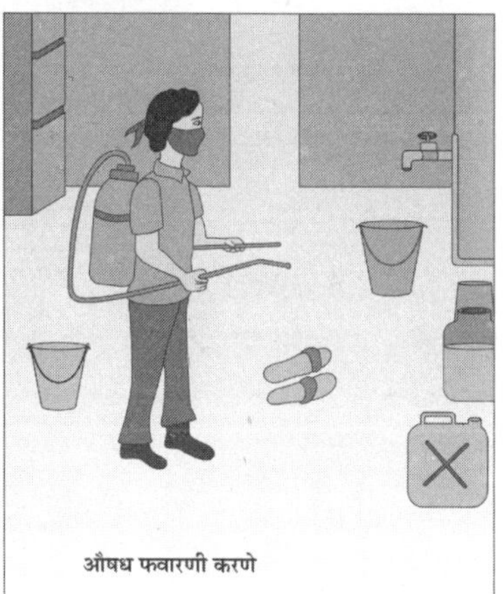
औषध फवारणी करणे

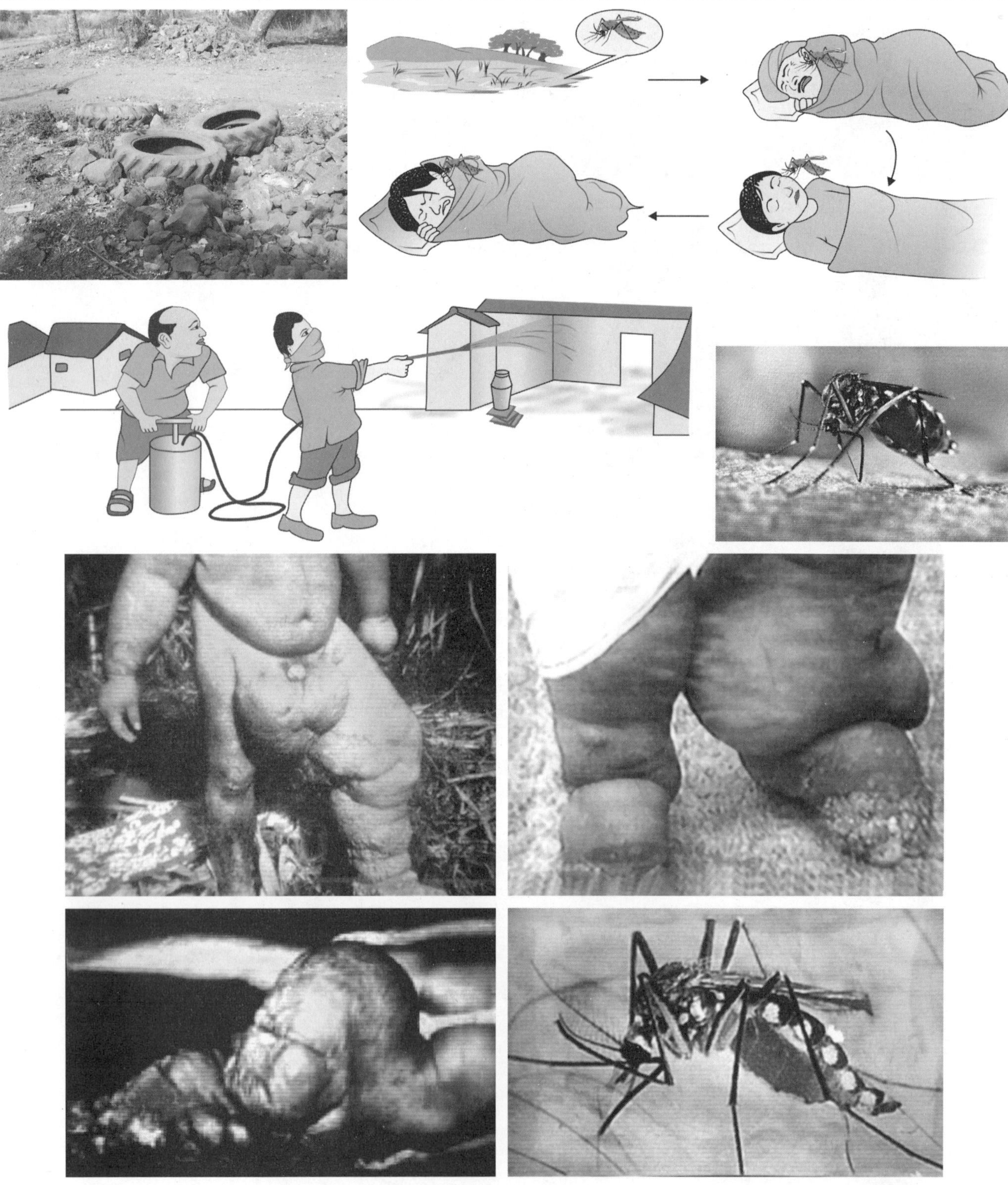

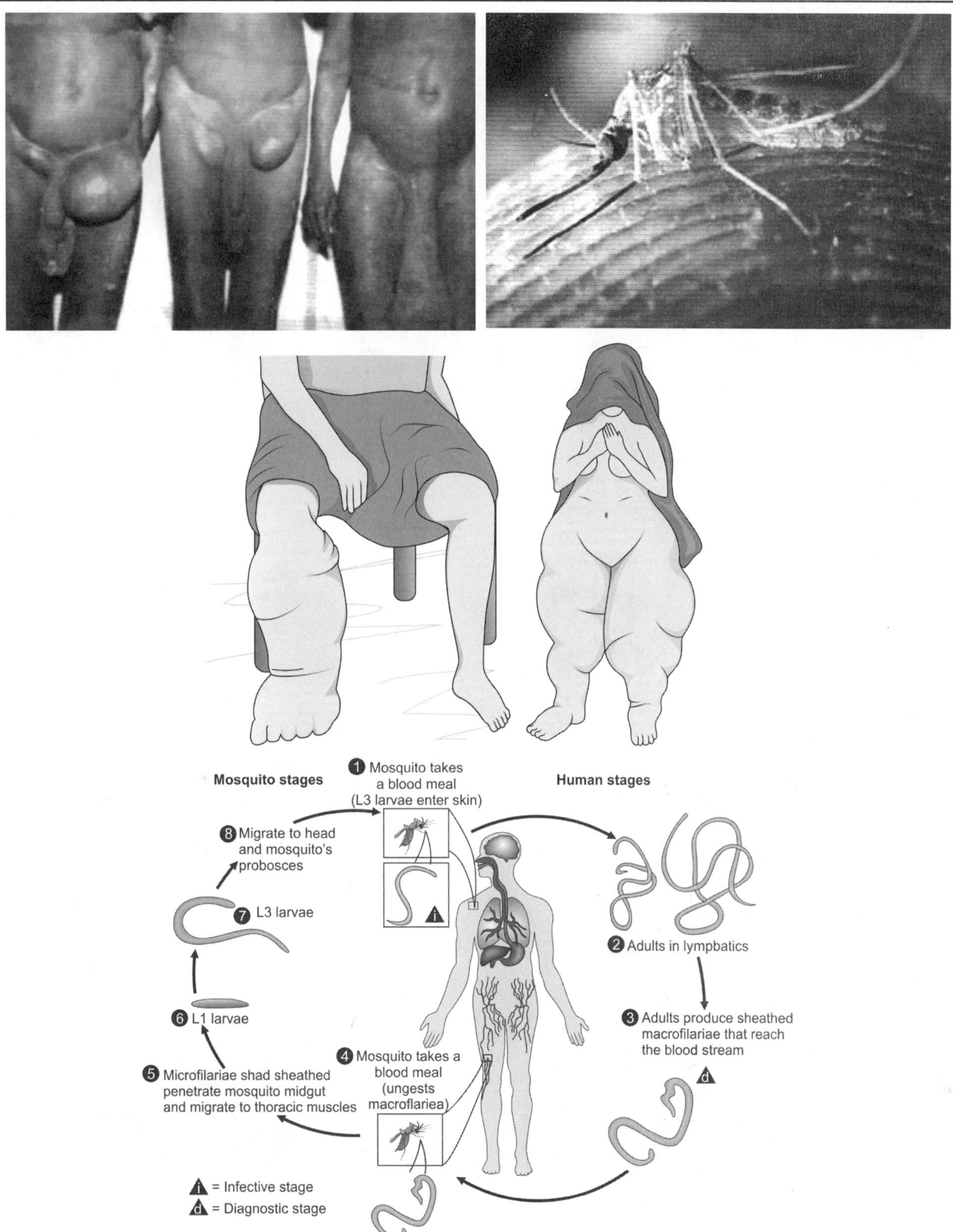
Mosquito stages
1 Mosquito takes a blood meal (L3 larvae enter skin)
Human stages
8 Migrate to head and mosquito's probosces
7 L3 larvae
2 Adults in lympbatics
6 L1 larvae
3 Adults produce sheathed macrofilariae that reach the blood stream
4 Mosquito takes a blood meal (ungests macroflariea)
5 Microfilariae shad sheathed penetrate mosquito midgut and migrate to thoracic muscles
= Infective stage
= Diagnostic stage

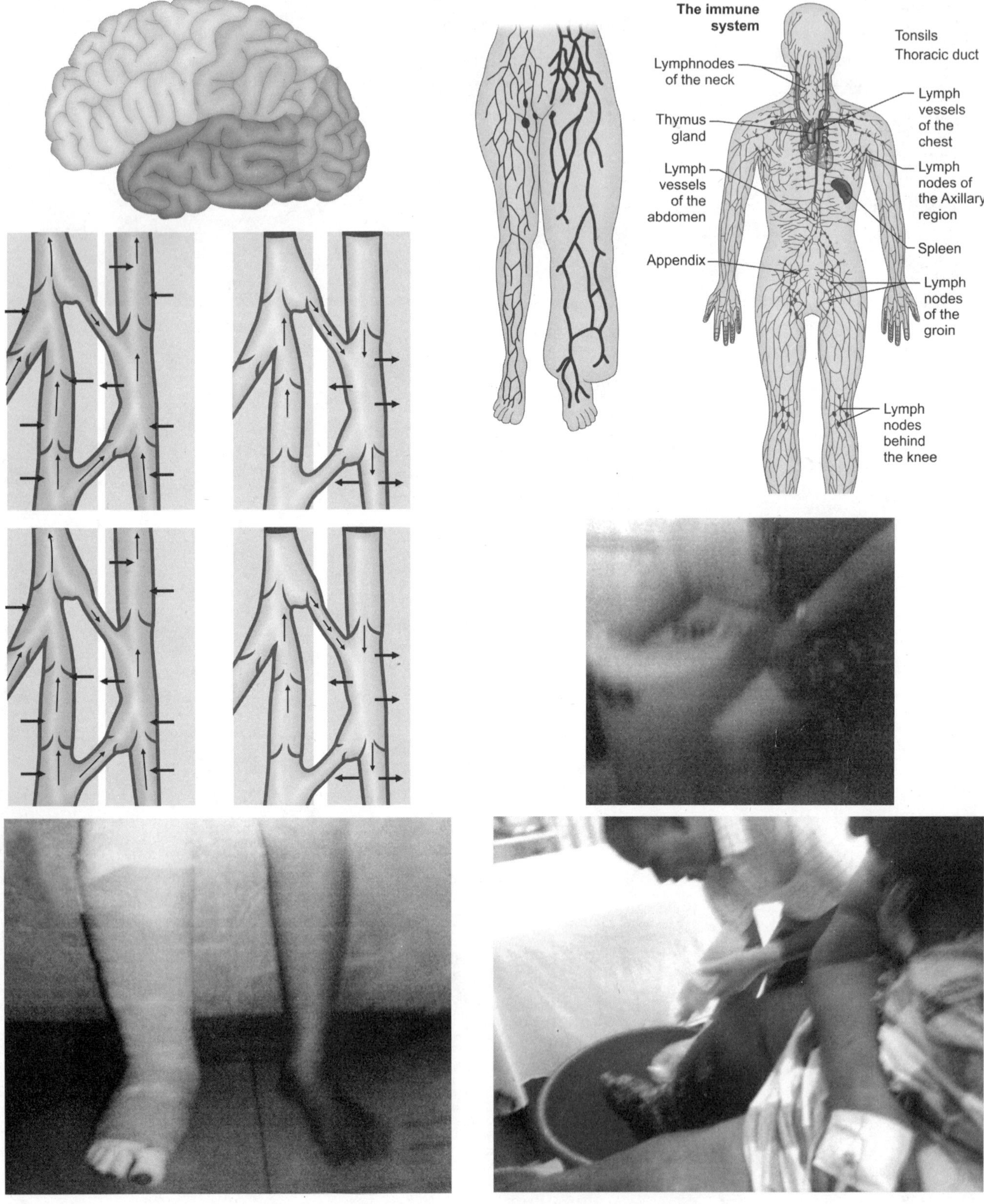
The immune system
Tonsils
Thoracic duct
Lymphnodes of the neck
Thymus gland
Lymph vessels of the chest
Lymph vessels of the abdomen
Lymph nodes of the Axillary region
Spleen
Appendix
Lymph nodes of the groin
Lymph nodes behind the knee

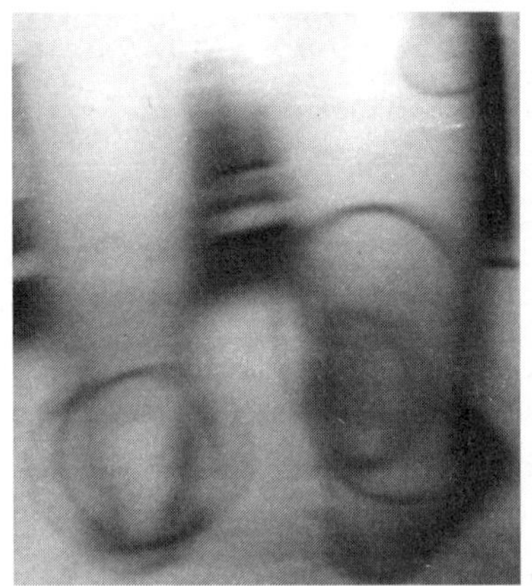

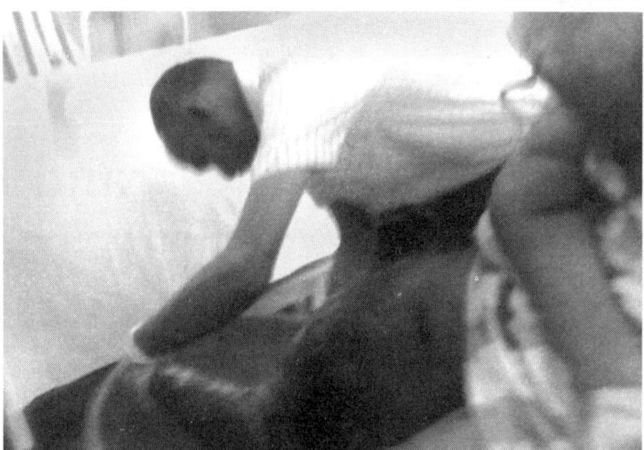

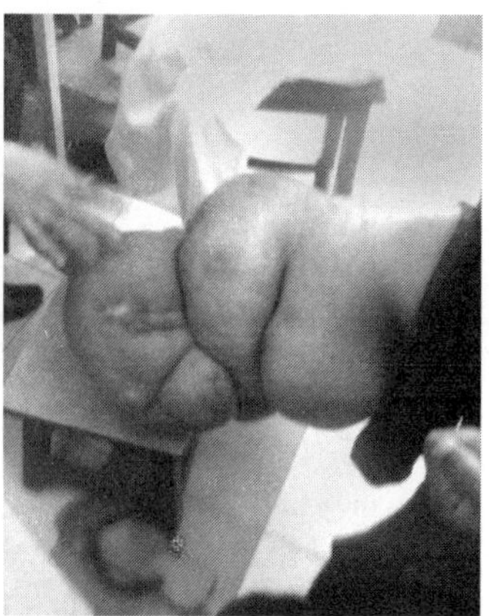

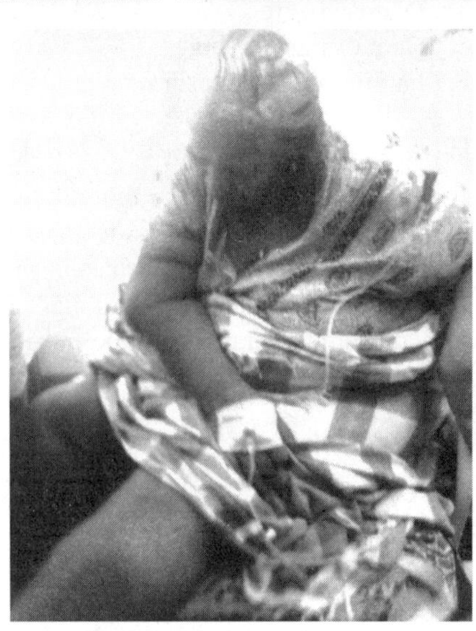

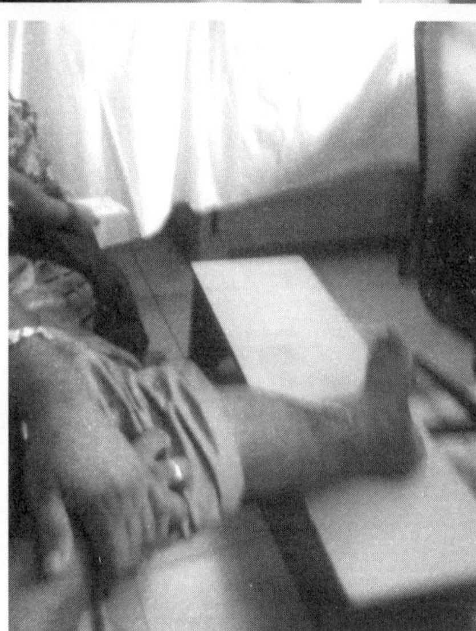

CHAPTER

55

MCH and Family Planning

INTRODUCTION

Pregnancy and **childbirths** are special events in women's life, and indeed in the lives of the family. This can be also a time of great hope and joyful anticipation. It also can be a time of fear, suffering and even death.

Although **pregnancy** is not a diseases but a normal physiological process yet it is associated with certain health risks and survival both for woman and the infant. Each pregnancy represents a journey into the unknown from where too many women never return.

What areas a nurse can give maternal health services?

1. Antenatal care
2. Diet in pregnancy
3. Postnatal care
4. Care of the new born.

What are the general fears of a mother?

They are as follows:
1. Pregnancy and childhood
2. Mother taught about balanced diet
3. Baby care
4. Infant feeding
5. Weaning
6. Immunization
7. Family planning.

What are the aims of mother and child health care?

1. To promote, protect and maintain the health and nutritional status of mother during pregnancy
2. To detect high risk pregnancies
3. To ensure that the mother receives the best available care during pregnancy
4. To prepare the mother physically, mentally and materially for the delivery
5. To reduce infant mortality rate and maternal mortality rate
6. Ensure safe delivery.

Other important factors to be stressed by a nurse are:
1. Breastfeeding—importance and principles of breastfeeding
2. Immunization
3. Supplementary feeding

What are the other maternal health services?

1. Pre-marriage counseling
2. Antenatal or prenatal care
3. Intranatal care
4. Postnatal care
5. Care of the new born
6. Family planning services.

What are the purposes of MCH services?

1. To reduce the maternal mortality
2. To eradicate the neonatal tetanus
3. To reduce the rates of babies born with low birth weight
4. To reduce the deaths due to diarrhea
5. To promote infant and child nutrition
6. Immunization.

What are the objectives of antenatal care?

1. To promote and maintain the health and nutritional status of a pregnant woman
2. To find out 'high-risk' pregnancies and give them special care
3. To ensure that the mother receives the best available care during pregnancy
4. To prepare the mother physically, mentally
5. To reduce maternal and infant morbidity and mortality
6. To have normal, healthy and living child
7. To teach mother craft and responsibility of motherhood
8. To foresee complications and prevent them
9. To remove anxiety and dread associated with delivery
10. To reduce MMR, IMR
11. To teach the mother elements of child care, nutrition, personal hygiene and sanitation
12. To sensitize the mother for the need of family planning.

What advice a mother needs?

1. Personal hygiene—need to bathe every day, to wear clean clothes
2. Rest and sleep—8 hours of sleep and 2 hours rest at mid-day, and small meals frequently advised.
3. Bowels—Constipation should be avoided—intake of green leafy vegetables, fruits and extra fluids
4. Exercise—Light household work can be done not lifting heavy weights especially during later part of pregnancy.

5. Dental care—give information about oral hygiene
6. Immunization- against tetanus two doses the first does at 16–20 weeks and the second at 20–24 weeks of pregnancy, the interval in between should be one month
7. Regular check up done—record of height and weight, blood pressure, urine for albumin, stool for intestinal parasite, blood for hemoglobin, grouping and Rh determination, VDRL test
8. Sexual intercourse restricted during the last trimester.
9. Care of the nipples—retracted inverted and flat nipples make breastfeeding difficult. Advice her to message the breast from the ribs towards the front and bring out the nipple.

What diet in pregnancy will you advise?

Pregnancy is a physiological process which requires considerable added nutrition for growth and development of fetus which helps in reducing LBW. Greater calories required in 2nd and 3rd trimester. Proteins 5 gm during the last 6 months of pregnancy, about 30 gm calcium deposited in fetus so 150 mg extra calcium during last 6 months. 540 mg iron found in fetus so about 2–3 mg iron/day during last 6 months vitamin A found in the liver of infant about 5400–7200 mg so additional requirement of 750 mg for a normal woman. Thiamin, riboflavin and multivitamins small quantities of it present in new born infant. The extra caloric allowances of 300 kcal/day, folic acid and ascorbic acid found in the infant too.

What are the different sources of nutrients she can take?

1. Protein—cereals, pulses, nuts, meat, fish, liver, egg, milk, leafy vegetables
2. Calcium milk and milk products
3. Iron green leafy vegetables, jaggery, meat,
4. Vitamin A—fish liver oil, mangoes, papaya, milk, eggs
5. Thiamin dried yeast, rice unpolished, whole cereals, soyabean
6. Riboflavin—liver, green leafy vegetables, cereals
7. Niacin—dried yeast, liver, unpolished rice
8. Folic acid—bajra, wheat, whole pulses, cabbage, spinach.

What are the ill effects?

Nutritional anemia obstructed labour, night blindness, simple goiter, low rate of weight growth. Pregnancy induced hypertension, abruption placenta due to deficiency of folic acid, still birth due to deficiency of nutrition, low birth weight.

What are the different types of anemia?

1. Iron deficiency anemia is most common form in many part of the world. The daily requirement is 1–2 mg for men and we get from highly colored vegetables. For women it is 3 mg daily requirement at she losses during menstruation and in pregnancy for growth of fetus. It is considered severe when hemoglobin level is below 9 g/dL
2. Megaloblastic anemia takes place when maturation of erythrocytes is impaired when deficiency of vitamin B12 or folic acid occurs
3. **Pernicious anemia** is most common cause of vitamin B12 deficiency. It is an autoimmune diseases in which intrinsic factor are destroyed in stomach
4. **Folic acid deficiency anemia** dietary deficiency, malabsorption
5. **Hypoplastic and aplastic anemia**—are due to varying degrees of born marrow failure, born marrow function is reduced it may be due to drug intake, ionizing radiation, some chemicals, viral diseases, etc
6. **Hemolytic anemia** occurs when red blood cells are destroyed while in circulation or are removed prematurely from the circulation because the cells are abnormal or the spleen is overactive
7. **Congenital hemolytic anemia**—genetic abnormality leads to the synthesis of abnormal hemoglobin and reduces oxygen carrying capacity
8. **Sickle cell anemia**—the abnormal hemoglobin molecule becomes misshaped when deoxygenated, making the erythrocytes sickle shaped. This tends to increase the viscosity of the blood, reducing the rate of the blood flow and leading to intravascular clotting
9. **Acquired hemolytic anemia** in which no familial or racial factors have been identified
10. **Normocytic norochromic anemia**—the number of cells are reduced and the proportion of reticulocytes in the blood may be increased as the body tries to restore erythrocytes numbers to normal this occurs.

How will you help mothers identify different signs?

1. Pallor, severe fatigue, malaise, weakness
2. Light headedness
3. Fever, exert ional dyspnea
4. Headache, vertigo
5. Sensitivity to cold, weight loss
6. Skin jaundice color, dry, brittle nails, spoon shaped concave nails
7. Blurred vision, scalar jaundice and retinal hemorrhage
8. Tinnitus
9. Smooth, glossy, brightened and sore tongue
10. Palpitation, heart failure
11. Anorexia, abdominal pain, tarry stool
12. Amenorrhea, decreased fertility
13. Back pain, sternal tenderness, joint pain
14. Confusion, loss of balance, depression anxiety.

Diet Rich in Iron

1. Apricot, beef, cabbage, dates, goose, peas, potatoes, radishes, raisins, tomatoes etc.
2. Oral iron supplementation therapy

MCH—Women of child bearing age 15–44 constitutes 22.2% of the population. Children under 15 years 35.3% of total population, therefore RCH/MCH is a major consumers of the health services. They are vulnerable or special risk group. The risk is connected with child bearing and survival in case of infants and children; 70% death occurring during 5 years of life. Undeveloped world MMR (Maternal Mortality Rate) is 13/1,00,000 live births. Much of the sickness and deaths are preventable by improving the health of MCH. Problems' affecting them is multifactor, today strand specialists in obstetrics and child health have joined hands and linked. That each mother has good health and every pregnancy may culminate in healthy mother and healthy baby. Child bearing, child spacing, family size, level of education, economic status, customs and beliefs, role of woman in society etc. influences her health.

Mother and Child is One Unit Because

1. During AN period, the fetus is a part of the mothers. Two hundred and eighty days fetus obtains all the building materials and oxygen from the mothers blood
2. Child health therefore closely related to maternal health. A healthy mother gives healthy baby and less chances of premature birth, LBW, still birth or abortion
3. Certain diseases of mother during pregnancy, e.g. syphilis, German measles, drug intake have their effects upon the fetus
4. The birth of a child dependent on mother 6–9 months child is on feeding; the social development also affect, e.g. maternal deprivation
5. Care cycle—inseparable
6. Mother is first teacher of a child, therefore called one unit.

Maternity cycle follows as below:

Fertilization
↓
AN or PN period
↓
Intranasal period
↓
Postnatal period
↓
Inter-concept ional period

MCH Problems Like Iceberg

1. Prenatal problem; congenital malformation; genetic and certain behavioral problem; malnutrition; infection; communicable diseases, unregulated fertility, socioeconomic condition
2. Direct malnutrition intervention cover wide range of activities that is supplementary feeding programme, distribution of iron, folic tablet, fortification and enrichment of foods, nutritional education etc.
3. Other—clean drinking water, food hygiene
4. Infection—may cause a variety of adverse effects such as- fetal growth retardation, low birth weight, embryopathy, abortion, puerperal sepsis
5. Education of the mother—good knowledge and practice of personal hygiene and appropriate sanitation measures in and around house to control common infection and parasitic diseases
6. Uncontrolled reproduction—LBW, severe anemia, abortion, hemorrhage.

In Domiciliary Care—a mother with normal obstetric history may be advised to have their confinement in their own homes, provided the home conditions are satisfactory. In such cases the delivery may be conducted by the health worker female or trained dai. This is known as domiciliary midwifery service.

Advantages

1. Mother delivers in the familiar surrounding of the home and this may tend to remove the fear associated with delivery in a hospital
2. The chances of cross infection are generally fewer at home than in the hospital
3. The mother is able to keep an eye upon the children and domestic affairs, this may tend to ease her maternal tension.

Disadvantages

1. The mother may have less medical and nursing supervision than in the hospital
2. The other may have less rest
3. She may resume her domestic duties too soon
4. Her diet may be neglected
5. Many homes in India are unsuitable for a home delivery
6. The arrangement that child birth is a natural event and should take place are home does not guarantee that everything will be normal
7. The FHW is a pivot of domiciliary care should be adequately trained to recognize the danger signal during labor and seek immediate help transferring the mother to nearest PHC
8. If sluggish pains or no pain after rupture of membranes
9. No progress
10. Prolapsed of cord or hand
11. Me conium stained liquor or a slow irregular or excessively fast fetal heart
12. Excessive; show; or bleeding during labor
13. Collapse during labor
14. PPH or temperature

15. Abnormally and difficult deliveries, has high risk cases it is difficult to conduct it at home, and when the normal delivery turns into abnormal need watchful alertness.
16. Rooming in is keeping the baby's crib by the side of the mothers bed, it helps to know her baby, better chance for bf, allays fear, baby not misplaced and it builds her self-confidence.

What is family planning?

Family planning is

1. To avoid unwanted births, to bring about wanted births
2. To regulate the interval between pregnancies
3. To control the time at which births occur in relation to the ages of the parents and
4. To determine the number of children in the family
5. To promote the adoption of small family size norm on the basis of voluntary acceptance
6. To promote the use of spacing method
7. To ensure adequate supply of contraceptives to all eligible couples within easy reach
8. To arrange for clinical and surgical services.

The term family welfare is much border its scope related to quality of life, education, nutrition. The health and happiness of families depends greatly on the family size, the number of children in family.

What is breastfeeding?

Breastfeeding is the nature's way to feed the young ones. Only in rare circumstances when the mother is taking certain drugs or infected with HIV/AIDS, or has active untreated tuberculosis avoided, human breast milk is the healthiest form of milk for babies. Babies have a sucking reflex that enables them to suck and swallow milk.

Breast milk is made from nutrients in the mother's bloodstream and body store, it has right amount of fat, sugar, water and protein required for the growth and development of the baby. During breast feeding antibodies pass to the baby, and it contains several anti-infective factors such as bile salt stimulated lipase that protects against micro-organism. It protects against allergies and decreases risk of cardiovascular diseases in later life. Mothers of breast feeding have been found to have less risk of breast cancer, ovarian and endometrial cancer.

Why family planning is important in India?

Currently India's population is the second largest in the world, next to china, over population has adverse effects on our per capital income. More than 4% of Indians populations live below poverty line which leads to sickness vicious cycle follows.

Population explosion has created various social problems like unemployment, overcrowding, illiteracy, low standards of living, urban deterioration, inadequate housing, and inadequate food, family not able to cope up with family demands as income does not increase comparing to family size, family disturbances, unhappiness and dissatisfaction, insecurity. Mother's general health gets impaired with increase number of pregnancies, repeated pregnancies have adverse effect on her and she becomes susceptible to infection. Children get less attention, negligence etc. To avoid all this problems it is necessary to have limited family.

Definition of family planning—"a way of thinking and living that is adopted voluntarily, upon the basis of knowledge, attitudes and responsible decision by individuals and couples, in order to promote the health and welfare of the family, group and thus contribute effectively to the social development of a country".

Other Definitions—according to WHO

1. To avoid unwanted births
2. To bring out wanted births
3. To regulate the interval between pregnancies
4. To control the time at which the birth occurs
5. To determine the number of children born to a couple.

Birth control means "children by choice and not by chance"

Contraceptives means

1. Prevention of the union of sperm and ovum
2. Suppressing ovulation
3. Interfering with implantation of fertilized ovum in the uterus.

All couples have the basic human right to decide freely and responsibly the number and spacing of their children.

It is said that population growth is like railway trains; are subject to movement. They start slowly and gain momentum, once in motion; it takes time to bring the momentum under control. The rampart population growth is greatest obstacle to socio economic advancement.

Ancient Ways of Family Planning

1. Ancestors believed that some kind of spirit entered the body and implanted the child
2. Women wore magic chains around their neck and waists to keep the spirit away
3. In Europe middle-aged women were instructed to rely on the ring made of precious stones
4. A woman was asked to take odd kinds of drink in order to become sterile. "Teas" made out of roots, weeds, leaves infusions of gun powder and pills made of quick silver were used. It was dangerous and unfortunately often it killed mother rather than prevented childbirth
5. In north Africa—froth from camels mouth was swallowed hopefully by women, sometimes they drank water that has been used to wash the dead
6. In Egypt woman were advised to eat the seeds of a castor oil plant after child birth, each seed said to give a years protection against pregnancy

7. Worlds 600 million Catholics and Jews oppose birth control
8. Abortion is legal and common in Japan and Soviet Union Russia
9. USA played pioneering role in discovering of steroid-new method of detecting ovulation sterilization by the hysteroscopic route; reversible surgical contraception' immunological and genetic engineering.

Development of Family Planning in India

1. 1877, Dr. Annie who raised the issue and introduced family planning service before the public
2. 1925, Professor Karve Mumbai started propaganda on birth control
3. 1930, Mysore government started the birth control clinic
4. 1935, Indian congress favored the family planning program
5. 1951, comprehensive program to check rapid population growth
6. 1953, 147 clinics were set up
7. 1969, millions of rupees allotted for family planning.

Scope of Family Planning

1. Advice of sterility education for parenthood
2. Screening for pathological condition related top the reproductive system, e.g. cervical cancer, genetic counseling, providing adoption services
3. Increasing female literacy rate
4. Enhancing child survival
5. Advancing the age of marriage of girls to 21 years through intensified publicity
6. Promoting the two-child family norm development of social consciousness.

Importance of Family Planning

1. Increased population—more than 40% lives below poverty line. Poverty leads to sickness and sickness into poverty
2. Population create various social problem like unemployment, overcrowding, etc.
3. Increase family size leads to insecurity
4. Adverse effect on mothers health
5. Causes malnutrition in children.

District family planning staff consists of:

District family planning officer	01
Medical officer	02
Extension educator	02
Information officer	01
Statistician	01
Administrative officer	01
Ancillary staff	01
Clerk	01

Family welfare services as follows—(according to marks you have to develop the answer writing on each point)

1. MCH
2. Marriage counseling
3. Nutritional guidance (anemia)
4. Premarital education
5. Sex education
6. Treatment of sterility
7. Improved quality of life
8. Employment and improvement in socioeconomic standards
9. Provision of safe environment
10. Institutional deliveries
11. Regular fixed dates clinic services
12. Domiciliary services
13. Community services
14. Regular follow-up
15. Provision of immunization (injection TT iron folic calcium etc.).

Family planning different methods—refer the text book for details

Tubectomy/TL—the tube through which the egg travels from sac to the womb is tied off and cut on each side. This prevents sperm/seed meeting the eggs. It is a female sterilization involves cutting and tying off the fallopian tubes.

1. This is the abdominal operation in which a small piece of each fallopian tube is removed and legated
2. The operation is done under GA/spinal anesthesia
3. Hospitalization is required for 5–7 days
4. Mostly performed immediately after child birth
5. Sterilization does not involve the removal of sex gland
6. 10 days woman can resume light work, not carry heavy weight
7. Female should not be less than 20 years or not more than 45 years
8. Couple must have 2 living children at the time of operation
9. Operation is irreversible
10. Consent obtained
11. It should not be with any outside pressure
12. They are done free of cost in government hospitals
13. 85% women go for it
14. It is simple, safe and cheaper with no side effects.

Mini-laparotomy—It is modification to TL. It is simpler procedure. It requires a small supra-pubic incision of 2.5–3 cm just above the pubic hair. The tubes are cut and ends are blacked. Then the incision is closed, less traumatic, done at PHC level.

Laparoscopy—It done by surgeon with use of laparoscope. The abdomen inflated with gas carbon monoxide, nitrogen or air to push away the intestine from the site of operation with laparoscope tubes are accessible, the fallopian ring/clips are applied. It is 100% effective, more popular method. It needs 48 hours stay in hospital. Small scar, it is contraindicated in woman who HB% less than 8%, or any heart diseases, HBP etc. complication could be puncture large blood vessels.

Vasectomy—It is male sterilization and is one of the most effective methods of contraception.

1. It is a simple, safe and relatively minor operative procedure. Performed under local anesthesia
2. It involves cutting and tying off the vas deferens/sperm tubes on each side
3. 100% effective if properly carried out
4. A small incision is made in the skin of the scrotum above the testicles and the ducts leading from the testicles and tubes from the gland on each side are tried off and cut. The incision is closed with a single stitch
5. Complete recovery takes place within a few days and the man experiences no changes in sexual desires
6. The age not less than 25 and not more than 50 years
7. After operation 30 ejaculation to be awaited or pregnancy takes place
8. To use contraceptives until aspermid has been established
9. Avoid talking bath for 24 hours after operation
10. To wear a "T" bandage or scrotal support for 15 days and keep the sight clean and dry
11. Cycling or lifting heavy weight avoid
12. Stitched removed on 5th day.

Complications

1. Pain and swelling
2. Scrotal haematoma
3. Local infection
4. Wound infection
5. Sperm granules that is accumulation of sperm common and troublesome
6. Blocking of the vas causes re-absorption of sperm and such circulation is harmful to physical health
7. Diminished sexual vigor
8. Impotency
9. Headache
10. Fatigue
11. Psychological effect.

What is MTP (Medical Termination of Pregnancy)?

MTP act was passed in 1971 that under following condition MTP can be performed:

1. **Medical**—endangers the mother's life or causes grave injury to her physical or mental health. Hazardous to pregnancy.
2. **Eugenic**—incurable hereditary mental or physical defect may be transmissible to the offspring
3. **Humanitarian**—pregnancy is the result of rape
4. **Socio economic**—could lead to risk of injury to the health of the mother.
5. **Failure of contraceptive** devices

What are the different methods used?

1. **Tube pipe** canula inserted via vagina into the uterus. The canula attached to suction machine and sucked out the contains up to six weeks of pregnancy, possibility of incomplete abortion
2. **D&C (dilatation and curettage)**—first 3 months under anesthesia different size cannula available inserted and open the mouth of a cervix and scrapped and sucked out the contains from the walls of the uterus
3. **Artificial labor**—16–20 weeks—withdraw contain amount of amniotic fluid from uterus and add some chemicals via syringe put back the fluid into uterus, the woman feels contraction and the child is killed and expelled out
4. **RU 486/PG**—combination of certain kind of drug prepared to prevent 9 weeks pregnancy. This prevents implantation or it up roots. It is a dangerous method complications like infection, hole in uterus, hemorrhage, rupture of uterus, continuation of pregnancy, irregular periods, psychological and social guilt and trauma.

What is abortion?

Abortion means killing a human being. (Nothing is more precious than life) Babies cruel and inhuman way murdered in mothers womb (womb becomes tomb).

1. **The vacuum suction method**—it works like a vacuum cleansers cleaning up dirt. The baby comes out in little pieces.
2. **The cutting method**—here the doctor just slices the baby to pieces inside the mothers womb.
3. **The surgical method**—the doctor takes the baby out by surgical opening. The babies then are generally used for experiments or else they are burned or drowned in water.
4. **A salt solution**—is injected into an amniotic sac and the baby is burnt.

What are the types of spontaneous abortion/ miscarriage?

1. Threatened—vaginal bleeding/spotting, mild cramps, tenderness over uterus, pelvic pressure, cervix slightly dilated.
2. Inevitable—bleeding more perfuse, cervix dilated, membranes rupture, painful uterine contractions, embryo delivered (D&C).
3. Habitual—spontaneous abortion occur
4. Incomplete—fetus expelled, placenta or membranes retained (D&E)

5. Missed—fetus dies in uterus or retained no symptoms of abortion.

Explanation

The figures will show the students how mother and child care is to be paid attention, and the important methods of controlling births. The importance of vaccination, breastfeeding, physical assessment and following health advice. The student during training time in practical rural and urban field is shown the different important aspects of MCH and FP care services provided. By the government health team.

Keywords
Purpose, objectives, fears, aims, advice, diet, signs, anemia, effects, problems, domiciliary care, advantages, disadvantages, family planning, operations, abortions, breastfeeding.

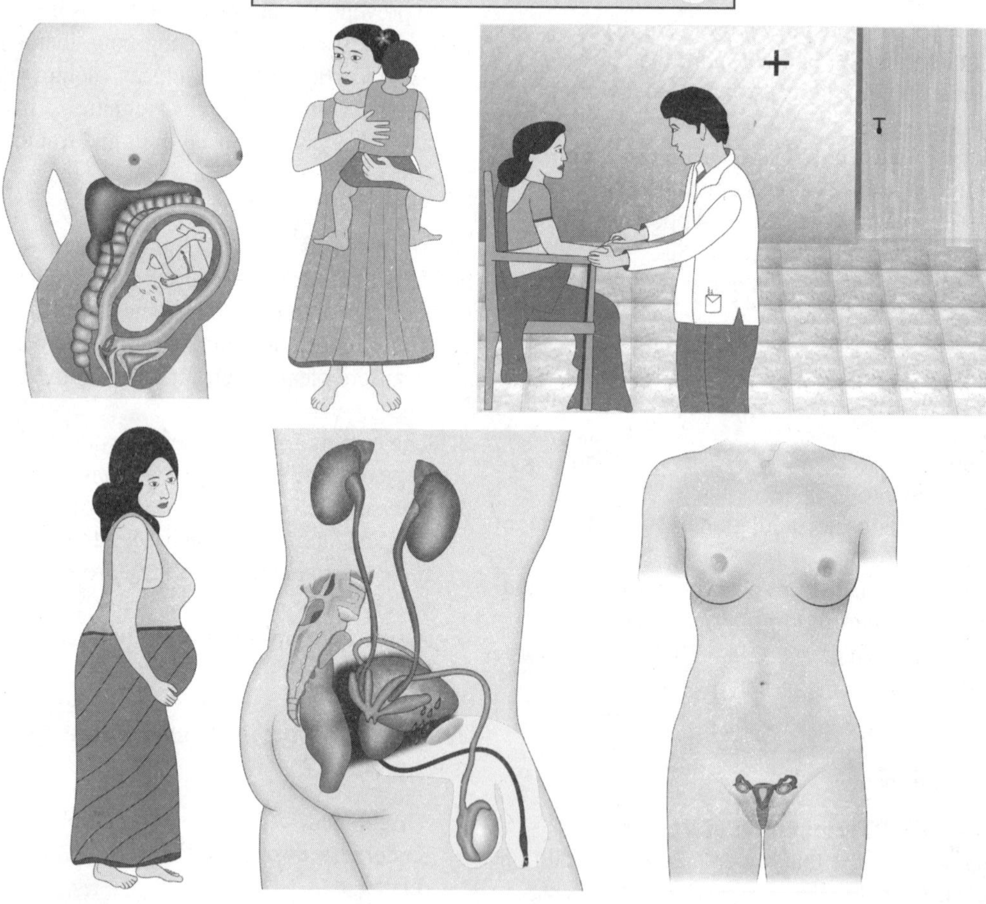

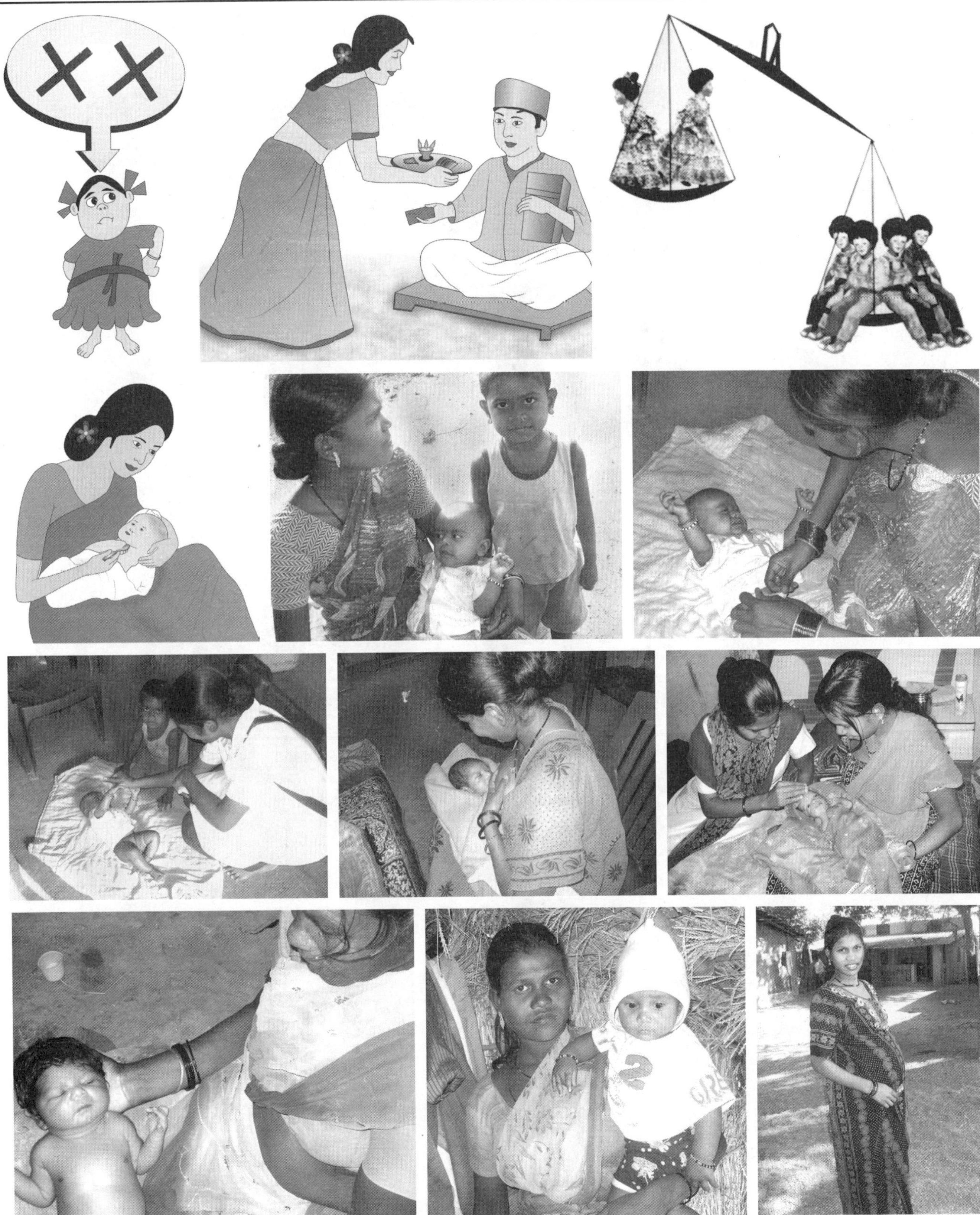

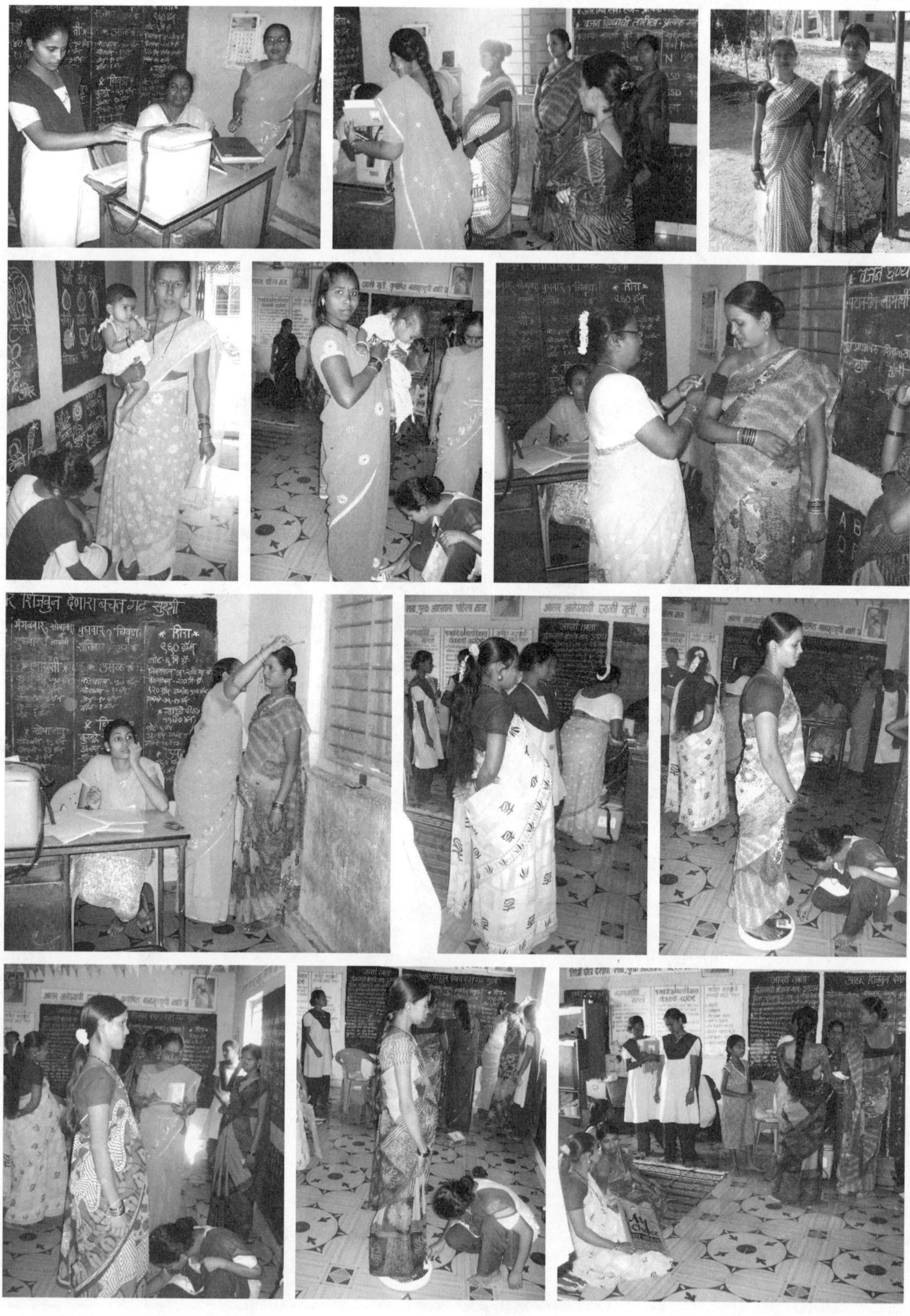

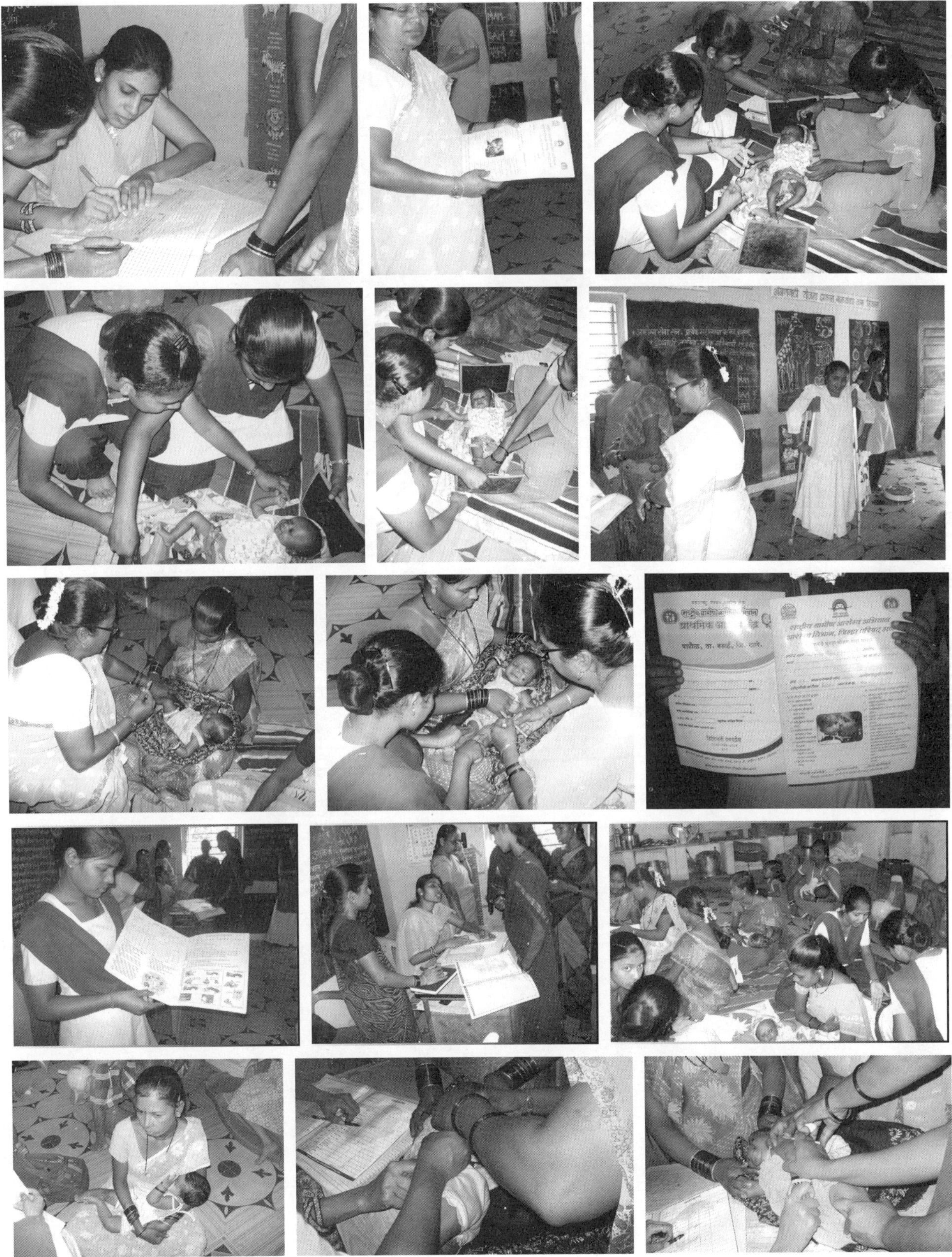

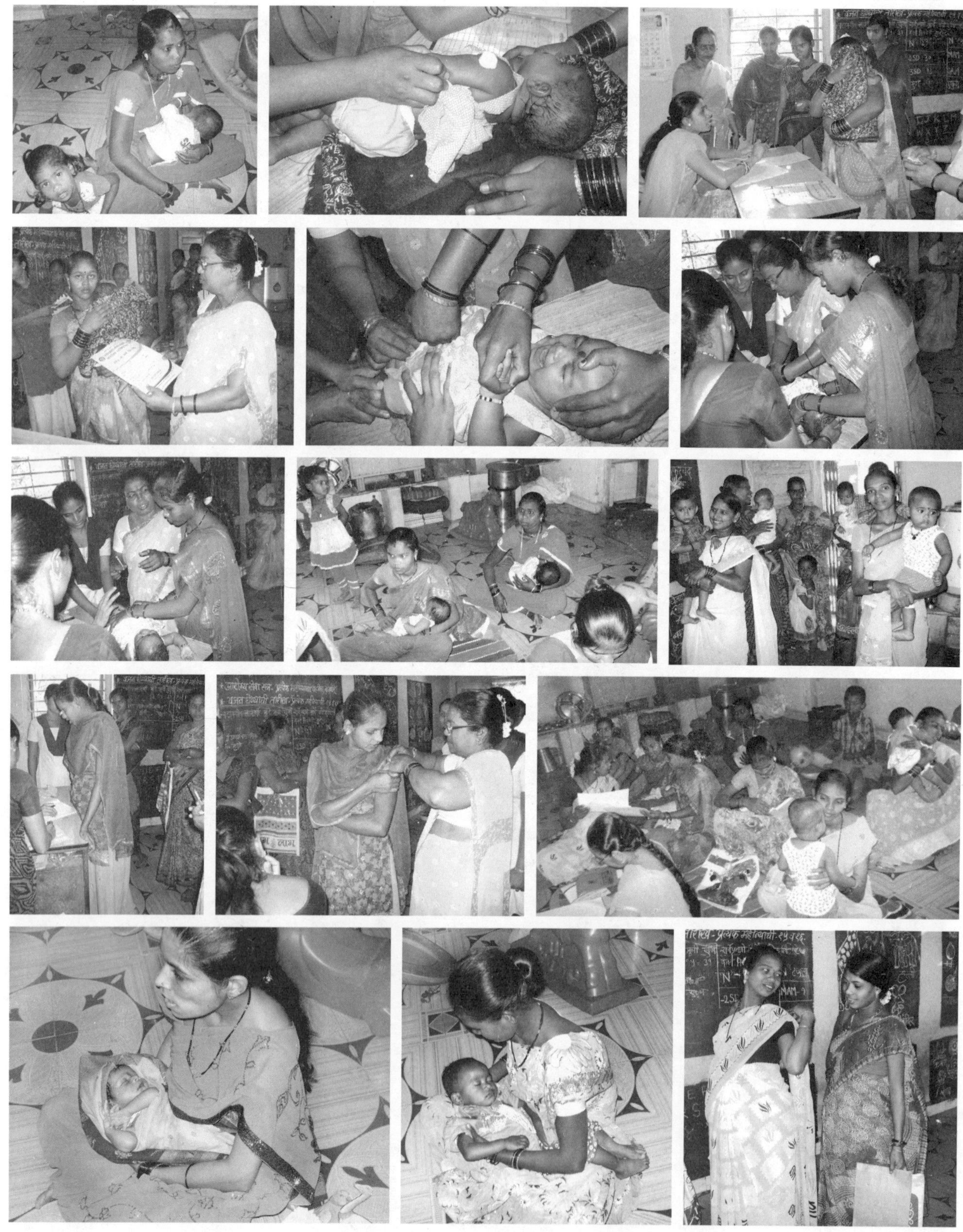

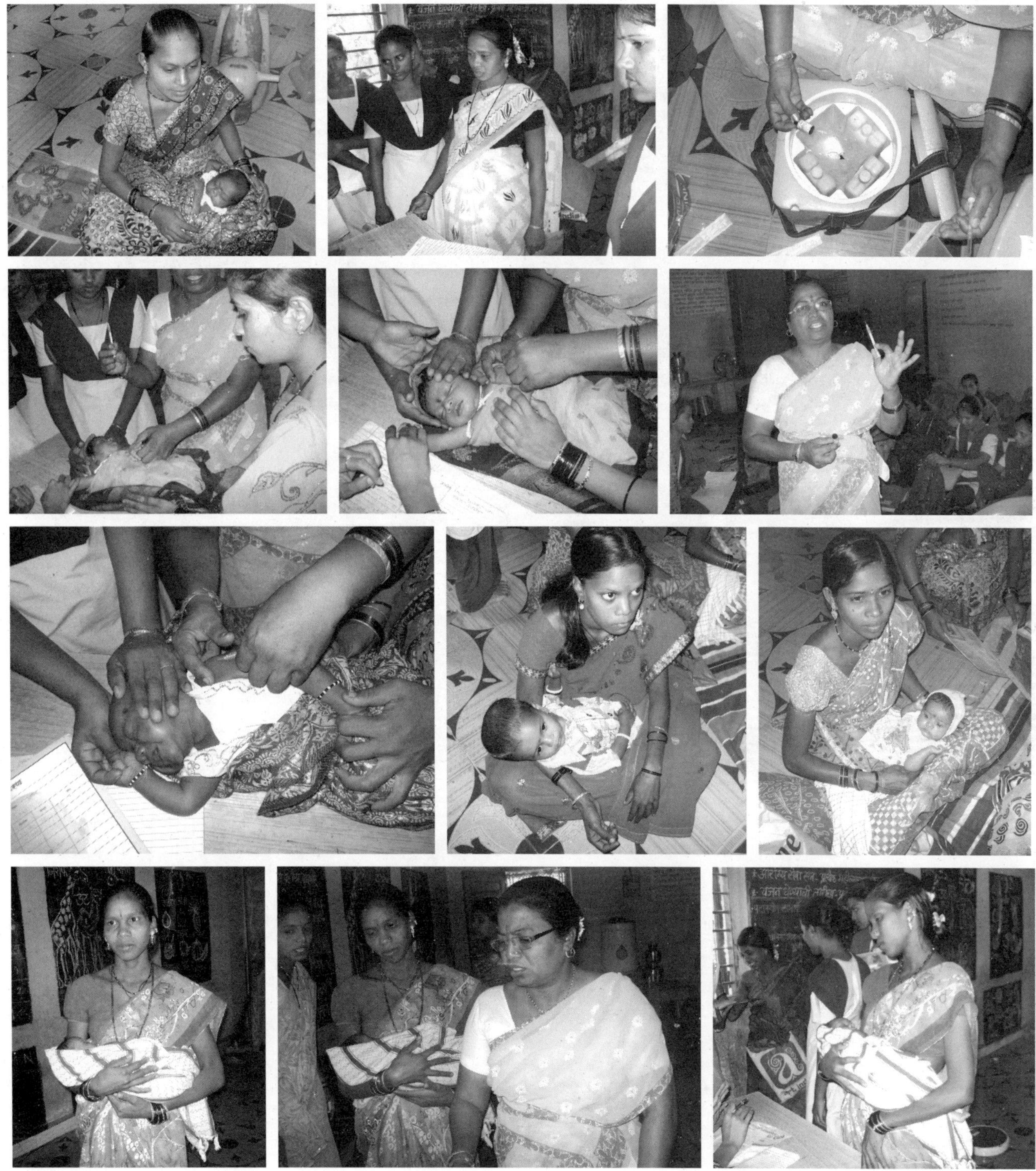

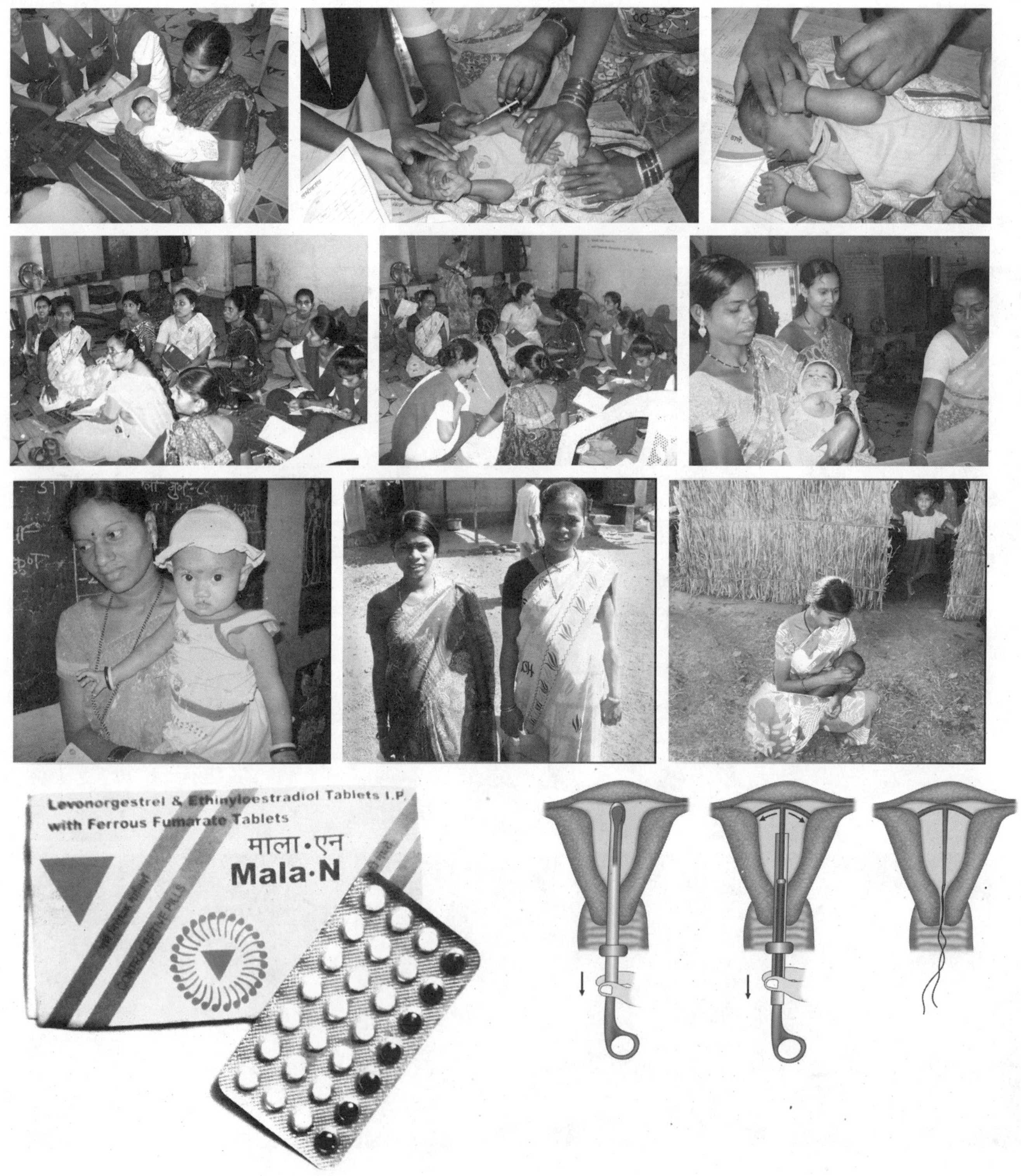
Levonorgestrel & Ethinyloestradiol Tablets I.P.
with Ferrous Fumarate Tablets
माला • एन
Mala•N

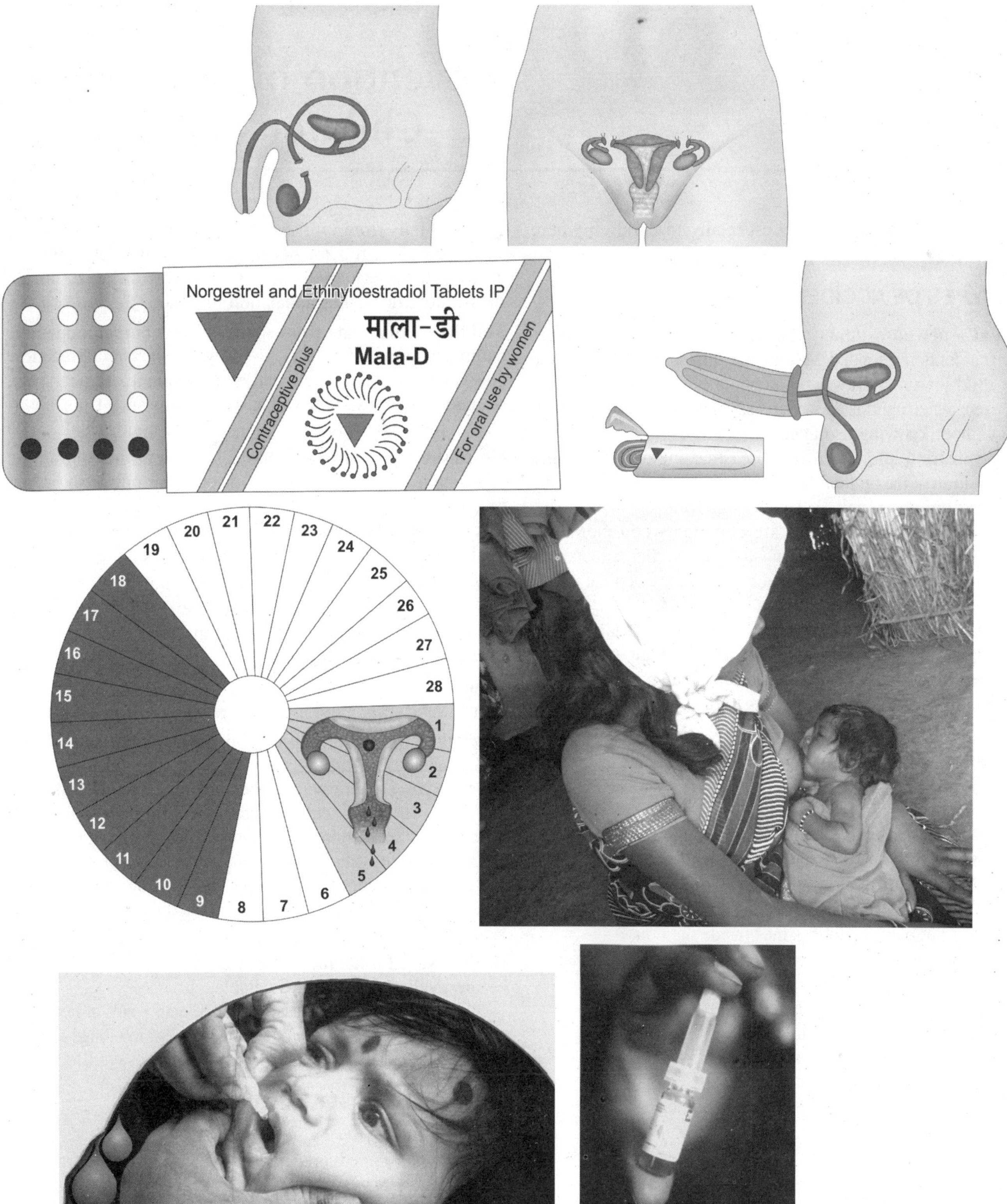

Norgestrel and Ethinyioestradiol Tablets IP
माला-डी
Mala-D
Contraceptive plus
For oral use by women
21
22
23
24
25
26
27
28
1
2
3
4
5
6
7
8
9
10
11
12
13
14
15
16
17
18
19
20

CHAPTER

56

Prevention of Accidents in Children and First Aid

An accident is an emergency especially in children where sudden death can occur.

TYPES OF ACCIDENTS

1. **Fall**—newborn infant who in crib relatively safe from accidents if attended. Accidental falls are common when child learns to crawl and attempts to stand and take few steps when child is active, and starts climbing up and down without knowing its danger.
2. **Aspiration and chocking**—breastfeeding done in proper position of the mother, do not give fluids, foods in sleeping position, do not talk or laugh while eating.
3. **Burns**—accidental burns are common when mother is cooking, or boiling water, unattained fire, hot objects left, electrical wire within the reach of a child. Keep the things on platform where child does not reach.
4. **Aspiration of foreign bodies**—child always puts almost everything in the mouth, such articles kept out of the reach of a child, or else he may put foreign body in mouth, nose, ear etc buttons, grains, pebbles, coins, nuts.

Prevention of accidents

- **Safety** education—Accidents in home/accidents in children
- Road
- Place of work.

The chief underlying factor is carelessness and the problem can be solved by health education

1. Indoor safety—keep away from loose electrical connections, hot iron, moving fans etc
2. Do not play outdoor games inside the house
3. Putting objects into ear or nose may lead to injuries
4. Handle knives and scissors with care
5. Watch TV from a distance
6. Playing with fire is hazardous
7. Keep a first aid box handy
8. Keep safe aid box handy
9. Keep safe distance while burning crackers
10. Always walk open foot paths
11. Cross the road at zebra crossing
12. Never play on the road
13. Never board or get off a moving bus
14. Avoid leaning out of a low terrace wall
15. Always use the bridge while crossing railway lines
16. Use a float while swimming alone
17. Always say 'no' to fights or sweets from strangers

Infants—falls from crib, bath, car, seats, rolling over, bath water temperature, hot beverages, kitchen safety, electric cords and outlets, medications, injury from toys, burns, suffocation, drowning, inhalation/ingestion, foreign bodies.

Toddlers—falls, cuts from sharp objects, burns, inquisitive nature, outdoor safety-cars, drive ways, parking lots, safety glass on doors, lock doors and windows, animal safety-pets, strange animals, storage of hazardous substances, poisonous plants, hot liquids, water safety-tubs, swimming pools.

Childhood poisoning—keep all medications and toxic products in original containers, keep them out of the reach of children, lock, do not take or give it in dark, do not mix common household cleaning products, destroy all old medicines, keep emergency poison control phone handy.

Pre-scholars—guns and rifles in the house, fire safety-prevention emergency measures, free drills, traffic, child abuse, bicycle, state boards, competitive sports, use of machinery-farm, lawn, cooling.

Adolescent—driving, drinking, motorcycle, competition sports, substance abuse, role modeling, stress and coping

Hazards outside the home—collection of refuse, garbage, broken glass, papers, a plastic, dead animal which give foul odor and gases and provides food and breeding places for flies and rates. Stray dogs, unprotected electrical installation, live wires, open fires, sharp instruments, badly contracted houses collapse, waste water soakage pits, collection of cow dung. Field accidents cuts and fractures, crushed injuries by tools, snake bits allergies and poisonous gases due to pesticides and fertilizers.

Basic first aid is the immediate treatment given in the victim before medical help made available.

Accidents can occur at any time, place, road, at home, at odd places where doctor is not available, e.g. in village school, picnic, first aid helps for immediate acton to save life.

Important of First Aid in the School

Types of emergency

1. Sports competition—injuries, falls, sprains and fractures
2. Rainy season—wet floor, slipped
3. Recess—running up and down, fight, pushing, stamping
4. Long assembly—fainting
5. Dispersal—all in a hurry to run home, pushing, stamping
6. Unknown disease—asthma, heat problem child suddenly collapses

7. Attention seeker—psychosomatic headache, abdomen pain, toothache, may or may not be real
8. Foreign body—chocks, swallowing unknown object, uncomfortable position, eating cooked potatoes, banana, soft rice, soft bread can help
9. Foreign body in the nose like popcorn, beans, marbles. Breath through mouth, make victim sneeze by snuff or pass thread into opposite nostril
10. Foreign body in the ear like insects—put war oil, water, insect float
11. Foreign body in the eye—slash water, clean with corner of handkerchief, put drops liquid parafine or castreroil
12. Sun stroke—starts with headache, vomiting, dizziness, fan, ice water bag, sprinkle cold water, tepid sponge
13. Convulsions—epilitic fit-due to high fever, low blood sugar, and changes in sodium level. Victim rolls the eyes, make body stiff, and becomes blue, froth from the mouth, unconscious. Turn the head outside, keep folded handkerchief between teeth, do not forcefully stop the fit, it can aggressive the stimulation, loosen cloth around chest and neck, do not give anything orally
14. Poisoning—keep the bottle out of reach, label it, do not pour in child's favorite drink bottle any poisonous liquids
15. Stings and bites—tourniquet, keep victim still an immobilized, wash bitten area, apply icepack
16. Fire—be calm and quick to find emergency exit, before opening the door, feel it that it is not very hot to touch, cover the nose from smoke, it can harm your eyes and face and produces respiratory problem. Do not jump from the window. Try to seek help from people standing below. If you have to cross the fire rap blanket or thick wet cloth, extinguish fire (petroleum) by sand, mud or soda.
17. Electrical circuit—pull main switch off, do not use bare wet hand to remove victim, use dry wooden stick or dry towel. Pull body from the distance for break the contact. Stand on dry wooden box or plastic mat or thick newspaper or use wooden chair table to push the victim. Start artificial resuscitation
18. Accidents fall from cradle, crossing road, climbing tree, drowning, touching electric instruments, shutting door, crushing fingers, bursting crackers, kite flying etc.

Conclusion—The slogan "safety first" does not mean that safety is the most important thing in life. Sometimes we may take risk yet we must stay alive to have a successful and happy life. Accidents are not planned, they can happen at anytime, and we should learn the accidents safety and first aids so it will equip us to act in emergencies. Due to rapid growth and development phase, children are vulnerable to such things. Teach them to keep hygiene, wash hands, wear neat and tidy uniform, wear shoes, and stay away from sick people. In school follow immunization schedule, regular periodic medical checkups, maintain medical first aid box up to date, have a camp and do blood group of children, provide prophylaxis like vitamin A, worms' tablet. Have regular health education. Drink safe water, eat hot cooked home food. Do not leave an infant unsupervised in the bath tub, keep the floor at home clean and dry, avoid scattered toys, do not rush up and down stairs, use a ladder or a stool to reach high places, do not wear nylon clothes in the kitchen they can catch the fire easily. Turn off the gas stoves when not in use, get then checked regularly to avoid leakage. Stale, spoilt and exposed food avoid as it can cause poisonous. Poisonous chemicals should be stored separately and away from eatables. Store all materials safety in labeled unbreakable containers rather than glass, cover when not used, do not use lammable materials near lame.

Keywords

Types of accidents, prevention, hazards, first aid, emergency, and conclusion.

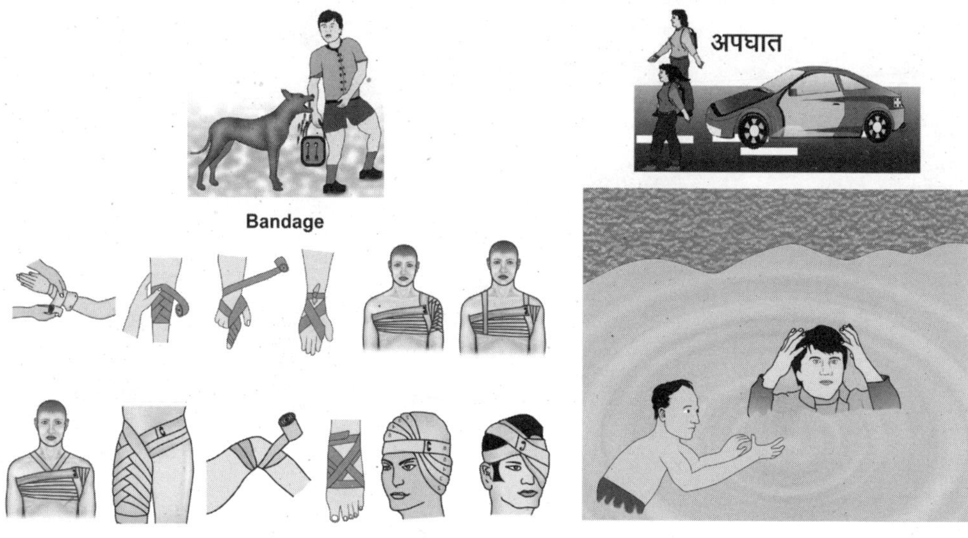

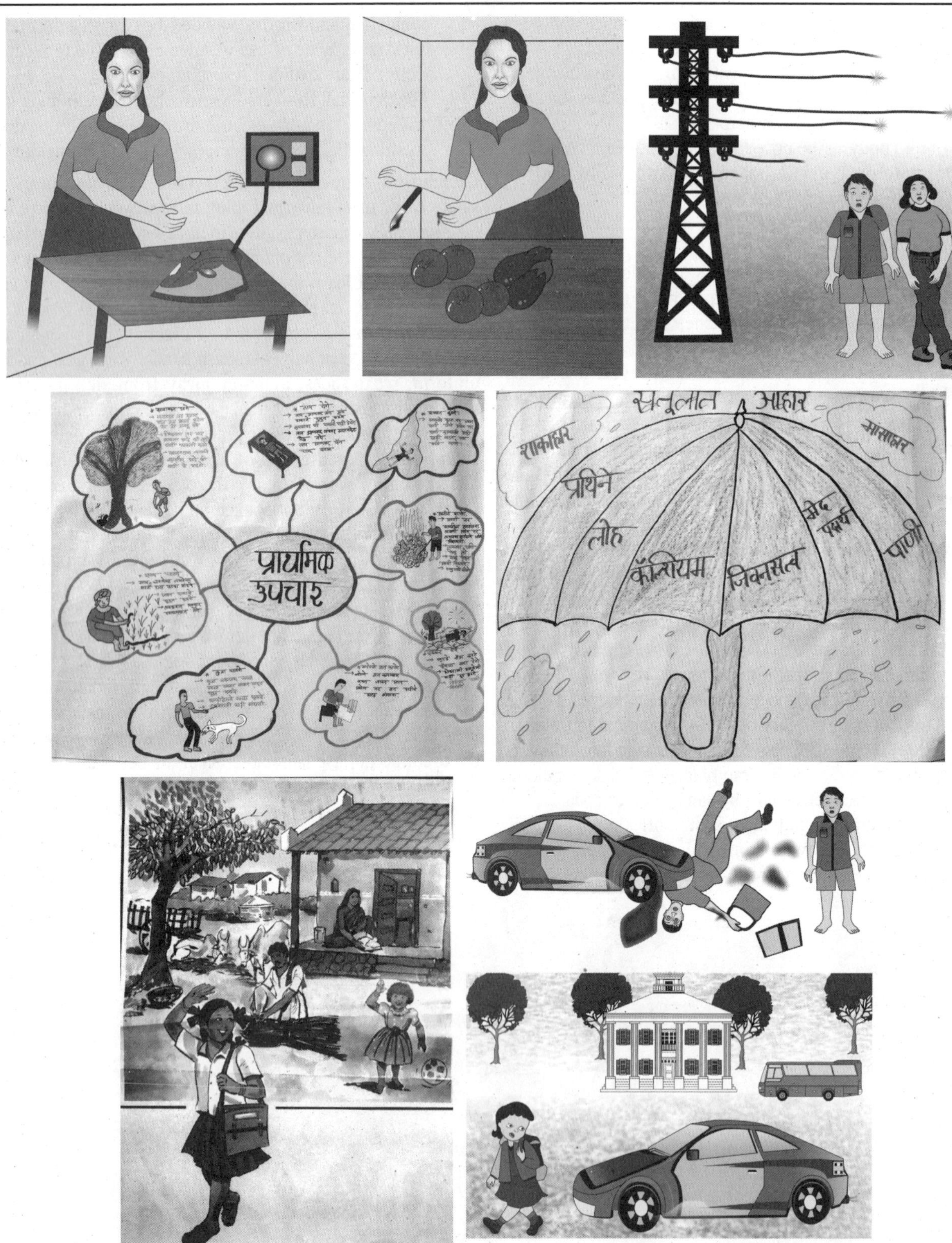

प्राथमिक उपचार
सन्तुलीत आहार
शाकाहार
मांसाहार
प्रथिने
लोह
कॅल्शियम
जिवनसत्व
मेद पदार्थ
पाणी

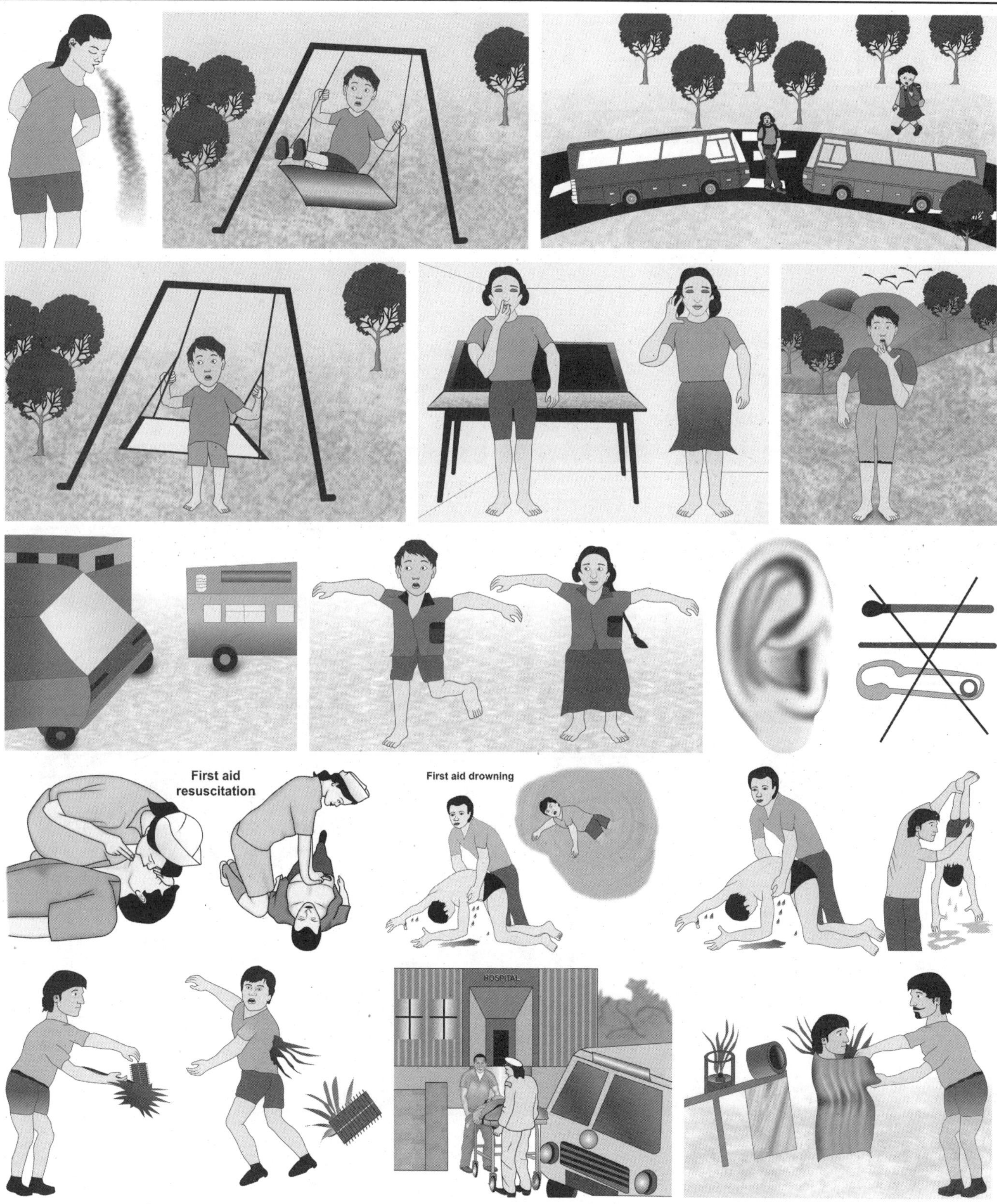
First aid resuscitation
First aid drowning
HOSPITAL

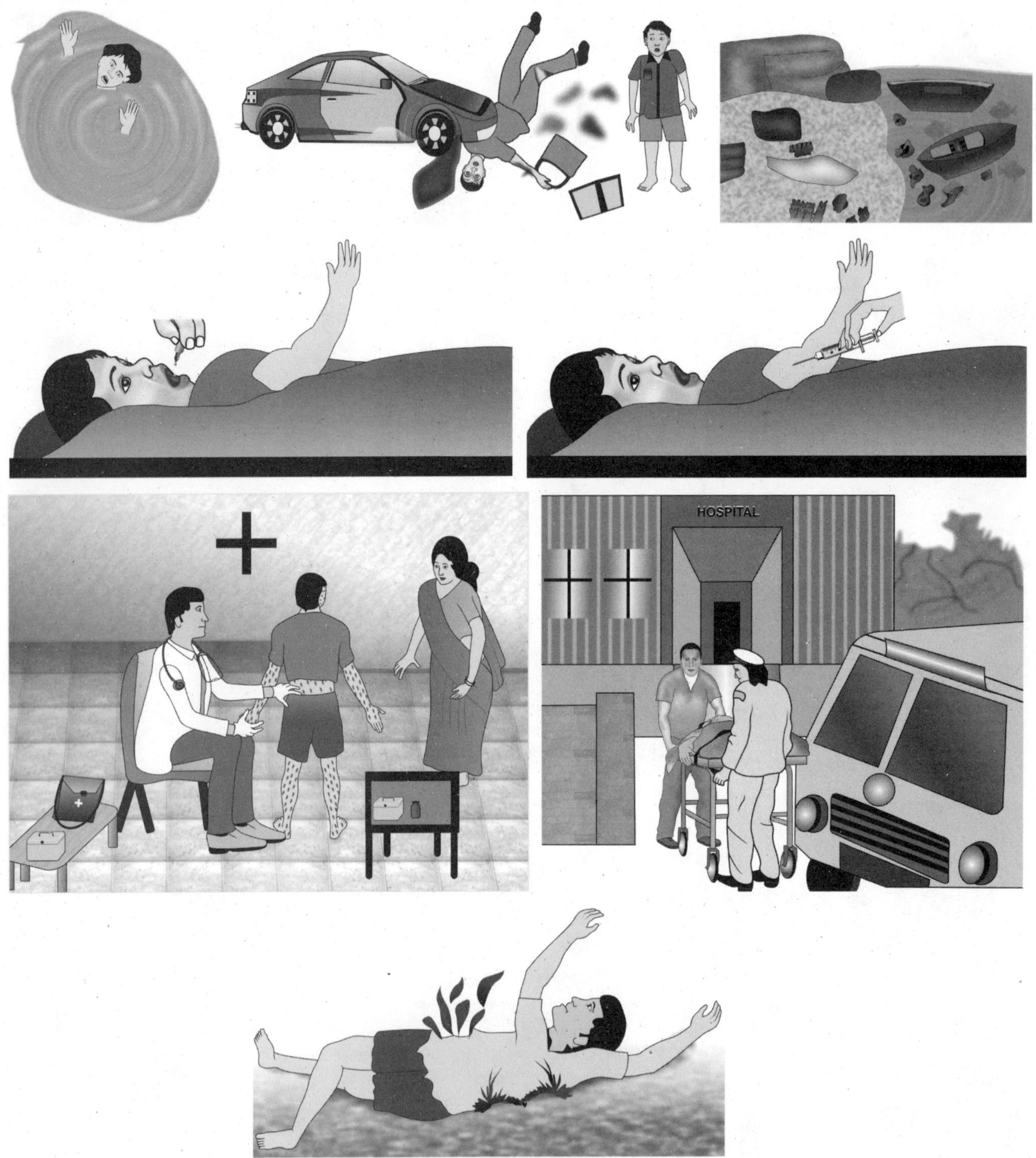
HOSPITAL

CHAPTER

57

Worm Infestation

SPECIFIC OBJECTIVES

1. What is meant by worm infestation?
2. Causes of worm infestation
3. Types of worm infestation
4. Sign and symptoms of worm infestation
5. Understand the life cycle of worm infestation
6. Common ways of finding and investigation
7. Treatment and complication of worm infestation
8. Aware of preventive method of worm infestation.

The term "amoebiasis" has been defined by WHO as the condition of harboring the protozoan parasite entamoeba histolytica with or without clinical manifestations.

The symptomatic disease occurs in less than 10% of infected individuals. The symptomatic group has been further subdivided into intestinal and extra intestinal amoebiasis only a small percentage of those having intestinal infection will develop invasive amoebiasis.

The problem of helminthes infestation is common in all tropical countries due to prevalent methods defecation and disposal of excreta. Intestinal infestation adds to the burden of the rapidly growing children whose health status is already compromised by illness, malnutrition and unsanitary living conditions.

There are round worms, thread worms, hookworms, tape worms, pin worms etc.

Round worms otherwise called as 'Ascariasis' it is more seen common in the children between the age of one to five years, in lower social economic status.

Thread worms other wise called as pin worm or seat worms. It is commonly found in children. It is transmitted through soil, finger and linen.

Hook worm or ancylostamiasis—they may occur as single or mixed infections in the same person found in all ages from 15 to 25 years.

More common in children of 1 to 5 years and found also in low socioeconomic group.

Threadworms found in children, in unsanitary living conditions, e.g. school, hostels, institutions and families.

Sign and symptoms of **round worms** is fever and Eosinophilia due to larva.

- Ascaris pneumonia due to larva in the lungs
- Abdominal pain
- Intestinal obstruction

General symptoms like diarrhea and high fever, pica, abdominal distension, sleeplessness, irritability and loss of weight.

Ascaris encephalopathy may occur with other infection.

Thread worms sign and symptoms is asymptomatic children may not have any complains, lack of appetite, loss of weight, grinding of teeth and abdominal pain, purities at the anal region, nocturnal enuresis may occur.

Sags and symptoms of **hook worm** is epigastric pain, fatigue and weakness, pica may be present, eosinophilia may be found.

Life cycle of round worms—they live in the upper part of small intestine. It resembles on ordinary earth worm. It measures up to 20 cm to 45 cm in length. The female lays eggs in large number which are passed in the Faeces. They contaminate the soil or vegetables. Given optimal conditions, the eggs take about 10 days to become embryonated. When the infective eggs are ingested, they reach the intestine where they hatch into larvae. The larvae penetrate the intestine and migrate to liver and lungs and then travel up the human host. They reach the small intestine where they become sexually mature in about 6 to 10 weeks.

There are two types of hook worms. They are found attached to the mucosa of the small intestine, particularly of the jejunum. Each worm measures about 8 to 10 mm in length. Adult are believed to survive for on an average of one to four years respectively. The worms are passed in the Faeces by infested persons.

The female parasite lays eggs which are passed in the Faeces. A single female may lay 10,000 to 20,000 eggs per day. The egg hatch into larvae outside the human body in the soil where they grow and develop into infective larvae. When a person walks bare foot on the contaminated soil the infective larvae penetrate the skin and enter the human host. They pass into the lymph and blood stream and reach the lungs; they travel up to trachea and the pharynx from where they are swallowed. The larvae finally reach the small intestine where they develop into sexually mature worms and start laying eggs in about 6 weeks.

1. Stool examination for ova or worms and microscopic examination of stool.
2. Piprazin citrate or tablet Mebendazole/Mebex bd, tablet Albendazone of a signal dose of 2.5 mg kg
3. It is advisable to treat the entire family at a time. Is given in health centers free of cost.

Can develop

1. Iron deficiency anemia
2. Edema
3. Heart failure

4. General fatigue
5. Cardiac failure
6. Appendicitis
7. Lymphadenitis.

Precautionary measures to be taken:

1. Develop hygienic habits of eating and washing hands with soap before and after eating and defecation
2. To prevent oral infections
3. Proper disposal of excreta is essential
4. Control of flies
5. Wash vegetables and eatables well in running or plenty of water
6. Keep the children's nail short
7. Use boil water for drinking.
8. Use of long pajamas to prevent auto infestation of pin worms
9. Antipruitic cream can be used to prevent itching
10. Detection early treatment of all infected persons can reduce soil contamination
11. Use of sanitary latrines helps to control spread so promote it
12. Efficient sewage disposal
13. Habits of using foot wear which prevents contact with contaminated soil in open field
14. Wearing shoos for personal prophylaxis
15. Health education directed towards raising the standards of personal and domestic hygiene.
16. Follow all sanitary measures as Ascariasis is disappearing spontaneously in certain areas as a result of improved sanitation
17. Mass treatment—periodic de-worming at intervals of two to three months may be undertaken in a place where protein energy malnutrition is highly prevalent.

Doctor finds 13-cm-long worm in man's eye—It was not only alive but moving and was visible by naked eye. It was coiled up underneath the conjunctiva, below the superficial layer of the eye, it is very rare that intestinal worms traveling to the eye. Doctor made a small opening in Krishnamurthy conjunctiva, and removed the 12.5 cm worm using a pair of forceps. The tricky procedure, which was video recorded, lasted for 15–20 minutes. The worm could have traveled deep into the eye or gone to the brain through the optic nerves, which could have been fatal. The live worm was pulled out from eye to see was horrified, as it kept moving and jumping, it was scary for a bit. It had traveled from his intestine.

Keeping worms away—wash hands before eating, eat only properly cooked food, drink boiled water, and take de-worming medication once in six month. Worms in the intestine eat up all the body's nutrition, so stomachache, irritable bowel syndrome do not ignore.

Summary—It has been estimated that about 45 million in India are infested with hookworm. The diseases are highly endemic. Roundworms too are widespread in India and 30% to 50% population are known to be infested. The parasite robs the human host of his nutrition especially in children. So let us take step to prevent control the ill effect of worm infestation. Each of us is responsible for our own health and so let us today count as number day one to make effort in practicing sanitary habits and get rid of this health problem and make our family free from worm infestation to enjoy health and well-being.

Keywords

Specific objectives, life cycle, threat worms, round worms, hook worms, summary.

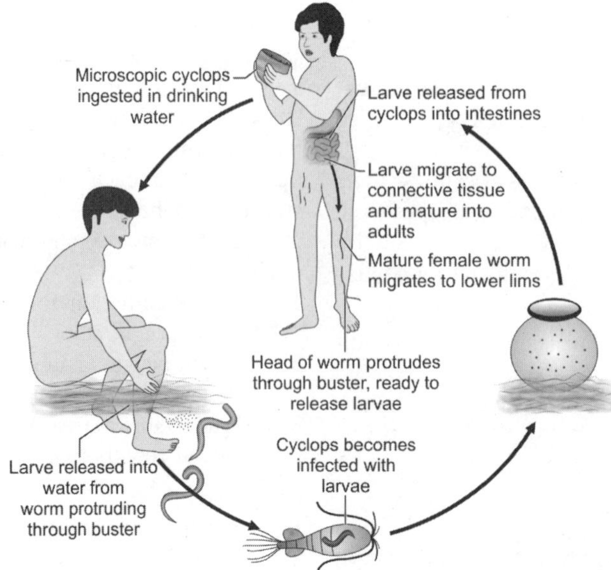

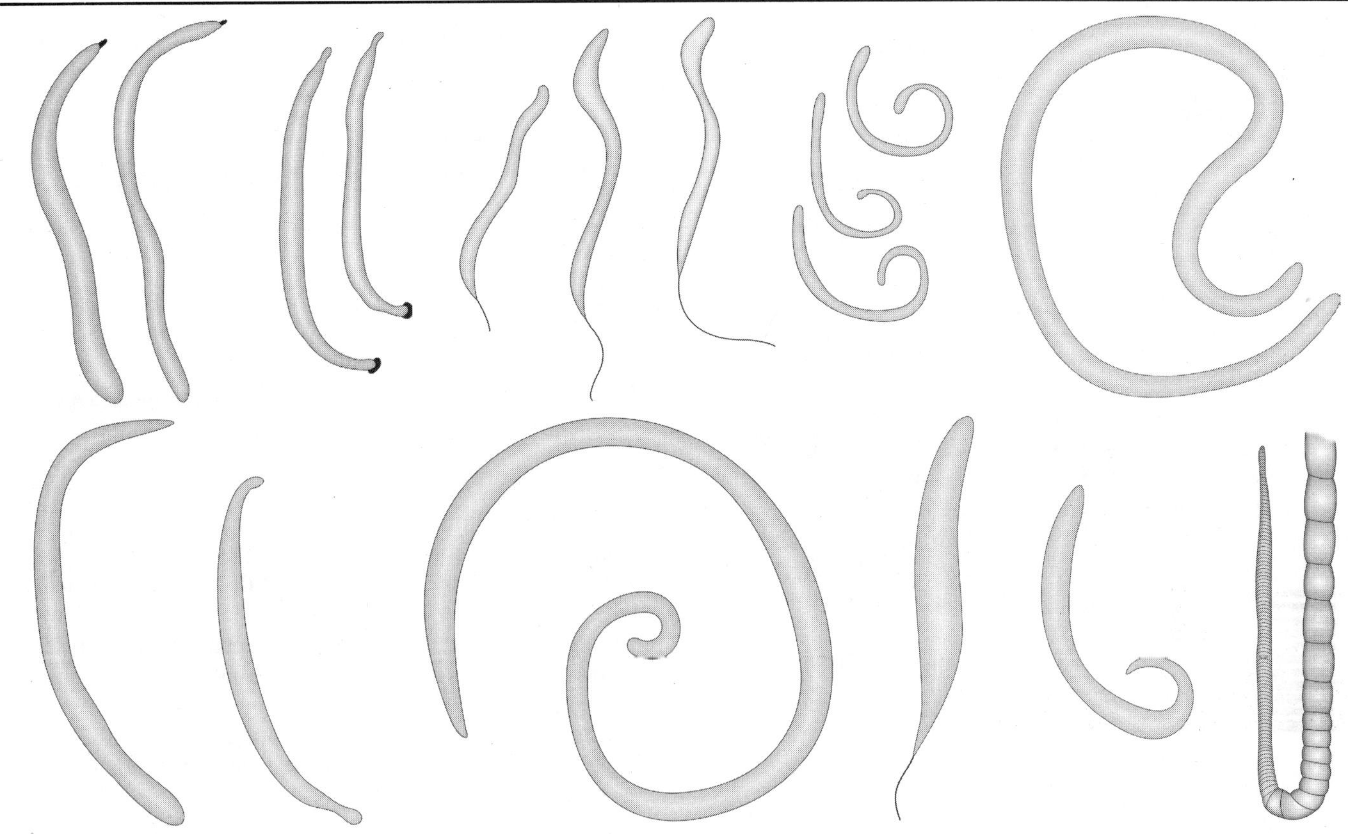

CHAPTER

58

Communication Methods

HEALTH EDUCATION/COMMUNICATION

1. Get the persons attention before attempting to talk or communicate
2. Stay in their field of vision, make eye contact
3. Establish the gist of what you are going to talk about
4. Your speech will be more easily understood when you are not eating chewing, smoking etc.
5. Keep your hands away from your face while talking
6. Do not talk too fast, pronouncing words clearly
7. Make them repeat the specifies back to you, many words sound alike
8. In case of failure in communication try to find a different way of saying the same thing, rather than repeating the original words over and over gain
9. Keep a note pad handy and write your words out and show them to the person if you have to
10. Use gestures and visual cues.

Methods of Mass Health Communication

Purpose of communication is to transmit information from one person or group of persons to other persons or groups with a view to bring about behavioral changes.

Or it is a direct or indirect exchange of information ideas as a means of understanding and education.

Process has a communicator, message that is clear, relevant, concrete, attractive, acceptable and specific. Channel by which the message is transmitted and audience who are consumers of this message.

Purpose of Communication

1. To educate public And to promote health and welfare
2. To transmit information from one person or group with a view to bring about behavioral changes
3. To help in effective communication
4. To minimize the barriers of language of distortion and of miss interpretation
5. To make there communication more lively, vivid so that the presentation is more realistic
6. To have the far reaching and more intense effort compare to their aids
7. To have the clarity in the reception of the message.

Importance of Communication

1. Exchange of information for study of a problem analyzing of a problem, solving it
2. It is an educational tool which can be used for general health population-gives opportunities in health field
3. It is helpful for understanding the patient
4. It is necessary for administration of programmed, supervision, guidance etc.

Barriers of Communication

1. **Physiological obstacles** is difficulty in hearing and expression, difficulty in visualization and speaking
2. **Psychological barrier** is emotional disturbances, mental tension, instability, lack of concentration, pre-occupation
3. **Emotional barrier** is over crowding, poor lighting, noise, thermal discomfort, bad odors, ill maintained, invisibility and congestion
4. **Sociocultural barrier** is poor knowledge of customs, practices, attitudes, habits, beliefs, languages, knowledge, confidence, level of understanding.

The barriers can be identified before embarking on communication through the study of selection of proper channel to reach easily.

For Effective Communication

1. One should be able to observe and listen properly
2. Not just presume and have visual contact
3. Observe while listening, expression on face convey non-verbal communication (body movement. Gestures)
4. Use familiar language of the people
5. Every word uttered distinctively and clearly
6. Avoid too fast or low tone talks and do modification according to the responses you get
7. Avoid repetition of words
8. Decide before hand the channel of transmission and the message you want to give.

Art of Observing and Listening in Communication

1. For effective communication one should be able to observe and listen properly because in the field of health, we rely more on individual contact.
2. The receiver should be understood by the art of observing and listening
3. Do not presume anything, listen and observe
4. The sender and receiver must be of face level to each other to facilitate visual contact
5. Which increases communication
6. Do not just listen, observe while listening the expression on face, convey a lot more than what is talked

7. Therefore facial expression, body movements, gestures can decide flow of communication. This establishes confidence, good repose and understanding.

Characteristics of good teaching aids—should be meaningful, purposeful, accurate, simple, cheap, large size, up to date, easily portable, motivates the learners, etc.

Criteria for selection should be the teaching objective, special group of learners, the age level, grade level, specific educational value, learning objectives and locally available material, proper presentation, educational level, socio-economic status, intelligence level. It also should have meaningful content, appropriate materials, and worth. It should be easy to see and understand, represent things that are common and understandable, neat, clear, visible, learner gets interest by seeing it, well planed in advanced.

Methods of Health Education

Classification

1. One-way
2. Two-way

One-way method—lecture, films, charts, flannel graph, exhibits, flash cards.

Two-way method—group discussion, panel discussion, symposium, workshop, role playing, demonstration.

Verbal communication—use of language, whether spoken or written.

Non-verbal communication—gestures, facial expression like smile, raising eye brows, wrinkling, staring, gazing, postures, bodily movements and even silence.

It has three approaches

1. Individual approach
2. Group approach
3. Mass approach

Radio, rape recorders, microphones, amplifiers and earphones are **auditory aids**.

Visual aids—black board, flannel graph, models, specimens, posters, slides, film strips, epidiascope and overhead projectors are visual aids

Sound films, slide tape combination, TV, computer and internet are **combined audio-visual aids**.

Lecture, films, charts, flannel graph, exhibits and flash cards are **one way methods**.

Group discussion, panel discussion, symposium, workshop, role playing, demonstration is **two-way methods**.

Tree charts, stream charts, table charts, flow charts are **projected and non-projected aids**.

Non-projected aids—Photographs are non-projected aids, it may be white and black or colored or mounted or un-mounted photographic prints. It can be used in personal teaching situations, as display type visuals in exhibitions or bulletin boards. For effective teaching it must tell story. Illustrations of drawing, paintings, sketching, etc.

Dramatization, puppetry, cartoons, comic strips, bulletin board, skit/diorama, mock-ups (artificial kidney demonstration dialysis) museum, field trip, experiment, kathas, bhajan mandalies etc. are **other methods**.

Conclusion—audio-visual aids work as effective tool in health education programme. A visual is what you can see and aural is what you can hear. In audio-visual aids, there is reproduction of sound and visual aids there is picture or image projected. More than one sense are affected and influenced in the audio-visual aids of communication. Auditory aids are tape recorders, microphones, amplifier and earphones. Visual aids are black board, flannel graph, models, specimens, posters, slides, filmstrips, epidiascope and overhead projector. Combined aids are sound films, slide tape combination and television. Its aim is to attract the audience, to impress, motivate and promote the acceptance and adoption of the message. For the purpose is to help effective communication, to minimize the barriers of languages, vivid and realistic and have clarity of the message. When you select aids, it must be well oriented with group of people, their culture, social, educational, psychological background and their location available, the educator should be a skilled communicator.

Explanation—audio-visual aids will help the students and they will come to know the intricacies of the phenomenon and how it can be used for the benefit of humankind.

Keywords

Health education, methods, purpose, importance, barriers, effective communication, art, criteria.

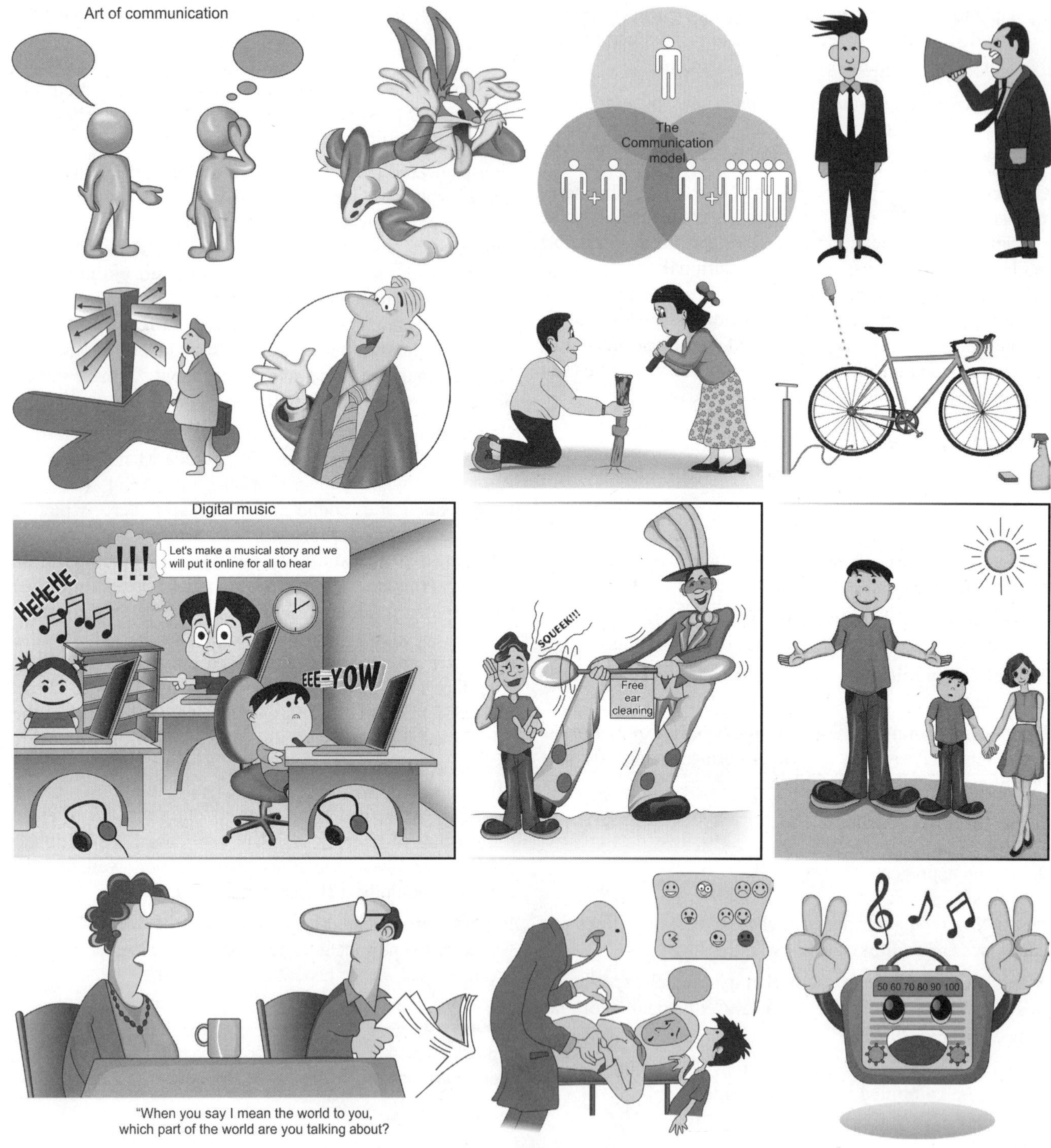

"When you say I mean the world to you, which part of the world are you talking about?

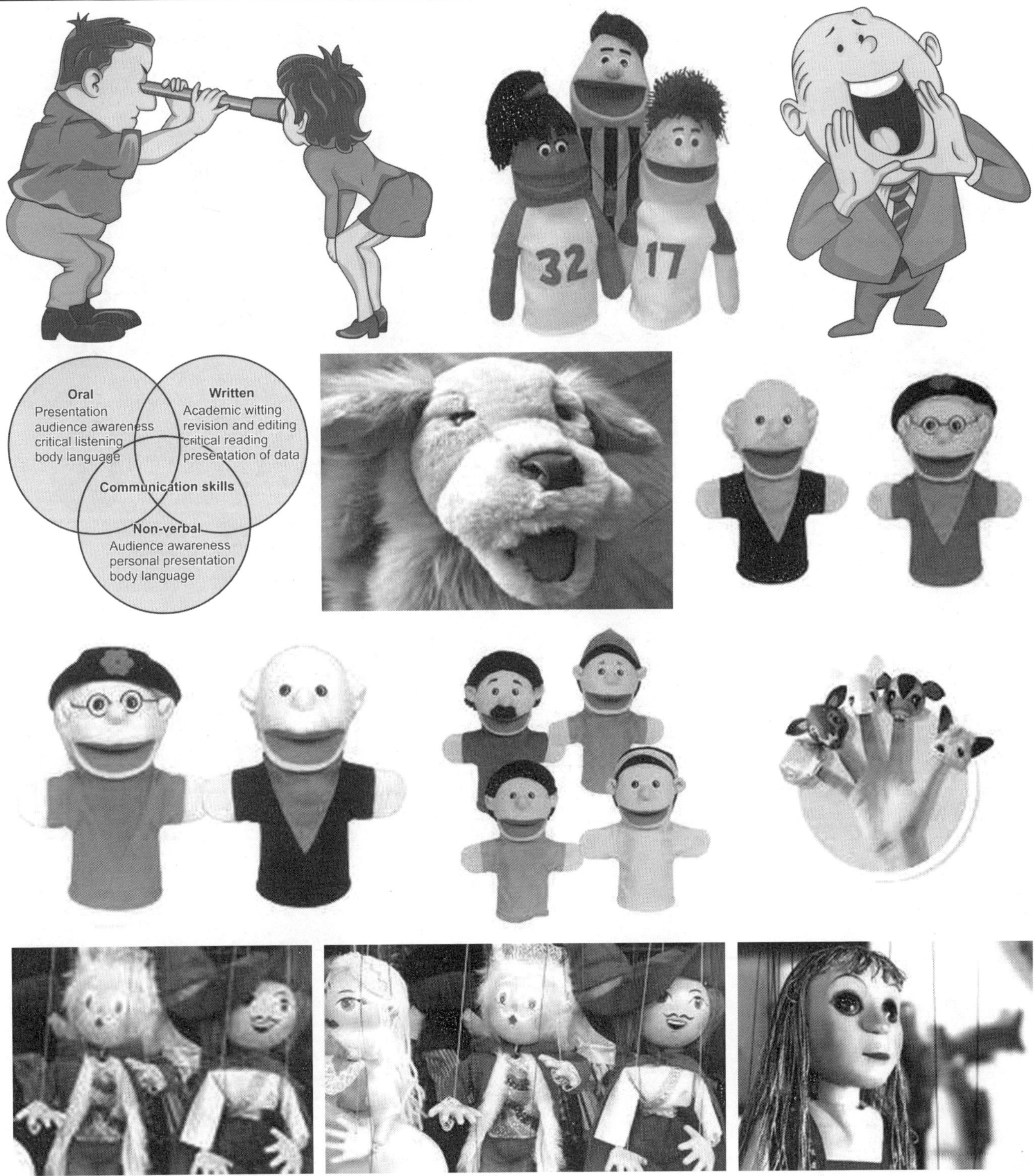
Oral
Presentation
audience awareness
critical listening
body language
Written
Academic witting
revision and editing
critical reading
presentation of data
Communication skills
Non-verbal
Audience awareness
personal presentation
body language
32
17

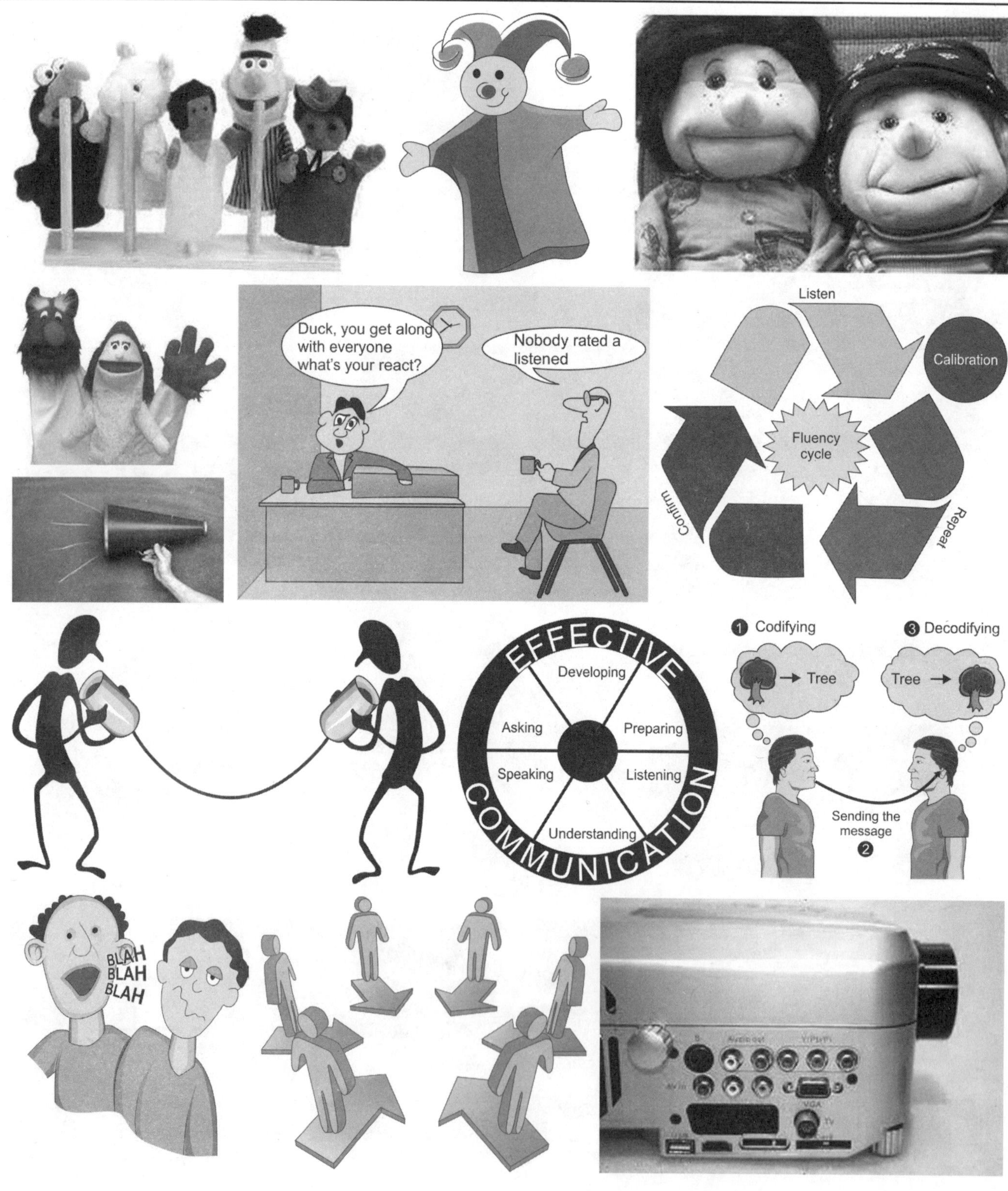
Duck, you get along with everyone what's your react?
Nobody rated a listened
Listen
Calibration
Fluency cycle
Confirm
Repeat
EFFECTIVE COMMUNICATION
Developing
Asking
Preparing
Speaking
Listening
Understanding
1 Codifying
3 Decodifying
Tree
Tree
Sending the message
2
BLAH BLAH BLAH
VGA

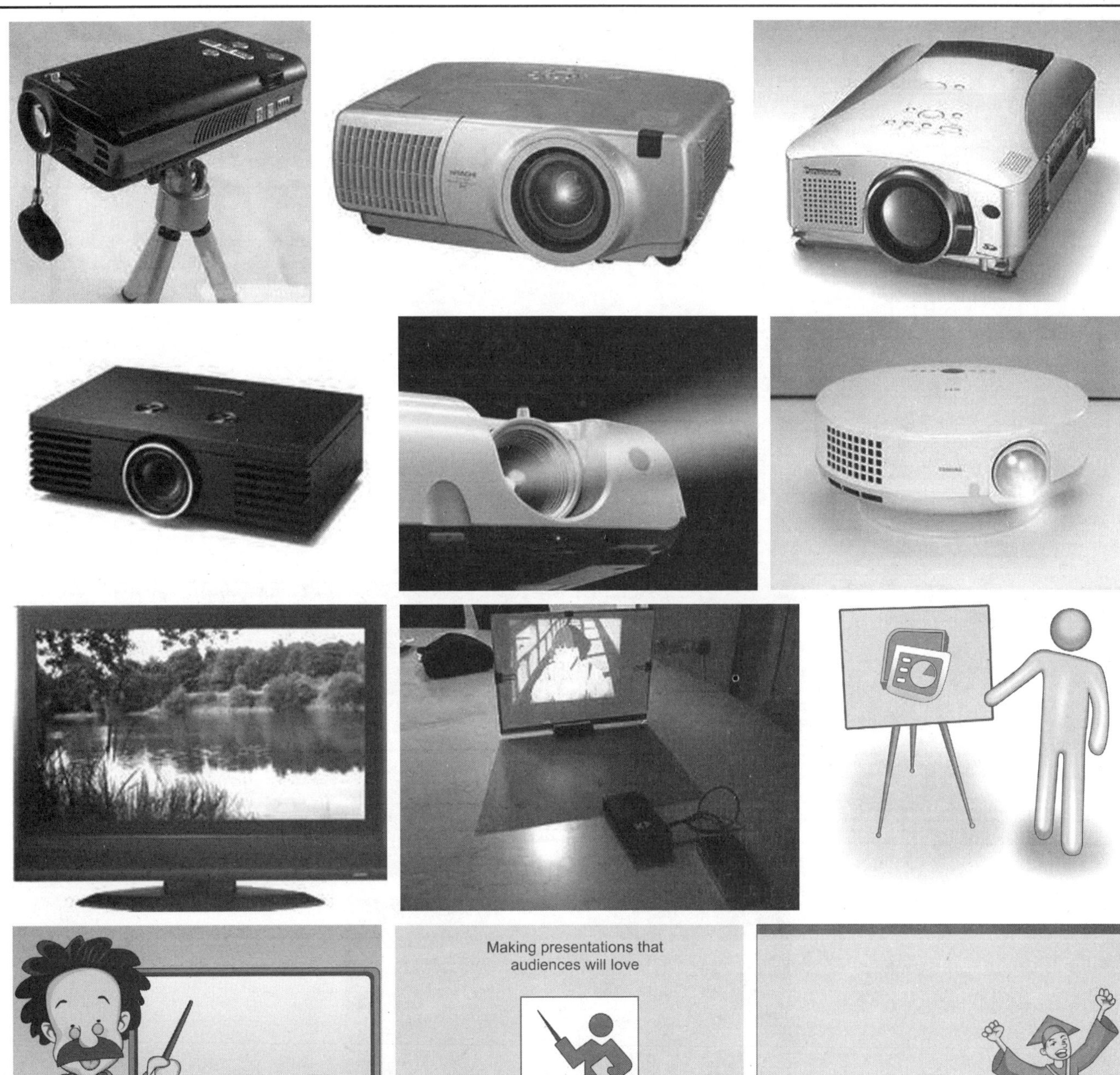
Making presentations that
audiences will love

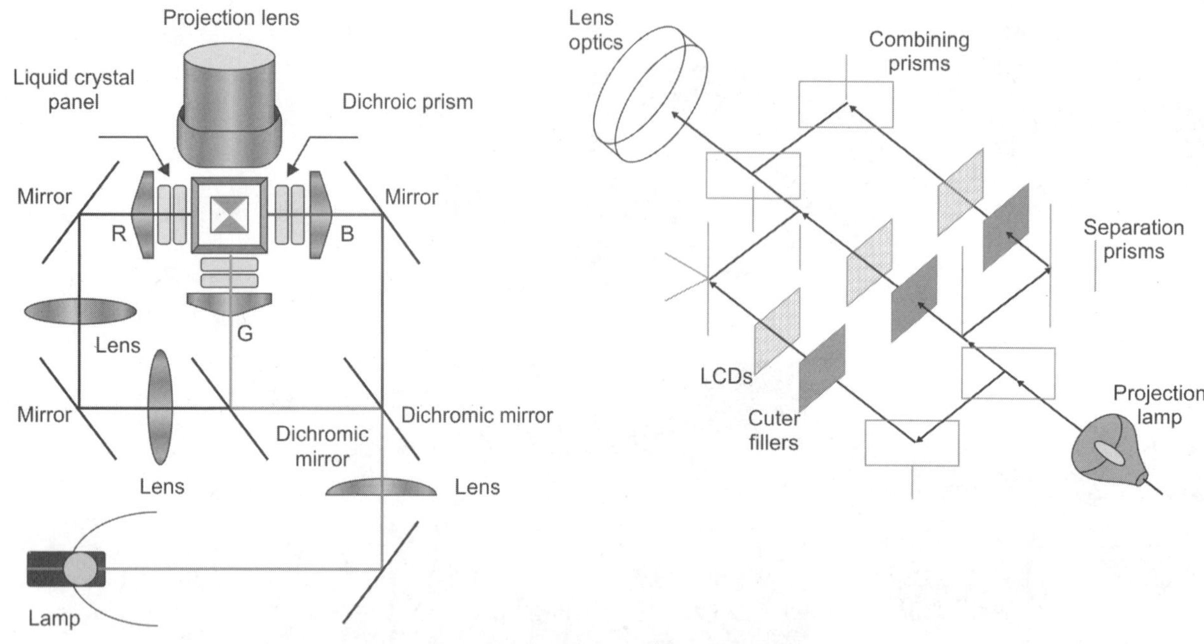
Projection lens
Liquid crystal panel
Dichroic prism
Mirror
Mirror
R
B
G
Lens
Mirror
Dichromic mirror
Dichromic mirror
Lens
Lens
Lamp
Lens optics
Combining prisms
Separation prisms
LCDs
Cuter fillers
Projection lamp

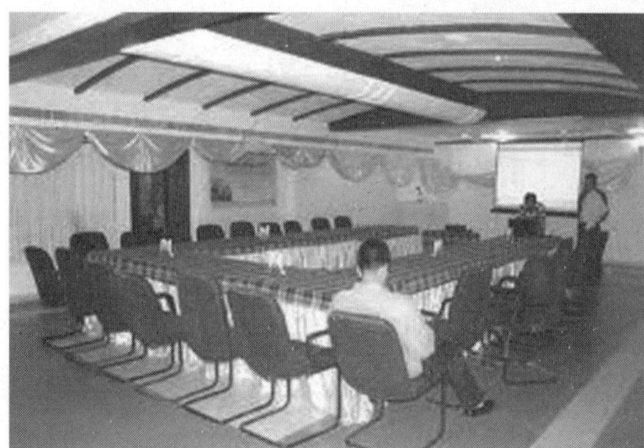

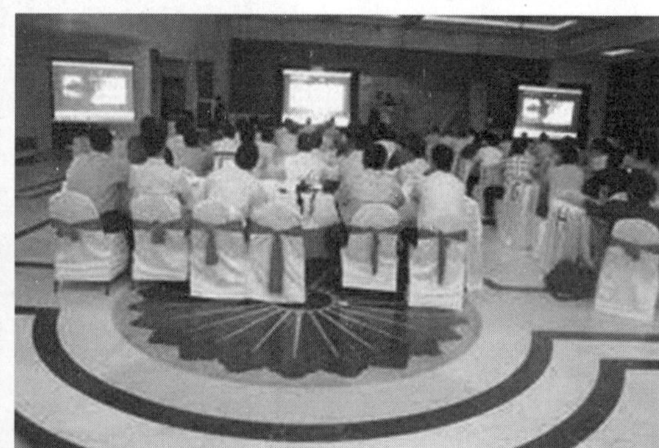

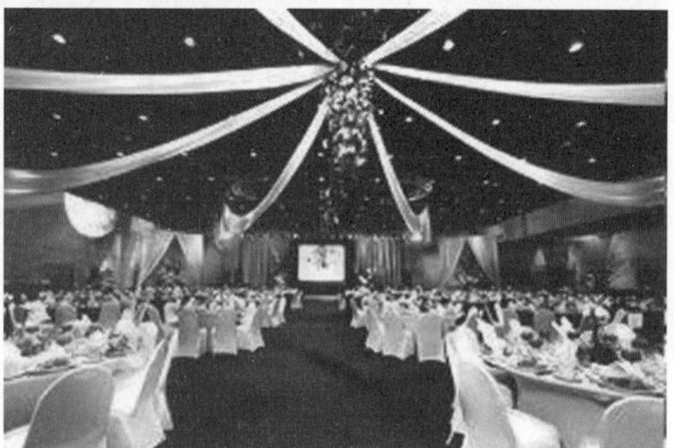

CHAPTER

59

Snake Bites

INTRODUCTION

Imagine in the home or outside when you see the snake, people take sticks and run with life behind the snake, isn't it? So much phobia in each of us incase the snake bits us then what I will have gone forever. In addition, because of this fear poor snake gets killed. In every country there, snakes exist. Total in the world there are 2,700 types of snakes found. Water snakes have tail like a fish flat that helps them to swim. Snake has such teeth inward that once he gets pray it cannot escape from his mouth. He attacks by catching with mouth of the pray.

In America there are certain kinds of snakes who swallow the whole baby chicken, and until the chicken reaches the stomach it does not know what is happening and the snake later vomits away the wings and all that he wants to throw later on separately. In monsoon you find more snake, pythons can sallow a huge goat and deer at a time by suffocating the animal and then after killing break the bones.

Land and water snake both can swim, snakes can not make hole to live by himself it lives in other animals house and in cracked places, female snake can lay from 10 to 100 eggs at a time, many enemies of the eggs even snake himself eats there own eggs, twice in a year the snake can lay the eggs. Soon after the birth of babies run away from them, every year the snake leaves a old skin and gets new skin, baby snakes contain six times more poison then the adult one, if two snake fight and bit each other they die, it does not drink milk nor keep watch over elders treasures, it is living as he is created.

Every year in India 3,15,000 people are bitten by poisonous snakes and among them around 10,000 people die. This is not accurate, as due to lack of notification many people who die are not recorded.

In India, we have 250 types of snake but only 50 types of snake are poisonous. Among from poisonous snake most of them live in the sea. On land, we have few poisonous snakes. Dangerous to human are cobra, krait, and russel viper and saw scaled viper.

Snakes do not have hair, and is cold-blooded animal, heat is not produced in his body, so it is not able to maintain its heat and therefore it likes warm places to hide, and in extreme heat and biting cold, it is not bale to survive.

Snake lives up to 12–15 years and python lives about 32 years from known facts. Snakes are non-vegetarians, if possible regularly drinks water, but if water is not available and easily cannot find water months, it can leave without it.

Reptiles that do not possess legs are known as snakes. All snakes can swallow animals thicker than their own bodes because they have amazing jaws. Stretchy ligaments link the upper and the lower half, and the lower jaw is made up of two bones also joined by elastic tissue.

Pythons have the biggest mouths and can even get to grips with a whole goat, pig or antelope. A python will seize its prey in its mouth and then tightly coil itself round the animal's chest, not crushing it but preventing it from breathing.

The king cobra is the longest of all poisonous snakes, reaching lengths of 5–4 m that is 18 feet. It injects so much venom in a single bite that it can kill an elephant in four hours. It is one of the few snakes that make a nest; the female coils on top of their eggs until the young snakes wriggle out.

Snakes do not have eardrums and so cannot hear sounds, but they can sense vibrations such as footsteps. Cobras do not move to the rhythm of the music of the snake charmer's pipe but are probably mesmerized by its movements.

Rattlesnakes can hunt in the dark because they are very sensitive to heat. They have two small pits just beneath their eyes, which are crammed with heat sensitive nerve cells. These can detect a temperature rise of a few hundredths of a degree centigrade. The rattlesnake can very accurately locate a small animal about a meter away. It then shoots its head forward at a speed of 3 meters a second, and its huge fangs inject its victim with a dose of deadly poison. Rattlesnakes are unusual snakes because they do not lay eggs.

Sea snakes come to the surface of the sea to breath but they can then stay under water for up to eight hours. They are able to do this because most of their body is lung; it even occupies space right into the tip of the tail. Sea snakes are about ten times more poisonous than the most poisonous land snake. They are found only in tropical waters.

The golden tree snake of Malaya can leap from a tree onto its prey. Once launched it can glide for more than 25 meter that is 80 feet. While in the air it keeps its body rigid and makes it into a hollow shape, which traps air, rather like a parachute.

Saw scale viper roams around in the night, among poisonous snake it is smallest 30–80 cm long and mouth triangle shape, when angers makes hissing sound, to bit it comes front running and bites, English alphabet 8 makes and bite.

Krait moves around in the night, and found in the bricks and stones also found on the roof of the house, one and a half meter long, color black, stomach white, and stripes on body.

We in rural areas of work where so many people work in field and forest are bitten by snakes and due to timely treatment lost their precious life. Through the health education, we can teach the first aid treatment and the recognition of different types of snakes that are poisonous and non-poisonous, the sings and symptoms of its bites.

Most snakes bite only if they are provoked. Not all snakes are poisonous. Even the bite of a poisonous snake is not always dangerous, because the snake bites in its defense; little or no venom is injected. The snakes have to be identified. No anti venom is necessary if snake is non-poisonous. If it is poisonous, its type must be identified so that specific antivenin can be administered. If the snake cannot be found or identified, it should be treated as poisonous, and general antivenin should be given.

Poisonous snakes are large, has belly scales cover entire breath of the bally. Vipers large with conspicuous pit between eye and nostrils, head scales present, where as the non-poisonous are small or moderately large, but not covering the entire breadth of the bally.

Symptoms of snakebites there will be fang marks, intense pain experienced at the site of the bite of a viper. Areas gets swollen and blackened, bleeding might be seen from different places.

Client vomits, collapse and coma follows the bite of cobra or similar snakes, neurological effects are seen, e.g. giddiness, lethargy, muscular weakness spreading paralysis, breathing becomes slow and labored. Respiration ceases it or without convulsions, that is 15 minutes to two hours later.

A bite from a sea snake is felt as a sharp initial prick, which subsequently becomes painless. After 1, 2 hours, generalized muscular pain and stiffness develop starting in the neck, shoulders and hips.

Urine becomes brown in color. Respiration failure may occur. No taste in the mouth, excessive salivation, cannot open the eyelid ptosis, drowsy, asthmatic, low blood pressure, fast heart bits, bleeding form nose, mouth sometimes, swelling of lymph nodes, bleeding from the sight of bit.

Lay the client down and reassure him, as he is usually very frightened, though most often his life is not in danger. Apply a broad, form crepe bandage above the bitten area. It should allow entry of a finger. Do not loosen it periodically like a tourniquet. Immobilize the bitten limb with splints to reduce lymphatic flow and spread of the poison. Leave bandage and splint in position till medical care is available; Wash bitten area with plain water or soap. Arrange for immediate transfer to a hospital with killed snake if possible. Should unconsciousness, respiratory arrest or cardiac arrest develop, give appropriate first aid.

If the bite is at a place where crepe bandage cannot be applied wash the bitten area and make 3 mm deep cuts through each fang mark with sterile razor blade, so as to cause bleeding and drainage of the venom.

Apply suction to the wound with a pump or mouth through a thin polyethylene sheet to avoid contacts between any cuts on gums and poison. Apply ice pack locally. Keep the client still. If needed give artificial respiration, for pain tablet aspirin or painkiller can be given, Arrange for transfer to the hospital. Do not suck the blood or go to superstitious doctor where time will pass and client can die, client is kept 24 hours under observation, ASV treatment will be started, if too much blood is lost then blood transfusion to be given, antibiotics, injection tetanus toxide, special care of a unconscious client.

Blood test—usually blood clots but if blood does not clot then it could be poisonous, urine for albumin test, if naked eyes if you see blood stain urine the snake is poisonous, blood uria/creatinin test as the poison spoils kidney, ECG if snake is poisonous it will affect the heart muscles so if needed take ECG can be done.

Prevent that no snake enters in the house, walk on clear clean ground, at night walk with shoos, tourch, and keep stick.

Their are so many blind beliefs existing about the snakes years hearing from one another and pass on to the next generation. If you kill female cobra male cobra takes revenge and vice versa. Rat snake if passes in between legs of buffalo buffalo dies. Snakes head there is a peal diamond. If snake lives 100 years it gets musthas, poisonous snake while biting turns up side done then poison is emptied. Do not go to the Bhagats to remove the poison.

Save yourself from snakes bit do not keep the hips of bricks, stones, grass bundles, holes of the rates fill, fire wood keep higher than the floor, crakes of the wall fill, and keep the surrounding clean.

Household water outlet cover it with net, so that snake is not able to enter in the house, if the house is build in the field then make the wall plaster smooth, and keep the nets to the windows. Do not put hand in the dark where it is not clean. Snake gets frighten of human beings, if you see the snake just stand still, fresh dead snake do not handle with hand but with use stick and try to learn the poisonous and non-poisonous snakes difference.

Snakes too are Gods creation in the nature, so do not simply kill them when you see them in distance places it passing when they do not harm you, take personal precautions as not to get a sting by it and save and prevent yourself by right treatment.

Explanation—how to recognize the stings of poisonous snake and simple snake.

Keywords

Reptiles, pythons, king cobra, rattle snakes, sea snakes, golden sea snakes, saw scale vipers, krait.

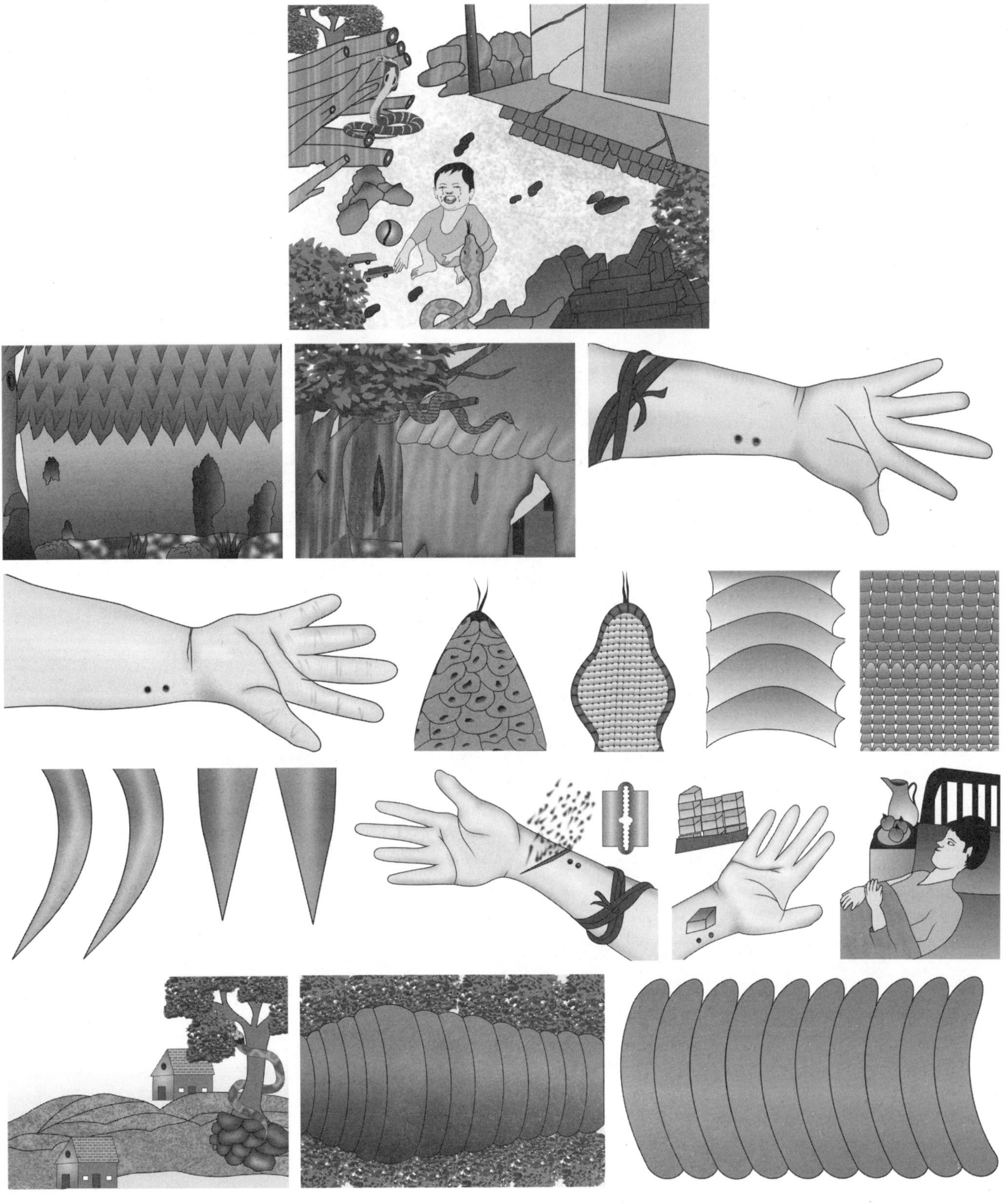

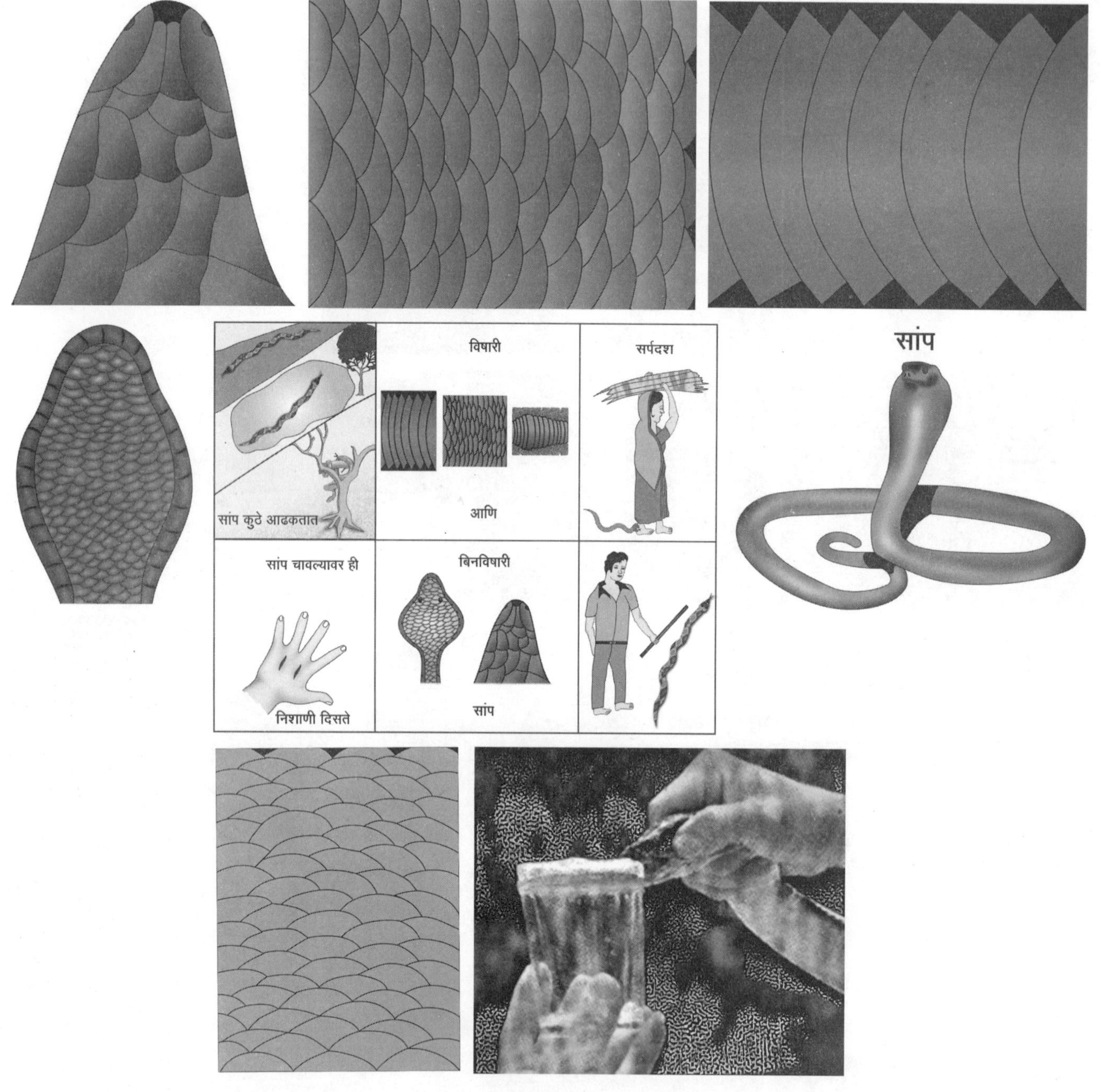
सांप
विषारी
सर्पदश
सांप कुठे आढकतात
आणि
सांप चावल्यावर ही
बिनविषारी
निशाणी दिसते
सांप

CHAPTER

60

Indigenous Medicines

INTRODUCTION

Strictly speaking, the traditional Indian medicinal system is synonymous with ayurveda. Doctors from alternative medicinal field look at the body, mind, spirit as a whole; they seek deeper cause of illness.

The basic foundation of alternative medicine is about harmony of the body, mind and spirit in order to promote health. They do not prescribe drugs or perform surgery. They believe in nature and the body's ability to heal itself. Consequently the focus is on illness prevention. Patients are counsel led in terms of required lifestyle changes that can reduce or eliminate the risk of illness.

Tibetan Yoga

When Buddhism spread through the Himalayas, it took with it yogic practice. Tibetan monk's condensed the 600 plus asanas which takes 15 minuets and results in a life time benefits. They balance the chakras and get them retaining, harmonizing the hormones. Muscles are toned, cardiovascular, respiratory digestive and nervous system are regulated, stress eliminated, concentration increased, energies flow of Prana regulates the hormones and increases the flow of CSF; as a result you sleep better and is extremely beneficial.

Message

To switch off and relax, recharge, reflect, detox and beautify is an health promoting experience. The healing power of touch therapy to slow down and de-stress, a message improves blood circulation which delivers oxygen and nutrients to the cells. It stimulates the body's waste products. It releases a hormone called serotonin that enhances as the body and minds "feel good" your mind body soul are in harmony. Easing muscles tension and cramps and relax every part of the body through deep tissue massages. Antenatal and postnatal benefits for women it can help in pain management in chronic condition such arthritis, sciatica and muscle spasms. You can remove extra pounds off your body in shape and beautify provides cellular renovation, refining pores and gives your skin uniform relief.

Heat treatment in the form of either warm dry air or warm, moist air heat the body to stimulate blood circulation, initially the purifying process.

In contras to heat treatments, **cold water** or ice applied to the body have been proven to stimulate the circulatory lymphatic and immune system.

Therapeutic mud's in either 'results' or 'serials; chambers exploiters dead skin cells, elimination of toxins and increase circulation.

Body wraps are exceptionally beneficial as a quick way to re-mineralize the body, replenish it with nutrients and elements lost on daily basis, thus boosting moisture in your skin, helping to rejuvenate and relax you.

Individuals want to look youthful and feel confident. Yoga and alternative therapies are noting new but people have begun to realize and understand the inherent benefits these things can provide to mind body and soul.

Ayurveda believes the basis of human body lays in dosha (humors that control functioning of the body), dhatu (serves types of body tissues) and mala (excretory products). Disturbances in the equilibrium of the dosha is believed to be responsible for diseases in the human body.

The **concepts of integrated medicines** use both ayurveda and allopathic often termed as mind body or holistic medicine has come long way both here and abroad. In chronic aliments where modern medicine or allopathic surrenders alternative medicines are sold to give patient hope. Prolonged intake of strong allopathic medicine could have a toxic effect; invasive therapy could lead to iatrogenic diseases or those caused by drug side effects. Alternative medicines has begun to gain acceptability in such circumstances.

Opponents say that there is little scientific research to show the success ratio of integrated approach. Imitated research or funding in integrated treatment makes it challenging to correct its actual healing power.

Go ahead and detoxify yourself—first detoxify your mind, rite it all evil thoughts and intentions. Do not harm others; some people tend to specialize in causing sorrow to others, use your faculties to fight the tendency of this negative thought, physical effect of negative thoughts. Over comes fear, afraid of what his mind projects have health fear not unfounded fears. Be self-confident and self-assertive in life. Transform ones emotions. There is higher energy residing right within us. Organize your and your receiver and connect it to the source of cosmic energy.

Vipassana—happiness seems to have become elusive for most. The constant chare for success has made us miserable. Our lives are ridden with stress and anxiety. We are always on run—chasing money, deadlines, targets and goals and overwhelmed with worry and restlessness.

Meditation offers a host of benefits—it is known to calm the agitated mind and help the mediator find peace and solace

Train mind to think healthy thoughts and lead a life free from anxiety and misery. Mind gets purified at the deeper level. You live a life you deserve to love, a life from hatred, ill will, animosity and mental unrest. Strive to live a life of love and compassion, happiness and liberation. Embark on the road to liberation from misery. Be a mental slave or a mental master, the choice is your.

A bowel of curds for a longer life, have several health benefits. It aids in smooth digestion, help insomnia, if massaged on the head will induce sleep, helps in several gastrointestinal disorders, prevents premature old age and osteoporosis, lose fat, curds is bone building food, it keeps wrinkles away.

Nimbu—lemon juice has more benefits than you ever though.

1. It has 5% citric acid, vitamin C, vitamin B, calcium, phosphorous, magnesium, proteins and carbohydrates.
2. Suffer from indigestion? Mix a few drops of lemon juice with warm water and sip on it. thus it is useful for treating nausea, heart burn, diarrhea, bloating and burping.
3. Since it is natural antiseptic, it is great to cure skin problems. It acts as anti aging agent by eliminating wrinkles, blackheads.
4. Toothache—applies fresh lemon juice in where it hurts. If bleeding gums, apply it, it stops bad breath.
5. A sore throat can be cured by gargling with lemon juice water regularly.
6. Nimbu panni controls high blood pressure, dizziness, nausea, reduces stress.
7. It also cures respiratory disorders like breathlessness and asthma.

Music—cleanses the soul; prayers coming from a pure heart can actually change the destiny

Kiwi fruit—this hairy, light brown fruit (Chinese gooseberry) when cut into half, looks very appealing because of its bright green color and a circle of black sesame like seeds in the center. Used in fresh cakes, fruit salad and other types of desserts. It is rich in vitamin, minerals ad falconoid, high amount of vitamin C, potassium, beta carotene, prevents asthma, wheezing and coughing specially in children, protects our DNA from mutations, provides a healthy amount of anti oxidants and vitamins. Consuming in daily diet is beneficial for maintaining healthy skin. It contains an enzyme that reacts chemically to break down proteins, contains lysine which helps in prevention of muscular degeneration or weakening on ones eye sights, glaucoma and cataract due to to aging. Having intake once daily diet helps to improve the cardio vascular health, prevents accumulation of deposits and plaques on the walls of the arteries

Jackfruit—nutrition facts

1. A 100g serving of ripe, cut and peeled fruit contains-energy-94 kcal, carbohydrates 24 g, protein 1.47 g, fat 0 mg, cholesterol 0 mg, dietary fibers 1.6 g.
2. It is a good source of vitamin C and antioxidants that helps strengthening of the immune system and enhancing the functioning of the WBC in the body. It is a good source of potassium regulates. Potassium helps to maintain the electrolyte balance in the body.
3. High fiber content—beneficial in reducing constipation and adding digestion. It said that it can do away with the carcinogenic chemicals in the colon. It slows down degeneration of cells. Healthy skin and vision.
4. Nature sugar like sucrose, fructose make good source of energy and easily digestible, it contains minerals like manganese, iron, vitamin B6, niacin, folic acid etc.
5. Required for optimum functioning of the body. Seeds are nutritious and good source of proteins.

Jaggery—unlike sugar, jiggery is a good source of iron and other mineral salts. In order to reduce anemia, eat one teaspoon jiggery daily. It aids digestion; therefore after a heavy meal one teaspoon will activate the digestion enzymes which speed up the process of digestion. It contains cleansing properties. Eating helps in relieve constipation.

Khatti mithi imli

1. Tamarind juice is a mild laxative.
2. It can be used to teat bile disorders.
3. Studies have shown that is can effectively cut on cholesterol levels.
4. The pulp leaves and flowers in various combinations are applied on painful and swollen joints.
5. Tamarind is used as a gargle for soar throat, and as a drink for relief from stroke.
6. The heated juice used to cure conjunctivitis. Eye drops made from tamarind seeds may be a treatment for dry eye syndrome. Its seed polysac chained is adhesive, enabling it to stick to the surface of the eye longer than other eye preparation.
7. It reduces fever and provides protection against colds. A home remedy suggest, make an infusion by talking one ounce of pulp, pour one quart of boiling water over this and allow it to sit for an hour. Strain drink it with little honey to sweeten, this will bring down the temperature several degree.
8. It helps the body to digest food better.
9. It applied to the skin can heal inflammatory problems.

High soy intake reduces risk of breast cancer. This soy intake during adolescence reduces the risk of breast cancer in pre-menopausal years by about 25–50% soy protein is a high quantity protein equivalent to the protein quality of egg, milk or meat, soybean that is functional food with complete protein package and containing essential amino acids that are required by the body.

Oats—contain soluble fiber called beta glucan which is known to help in reducing cholesterol by blocking of re-absorption of cholesterol when it passes through the digestive system.

Regularly having oats lowers the cholesterol level in body. Oats contains low level of sodium. This reduces risk of hypertension.

The soluble fiber presents in oats tends to slow down to digestion of carbohydrate thereby reducing the spikes in the blood sugar levels, makes you much fuller, good for these trying weight reduce. It contains less amount of fat and lesser calories, good fiber reduce constipation. It is also known to contain compounds called phyto chemicals that ca reduce ones risks of cancer.

Fast—to fast to abstain from something that gives us pleasure and enjoyment, it is a way to spiritual fitness; it helps develop self-discipline to transcend sensual and physical gratification. Fasting is fuel for soul that ignites faith. Fasting has a social significance. In India it is rural women who fast more than men. They seem to gain tremendous inner strength and power to overcome suffering, alleviate the pain of others and thereby become life givers. True fasting will remind us of the bounty we enjoy on a daily basis, and sensitize us to the reality of force hunger too of people in our planet g through day after day.

Telemedicine—is the use of electronic information and communication technologies to provide health care irrespective of physical proximity between doctors and patient.

Such as facility required software to enhance doctors pt communication, high resolution cameras, as well as video conferencing facilities. The cost of setting up one such centre can range from Rs. 60.000 to several crores depending on the technology installed.

Pan African E-network project-funded by Indian government as Rs. 1.200 crores. Eleven super specialty hospitals from India will reach out to 53 nations across Africa.

India will provide online medical consultation to each country for a specified number of hours daily. Advice will be given to 5 patients per day per country. 10,000 African students will be able to work with 7 universities in disciplines such as medicine, cardiology, neurology, oncology disease, etc.

There are 31 telemedicine centers set up under the NRHM at district hospital. Each centre has an ECG scanner, satellites connections. Whenever a district hospital is faced with a complicated case, doctors can consult their urban counterparts and specialists, consulting doctor's examination patients medical history and advice accordingly.

Chinese abdominal massage—release tension and relieve energies through message. This is one message technique that leaves you not only relaxed from outside, but rejuvenates from deep within. You have to be frees from daily stress of life. It is holistic adopted by Taoist Chinese—by working only on stomach area and manipulating the internal organs with soft, gentle but deep and soothing strokes, the therapist releases patient's mental and emotional tension. It is very true that the body's natural ability to heal itself is real. It last 40 minutes incorporated with reflexology points of foot. Tension, stagnation, toxins, spasms, bloating accumulation fat.

Yoga should be practiced with firm determination and perseverance, without any mental reservation or doubts. Yoga teaches us to cure what need noble endured and endure what cannot be cured. The word yoga literally means to join up, or to yoke together. What were trying to join together in yoga is body, mind and spirit.

Get the glow with yoga—yoga can help one slow the aging process. Practicing yoga can raise your metabolic rate, which helps in achieving ideal body weight. It is not enough to be slim, toning and strengthening of the muscles make the body firm and supple. This makes you fit and youthful. Real cleansing or detoxification happens from the inside. Powerful yogic techniques clean out the entire system from inside out. Yoga also provides nutrition at the cellular level and helps optimize the functioning of the endocrinal system, thereby reducing stress levels considerably. All this results in glowing skin.

Stress and pollution causes deterioration of the body resulting in aging, yoga, asana, pranayama helps improve blood circulation detoxify the body ad restore proper functioning of the body consequently slowing down ageing.

It is like Katha-Vartha, Prabhat Pheries, songs and drams have roots in our culture.

Health messages can be carried through these media.

Home remedies

Irritated by black heads

1. Make a paste of fresh Methi leaves and apply it on your face for 10–12 minutes every night. It dries the oil from the blackhead reducing the swelling around it
2. Grind reddish seeds with water to form a thin consistent paste. Scrub it gently on your face, this help blackhead removing completely
3. Orange peels can be ground with water to form a thick paste. Apply and leave it over night on the affected area
4. Mix mint juice with haldi powder and apply to affected areas, keep it on for 30 minutes and wash off with lukewarm water.
5. Put a small bit of toothpaste on the blackheads, if dries them cut.
6. Beat an egg white and add 2 teaspoon of fresh honey to it. Apply the mixture on your face and let it dry for 20–30 minutes. Rinse it off with warm water
7. To sooth backache, rub garlic oil and take a warm bath 3 hours later. To make the solution, fry 10 cloves in 60 ml of mustard oil till it turns brown.

Complementary therapies:

1. Psychotherapy
2. Physical exercise

3. Massage therapy
4. Light/phototherapy
5. Meditation and yoga
6. Relaxation technique and visualization
7. Counseling
8. Family and marital therapy
9. Milieu, hypnotherapy
10. Bio-feedback
11. Herbal and nutritional therapy
12. Acupuncture
13. Therapeutic touch
14. Aroma therapy—using essential oils extracted from plants for therapeutic effect. It can be used as room perfumes for inhalation; the oils can also be absorbed through the skin when added to vegetables oils for message, dropped in a bath tub. It helps to reduce stress, anxiety and depression
15. Autogenic training—a psycho physiologic form of psychotherapy, in which the patient carries out himself by using passive concentration upon certain combinations of psycho physiologically, adapted verbal stimuli. Humor and laughter therapy amusing interventions used by health care professional or patient to produce a beneficial response in short/long yet reduces anxiety, relief hostility, aggression, provides deep relaxation and influences hopefulness
16. Reflexology—is potentially a valuable therapeutic nursing skill and could have cost effective benefits in health care. It is a treatment which applies in health care. It is treatment which applies verifying degree of pressure to different parts of body usually the hands and feet in order to health and well-being. General pressure is thought to facilitate the breakdown and elimination of crystalline deposits—if calcium and uric acid on the nerve endings of the feet. All systems and organs of the surface of the skin, in particular on to the hands and feet. Thus, by applying gentle pressure to these areas it is possible to effect a change in another part of the body in order to promote well being relaxation.
17. Home an herbal medicines
18. Hydrotherapy
19. Magnetotherapy
20. Homeopathy and bio-cemetery
21. 12 salt therapy
22. Drugless alternative system of medicine

Conclusion—indigenous systems of medicine are known by such names as traditional medicine, alternative medicine and complimentary medicine. Is of medicine is the name applied to healing philosophy approach and therapy outside the institutions where scientific medicine is taught. Many of the modalities employed by the indigenous system of medicine and they are not scientifically tested able. The Indian system of medicine practitioner treats the whole patient rather than the diseases structure/organ/system. The diagnosis and treatment are individualized. Number of patients receives the same treatment even if they have the same clinical features. A spiritual element is often incorporated in indigenous system of therapies. The practitioner believes in the same values, spiritual philosophy and religious belief as the system is less authority and more approachable than all allopathic doctors and cost is less than allopathic, danger is it may of may not be safe. Many of them contain harmful ingredients such as arsenic, lead, mercury and corticosteroids.

Explanation—many different Indian medical plants figures given for students to recognize and understand how home and herbal medicines are used and grow in India.

Keywords

Tibetan yoga, message, heat treatment, mud, wraps, vipasana, music, detoxification, nutritional facts, abdominal message, yoga, fast, telemedicine, home remedies.

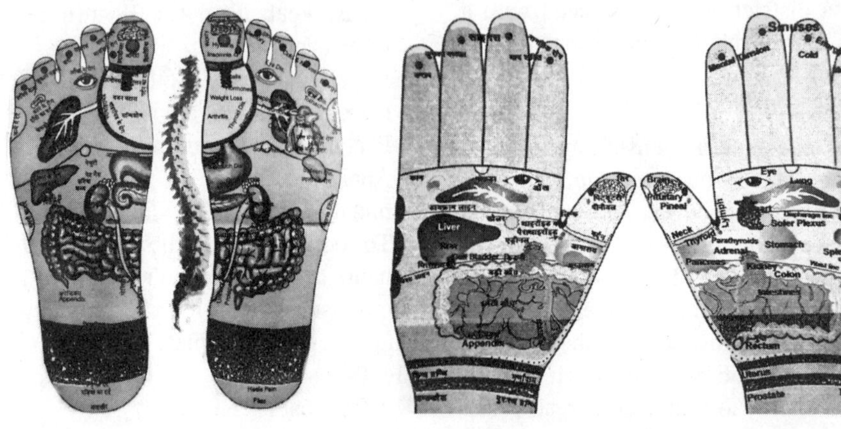

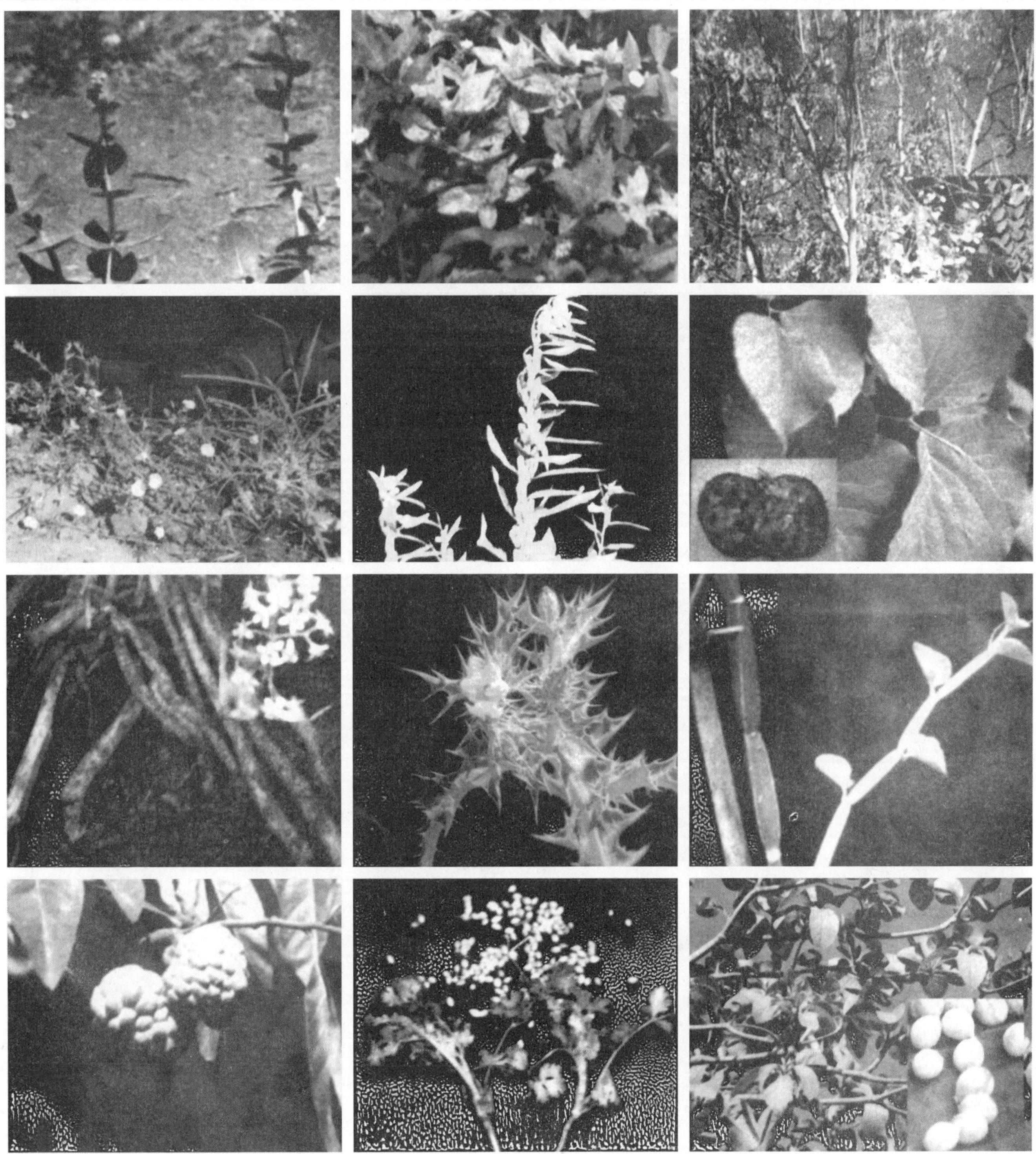

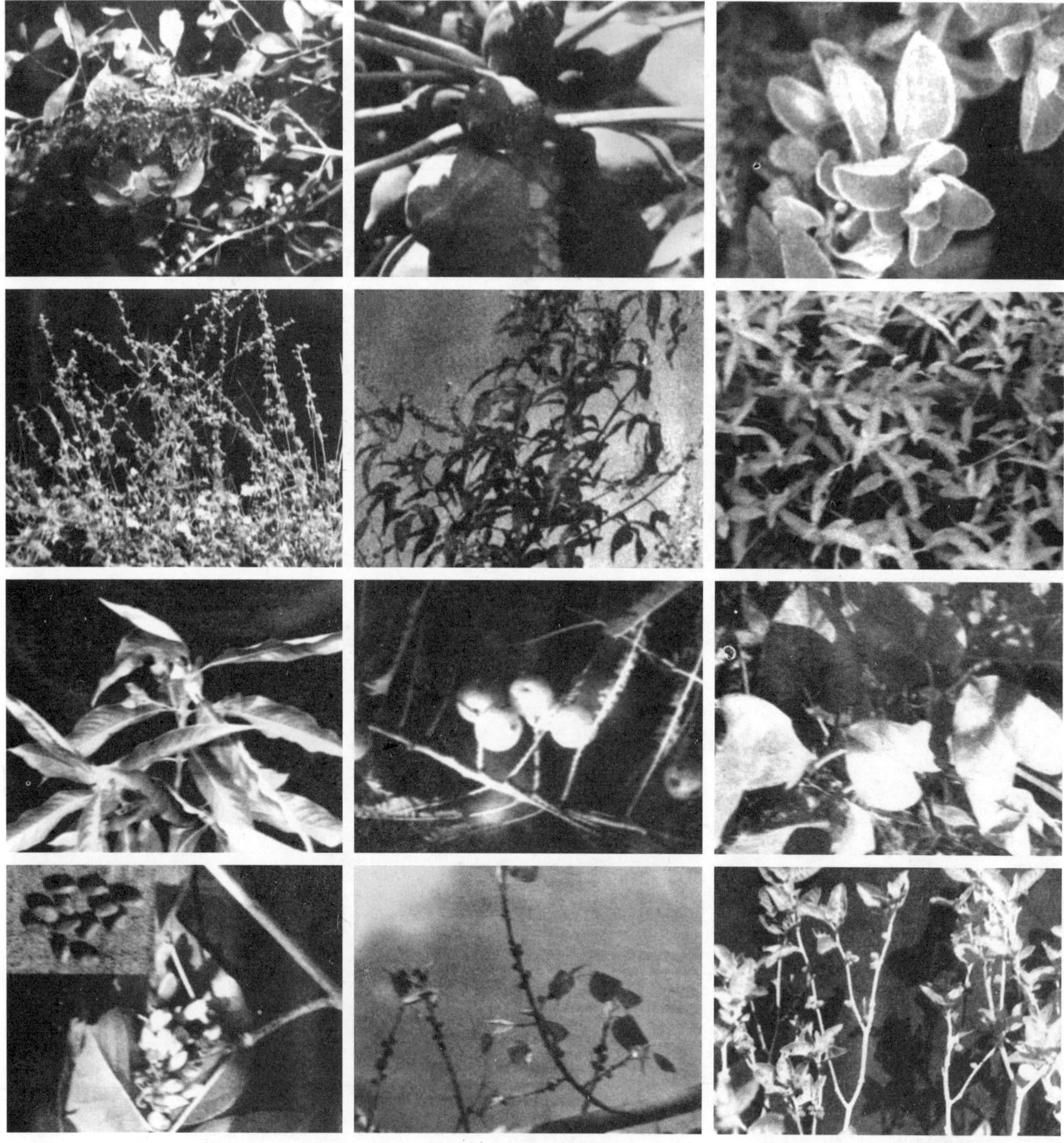

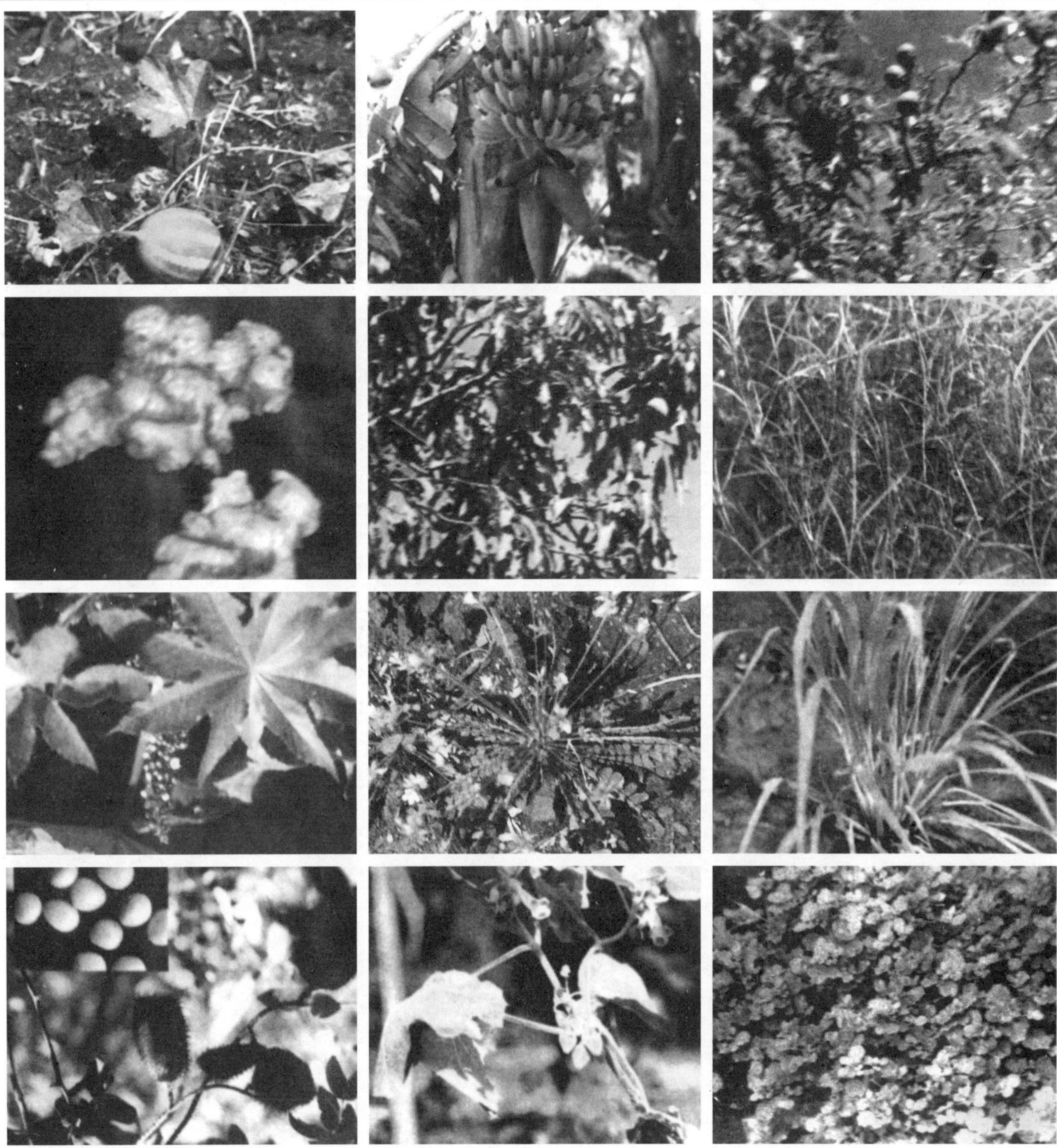

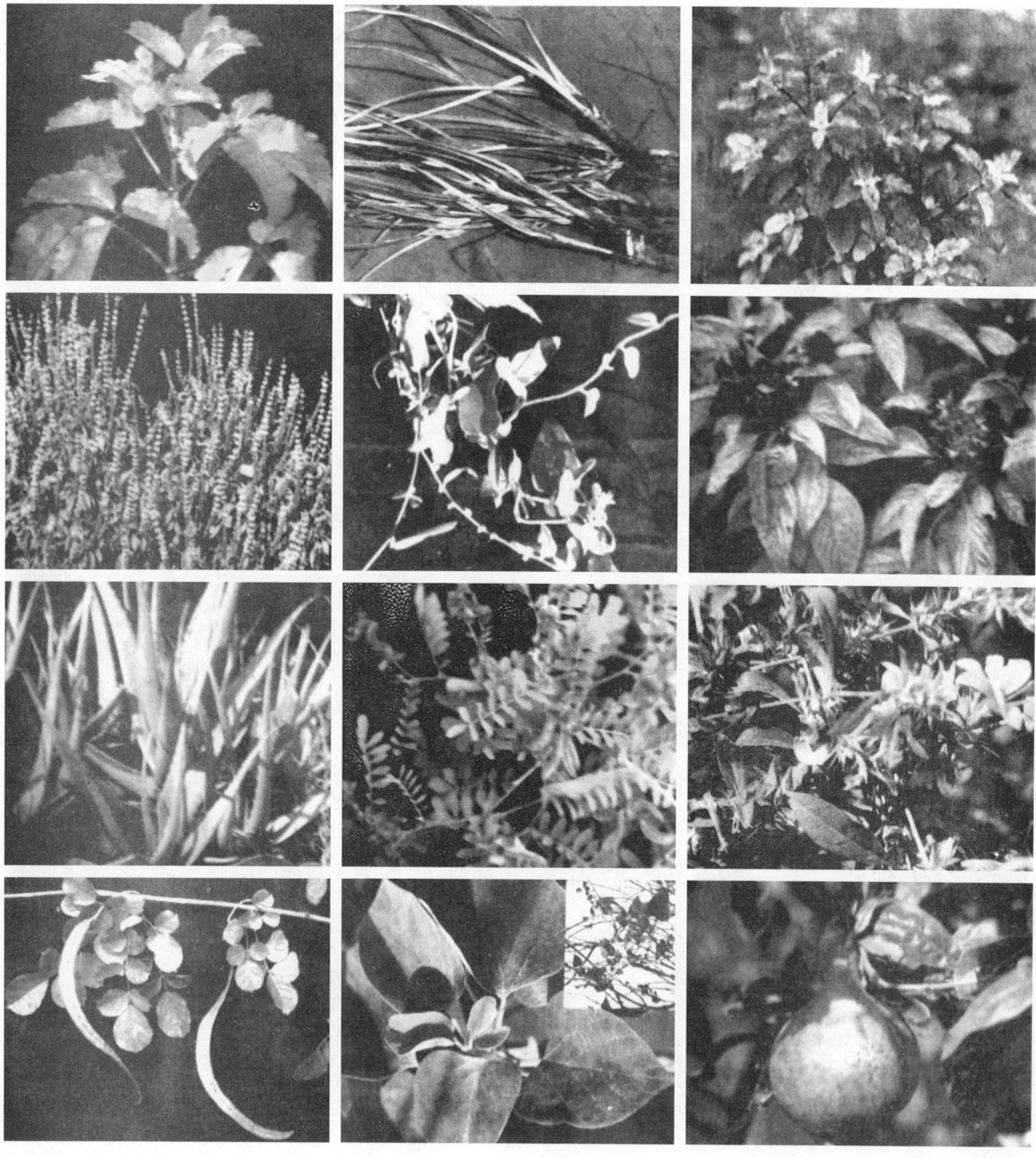

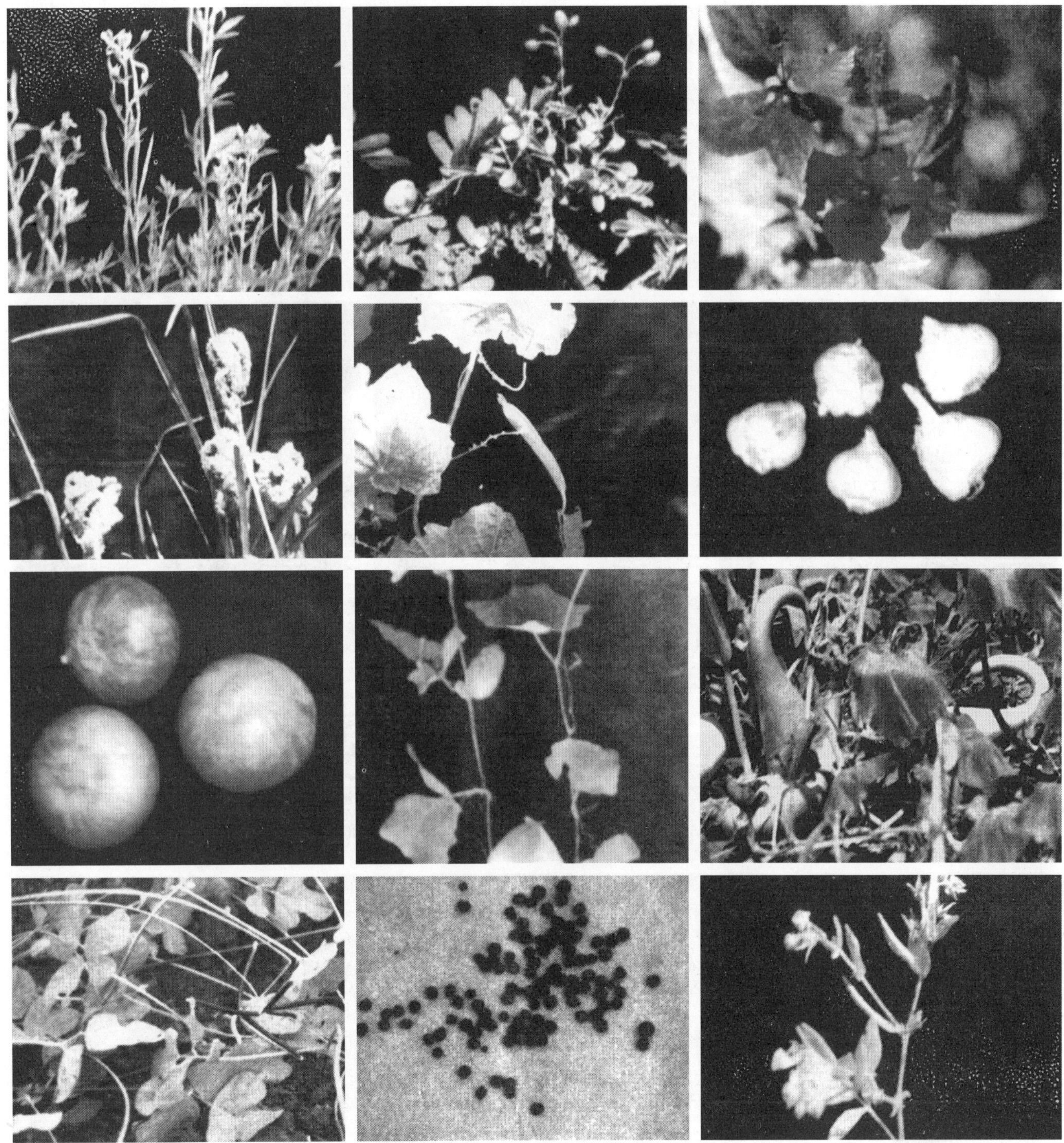

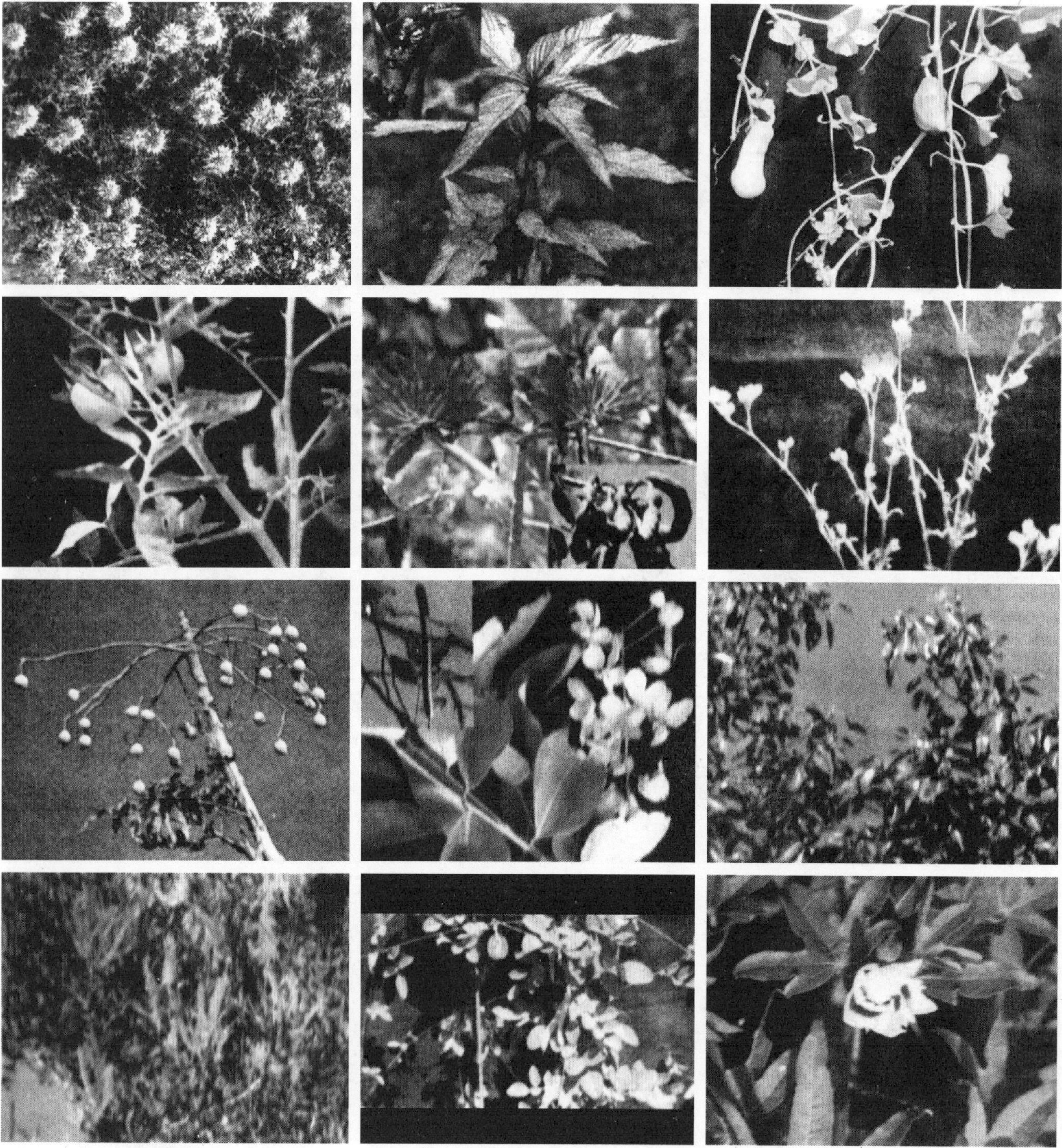

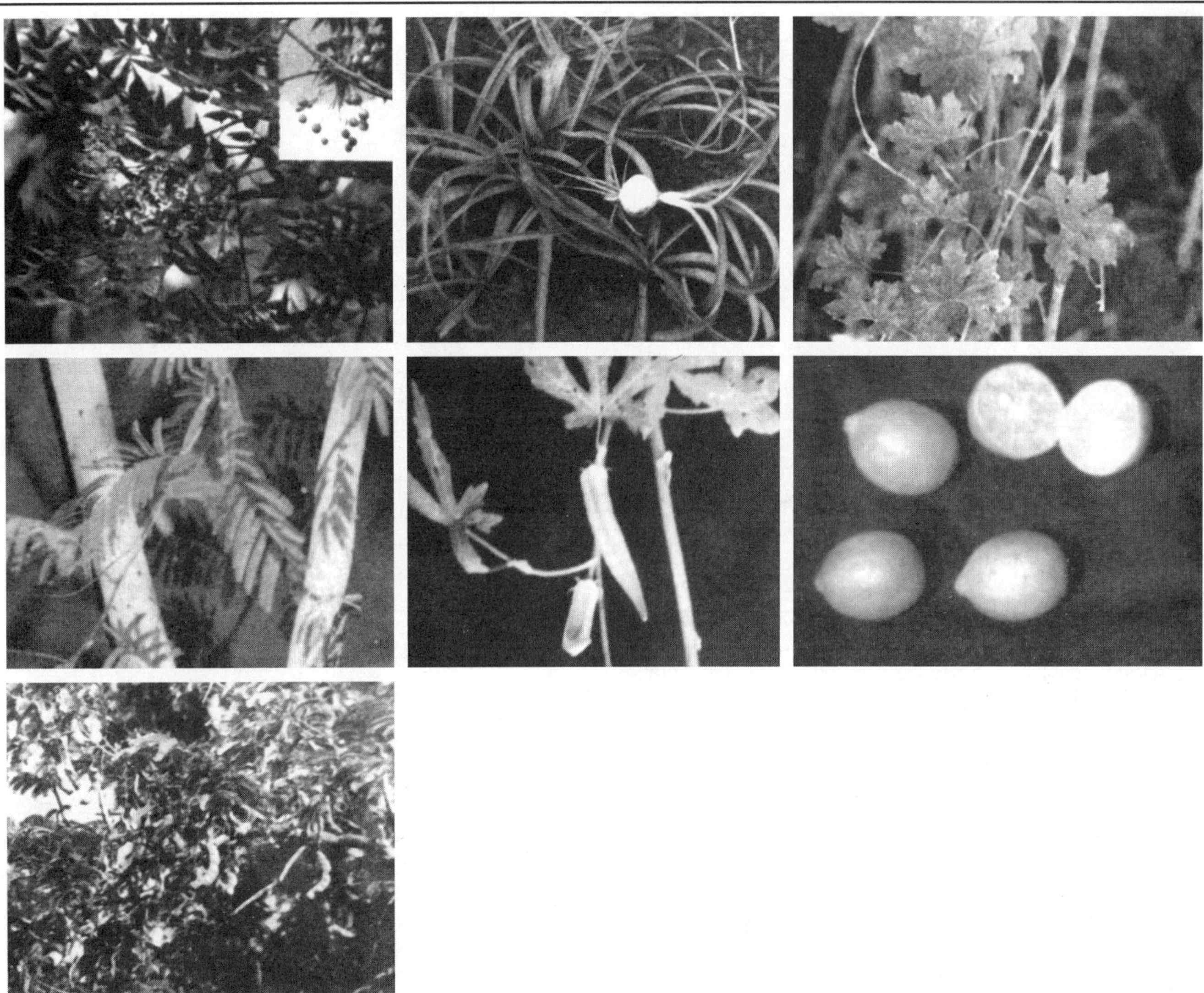

CHAPTER

61

Invisible India

MOBILIZING THE OTHER INDIA

Looking back looking ahead

- Is a person more than a bio-physiological system?
- Is health more than the absence of diseases symptoms?
- Is health solely the result of the interaction between host-agent and environment?
- Is health the ability of an individual to perform work?
- Are health and wellness same? Are diseases and illness different? Are there levels of health?
- Do you realize that India has the world's largest constituency of invisible people? They are in hundreds of millions, yet no one notices them. They are a blind spot for us. They have voter IDS, some have PAN cards, cell phones, banks have opened accounts, ATMs in remote areas, despite all this, they remain the lost children of this republic. Most of them are young, unemployed, others are old unemployable. They are all part of an Indian that has been left behind. No, they do not make that choice, they do not belong to the mainstream, they are not part of technology revolution, and cell phones are not a substitute for electricity and drinking water.

They have not heard of the economic reform nor benefited from them. They do not even know that the India they live in is one of the fastest growing economies in the world. They won't believe if you told them, for it has not made the slightest difference to their lives. They would not know to count cores. They have not heard of common wealth games, housing scam. Justice is simply not affordable so they live their lives without any expectations. They may not know the President of India, they cannot name cabinet minister, most of them are poor, so poor that it may perhaps will embarrass you to know; to the extend of poverty. Sixty-five percent go hungry, 75% have no access to health care.

Our drives shoo them away, cops pick them up and throw them out, and they embarrass us by just being there. We wish they would disappear, we ignore them. Schemes do not reach them. The money vanishes long before it can reach them. What is worse, no one cares. That is what makes it easy to steal there funds. The urban poor are even worse off, no one cares, no one event wants to help them as they are labeled as unwanted migrants.

They are from same country, driven by poverty and loss of their land. They are the unwanted insiders whom we want to hide from the world, as well as from ourselves. We are ashamed of our poor. They remind us of our failures, we want to talk to the world today about our ambitions, space programme, our nuclear expertise, our defense, capabilities, our economic power, our IT genius, the amazing steps we have taken in biotech.

We want to boast that 4 of our top 10 richest men in the world are Indians. For if we keep ignoring them forever. There is limit to which people will tolerate the indifference of their government.

The nameless, faceless, roofless fellowman of our country.

There is another India with which many of us have only a passing acquaintance. It is an India of the several hundreds million people who barely make a few rupees a day. They live without a roof over their head and die without medical treatment. They cannot write or spell their names.

It is time we gave the other India hope of a better life, not just because it is right thing to do, but also, because, if we do not our India would not grow and prosper in long run.

Can the one eye weep while the other sleeps? To wipe every tears from every eye will take time, but let us start today with one at a time.

Bible says 'what so ever you do unto this little one you do unto me' give food to the hunger, water to the thirsty, aid to ailing, visit to the lonely.

Blessed are the poor, the kingdom of God is theirs. Be pure of heart, be merciful and compassionate. Beget love not hate, you shall see God. Because they are the burning bush of the author and creator of this universe.

Remove your saddles before poor, because God resides in them. You are called to set them free, all bonded and mend their broken bodes. That is your nursing profession. Fullness of life as fullness proceeds fullness. As Bible says God has come to give life that is in abundance.

Love is enough enkindle them. Give that smile and healing touch as you pass by this world you may not get chance again

No historic transformation can occur with only gains and no losses. There is other India, the India of the small farmers, of tribal clinging to their disappearing forests, landless Dalits living in the shadow of the upper caste, atrocities. It is another world, untouched by globalization. Today global competition and insatiable hunger for profits are driving globalize India into a headlong collision with this other India.

We do not need rocket science, to see the underlying arithmetic mobilization of the other India within the democratic space is probably the single greatest political change of out times. India also marks the dividing line between the politic of violence the path of non violence.

Today when we are engulfed by the dark forces of corruption, consumerism and careenage in our country, need our nation to freedom from the bondage of oppression of evil

What is our contribution towards corruption? Are we not equally responsible for the situation we find ourselves in today? We are on the shortcuts and find ways to hoodwink the law.

What is India?

1. A nation where pizza reaches home faster than an ambulance or the police.
2. Where we get car loan at 5% but education loan at 12%.
3. Where people worship Durga, but want to rape and kill their daughters.

The last survey conducted by the health ministry-reveals that:

1. There is a short fall of over 20,500 sub-centers and 4,500 PHCs;
2. 2,135 community health centers
3. There is short fall of over 12,000 specialists' surgeon, gynecologist, pediatrics and physicians even at CHC level;
4. About 10% PHCs have no doctors; lab technetium's making impossible doctors to make any investigations and forcing the patient to get tests done in private labs;
5. Almost a 3rd of sub-centers and 10% of PHCs have no electricity or water;
6. 70,000 deaths/year=maternal
7. 30% hemorrhage and excessive bleeding;
8. 16% sepsis and infections;
9. Despite JSY= 47% Institutional delivery 5% assisted by skilled health personnel and coverage of JSY is 13%;
10. 17.26 L/children die IMR 50/1000;
11. 54% children fully immunized,
12. 34% receive ORT.

Poor facilities and rising cost of healthcare even at govt. hospital are pushing people towards more expensive private setups; large sections are bankrupted or go without treatment. Mobilizing local communities to demand better services from public health facilities have been found to be successful in ensuring better services delivery and improved accountability.

Crippling Numbers

Vulnerability factor

1. Married women aged 15–49—56% ½ who are anemic
2. MMR 230 deaths/1,00,000 live births
3. Institutional delivery 47%
4. Malnourished children 46%
5. Children 6–35 months anemic 79%
6. IMR 50 death ga/1,000 live births
7. Children 12–13 months fully immunized 54%.

Expenditure on Health

1. 1950–1951 = 0.22% GDP
2. 1960–1961 = 6.63% GDP
3. 1970–1971 = 0.74% GDP
4. 1980–1981 = 0.91 % GDP
5. 1990–1991 = 0.96 5 GDP
6. 2000–2001 = 0.9% GDP
7. 2009–2010 = 1.09% GDP

Looking back looking ahead—India has witnessed a remarkable transformation in the last 100 years from being a much exploited part of the British empire to an emerge global powers. From a poor nation ravaged by a bloody partition and four wars, to one of the fastest growing economies from a land of snake charmers to an IT superpower whose talent runs the computers of the world's largest corporation? Every ending is a new beginning, as the years pass, all we need to achieve is in the beginning ready to rediscover, our very existence, the essence of our being, our soul, out heart, our previous breath, this precious moments. No body can go back and stat a new beginning, but everyone can start today and make a new ending.

Shoulder responsibility—Most of the health problems are preventable or controllable if anticipated, recognized and treated early.

Indian companies are now targeting rural India with a variety of innovative and cost effective tech solutions that attempt to solve to everyday problems in our remotest villages

Indians hunger for new technology is as sharp in its countless small villages as in its shiny office towers or shopping malls and business are walking up n area of massive potential growth.

Specific include being aimed at Indian villages include a mobile phone cash transfer systems, robust low energy refrigerators and a clever twist on the humble kitchen stove cash transfer to family has become easy.

Solar batteries powered ATM also heralding a technological revolution in rural communities has overcome power cut shortage. Villagers are not affluent but they do have money. What they do not have is way to have money.

You learn more from your mistakes than from your triumphs. Walk a path and leave imprint.

Today the private sector accounts for 80% of persons expenses on health inadequate funding of public health and consequence deteriorate in the share of public health expenditure.

ICDS—hunger kills—46% of infants are malnourished,49% of women anemic

ICDS now the world's largest infant feeding programme is doing on the ground, **Anganwadi** without drinking water, without toilet, staff shortage. Thousand of cores of rupees ca spent on these schemes every year. Food is a daily needy you can not skip nutrition for a week and resume, inadequate nutrients at early age has permanently impaired physical and mental capabilities it is like nut and bolts.

Malnutrition kills 56,000 children annually in urban slums. What is the reason for the frequency in deaths from malnutrition in Mumbai? These deaths occurred in the community of a rag pickers that live on garbage dump. If they do not spend their day sorting out and selling garbage, they can not eat. The women are anemic, their children are born under weight and often do not survive beyond 2 months. Among those that do, their nutritional status keeps going down because they live only on breast milk. Whenever communities exist in such condition with no access to electricity, clean water and sanitation, malnutrition and related diseases exists.

Want a ration card—pay a cop, want a passport, illegal water connection, want electricity line, pay a bribe and get connected. India's problem will get worse—there will be no peace until there is justice. And there will be no justice till the honest are allowed to live honestly.

1. It is estimated 70 million people with disabilities in India
2. Almost 95% have no axes to education or employment opportunities
3. That is the equivalent of denying education or employment to the population 52% of the disabled over 36 million are illiterate
4. Despite 1995 legislation that secures the rights of the disabled. India is accused of having welfare based approach rather than a right based approach to the whole problem
5. Of the 70 million Indians with disabilities 95% have no access to education or employment. The problem lies with the welfare based approach of the goverment.

India on Sick Bed

1. Public spending on health 0.94% of GDP among lowest in the world
2. Indians have to pay 80% of their medical expenses from their pockets
3. 74% of this expenditure incurred for out pt treatment, not hospital care
4. Drugs accounted for 72% of the total private out of pocket expenditure
5. 30 mm Indians pushed into poverty from ill health every year
6. 30% rural Indians do not go for treatment for financial reasons
7. 47% of hospital admissions in rural India and 31% in urban India fiancé by loans and the sale asset.

2010 research shows that millions of Indian population still face hunger despite the growth.

Hunger continuous to stalk over 300 million citizens.

India slipped to 67th the place among 122 countries in the global hunger.

NREGA—plug the hole in the bucket poorly designed welfare program make goverment throw good money after bad. If public funded welfare program well designed they will be more effective in reaching the poor and leak less. Monitoring evaluation and re-designs program is must. All that happens is hat the names of welfare program change when a new government come to power—with very little fundamental in programme design. 2005 NEREGA was well-designed programme that the reached the self targeted beneficiaries, minimize leakage and has had a major impact. There is a need for program to be monitored well using an online publicity available data to minimize-provide feedback online publicity MIS management information system. The speed with which the data reaches the ministry from block levels.

Nurses must be able to grow and evolve in order to meet the demands of a dramatically changing health care system. The goal of nursing education is to prepare today's nurses to meet the challenges of tomorrow. Nursing knowledge is a fusion of theoretical, practical, self, ethical knowledge. Nurses must become increasingly futuristic in developing roles and responsibilities. They need to be equipped for success.

Nursing practice—taken place in many forms and in many different settings. The knowledge explosion has let some to specialize their roles in various fields. These factors have added complexity to describing the role of a nurse. The practicing professional nurses work continually to re define an refine ideas about the nursing role. Role conflict occurs when she is expected to perform two or more incompatible roles in given time. She must learn to set priority and can effectively budget time. Her role like advisor, caregiver, educator, good observer, leader, planner and manager.

Public health—it is science and are of preventing diseases, prolonging life and promoting health and efficiency through organized community efforts for the sanitation of the environment, the control of communicable infections, the education of individual in personal hygiene, the organization of medical nursing services for early diagnosis and preventive treatment of diseases and the developing of social machinery to ensure for every individual a standard of living adequately for the maintenance of health, so organizing these benefits as to enable every citizens to realize the birth right of health and longevity.

How and whom the health-care services would be provided—health is influenced by a number of factors, such as adequate food, housing, basic sanitation, protection from environmental hazards and communicable diseases. Health care implies more than medical care. It embraces multifactor services provided to individual or community for the purpose of promoting, maintaining, monitoring and restoring health. Health care is a public right and it is the responsibility of govt. To provide this care to all people in equal measures. Health services should be organized to meet the needs of entire population and not merely selected groups. It is realized the needs of vast majority or deserved poor rural and urban people should be supported by appropriate referral system. Provide primary care that is close to the people where most of their health problems can be dealt and resolved. More complex problems could be dealt in district hospitals and the others to specific facilities and attention of highly specialized dealt with The purpose of health care services is to improve the health status of the public. The parameters should be food production, reduced poverty, increased education and employment, improve sanitation, stabilize population, and improve quality and standards of life, etc.

Getting the basics rights—universal health coverage proposal may become reality as early as the best five year plan. When it is implemented this measure will reduce private health expenditure across categories, especially from the high middle clan down to the poorest. This will have a better run. The very poor are nearly always mute spectators of a process outside their control.

When we went door to door and house to house visits we found many laborers were migrated from different parts in search of job where they stay abut six months in open fields. You can see in pictures they are preparing hand bread in cold winter or in hot sun scourging in the afternoon. They come along with full family along with animals too. Children do not go to school as no one remains at home to feed and take care of them. They play in mud and live very unhygienic surroundings. They word very hard to get hand to mouth food. They are making brinks whole life but never have they had their own house to live life through.

Health statistics in India are grim beyond belief. About half of the admissions in rural hospital are paid for with borrowed money. Little less then a third of the sick in rural India do not seek medical help at all because they cannot afford it. Public hospital, the services are poor. Roughly 71% of the sick go to private health providers. The planning commission has provided the compass, but politics must have the strength to undertake the journey.

Poverty line—is required because we need to compare their relative numbers, which states are reducing poverty at what rate. Forty-one crore people are BPL today, living a sub-human existence. Because govt. Schemes are not working. In the cities the poorest are those sleeping on the road. The government does not give them ration cards; it says you do not have an address. We have anti-poor municipalities and police. They want to get rid of the poor, not the poverty.

Food safety and standards ACT 2006 has established Food Safety and Standards Authority of India (FSSA) under administrative control of minister of health and family welfare govt. of India regulates their manufacture, storage, distribution, safe and import to ensure availability of safe and wholesome food for human consumption.

The cabinet clearing the food security bill takes India a step closer to introducing a major welfare scheme. Extending subsidized food to will benefit the poor across the social board, covering 50% of the urban and 75% of rural population. BPL family identification of beneficiaries ought to be linked to the adhered project.

Government claims the scheme will need 61 million tones grain which is higher than the 56 million tones estimated. While the maximum grain produced in a single year is 57 million tones, may need to buy costly import of grain if production falls. Apart from hugh funds needed to increasing agricultural production or to build storage space. Therefore need to prepare the ground before launching food security plan, to clear the bill.

Some Hope for Indian Hungry

1. For priority group B PL—7 kg grain/month/person—rice at rupees 3/kg, wheat at rupees 2/kg and coarse grain at rupees 1/kg.
2. For general group—3 kg/person/month at half of minimum support price given to farmers.
3. Beneficiaries under priority group—minimum 46% of rural population and 28% of urban population.
4. Meals for vulnerable communities—mid-day meal scheme and I C DS, brought under bill, other schemes to be made legal entitlements.
5. Total fiscal bill rupees 1.5 lack crore roughly concluding states to share.
6. Existing nutrition and selected social security scheme would also be brought under the legislation as an entitlement.

Global hub

1. India should ride on this advantage and open its **education sector** to foreign investors. India can involve both public and private partners especially at college and university levels and attract foreign investors. We need to imbibe a flexible approach in choosing our streams at the college level, like the west to tap foreign talent.
2. **Medical tourism**—inexpensive medical facilities coupled with talented doctors make India a viable option in near future, as it is already doing well in this area, we need to keep the momentum going and not compromise on quality to keep that tempo intact. It important for Indian medical fraternity to keep itself updated.
3. **Service industry**—apart from IT industry that has led the nation in the global market, telecom is one sector where

India can become a major player with mobile levels across the country. We bring about positive change will have far reaching effects.

4. **Ayurveda and yoga**—a country that gave birth to yoga and Ayurveda is fighting to keep its own child in its own fold. India should make an attempt to encourage its education in school level so as to get popular years to come and foreigners come to India.

The age of urbanization—India is facing an unprecedented scale of urbanization with 700 million people likely to move to cities by 2050. To plan, develop and to build a new India which is ecologically and economically sustainable. Urbanization is accompanied by unprecedented consumption of natural resources; cities occupy 3% of the earths land surface use 75% of the resources and accounts 2/3rd of all energy and greenhouse gas emission. Hoe India manages its urbanization is coming decades will determine its future. This requires political leadership, vision, capacity building and institutional reforms to make tomorrow smile.

The future of any nation lives in the hands of its people. And it is the people from the rural hinterland who are actual backbone and drivers of the development of any country.

Explanation—pictures showing Incredible India and its people and how India still lives in villages. It also shows where we are in this 21st century with ultra modern life style at one side and at the same time other world where people live hand to mouth. How in technological world they still far behind primitive ways living even today.

Keywords

Mobilizing, vulnerability, expenditure, survey, responsibilities, malnutrition, sick bed, ICDS, food safety, NREGA, hunger, statistics, global hub.

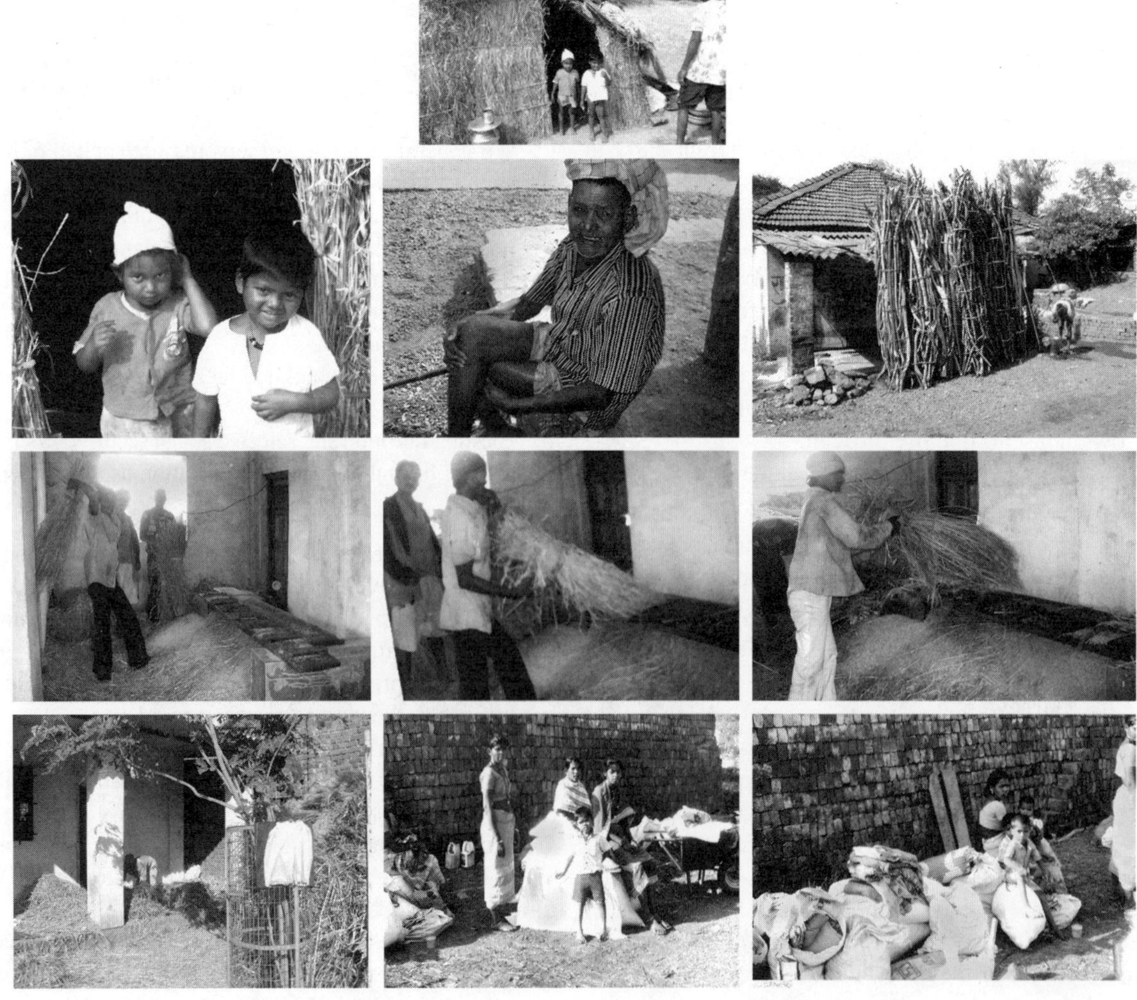

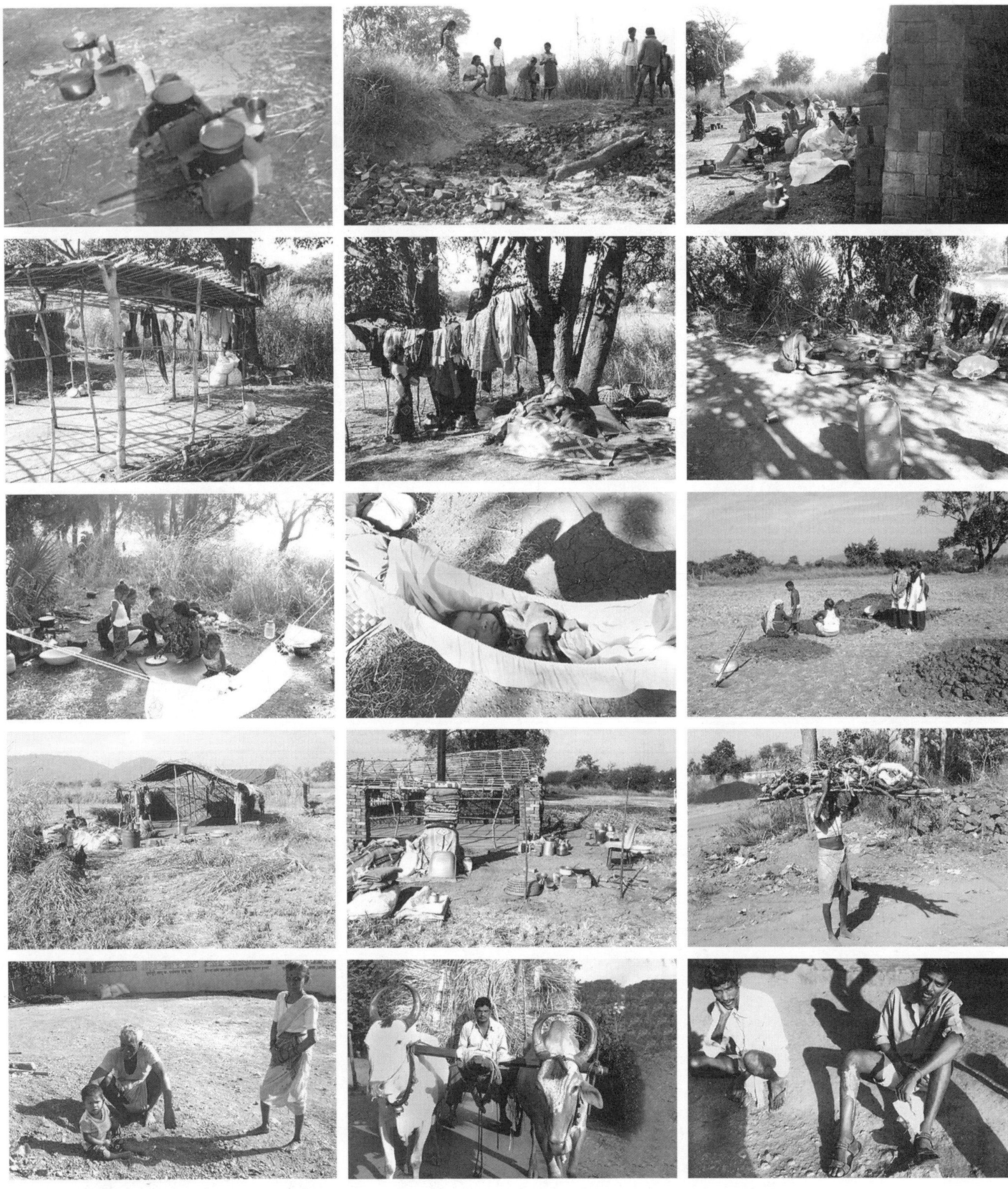

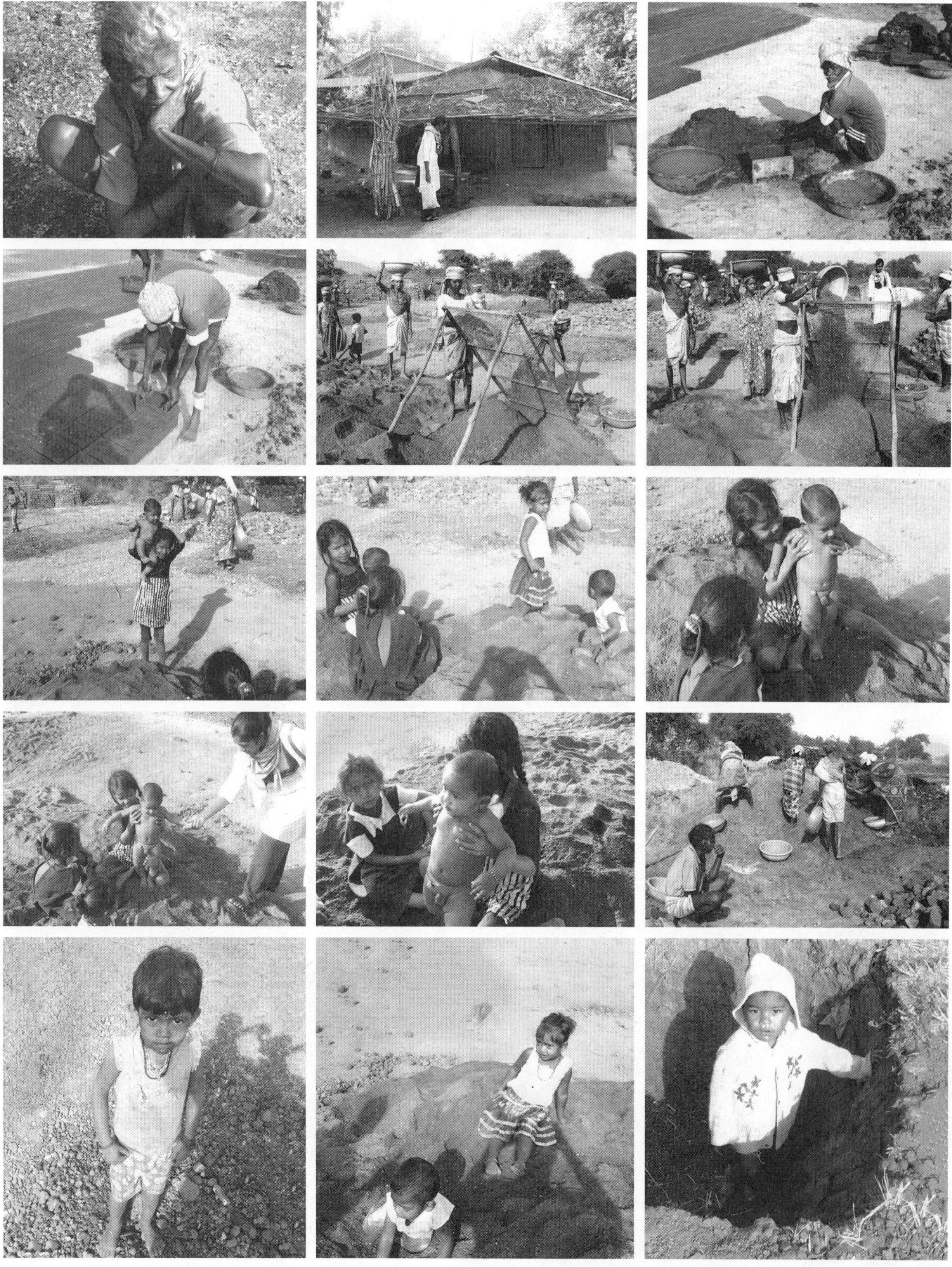

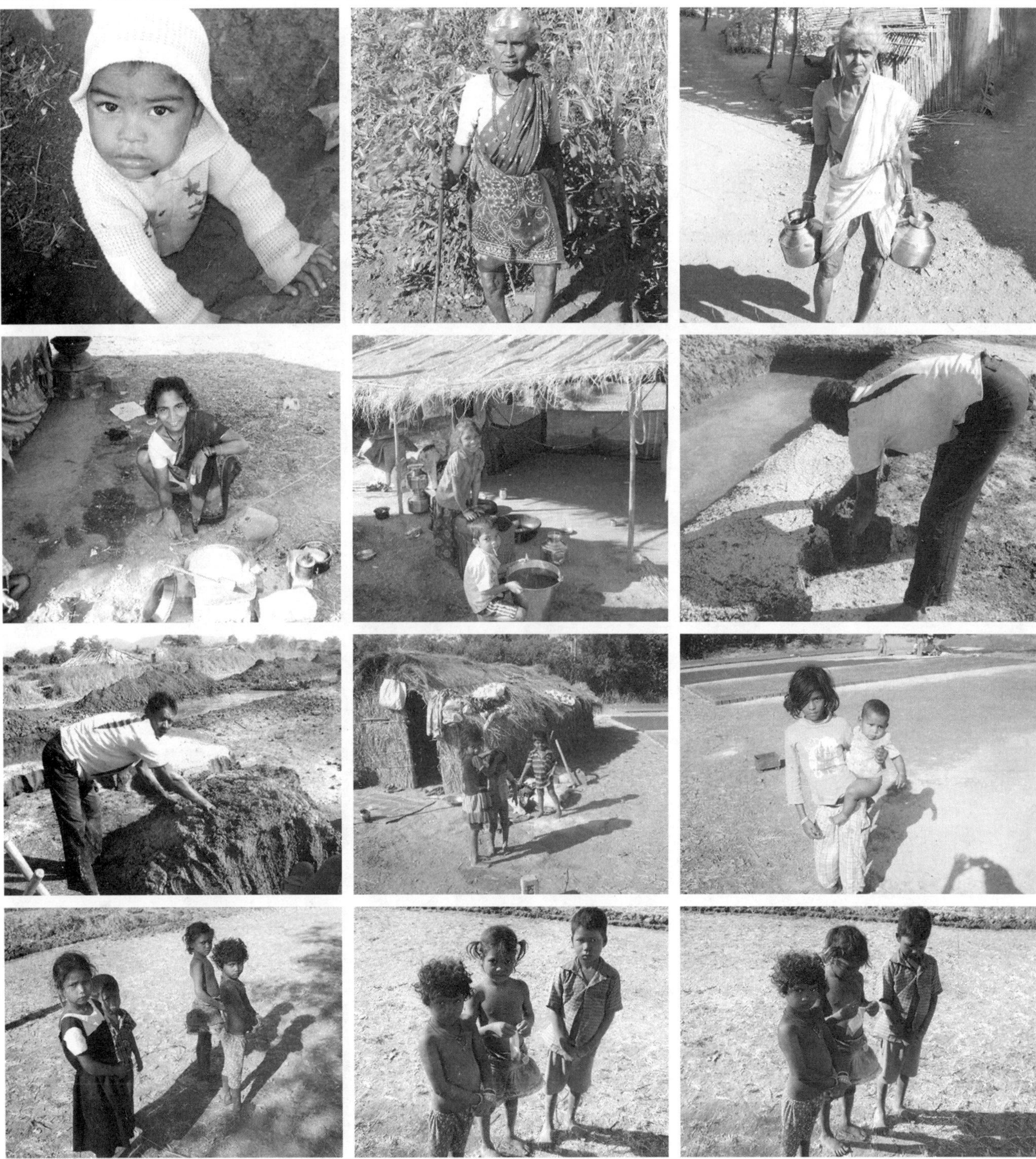

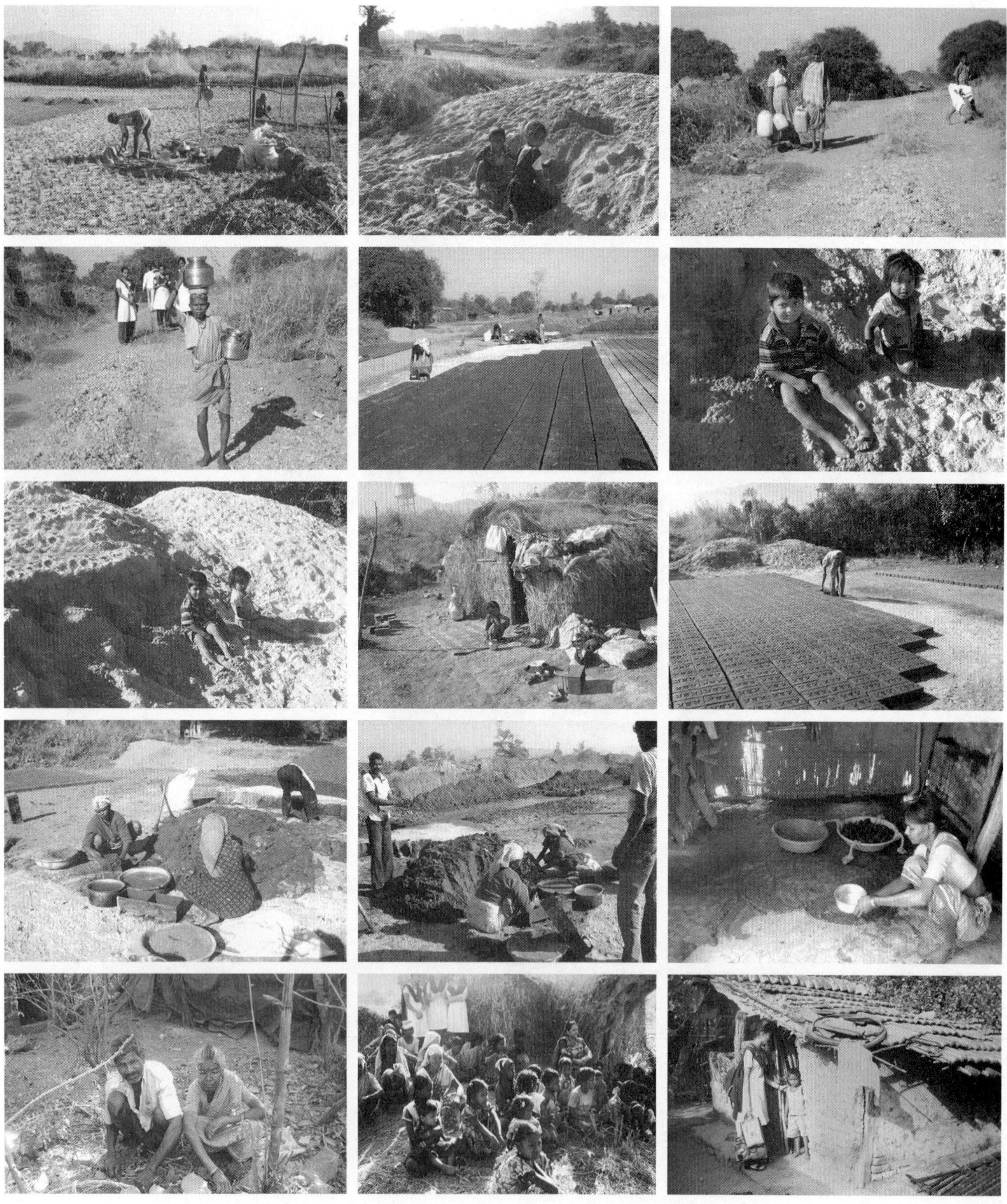

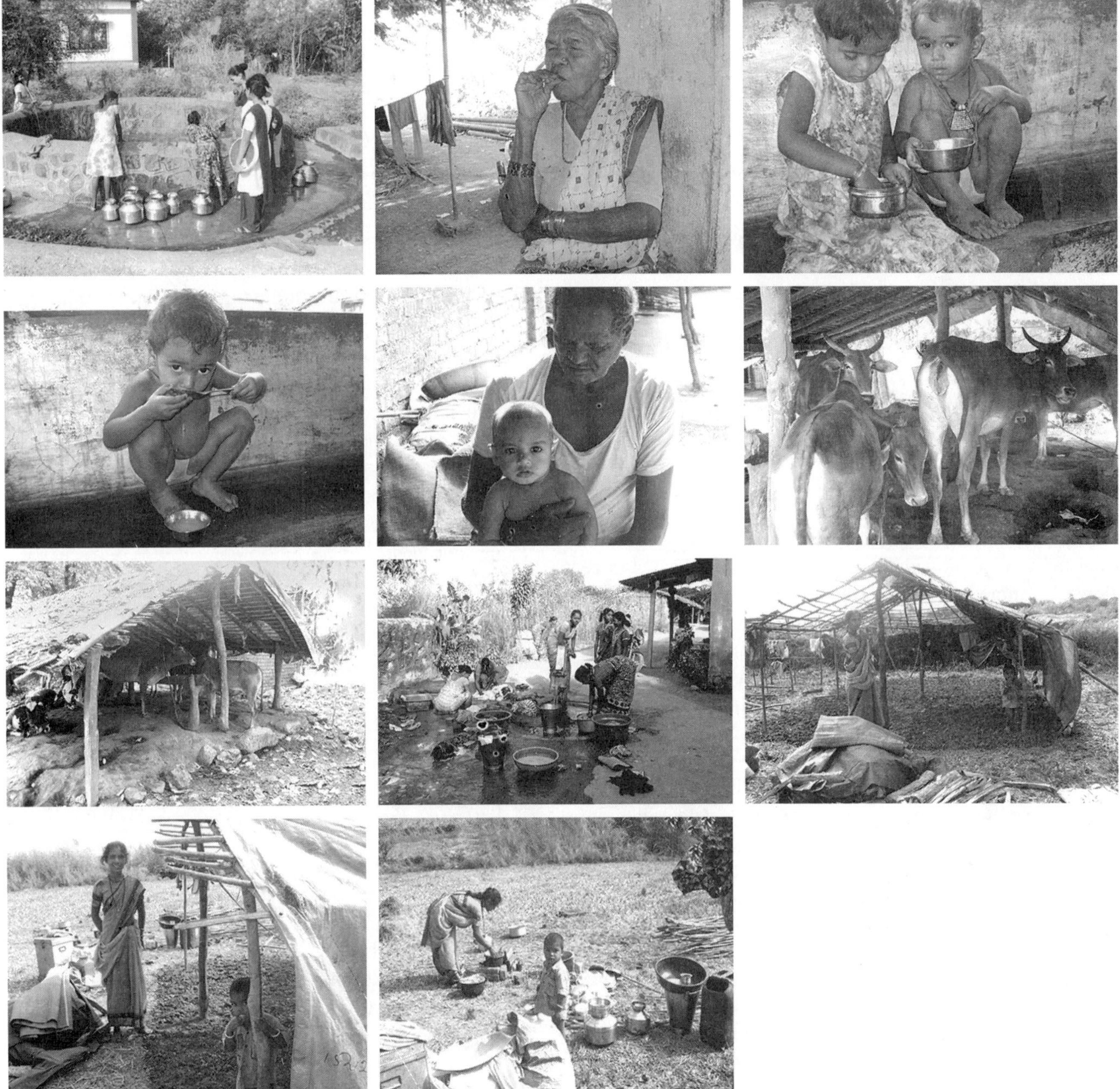

CHAPTER 62

Revision at a Glance

Believe in the best, think your best, have a goal for your best, never satisfied with less than your best, try your best and in the long run things will turn out for the best, always add up the best.

This chapter will help the students to prepare in some extend the viva examination by reading these questions and revising her syllabus in gist.

Viva examination is the commonly used evaluation process for measuring educational outcomes. There are different ways of performing examinations. In professional education, oral examination is often combined with practical examination. In viva examination, the students are asked series of questions on the selected topic and student is expected to give immediate response verbally. They can be focused on practical/clinical situations; it is valid methods of deep learning, application theory into practice, and problem solving skills. The viva questions a redirected towards the knowledge related to the skills, which the student has just demonstrated, also knowledge, which cannot be accessed through skill presentation, can be done through oral viva. Here teachers get excellent opportunity to assess abilities, assess verbal and nonverbal skills, and see the level of confidence, tone of voice, facial expressions, vocabulary and teacher can correct the wrong concept in relation to client care practice. Helps in direct testing of knowledge, students can be guided face to face wrong concept can be corrected. Students feel tensed and they try to study all that they feel is important, the examiner also have to prepare themselves in terms of questions to be asked and get acquainted to tools and techniques of viva examinations. The purpose is to find out what the students know, know the objective, know the syllabus, and remember the points of viva examination.

Examples of revision and likely asked questions in exam they are as follows:

1. **What are the functions of education?** The functions of education are to compete the socializing process, to transmit the cultural heritage, and formation of social personality. It also aids in reformation of attitude, and for occupational placement an instrument for livelihood. It confreres individuals status in society with kind and type of education received. It encourages spirit of competition and train for skills that are required in economy. It forester participant democracy, impart values, therefore education is an integrative force.
2. **What is the aim of education?** It provides knowledge and skills, vocational to earn livelihood, to be productive in life, to acquire intelligent, knowledge, thinking, reasoning and judgment, to grow as productive citizen, to provide knowledge to keep well being and healthy life, to develop character, human values, attitudes and habits, to develop moral values of honesty, truthfulness, goodness, courage etc, its aim is to respect for other culture, recharge depleted energy level, to self realization of strength and weakness, to give international understanding, and to ensure harmonious development.
3. **What are the types of education**—there are formal education, non-formal education and informal education.
4. **What are the good qualities of education**—increasing opportunity for higher studies, inculcating right attitudes, professional development, development of high-tech–high-touch approach, cultivation of spiritual values, forward looking value.
5. **What are the teaching methods**—learning by doing, play way method, observation and experimentation, self-education or self-effort.
6. **What are the levels of knowledge**—level of comprehension, level of application (ability to use learned concepts) level of analysis (break down information) synthesis, evaluation.
7. **Steps of education**—are to receive, respond, value, organize, and to adapt.
8. **Qualities**—is to be relevant, feasible, measurable, observable, logical.
9. **What is the mark of good teaching**—good teaching recognizes individual differences, it causes to learn, it provides opportunity for activity, it is kind and sympathetic, it reduces distance between teacher and students, it is flexible, it incorporates cooperation, it is democratic, it gives desirable and selective information, it helps to adjust to environment, it is progressive, it considers level of students, it is diagnostic and remedial, it stimulating, it develops initiative, independent thinking and doing, infuses confidence in students, it is carefully planned, it gives clarity and good feed back, it is effective teaching and learning method.

10. **What is good nursing education?** Good nursing education has good interpersonal relationship with students, it has a professional competence, it is student friendly behaviour in clinical area, its methods suit to the level of student, it uses creativity, it considers available resources, it motivates and guide in knowledge, it arouses students interest, it introduces new areas of learning, it clarify difficult concepts, promotes critical thinking, it prepares them for discussion, it makes lectures interactive, it emphasis higher level of intellectual skills, it gives clear direction, it assist students to develop, it clarify concepts, shares information, it fosters democratic values, it develops team spirit, it builds social skills and right attitudes, it arouses interest, it builds gap between theory and practice, it develops critical thinking, it provides feed back, it enables students to empathies with real life situation.
11. **What you mean by nursing education?** What are the objectives of nursing education? What is the general purpose of education? Which factors influence learning? Can you explain the teaching responsibilities of a nurse? What preparation needed before lecture? State characteristic of education, describe various types of AV aids, explain demonstration method, describe characteristic of good leader? Describe the steps in developing lesson plans. Aims and objectives of education. Advantage and disadvantage of project method, define various types of learning, and write basic types of learning? Describe the qualities of a nurse educator? What is the distance education, its importance and implementation in nursing? Describe the importance of clinical teaching?
12. AV aids should be cheap and easily available.
13. A small scale trial study is termed as pilot study.
14. The best method to impart and acquire knowledge in teaching and learning process is discussion.
15. Education increases social efficacy and productivity.
16. Realizing ones own physical, moral, intellectual, emotional abilities is self-expression.
17. To produce well qualified and competent professional nurses one of the purpose of education.
18. Education brings about transformation of rational behavior to impulsive behavior.
19. Testing the learning product through usage is known as evaluation.
20. 'Educatum' means the art of teaching or training.
21. Educate means to raise or being up to nourish, to take care.
22. The creation of a sound mind in a sound body defined by Aristotle.
23. The person who impart education is educator.
24. Philosophy and education are tow sides of coin
25. All round development of client is to be physically strong and economically sufficient
26. Assimilated knowledge is called self-expression
27. Field trip is a self-instruction steps to enables students to learn by self
28. Discussion method involves interaction in group
29. Education creates awareness
30. Projected method is learning by doing
31. In lecture method student is in passive state
32. Role play method improves communication and leadership abilities
33. Student in their problem need advice and guidance.
34. For staff development in-service education is important factor.
35. Education is tri polar process.
36. Learning needs motivation and interest.
37. Language can be barriers of communication.
38. Self discipline and honesty is important characteristic of a nurse.
39. Visualized explanation facts concepts and procedure is demonstration.
40. Teaching learning is an interaction between teacher, pupil and environment.
41. Av aids supply a concrete basis for conceptual thinking, there by reduces measuring words.
42. Education is a transmitter and preservers of culture.
43. Seminar is defined as assembled group of 10 to 25 person who share a common leadership.
44. Motivation plays an important role in student nurse development.
45. Project method student learns by doing.
46. Selected sources of review of literature are journal.
47. The formal agency of education is school.
48. Learning helps student in modifying behavior
49. Student can prepare before viva revision by going through following matter
50. Cell is a functional unit of the body
51. The life span of RBC is 120 days
52. Hypothalamus is the heat regulating center
53. Urinary bladder has capacity of 300–400 ml
54. Pyloric sphincter is situated at stomach
55. The study of virus is called as virology
56. Human body develops from a single cell called as Zygote
57. Sperm x + ovum x gives birth to female child
58. Catabolism is breaks down large molecule
59. Oteoblasts is born forming cell
60. Suprarenal glands is also called as adrenal gland
61. Vagus nerve is the 10th cranial nerve
62. Largest and strongest bone in the body is known as femur
63. Epidermis is called a superficial layer of the skin

64. Shoulder joint is synovial joint
65. Right side of the heart deals with deoxygenated blood
66. Bowmans capsule is also called asglomerula capsule
67. Pituatory gland situated at brain
68. Total number of ribs in the body is 12 pairs
69. Foamen means opening
70. Mastication means chewing
71. Iris is the visible coloured part of the eye
72. Roughtly triangulat shaded seasnoid bone in the knee joint is patella or knee cap
73. Sciatic nerve is the largest nerve in the body
74. Louis pasture is the father of microbiology
75. Olfactory nerve gives sense of smell
76. Retina is the inner layer of the eye
77. Largest gland in the body is liver
78. Artery which supply blood to the eye ciliary's artery
79. Normal number of cardiac cycle per minute 60–80
80. SA node is also called as pace maker of the heart
81. Brain is situated in the cranial cavity
82. 31 pairs number of spinal nerve
83. Parathyroid gland secrete parathyroid hormone
84. Lacrimal glands secrete tears from the eye
85. Zygomatic bone is also called as cheek bone
86. Axillary artery in upper limb
87. Blood is a straw color fluid
88. Mitrochondriya is the power house of the cell
89. Blood is connective tissue
90. Membranous covering of brain and spinal cord is known as meninges
91. Breasts is the accessory gland of female reproductive system
92. The immunity develops after birth is called innate
93. Pancreas is both exocrine and endocrine gland
94. Luckocytes are also called as WBC
95. Pulmonary Artery Contains Deoxygenated Blood
96. Flagella is made up of protein material called flagellin
97. Coccyx is terminal vertebrae
98. Hnig joint distal end of tibia
99. Diaphragm is dome shaped
100. Liver-hexagonal
101. Heart-atrium
102. Dettol is common disinfectant used in hospital
103. A germicide disinfectant
104. Bicuspid valve is also knows as Mitral valve
105. The functional unit of kidney Nephrons
106. Breast bone is also called sternum fat is synthesized from carbohydrates and proteins
107. Daily secretion of gastric juice is 2 liter
108. Trachea is also called wind pipe
109. Passage for food and air is Phyrax
110. Child birth is also called as pariturition
111. The weight of the vireus 30–40 gm
112. Daily secretion of bile is 500–1000 ml
113. Largest serous membranes of the body peritoneum
114. Prolactin is the hormone that stimulates lactation
115. Sound wave travel at a speed of 332 meters/1088 feet
116. Respiratory centre is stimulated in the medulla oblongata
117. Tongue is a voluntary muscular structure which occupies the floor of the mouth
118. Daily secretion of saliva is 1.5 liters
119. Tuberculosis is caused by Mycobacterium Tuberculi
120. Laryngeal prominence is also called as Adams apple
121. Degtution is also called as swallowing
122. Light waves travel as a speed of 186,000 miles/300,000 km
123. Formation of new suga is Gluconeogesis
124. Surfactant is a Phosphoilipid fluid which prevents the alveoli from drying out
125. Arterial blood pressure is measured with sphygmomanometer
126. Cholecystitis means inflammation of gallbladder
127. Total number of bones in human body are 206
128. Covering layer of lung is pleura
129. Skin is Integermentary system
130. The femur is thigh bone
131. The gullet means stomach
132. Cardiac muscle is involuntary
133. RBC are developed from red bone marrow
134. Bile is stored in gall bladder
135. Ball and socket joint is freely moveable
136. Islets of largerhans situated in pancreas
137. Splenomegaly means enlargement of spleen
138. Cardiac muscle is found in the heart
139. Testosterone is male sexual hormone
140. Trachea is a 'C' shaped cartilaginous ring present
141. Bile is necessary for digestion of fat
142. Mandible is moveable bone in the skull
143. Colostrums is a thin fluid which is rich in protein
144. Sterilization include autoclaving
145. The normal serum sodium level is 135–145 meg/l
146. Estrogen is female sexual hormone
147. Invasion of the body by microorganism leads to infection.
148. Ptyalin is an enzyme present in saliva
149. Disorder caused due to deficiency of ADH hormone diabetes insipid us
150. Effective method to destroy spores through sterilization is steam under pressure
151. Intelligence is the total quality of an individuals behaviour
152. Unconscious conflict is mental conflict below the level of conscious awareness
153. The process of socialization states from norms, habits and ideals

154. Rationalization is a defense mechanism
155. Personality is a key word in psychology
156. Controlled thinking is the force that initiates sustains and delivers the activity of an organism
157. Hyperesthesia is an excessive response to stimuli
158. Illusion is a false perception
159. Drug dependency is a social problem
160. Factors that control attention is intensity reasoning and problem solving is the best form of controlled thinking
161. Frustration is a condition of extreme tension
162. Day dreaming is an example of free thinking
163. Skills help in development of integral personality
164. Imagination is type of free thinking
165. Habit is a form of learned behavior
166. Learning is self-active process
167. Cultural factors influence social change
168. Emotion is a conscious stirred up state of our organism
169. An emotion is strong feeling
170. Anesthesia is a sensory abnormality
171. A study of human behaviour is called psychology
172. Motivation is effective factor of learning
173. Age is not a factor of intelligence
174. Habit is acquired through repetition
175. Some individuals adopt what is known as defense mechanism to over come failure or defect
176. Conflict is the tug of war between two different opposite ideas and it is the course of action
177. Reasoning is a mental process in which we deal with thoughts and ideas
178. Marriage is a mode of action as well as a system of beliefs\perception is a mental process which gives meaning to the sensation
179. Emotion is a strong feeling
180. False perceptions are called illusion, hallucination
181. Introspection is the examination of ones own thought
182. Curiosity is also social motive
183. Children by choice and not by chance is family planning
184. 90–120 is the IQ of the normal individual
185. Euthanasia is medical termed used for mercy killing
186. Hydronephrosis is dilation of renal pelvis
187. Pneumothorax is accumulation of air in pelvic cavity
188. Gastrostomy is a surgical procedure to create opening in stomach through the abdomen
189. Nitrous oxide is called as laughing gas
190. Susrutha is a father of Indian surgery
191. Inspection is initial assessment in abdominal examination
192. Metabolic acidosis a patient develops late shock
193. Oliguria is a sign of progressive Hypovolemia
194. In pernicious anemia to absorb vitamin B12 schilling test is done
195. Decreased oxygen supply to the tissues known as hypoxia
196. An increased temperature and pulse rate is possible complication of thyroid crisis
197. Hital hernia is hernia ion of the portion of the stomach through an opening in diaphragm
198. Portal hypertension increased pressure in portal vain
199. A rigid board like abdomen indicates perforation of ulcer
200. R L, D5 are hypotonic solution
201. Achaiasia isabsent or impaired peristalsis of esophagus
202. Hump back is called kyphosis
203. Angioma is a tumor arising from blood vessel
204. GERD is back flow of duodenal or gastric content
205. Convulsions also called epilepsy
206. Kernig's signs is early clinical manifestation of Meningeal irritation
207. Aneurysm is called dilation of artery
208. Disalysis is a removal of waste products from body by an artificial kidney
209. Normal intracranial pressure is 5–15 mm of Hg
210. Aphasia is absence of speech
211. Hypokalemia is decreased potassium level in blood
212. Hypernitrimea is increased sodium in the blood
213. By fumigation sterilization of OT is done
214. Accumulation of fluid in plural cavity is called plural effusion
215. Reeducation in the O_2 carrying capacity of the blood is called anemia
216. Immunity is the body's first line of defense against an invasion by microorganism
217. Diabetes mellitus is a chronic disorder of carbohydrate metabolism
218. Water aids in excretion of waste
219. Normal serum cholesterol level is 150–200 mg. dl
220. Hyper apnea means excessive CO_2 in the blood
221. High risk consent to be taken from a patient who is under going Thoracotomy
222. In nursing physical examination is necessary in assessment phase
223. Auto immune disorders is illness due to immune responses against self antigens
224. Comparison of clients health status with the outcome is the final nursing process
225. Substance used to counteract the effect of a drugs or poisons is called antidote
226. Administration of injection TT is an example of passive artificial immunity
227. Blood urea and serum creatinin values indicate renal function
228. Phosphorous is essential for the formation of bone and teeth
229. Tonometry is used to measure IOP
230. The radiation therapy helps to delay or destroy the growth of malignant cells

231. Shock occurs due to administration of penicillin
232. After Traceostomy the most important point in nursing care is prevention of infection
233. Dick test is done to detect the susceptibility of scarlet fever
234. When ever Digoxin is given the nurse has to make sure that the pulse is above 40/minute
235. The purpose of surgical asepsis is to prevent infection
236. Another name for tetanus is lock-jaw
237. Lymphadenitis is an inflammation of adenoids
238. Ptosis is dropping of eyelids
239. Most important objective during the early post burn phase to replace fluid volume
240. ECG helps to establish the diagnosis of function of cardiac muscle
241. Nystagmus is defined as rapid involuntary movement of the eyeball
242. Cataract is called blurred vision
243. Abnormal dilatation and tortuous subcutaneous veins is called varicosities
244. Rheumatic fever is caused by group a Beta hemolytic streptococci
245. Human immune virus destroys CD4 cells
246. Occult blood means hidden blood
247. The causative organism of syphilis is Tripanoma Pallidum
248. Bleeding disorder is due to deficiency of fibrinogen
249. Schizophrenia is an example of functional psychosis
250. Mental health is a balance between body, mind, spirit and environment in which a person lives
251. Delusion is an abnormal thought
252. Causes of mental illness can be biological, psychological, sociological and biochemical
253. A person with paranoid personality suspects that other people will harm them
254. Gloomy, submissive, quiet and kind people will have melancholic personality
255. Illusion are misperceptions of external stimuli
256. Mania or depression is an example of disorders of emotion
257. Antasy is imagined achievement of ones unmet needs
258. Duration of ECT is 1 to 8 second
259. ECT contra indication in increased intracranial pressure
260. Delusion is a firm false belief, opposed to reality
261. Amnesia loss of memory or inability to recall past experience
262. Schizophrenia is an example of schizoid psychosis
263. Echopnexia is the repetition of words
264. Catatonic schizophrenia is a indication of ECT
265. Peptic ulcer is an example of psycho somatic disorder
266. Milliu therapy is a scientific manipulation of the environment
267. Lithium carbonate is a drug of Mania choice
268. Bipolar mood disorder is the lesser degree of mania
269. Psychotherapy is the treatment of emotional bodily problems by psychological mean
270. Tricylie is a drug known as anti depressants
271. Suicide is a psychiatric emergency
272. Stupor is a condition in which the patient is immobile
273. Suicide is a self destruction
274. Violence is an expression of aggressiveness
275. Addiction seems to result from social isolation
276. Diazepam is an example of Benzo diasepines
277. Phobia is an unreasonable fear of an object or situation
278. Schizoid personality is characterized by feeling of loneliness, isolation
279. Paranoid personality is suspicious, stubborn, unhappy, sarcastic
280. Zoo-phobia is a fear of animals
281. Voracious apatite may be seen in Hypomania
282. Haloperidol is a anti psychotic drug
283. Eptoin is an anti-epileptic drug
284. Mental Health Act was passed in 1987
285. Parole is a method of discharge procedure
286. Phenobarbitone is a sedative
287. Repeated washing of hands is an example of Echopraxia
288. The first stage of convulsion is Aura
289. Diazepam is a anti anxiety drug
290. At two year the child can speak 1-worded sentence
291. At 3 month an infant can hold the head
292. At one year child has 6–8 teeth
293. At 4 years child has bowel and bladder control
294. 120–140 is a normal heart rate of an infant
295. Injury to 5th and 6th cervical spinal nerve causes Erb's palsy
296. Neonatal Hyperbilirubinemia is also called as Icterius Neonatrum
297. MMR vaccine is given between 15–18 months
298. Foul smelling ribbon like stool found in infant with Hirschprung's diseases
299. The most common respiratory infection in infancy is acute nasopharyngitis
300. Urethra opens on the dorsal surface of the urethra is Epispodiasis
301. The children with cerebral palsy have borderline intelligence
302. Megaloblastic anemia refers to the abnormal development of red cells
303. Normal portal pressure is 5–10 mm of Hg
304. Amebiasis is treated with Metronidazole 20–40 mg/kg
305. Sun set eyes is typical characteristic of Hydrocephalus
306. Absence of anal opening is imperforated anus
307. Involuntary bed wetting after 4 years of age is known as Cryrasis

308. Deficiency of sodium causes muscular cramps
309. Daily requirement of sodium in the diet is 1-15 g ms
310. Daily requirement of proteins for adult weighing 45 kg is 45 g ms
311. Basal metabolic rate is checked in thyroid disease
312. Mono Saccharides, Dia saccharieds and Polysaccharides are the type of carbohydrates
313. Kwashiorkor is caused by protein deficiency
314. Constipation is caused by lack of roughage
315. Water born diseases are cholera, jaundice, typhoid and poliomyelitis
316. Lactating mothers require 27000 to 3000 calories per day
317. Due to deficiency of vitamin D children suffer from rickets and adults from Ostomalisia
318. We need food rich in calcium and phosphorus for health of the teeth and bones
319. Food is classified as a energy producing foods, body building foods and protective foods
320. Functions of food are to provide energy, to build and repair of tissues, to carry out various body processes, to help in physical and mental development of the body and to develop resistance against disease
321. End product of protein is called amino acids
322. The essential amino acids are lysine, leucine, isoleucin, methonine, phenylanine, threonine, tryptophance and valine
323. Proteins are classified into animal proteins and vegetable or plant protein
324. Main function of protein are for growth and development, for repair of tissues, for synthesis of hormones, antibodies, enzymes
325. The daily requirement of carbohydrate should be 350 to 400 g ms
326. Functions of carbohydrates are to provide energy and to oxidize fats
327. Fats are classified into a saturated fat, and unsaturated fat
328. Main functions of the fats are to provide support to internal organs, provide energy
329. Vitamins are classified into fat soluble vitamins and water soluble vitamins
330. Water soluble vitamins are B and C
331. Fat soluble vitamins are A, D, E and K
332. All vitamins work as catalysts in various body process
333. Vitamins D is necessary for absorption of calcium and phosphorous
334. Vitamin B/thiamin deficiency causes beriberi
335. Deficiency of vitamin C causes scurvy and vitamin B deficiency causes pernicious anemia
336. Folic acid is essential for synthesis of DNA
337. Daily requirement of vitamin C is 50 g ms
338. Iron is required for formation of hemoglobin in the blood
339. Calcium is absorbed in the intestine
340. Daily intake of sodium is 10 to 25 g ms
341. Deficiency of fluorine results in dental carries
342. Methods of group teaching are one way method and two-way method
343. Min types of communications are verbal and non-verbal; formal and non-formal, one-way and two-way and face to face and mass-communication
344. Basic skills required for communications are human relations skills, listening skills, writing skills and drawing skills
345. The atmospheric air contains 20.93% of oxygen
346. Tuberculosis is air born disease, BCG vaccine is given to prevent it
347. Deficiency of calcium causes Tetany
348. Two methods of group teaching are one way or didactic methods and two way or Socratic methods
349. Most important objective of antenatal care is to promote and maintain the health of the mother during pregnancy
350. Vitamin k is called as coagulant vitamin
351. School health services are considered to be very important and integral part of the total community health services
352. Soft water produces good leather with soap
353. Communication is most important key factor in family planning programme
354. Immunization is given to prevent the disease so it should be given at regular intervals
355. Health education can be given to each and every person
356. Plain water is given to an acid poisoning
357. The period from entry of germs in the body to the occurrence of signs and symptoms is called ‘incubation period’
358. Egg flip is given to diarrhea patient
359. Children must be vaccinated before being admitted in the school
360. Typhoid fever is transmitted by typhoid bacilli and malaria is transmitted by bite of female anopheles mosquito
361. Puppet show is the best method for teaching illiterate people
362. Excessive vitamin is stored in the liver
363. Pasteurization is the safest method of human consumption
364. Clostridium Botulinum is the causative organism of food poisoning
365. Larvae of anopheles mosquito rest parallel to water surface
366. Chlorination is most important step in water purification
367. Destruction of forest is hazardous to health
368. Barley water is given in the patient of urinary infection

369. The articles used for the infectious patients are called Fomites
370. Boiling point of water is 100°C
371. Cold chain should be maintained for polio vaccine
372. Presence of Bitot's sport in the eyes are the signs of vitamin a deficiency
373. Water helps in regulating body temperature
374. Measles vaccine produces active immunity
375. Bad oral hygiene causes pyorrhea
376. OT test is done for detection of chlorine in water
377. Vitamin C is essential for healing of wounds, Amla is riches in vitamin C
378. Vitamin B1 is known as riboflavin
379. Tea contains tannic acid
380. Tab vaccine is given to prevent typhoid
381. The nutritive value of protein depends upon types of pulses and cereals eaten
382. Iodine is required for synthesis of hormone thyroxin
383. A Mid-day school meal must supply at least ½ or 50% of the protein required
384. Hookworm infestation may occur to the people walking bare foot. Worm infestation causes anemia
385. Excessive ingestion of fat may result in obesity
386. The best method of refuse disposal is burning
387. 3 grams of fat contain 27 calories
388. Saffola is good source of unsaturated fat
389. Sugar is good source of carbohydrate

You can do research on following examples and many more examples that you will come across in your clinical settings

1. Study on incidence of constipation among patient admitted in orthopedic ward
2. Sleep disturbance of patient admitted in emergency unit
3. Learning need of high blood pressure patient visiting cardiac OPD
4. Assess the factors of health seeking behaviour of people staying in the rural community
5. Alcohol consumption pattern among patient diagnosed with alcoholic liver cirrhosis
6. Diabetic complication
7. End stage of renal disease
8. COPD patient
9. Perception of different patient assignment method for providing nursing care
10. Women living with chronic alcoholic husbands
11. Socio-cultural beliefs of people in tribal of antenatal, postnatal
12. Adaptation process of patient diagnosed with cancer
13. Adaptation level of people with post injury permanent physical disabilities
14. A case study on the available and utilization of energy services in civil hospital
15. Psychological needs of ICU patient
16. Social problems—sexual harassments (suffers range of consequences, withdrawal from social interaction, changed career goal, decreases loss of self-confidence) reaction of male and female towards this
17. A descriptive study of level of satisfaction with nursing care
18. Descriptive study of existing mouth care practice in critically ill patient admitted in ICU
19. Descriptive study on prevalence of backache among nurses working in critical care unit
20. Varicose vein problem in nurse's in prolonged standing in ward or operation theater
21. Prevalence of hospital acquired infection among patients admitted in icu
22. Descriptive study of women who have underwent female feticide
23. Understand the process of adaptation of stress in rural tribal population
24. Pin site infection with external skeletal fixation

Examples of critical thinking—nurses can do while with different patients in different situations in different diseases conditions

1. What are the priorities during the emergent phase of burn care?
2. What assessment parameters would you monitor closely?
3. What are patients immediate care needs what should you do immediately?
4. What important factors need to be addressed as part of his discharge plan?
5. What immediate concerns would you have for his airway?
6. What strategies would you use to relieve his pain?
7. What are the psychological and emotional need to be addressed?
8. Is their need to be alarmed?
9. What initial measures are you planning?
10. How would you determine whether your intervention were effective in alleviating the increased ICP?
11. What patient and family teachings is important, how would you modify your teaching?
12. What is the evidence base for treatment practice?
13. What is your rationale for these assessment and actions?
14. What intervention can the nurse implement to address his concerns?
15. What teaching would be indicated to prevent another stroke?
16. What addiction test do you think will be necessary?
17. What could be the etiology of her complaints?
18. How can you make the patients environment safe?
19. What critical information do you need to provide to the emergency physician?

20. How do your finding affect your care?
21. What nursing observations and assessment are indicated?
22. What safety precautions are essential and why?
23. What type of medical treatment might he under go?
24. What do you suspect is happening?
25. What are the possible causes of his condition and how would you intervene?
26. What resources may be needed to enable her to be successful?
27. What are the possible medication regimens that may be used to treat disease?
28. What is you priority in nursing diagnosis and intervention?
29. What specific questions would you ask him to determine the status of his health?
30. What support systems would you mobilize for this patient?
31. What would you instruct her to do, provide rationale for your interventions?
32. What resources and referrals would you make available?
33. How would you prepare him for health screening test?
34. What criteria would you use in this patients care?
35. What type of palliative care services may be helpful for this case, why?
36. What initial lab test would you anticipate to be ordered?
37. What test do you think would be respected at this time, why?
38. What you can do to aid him during the treatment?
39. What is his options?
40. How would you discuss these issues with him?
41. What risk factors modifying would you want to address with this patient?
42. What evidence base information supports you r actions?
43. What should nurses in different roles in the community do to replace the risk of new infection and to reduce peoples anxiety?
44. What steps should be taking to reduce the risk of further outbreaks?
45. How do the actions, uses and indications of these medications differ?
46. What documentation and reporting is needed?
47. What testing, treatment and counseling are indicated?
48. What nursing care is important to minimize the risk of complications?

To improve the nursing care nurse needs to add new knowledge. Without new knowledge, nursing care can't be improved. It propels the nurses towards professional growth. Thus, research helps to bring new facts out of the unknown. What is the nature of knowledge? It is not a book, pass on examination and finish with education. The whole life from the moment you are born to the moment you die is a process of learning.

Index